MEDICAL PROCEDURES, TESTING AND TECHNOLOGY

HYPOTHESES IN CLINICAL MEDICINE

MEDICAL PROCEDURES, TESTING AND TECHNOLOGY

Additional books in this series can be found on Nova's website under the Series tab.

Additional e-books in this series can be found on Nova's website under the e-books tab.

LABORATORY AND CLINICAL RESEARCH

Additional books in this series can be found on Nova's website under the Series tab.

Additional e-books in this series can be found on Nova's website under the e-books tab.

MEDICAL PROCEDURES, TESTING AND TECHNOLOGY

HYPOTHESES IN CLINICAL MEDICINE

MOHAMMADALI M. SHOJA
PAUL S. AGUTTER
R. SHANE TUBBS
MOSTAFA GHANEI
KAMYAR GHABILI
ALON HARRIS
AND
MARIOS LOUKAS
EDITORS

New York

Library of Congress Cataloging-in-Publication Data

ISBN: 978-1-62257-276-2

Published by Nova Science Publishers, Inc. † New York

Dedication

To the memory of Prof. *Mohammad Reza Nasizadeh,* who was a light in the life of his pupils; to Prof. *W. Jerry Oakes*, and Prof. *Khalil Ansarin* for their profound knowledge, excellent mentorship, dedication and spontaneous encouragements; and to Mr. *Douglas Huntley* for his adventurous life and wonderful friendship.

Mohammadali M. Shoja, MD

To *Alun H. Maddy*, who taught me to think scientifically and to question what is commonly assumed; and to *Lewis Thomas*, who taught me how to balance caring with common sense.

Paul S. Agutter, MD, PhD

To my wife *Susan* and son *Isaiah* for their support and love, and to *W. Jerry Oakes* for his encouragement and perseverance.

R. Shane Tubbs, PhD

To my students

Mostafa Ghanei, MD

To my parents, *Naiyer* and *Samad*, and my brother and sister-in-law, *Shahrokh* and *Aida* whose words of encouragement and push for tenacity ring in my ears; and to *Prof. Khalil Ansarin* and *Prof. Mohammad Reza Ardalan* whose encouragement and advice have shed light on my academic life.

Kamyar Ghabili, MD

To my precious children, *Danielle* and *Jonathan*, who are truly my inspiration and continually fill my life with love and joy.

Alon Harris, MS, PhD, FARVO

To my parents *Anastasia* and *Christos* who taught me to develop hypotheses and initiate research in order to find an answer.

Marios Loukas, MD, PhD

Contents

Preface

In 1999, Alvan Feinstein published an article in the *American Journal of Medicine* lamenting the loss of contact between bedside and bench, research and practice, and arguing for a greater emphasis on pathophysiology in medical education to bridge the gap (Feinstein 1999). Feinstein's observations were wise, but in some respects the gulf between research and practice is fundamental. Biomedical research and clinical practice entail different values, attitudes and mind-sets. The researcher, who is not usually medically qualified, is mainly concerned with *explaining general phenomena*. The MD, who is not usually trained in scientific research, is mainly concerned with *predicting* the course of illness in *individual patients* (Kassirer 1983). Both the researcher and the physician employ hypotheses but they use them for different purposes.

In biomedical research, broad hypotheses are formulated - a creative act - and experiments are conducted to test them critically. The experimental data must be 'hard'. Scientific investigations that accord with these principles lead to reliable, or at least plausible, explanations of phenomena that would otherwise remain mysterious (Feinstein 1983). In contrast, although medical decisions about patient care may be (and in the best circumstances are) informed by biomedical research findings, they also depend - crucially - on 'soft' data about the clinical and personal circumstances of the individual patient. For the physician, 'hypotheses' are ephemeral matters of differential diagnosis and choice of treatment. Physicians have to think on their feet; researchers usually have time to ponder.

Nevertheless, there is commonality between these two kinds of hypothesis. Psychology students (i.e., novices) asked to formulate diagnoses on the basis of ECG data were significantly more successful if they were able to propose hypotheses and test them against the data than if they followed prescribed rules of inference (Norman *et al.* 2000); this study reflects common experience in clinical practice. Just as research scientists formulate preliminary explanatory hypotheses on the basis of minimal information, so physicians formulate preliminary diagnostic hypotheses on the basis of minimal clinical findings (Kassirer 1983). In both cases, the hypotheses provide a basis for further data-gathering (by experiments in the one case and by examinations and laboratory investigations in the other). In both cases, successive hypotheses become increasingly detailed and specific until they attain the status of 'reliable understanding'. This general model of problem-solving (clinical and scientific) is supported by a considerable body of research in cognitive psychology and other fields and is generally acknowledged (Fransella and Bannister 1986; Hulley *et al.* 2006; Vance 1995; Wisenberg 1993). Regrettably, undergraduate training in both science and medicine seldom emphasizes problem-solving; in many medical and science faculties there is still a near-exclusive reliance on book learning and memorization that is in many respects counterproductive.

Of course, tenacious adherence to a favourite hypothesis is also counterproductive: in research, it delays or even prevents the progress of understanding; in clinical practice, it can cost lives. The 19th century geologist Thomas C. Chamberlin (1843-1928) epitomised this infelicitous tenacity as 'the method of the ruling theory' and gave examples of its unfortunate consequences (Chamberlin 1890). He advocated an alternative, 'the method of multiple working hypotheses', as a prophylactic against its dangers, and Davies and others have argued that 'the method of multiple working hypotheses' is valuable in clinical medicine as well as in basic research (Davies 1997). At both bench and bedside there is a strong argument for a policy of considering two or more hypotheses concurrently. Querying an initial hypothesis from the outset has been shown to enhance the ability of medical students to arrive at accurate diagnoses more rapidly, and its value in research is well known (Corderre *et al.* 2010; Fransella and Bannister 1986). There is a tendency in the medical and biomedical literature, and in clinical practice, to yield to 'the method of the ruling theory'. Davies proposed that the current 'pharmacodoxy' might exemplify it, and invited his readers to adopt the more intellectually developed, sophisticated, efficient and reliable 'method of multiple hypotheses' in their work (Davies 1997).

This book may be seen as a response to Davies's invitation. We offer a number of novel, non-mainstream hypotheses – in various states of development – from authors with relevant expertise and experience; our first aim is to challenge the 'ruling theory' in each field concerned. Our second aim is to address Feinstein's concern by attempting, in the areas of clinical medicine and biomedicine that we cover, to restore some part of the pathophysiological bridge between bench and bedside (Feinstein 1999). We also have a third aim, which we believe to have overriding importance. Throughout the book, the human diseases and health issues of most recent importance are covered. A "slow motion" cancer epidemic is sensible worldwide (Nelson 2011). It is expected that without a program of research and action, "an epidemic of neurologic [neurodegenerative] diseases on a global scale" is inevitable over the next four decades (Jessen 2010). Autoimmune diseases are on rise and the causative link with the modern lifestyle is obscure. There is an urgent need for new ideas and new research in these areas. By promoting the hypotheses that we include in the book, we hope to contribute to meeting that need.

Finally, hypotheses are fundamental to all sciences, including medicine. They play a critical role in motivating the development of science, since interesting and important hypotheses foster the diversity and debate upon which the scientific process depends. It is not feasible to regard a hypothesis as intellectual property before it has been practically tested and published or patented. This consideration may discourage many from expressing their ideas and thus prevent future innovations. Some radical hypotheses would be rejected by most conventional journals. It is necessary to learn and understand how to assess a process, realize and discuss details and consequently launch a hypothesis. An ideal hypothesis/theory reported in the biomedical field should have at least the following characteristics: (i) it should be supported by indirect evidence; (ii) it should be novel but relevant in the context of available scientific knowledge; and (iii) it should have the potential to be experimentally verified. This book introduces readers to examples of such innovative thinking. A sentence by David Horrobin (1975), referring to the journal *Medical Hypotheses*, summarizes this perspective:

"The history of science has repeatedly shown that when hypotheses are proposed it is impossible to predict which will turn out to be revolutionary and which ridiculous. The only safe approach is to let all see the light and to let all be discussed, experimented upon, vindicated or destroyed."

References

Chamberlin, T.C. (1890) The method of multiple working hypotheses. *Science*, 15, pp. 92-96.

Corderre, S. *et al.* (2010) To think is good: querying an initial hypothesis reduces diagnostic error in medical students. *Academic Medicine*, 85, pp. 1125-1129.

Davies, S. (1997) T. C. Chamberlin and 'the method of multiple working hypotheses': its relevance to clinical medicine today, 100 years after publication. *Journal of Nutritional and Environmental Medicine*, 7, pp. 233-235.

Feinstein, A.R. (1983) An additional basic science for clinical medicine: I. The constraining fundamental paradigms. *Annals of Internal Medicine*, 99, pp. 393-397.

Feinstein, A.R. (1999) Basic biomedical science and the destruction of the pathophysiologic bridge from bench to bedside. *The American Journal of Medicine*, 107, pp. 401-407.

Fransella, F. and Bannister, D. (1986) *Inquiring Man: the Theory of Personal Constructs, 2nd Edition*. London: Routledge.

Horrobin, D.F. (1975) Ideas in biomedical science: reasons for the foundation of medical hypotheses. Medical Hypotheses, 1, pp. 1-2.

Hulley, S.B. *et al.* (2006) *Designing Clinical Research, 3rd Edition*. Philadelphia, PA: Lippincott Williams & Wilkins.

Jessen, W. (2008) *Neurodegenerative Disease and the Coming Epidemic* [WWW] Highlight Health Website. Available from: http://www.highlighthealth.com/neurological-disorders/neurodegenerative-disease-and-the-coming-epidemic [accessed 2/2/2012].

Kassirer, J.P. (1983) Teaching clinical medicine by iterative hypothesis testing. Let's preach what we practice. *The New England Journal of Medicine*, 309, pp. 921-923.

Nelson, R. (2011) *Global Cancer Epidemic - A 'Crisis in Slow Motion'* [WWW] Medscape Today Website. Available from: http://www.medscape.com/viewarticle/744973 [accessed 2/2/2012].

Norman, G.R. *et al.* (2000) The benefit of diagnostic hypotheses in clinical reasoning: experimental study of an instructional intervention for forward and backward reasoning. *Cognition and Instruction*, 17, pp. 433-448.

Vance, M. (1995) *Think Out of the Box*. Pompton Plains, NJ: Career Press.

Wisenberg, R.W. (1993) *Creativity: Beyond the Myth of Genius, 2nd Edition*. New York: W.H. Freeman & Company.

About the Editors

MOHAMMADALI M. SHOJA, MD is affiliated with Division of Neurological Surgery, Department of Surgery, University of Alabama at Birmingham, and Section of Pediatric Neurosurgery, Children's Hospital, Birmingham, Alabama, US, and Tuberculosis and Lung Disease Research Center, Tabriz University of Medical Sciences, Tabriz, Iran.

PAUL S. AGUTTER, MD, PHD is affiliated with Theoretical Medicine and Biology Group, Glossop, Derbyshire, UK.

R. SHANE TUBBS, PHD is affiliated with Pediatric Neurosurgery, Children's Hospital, Birmingham, Alabama, US,

MOSTAFA GHANEI, MD is affiliated with Deputy of Research and Technology, Ministry of Health and Medical Education, Tehran, Iran.

KAMYAR GHABILI, MD is affiliated with Medical Philosophy and History Research Center, Tabriz University of Medical Sciences, Tabriz, Iran.

ALON HARRIS, PHD is affiliated with Department of Ophthalmology, Indiana University School of Medicine, Indianapolis, Indiana, US.

MARIOS LOUKAS, MD, PHD is affiliated with Department of Anatomical Sciences, St. George's University, Grenada, West Indies.

In: Hypotheses in Clinical Medicine
Editors: M.M. Shoja, P.S. Agutter et al.
ISBN: 978-1-62257-276-2

Chapter 1

From Hypothesis to Evidence-Based Medicine: Connecting the Dots

Bradley K. Weiner*[*1], Joseph Fernandez-Moure[2], Ennio Tasciotti[2] and Mohammadali M. Shoja[2]

[1] Weill Cornell Medical College, Orthopaedic Surgery, Spine Advanced Technology Laboratory, and The Methodist Hospital
[2] The Methodist Hospital Research Institute, Houston, Texas, US
[3] Division of Neurological Surgery, Department of Surgery, University of Alabama at Birmingham, Birmingham, Alabama, US, and Medical Philosophy and History Research Center, Tabriz University of Medical Sciences, Tabriz, Iran

Abstract

In this chapter, an attempt is made to highlight the differences between *evolutionary* and *revolutionary* hypotheses. Most hypotheses about etiology or novel therapies are *evolutionary* in nature and advance the field of medicine incrementally. *Revolutionary* hypotheses, on the other hand, are received with skepticism, but they advance the field enormously if corroborated. Viewing truly *revolutionary* hypotheses from an *evolutionary* perspective is misguided and dangerous. If an unusual hypothesis is presented reasonably, is founded upon solid science, and addresses important aspects of pathology that currently lack a clear explanation or solution; then it should be listened to and given a reasonable consideration. Medical hypotheses and evidence-based medicine represent a continuum, one complementing the other, and any separation between the two remains artificial as far as the patient care and advancement of knowledge are concerned.

---

[*] E-mail: BKWeiner@tmhs.org

Introduction

Medical hypotheses are sometimes opposed to evidence-based medicine. This view is non-scientific, and amounts to a dogma with potentially serious consequences as far as patient care and advancement of knowledge are concerned. In this chapter, we emphasize that these two entities should be regarded as a continuum, one complementing the other, and any separation between them is artificial.

I. Evidence-Based Medicine

Over the past half century, the practice and business of medicine has expanded exponentially and the overall costs of healthcare have escalated commensurately. Using the United States as an example, health spending was $14 Billion in 1950, $75B in 1970, $714B in 1990; and in 2011 it approached $2.6 Trillion. The share of gross domestic product (GDP) represented by this spending was 3% in 1950, 7.2% in 1970, 12.3% in 1990, and is now nearly 20%. The percentage of personal expenditure devoted to medical care has risen from 5% in 1950 to nearly 16%. Perhaps most importantly, the relative price of medical care has also risen exponentially - the Consumer Price Index (CPI) for medical care is rising 64% more quickly than the CPI for all other goods and services (Weiner 2011).

Consequently, payers - government (Medicare and Medicaid in the US; National Health System in England; etc.) and corporate (via their purchase of health insurance for employees) - have become progressively more concerned about their ability to cover these escalating costs. When this is coupled with the potential impact on national competitiveness, the natural response has been to control spending and limit services. We are told that healthcare costs are at crisis levels and intervention is deemed financially necessary.

However, who should intervene to control the spending and use of services? Logically, the ideal people to do so are the physician and patient. Unfortunately, multiple factors have rendered physicians and patients either unable or unwilling to address cost issues. These factors include:

1. The inextricable, unshakable contextual physician / patient factors: Financial incentives for physicians to treat and treat aggressively, patients' secondary gains in the sick-role (worker's compensation, etc.), intrusion of pharmaceutical and device companies into the medical decision-making process, etc.
2. Lack of expertise: Physicians are trained to be experts in anatomy, physiology, pathology, pharmacology, surgery, etc. but not cost control. They are not taught how to factor the financial impact of medical treatment into the clinical decision-making process.
3. Ignorance: Physicians and patients generally have little idea what their diagnostic and therapeutic decisions actually cost. There has been little need. Payers cover most of the costs and these payers have thrived. Health insurance companies measure their profits in billions and governments have a broad tax base of support - the largest sector of which, in several countries, is healthcare itself.

4. Etiquette: The inclusion of cost considerations in medical decisions has been considered 'unseemly' or 'inappropriate' - rapid diagnosis and treatment have been the focus; the costs are often considered worthwhile (quite often, no matter how high).

If physicians and patients are unable or unwilling to address these issues, how about the payers themselves? To date, direct efforts by payers to decrease costs via decreasing reimbursement have made surprising little impact (and only in individual cases). Continually rising utilization of services and the introduction of ever more costly new technologies have rendered these efforts moot. As can be seen in the cost numbers above, lowering payments has withdrawn (at most) a cup of water from the rising ocean tide of medical expansion.

Recognizing that simply decreasing reimbursements was insufficient, payers have tried at various times to control utilization directly via rationing (although the word 'rationing' is seldom used explicitly). These attempts have faced remarkable resistance; the public response to tightly 'managed care' by insurance companies or *explicit* rationing by government payers (such as that attempted in Oregon in the US or national health systems in Europe) has been one of disdain. Payers, it is thought, should *not* be the primary medical decision-makers regarding medical care, nor should they have absolute veto power over such decisions.

But if costs and over-utilization are problems or crises that need to be addressed, *and* physicians and patients are unable or reluctant to address them, *and* payers' direct attempts to intervene have been ineffective; who, then, should do so? Who should fill the void? The answer over the past 30 years has been a discipline that merges social science and medical economics under the umbrella 'Health Services Research' (HSR). This discipline was 'new' in 1980 but has matured at a remarkable pace. Nearly every medical school in the US and Europe now has divisions or departments aimed at the study of some of these issues. Payers, government and private, have redirected their efforts, dedicating significant resources to the study of these issues, and researchers - as they most often do - have followed the money. In their failure to impact the situation directly, payers have turned to this new branch of research / science to discover novel and alternative ways to 'get it done' *for* them.

What began as an exercise in auditing - researchers cataloguing the products of biomedicine; number of tests performed, number and types of services provided, length of stay in hospitals, dollars spent on care, etc. - has evolved into the application of specific social scientific and medical economic methodologies to obtain better documentation of the situation and, far more importantly, to *alter* the delivery of health care often with cost controls at the front end of service provision (Frankford 1994). The threads of these methodologies have been sewn, tightly and ubiquitously, throughout the fabric of health care.

An alphabet soup of concepts and methodologies has emerged from HSR and nearly all players in healthcare - payers, hospitals, physicians, scientists, and patients - are at least superficially (and often deeply) familiar with many of them: EBM (evidence-based medicine), CEA (cost-effectiveness analyses), RCTs (randomized clinical trials), DRGs (diagnostic related groups), QALY (quality adjusted life years), etc. These concepts and methodologies have become so well entrenched that they are now a routine part of daily life in medicine and healthcare. The way clinical data are collected has shifted from physician-assessed objective measures of biomedical outcomes to patient-centered questionnaires that assess quality of life via bio-psychosocial parameters. Therapeutic interventions - choices that were based on experience, training, and expert opinion - are now expected to be based upon the medical literature. And with RCTs as trump cards, the literature is now graded for quality on the basis of limiting potential bias. The day-to-day practice of medicine, once an art emerging from basic science, is now meant to be guided by evidence-based principles and guidelines. Methods of cost-effectiveness analysis now determine what health care services are reimbursed.

II. Hypothesis

So, in an age where care is guided by randomized trials and cost-effectiveness analyses, where do novel hypotheses regarding etiology and therapeutics fit? How does a hypothesis 'mature' to the point where it might make an impact on patient care when such care is controlled by health services research and its reliance on evidence-based medicine?

III. Hypotheses of Etiology

Medical hypotheses in general can be divided into two basic types: Those putting forth novel concepts of *etiology* and those putting forth novel concepts of *treatment.* Both of these can be further subdivided into concepts that are *evolutionary* and those that are *revolutionary.*

a. *Evolutionary hypotheses of etiology* are characterized by their presentation of novel concepts of cause that are clearly in line with the currently accepted theory. An example would be an hypothesis that a particular breakdown product of cartilage cell death results in acceleration of further cell death. If corroborated at the basic science bench, this supported hypothesis might lead to greater understanding of the pathophysiology of arthritis (an *academic* benefit) and might also lead to a novel therapy aimed at preventing the breakdown product's action on viable cartilage cells (an *academic* and *therapeutic* impact). In either case, the new hypothesis put forth or the potential knowledge gained is in line with current understanding and therefore much more likely to be accepted in the literature and eventually into part of accepted evidence-based care. Remember - evidence-based medicine rests on the principle that care should be guided by the best available evidence *in the medical literature*, and novel hypotheses are far easier to accept in the literature when they are evolutionary in nature.

b. *Revolutionary hypotheses of etiology* are often viewed with suspicion because they contradict the currently-accepted basic science evidence-base. Exceptions occur when a 'new' disease emerges and the potential theories on etiology are wide-ranging - an 'open' field - as in the early phases of emerging infectious diseases. Far more commonly, when a solid current evidence-base is available, wholly novel concepts of etiology are viewed with skepticism. It is assumed that the proposer simply does not understand the underlying basic science. Most of the time, frankly, this is true. A brief review of etiological hypotheses put forth over the years in the journal *Medical Hypotheses* (for instance) suggests that hypotheses that are a considerable distance from the mainstream rarely end there. That said, such a hypothesis does occasionally ring true and, when this eventually occurs, entire new branches of basic science aimed at the disease and entire new programs aimed therapeutic interventions emerge, often resulting in novel treatments that radically alter the trajectory of disease, greatly decreasing morbidity and/or mortality. The medical specialties of infectious disease and rheumatology are perhaps the brightest examples, where revolutionary hypotheses of etiology have panned out and lives have been saved or greatly improved in quality. What killed and maimed many of our predecessors is now often just controlled by a pill in western societies with reasonable health infrastructures.

IV. Hypotheses of Treatment

a. *Evolutionary hypotheses of treatment* are proposed novel therapies that fall in line with current treatment modalities. Examples could be a new antibiotic or a new anti-inflammatory drug that differs slightly from those currently employed. A modification of current gold-standard surgical intervention such as decompressive laminectomies for lumbar spinal canal stenosis would be another example. In order for these therapies to be employed, they must (and should) pass through the evidence-based mill. They should have a solid basic science foundation confirming that they are likely to succeed both from the bench and in vivo. If appropriate they should have passed through 'Phase I' trials. They should be tested in randomized trials or quality matched cohort studies to determine that they are at least as effective as the current gold standard. From the same studies, they should be demonstrated to be at least as safe. And if the newly introduced therapy is equivalent to the gold standard in regards to efficacy and safety, it should be more cost-effective. Such developments, adding an additional branch to a mature tree, are common and make up the bulk of RCTs currently published in the literature, establishing our evidence-base and appropriately guiding the bulk of patient care.

b. *Revolutionary hypotheses of treatment* are often viewed, like their etiological counterparts, with skepticism. Because they are not in line with current thought regarding therapy they are often not taken seriously, and with good reason - most such proposals turn out to be misguided. However, those that turn out to be true (perhaps 'remarkably useful' is a better term) represent many of the major advances in medicine. In these cases, the findings of simple case series reports are often so compelling that putting the therapy through the evidence-based mill would be unethical - would lack the equipoise required for randomizing patients into the non-treatment group. It would be wholly inappropriate to include someone in the control arm of the study knowing, on the basis lesser quality studies or reports, that the new treatment is superior. The introduction and use of antibiotics for bacterial meningitis is a classic example.

There are important prerequisites: (a) The hypothesized therapy must rest on an excellent foundation of basic science. It must make solid scientific sense. We are all well aware of unusual, non-scientific therapies that have been shown to be temporarily effective because of the placebo effect alone. (b) The disease/process being treated must be a major cause of mortality, morbidity, or have no viable treatment options available. Many of our major advances in medicine - novel chemotherapeutic agents and radiation therapy for cancer, nearly all antibiotics, life-saving surgical techniques such as appendectomy - came about *without* RCTs; but were found so compelling that immediate implementation was undertaken. Subsequently, entire new lines of research developed 'on the backs' of these revolutionary discoveries and persist to this day. These subsequent new lines of research, treatment, theories of etiology are *evolutionary* in nature, representing modifications of the previously revolutionary finding.

V. Summary: From Hypothesis to Evidence-Based Medicine: Connecting the Dots

It is clear from the recent history of medicine that the bulk of hypotheses of etiology or novel therapies are *evolutionary* in nature. They rest on a solid foundation of basic science and clinical background knowledge. While not earth-shattering, they advance the field of medicine incrementally and - importantly - most often safely. Accordingly, they are greeted within the medical community with an open mind, are more likely to be published in quality journals and textbooks, are more likely to be evaluated with equipoise in quality RCTs, and are consequently more likely to become part of the established evidence-base, which will be used to establish guidelines of treatment.

Revolutionary hypotheses, however, face a far more difficult road from idea to evidence-base. They are envisioned by the medical community with suspicion. They don't follow. They aren't branches of the tree, but entirely new plants. Most often, this suspicion is justified. Novel concepts are often high-risk and there must be demonstration of high reward before they are taken seriously. Most proposed revolutionary hypotheses fail to produce such rewards.

There are, however, notable exceptions. Not all are historical in nature (such as the discovery of antibiotics for infections, radiation therapy for tumors, or appendectomy, discussed above). A more recent example is the use of extracorporeal membranous oxygenation (ECMO) for the treatment of neonatal persistent pulmonary hypertension (PPHS) (Worrall 2007). Historically, prior to the 1980s, the mortality rate of PPHS exceeded 80%; eight out of ten newborns died regardless of treatment. In 1982, a physician named Bartlett and his co-workers in Michigan published a paper outlining a *revolutionary* hypothesis of treatment, demonstrating that the mortality rate for PPHS could be reduced to less than 20% with ECMO - only two out of ten babies died. Their use of ECMO was founded upon some solid background information (a prerequisite noted above): PPHS results from immaturity of the lungs, which are unable to allow properly for the transfer of oxygen to the blood stream in afflicted neonates. Otherwise, babies with PPHS are healthy, but the lack of oxygen in the blood leads to a cascade of injured tissues ultimately resulting in death. It was known at the time that if the babies could be kept alive long enough to allow for maturation of their lungs they might recover significantly. This background information led to the development of ECMO and its use for PPHS. ECMO, essentially, replaces the lungs temporarily (Bartlett *et al.* 1982). Blood is removed from the babies' veins prior to getting to their lungs and runs through a machine that affects the transfer of oxygen to the blood, and the newly oxygenated blood is returned to the baby via the carotid artery. The immature lungs are 'bypassed', allowed to mature, and once they have done so and have begun to function normally, ECMO is discontinued and the majority of babies are able to survive.

Unfortunately, the original study by Bartlett and his colleagues was viewed with skepticism because of its revolutionary status and because the information was presented within a poorly controlled historical cohort study, about two layers below randomized trials on the accepted hierarchy of evidential quality. From the HSR perspective, historically controlled cohort studies carry very little weight in comparison to RCTs. In consequence, Bartlett and his team felt compelled to conduct a prospective randomized trial to support their findings further. That is, despite a firm belief that ECMO was far more effective and safe than other treatments, they pushed forward with an RCT. Needless to say, *they* were not *unclear*; but their personal lack of equipoise was trumped by disagreements among accepted experts within the wider community and, oddly, these disagreements centered primarily on research methodology as opposed to underlying physiological/medical understanding. In other words, this *revolutionary* hypothesis, which appeared to be true/remarkably useful, was initially *rejected* by the broader medical community and forced to go through the evidence-based mill which, as was noted previously, is only appropriate for *evolutionary* developments (or for those diseases that are not life-threatening, terribly morbid, or without available options). This proved to be a mistake.

The results of the subsequent RCT, which compared survival rates between ECMO-treated babies and those treated by conventional therapies, were impressive. Of twelve babies enrolled, all eleven treated with ECMO survived while the one child treated with conventional modalities died (Bartlett *et al.* 1985). Given these findings, coupled with the historical 80% mortality rate and the findings of their 1982 study, Bartlett and his co-workers halted the study. Clearly, the point was made: ECMO saved lives and was a superior treatment option.

Sadly, however, there is more to the story. While those with an ethical bent might be asking 'Why did we have to lose the one child randomized to conventional treatment?', several health services researchers at the time were asking a quite different question: 'Why were eleven randomized to ECMO and only one to conventional treatment?' It turns out that the authors used an uncommon type of randomization called 'play the winner', wherein the results of each iteration in the study impact the randomization. That is, if the first baby survived, it became more likely for the next baby to be randomized to that treatment, and if the first baby died it became less likely for the next baby to be randomized to *that* treatment. Thus, as it turned out, the first baby in their study died and had been treated by conventional therapies, and the next set of babies survived and had been treated by ECMO. Accordingly, given their methodology, subsequent babies were much more likely to be randomized to ECMO with increasing frequency as ECMO racked up successes. The end result was an 'unbalanced' randomization - and, according to HSR, not true randomization (which results in each iteration having a 50 / 50 chance of assignment to either treatment group if there are two groups). The following quotations followed the publication of their paper (Worrall 2007):

> "...the results are not convincing because only one patient received the standard therapy."
> "Further randomized clinical trials using concurrent controls and randomization will be difficult, but remain necessary."

Viewing truly *revolutionary* hypotheses (that have been shown to be remarkably effective in case series reports) from an *evolutionary* perspective is misguided and dangerous. Further RCTs were carried out. O'Rourke and co-workers in 1989 reported their results using 'proper randomization' and standard methodologies (O'Rourke *et al.* 1989). Nineteen patients were enrolled. Nine received ECMO and all survived. Ten received conventional therapies and four died. The trial was stopped and those on the trial waiting list were then all placed into the ECMO group (twenty additional babies) and all but one survived. Established resistance to revolutionary hypotheses and the call for a second randomized trial had won; methodology had trumped observational background knowledge; and four more babies had died in the name of misguided randomization.

Conclusion

The lesson here is that the principles of evidence-based medicine and the demand that hypotheses be confirmed in a rigid scientific fashion culminating in randomized trials, while *absolutely appropriate in the great majority of cases*, has the occasional exception and these exceptions often represent truly revolutionary findings. We all - even those us who are 'true believers' in the benefits of the principles of evidence-based medicine - are best served by keeping an open mind. If an unusual hypothesis is presented by a reasonable source, is founded upon solid science, and addresses an important aspect of pathology that currently lacks a clear solution; then we should listen and give the hypothesis reasonable consideration.

But how do we weed through the numerous hypotheses that rest on shaky basic science foundations, or address minor problems, or are from unreliable profit-driven sources? How do we get to the good stuff? The answer, I believe, rests in simple, open-minded, quality *editorial* work. A wide-open, all-comers-welcome philosophy indeed welcomes all-comers. You get what you ask for. And readers of journals and books and the media are overwhelmed by foundationless hypotheses supported by weak studies resting on the placebo effect and pseudo-science to demonstrate supposed efficacy. We can do better. From an editorial perspective, we cannot *only* rely on the products of formal evidence-based medicine to determine what is publication-ready. We must also have an open mind regarding potential novel theories of etiology or therapy that meet the prerequisites for quality described above. Our journals and books might then prove to be a valuable resource for those looking to publish promising ideas and those aiming to learn about them or independently test them. And patients will be better off for it.

References

BARTLETT, R.H. *et al.* (1982) Extracorporeal membrane oxygenation for newborn respiratory failure: forty-five cases. *Surgery*, 92, pp. 425-433.

BARTLETT, R.H. *et al.* (1985) Extracorporeal circulation in neonatal respiratory failure: a prospective randomized study. *Pediatrics*, 76, pp. 479-487.

FRANKFORD, D.M. (1994) Scientism and economism in the regulation of health care. *Journal of Health Politics, Policy and Law*, 19, pp. 773-799.

O'ROURKE, P.P., *et al.* (1989) Extracorporeal membrane oxygenation and conventional medical therapy in neonates with persistent pulmonary hypertension of the newborn: a prospective randomized study. *Pediatrics*, 84, pp. 957-963.

WEINER, B.K. (2011) Necessary and potentially evil. *The Spine Journal*, 11, pp. 715-717.

WORRALL, J. (2007) Why there's no cause to randomize. *British Journal of the Philosophy of Science*, 58, pp. 451-488.

In: Hypotheses in Clinical Medicine
Editors: M.M. Shoja, P.S. Agutter et al.
ISBN: 978-1-62257-276-2

Chapter 2

Paradigm Shifts and Explanation in Clinical Medicine: The "How" of Reality and the "Why" of Truth

Alireza Ghaffari[1], Mohammadali M. Shoja[2*], R. Shane Tubbs[3], Marios Loukas[4], Paul S. Agutter[5], Kamyar Ghabili[6], Jalal Etemadi[6], Aaron A. Cohen-Gadol[7] and Bradley K. Weiner[8]

[1]Tuberculosis and Lung Disease Research Center,
Tabriz University of Medical Sciences, Tabriz, Iran
[2]Division of Neurological Surgery, Department of Surgery,
University of Alabama at Birmingham, Birmingham, Alabama, US
and Medical Philosophy and History Research Center,
Tabriz University of Medical Sciences, Tabriz, Iran
[3]Pediatric Neurosurgery, Children's Hospital, Birmingham, Alabama, US
[4]Department of Anatomical Sciences, St. George's University, Grenada, West Indies
[5]Theoretical Medicine and Biology Group, Glossop, Derbyshire, UK
[6]Medical Philosophy and History Research Center, Tabriz University of Medical Sciences, Tabriz, Iran
[7]Goodman Campbell Brain and Spine, Department of Neurological Surgery,
Indiana University, Indianapolis, Indiana, US
[8]Weill Cornell Medical College, Department of Orthopaedic Surgery,
The Methodist Hospital, Houston, Texas, US

Abstract

The philosophy of science in general, and the philosophy of biology in particular, are relevant to scientific medicine. However, contemporary medical understanding raises distinct and perhaps unique ontological and epistemological issues that merit separate

[*] E-mail: shoja.m@gmail.com.

consideration, not least because they can have implications for practice. In this paper, we identify some of these issues, using the current controversy surrounding the treatment of anemia in cases of chronic kidney disease as exemplar. The preliminary inferences drawn from this discussion are presented as starting points for more detailed exploration by philosophers, as well as matters for attention by clinicians.

Introduction

Medicine, in both practice and research, presents ethical problems that have rightly engaged the attention of moral philosophers. However, it also presents distinct metaphysical problems that have been less widely considered. In so far as mainstream medicine today has a scientific basis, the philosophy of science in general is pertinent to its epistemology and ontology; in so far as medicine is related to biology, the philosophy of biology is also - and in some ways more directly - pertinent. However, as we shall show in this article, not all metaphysical issues in medicine can be elucidated fully by reference to either of these disciplines. Our aim is to identify some of these issues, illustrating our argument with a controversial example from current medical practice, and to argue that detailed philosophical analysis of those issues could be beneficial to physicians.

The article is organized as follows. The first section is a brief overview of the nature of scientific thought. The second and third sections review two topics in the philosophy of biology that are particularly relevant to medicine. This is followed by a short review of the literature relating to the treatment of anemia associated with chronic kidney disease (CKD), and then an analysis of the philosophical issues arising from this example. The concluding section seeks to generalize the inferences from this analysis.

Scientific Thought

Human understanding depends not only on information obtained through the senses (with or without the aid of special instruments) but also on the way in which the mind is predisposed to organize and interpret that information. In its general sense, this assertion has become a commonplace, and does not necessarily entail commitment to Kantian epistemeology (Guyer 1987). Indeed, the picture of "man as scientist" in Kelly's personality theory (Fransella and Bannister 1986) emphasizes the provisional structuring of everyday knowledge; the "theories" we construct about the world are tested by further observation and are refined accordingly. In scientific disciplines, this process is more formalized, but - in broad terms-it is qualitatively similar to the everyday; as Popper observed, science is "common sense writ large" (Popper 1959).

Nevertheless, closer scrutiny of this formalization reveals ways in which scientific explanations are distinctive (Agutter and Wheatley 2008). For example:

- They are naturalistic rather than supernaturalistic.
- They are mechanistic rather than teleological.
- They are general rather than particular, and seek to be comprehensive.
- They tend to be abstract rather than concrete, and (where possible) mathematical.
- They are expressed in 'value-neutral' terms.

Some of these characteristics (such as naturalism as opposed to supernaturalism) can be traced to ancient Greek roots (Lloyd 1991), or at least to the scholars of the Islamic golden age (Bakar 1999), and were developed in medieval Europe (Grant 1996), but they became formally established during the 'scientific revolution' in Europe, particularly in the contributions of Bacon, Galileo and Descartes (Henry 2002; Pitt 1997; Scott 1979) and the achievements of Newton (Buchwald and Bernard 2001). Broadly, they apply to scientific medicine today, though medical explanations are limited in generality because of the breadth and complexity of the subject matter; they become concrete rather than abstract when individual patients or groups of patients are considered; and they are mathematical only in respect of certain modeling exercises and in the statistical evaluation of clinical trials or of epidemiological evidence.

The Newtonian system of thought became an ideology of reductionism and mechanistic causal explanation after the 17th century, granting a central role to observation and measurement. That ideology survives in modern science, though it can take on many forms, determined by the possibilities afforded by new methods and instruments and exemplified by landmark experiments; these forms were labeled "paradigms" by Kuhn (1970). Paradigms profoundly affect attitudes and practices in all natural sciences, and they have a significant role in medicine, though they have been less thoroughly explored in biology and medicine because most philosophers of science have focused their attention on physics. Biologists often deny the "sovereignty of ideology" in their decision making, stressing methodological approaches to problem solving, but the human mind cannot process information without an operating system of ideology (cf. Fransella and Bannister 1986).

Notwithstanding the particular attention that philosophers have paid to physics, there have been major contributions to the philosophy of the life sciences, and these have highlighted certain distinctions between the physics-related and biological disciplines. Two of these distinctions are directly relevant to the present paper: the "problem of purpose", and the very complicated character of living systems. We will now consider these two distinctions in relation to medical understanding and practice.

The "Problem of Purpose" in Biology

The constituents of an organism (organs, tissues, cells, molecules) have *functions* within that organism. It is scientifically legitimate, and indeed necessary for adequate description, to say what e.g. a hemoglobin molecule or a kidney in a mammal is *for*. Thus, a function of hemoglobin is to bind oxygen at the lungs and release it in the capillary beds of respiring tissues; a function of the kidney is to ensure that the water content of the body remains within certain limits. (We write 'a function' rather than 'the function' because the objects in question may serve more than one physiological purpose.) These functions are defined 'from within'; they serve the needs of the organism that contains the objects in question. This is in contrast to the products of technology, which serve the needs or purposes of their makers and users. (A washing machine does not wash clothes for itself, but for its operator.)

This characteristic of organisms, that their parts are 'endowed with purpose' - for which Monod (1970) coined the term *teleonomy* - is on the face of it alien to the Newtonian ideology of science; it seems to entail teleological as opposed to mechanistic explanation.

Rocks, rivers, stars and clouds are not teleonomic; it makes no scientific sense to ascribe 'functions' to them. Our scientific accounts of such objects are unproblematic; cause is the temporal antecedent of effect. Teleonomy, however, appears to invert this linear chronology of mechanistic causality; the 'teleological cause' (function) of hemoglobin (i.e. oxygen transport) succeeds, not precedes, the 'teleological effect' (the organism must contain hemoglobin). However, several writers have shown that this problem is soluble by reference to the theory of evolution (Agutter and Wheatley 1999; Mayr 1972; Monod 1970; Nagel 1979). For example, in the case of hemoglobin, we can write:

- Mammals do, as a matter of fact, contain hemoglobin. (An empirical generalization.)
- Hemoglobin binds oxygen at the lungs and releases it in the capillary beds of respiring tissues. (Another empirical generalization, a matter of experimental physiology, and essentially 'causal' in the mechanistic sense.)
- Nothing other than hemoglobin ensures adequate oxygenation of respiring tissues. (A third empirical generalization, enriched by comparative biological studies.)
- Unless adequate oxygenation is ensured, the mammal will not survive to reproductive age and leave offspring. (The assertion that adequate oxygenation is a necessary condition for survival and reproduction evokes the principle of evolution by natural selection, and it is the key to this analysis. It entails the belief that hemoglobin has been functionally perfected by natural selection, making it a *consequence* of the requirements for survival and reproduction.)

Thus, mechanistic sense can be made of teleonomy by virtue of the theory of evolution. This illustrates the central importance of evolutionary theory to scientific biology, and, by implication, to medicine, which is an applied aspect of biology. Indeed, the need for medical practitioners to comprehend the theory of evolution has been highlighted by several authors (e.g. Domazet-Lošo and Tautz 2008; Lappe 1994; Nesse and Williams 1994), though their concerns have mostly been practical rather than metaphysical.

There is one sense in which teleonomic propositions differ between basic biology and an applied discipline such as medicine. In basic biology, we can easily show that 'function' does not mean the same as 'effect', by (for example) examining the statements:

- An effect of hemoglobin is to make blood red.
- A function of hemoglobin is to make blood red.

The first statement is common knowledge but the second makes no sense. In contrast, consider this pair of statements:

- An effect of aspirin is to inhibit platelet aggregation.
- A function of aspirin is to inhibit platelet aggregation.

In this case, the former statement is an empirical generalization from applied pharmacology, while the second makes good sense in the context of treatment of e.g. patients at risk for thrombosis. In medicine, therefore, as opposed to basic biology, function-statements applied to drugs are as intelligible as effect-statements, and are closely related to them in meaning.

One inference from this discussion is that while much of the philosophy of biology is pertinent to the philosophy of medicine, some aspects of the philosophy of medicine are distinctive. Therefore, we cannot look to the philosophy of biology for answers to all our questions about medicine.

The Complexity of Living Systems

Everything in an organism obeys the laws of physics and chemistry and nothing else. Living matter differs from non-living matter only in the way it is *organized.* Such organization is responsible for the distinctive properties of organisms and is the root of the teleonomic character of their parts. This position was made explicit in Bichat's *General Anatomy* (Bichat 1801), while scientific physiology was in its infancy, and was stated succinctly half a century later by Lister (1863): *'Living matter has properties distinct from, albeit not inconsistent with, those that are traditionally addressed by physicists'.*

A great deal has been written on this subject, but only one point is important in the present context. In contrast to physical systems, events within living organisms can seldom be explained in terms of simple linear cause-effect relationships. Rather, there is a network of causal connections, exemplified (and symbolized) by the signaling pathways activated in target cells by multiple effectors, and the multiple changes brought about by those pathways. Typically, many causes and many effects surround any event in an organism, and the cause-effect linkages are interdependent. Moreover, such networks generally include feedback loops that modulate the flow of events; on the more macroscopic scale, such regulatory mechanisms provide the basis for homeostasis. The identification of homeostatic mechanisms forms the root of a dominant paradigm in modern biology and medicine.

One consequence of this characteristic of biological causality is that much of the vocabulary of biology - and medicine - is more akin to that of control engineering than physics: terms such as control, regulation, transcription, code, feedback and signal are not to be found in physics or chemistry texts, but are part of the language of engineers. This observation is no more than an updated version of what Bichat (1801) and Lister (1863) wrote in the 19th century, but it suffices to show that their insights remain valid, despite the advances in knowledge during the past 150-200 years. It constitutes a serious challenge to radical reductionism and to strict adherence to the Newtonian ideology in medicine and biology.

The practical implication is straightforward, though it is often overlooked: any action that interferes with a particular 'cause' of events in a biological system is likely not only to alter many 'effects' but also to affect other 'causes'. Blocking a single receptor on a single cell type can disrupt many aspect of that cell's activity, with consequences for the activities of other cell types and potentially for the body as a whole. The significance of this for medicine is obvious: all drugs have side effects, some of which may be unforeseen despite rigorous testing, and they might not exert the desired effect(s) on some patients.

To explore this simple generalization in more depth, we now consider an example from contemporary medical practice that is beset with uncertainties, as the literature reveals.

Example: Anemia and Chronic Kidney Disease

Anemia is a major complication of chronic kidney disease (CKD), despite recent advances in therapy, and it tends to become more severe with increasing deterioration of kidney function; some 50% of stage 4 CKD patients and almost 100% of stage 5 patients are affected (Gillespie *et al.* 2007). Anemia in such patients can have many causes, notably impaired erythropoietin output consequent on deterioration of the renal parenchyma, but iron deficiency is also common in this population (Lankhorst and Wish 2010) and secondary hyperparathyroidism, dyslipidemia, vascular calcification and reduced erythrocyte life span consequent on uremia can also be relevant factors (Brosnahan and Fraer 2010; Dowling 2007; van der Putten *et al.* 2008). Therefore, careful evaluation of each individual patient is required. Anemia is especially problematic in end-stage renal disease patients who are subjected to chronic hemodialysis. Treatment is required because the anemia entails a significant risk for left ventricular hypertrophy, angina, congestive heart failure (Dowling 2007; Gillespie *et al.* 2007) and accelerated progression of renal failure as well as a decrease in quality of life (impaired oxygen delivery and utilization, poor cognition and decreased immune function), and there is general improvement if it is corrected. Erythropoiesis-stimulating agents (ESA), a range of biotechnological products (Goldsmith 2010), constitute the standard therapeutic approach to the correction of anemia in these cases, and the development of new ESAs is continuing (Del Vecchio *et al.* 2010).

However, ESA use and alternative therapeutic approaches are associated with unexpected problems and have become controversial. Debate about the stage of disease at which interventions to correct the anemia should be commenced, and about the appropriate target hemoglobin level, began in the 1990s (Roger and Levin 2007); there were no placebo-controlled trials for several years. Remarkably, the findings concerning renal function, cardiovascular dysfunction, diabetes etc. were discouraging (Drüeke *et al.* 2006; Ritz *et al.* 2007; Singh *et al.* 2006). These studies showed that normalization of hemoglobin levels is not necessarily effective and can sometimes be associated with worse outcome (Weiner *et al.* 2005). A target hemoglobin level of 11-12 g/dl in patients treated with ESA has been recommended as a result of several trials and working group considerations (Locatelli *et al.* 2010), but this cannot always be attained (Kanbay *et al.* 2010); the cause of ESA-resistant anemia remains uncertain. ESA use appears to be contraindicated for diabetic patients and needs to be closely monitored in cases of cardiac insufficiency because of the increased risk of stroke (Locatelli *et al.* 2010; Singh 2010).

It is widely held that because CKD is associated with an enhanced inflammatory response and increased levels of inflammatory cytokines such as hepcidin and IL-6 (Malyszko and Mysliwiec 2007), the anemia of CKD is the result of an inflammatory disorder (Koury and Ponka 2004). Hepcidin down-regulates ferroportin, the iron efflux channel in enterocytes and macrophages (Nemeth *et al.* 2004), and therefore impairs iron loading on to plasma transferrin; and erythropoietin action depends on the effective mobilization of iron stores, along with an intact signaling pathway involving the erythropoietin receptor and the JAK/STAT system. Hepcidin may also inhibit the survival and differentiation of erythroid progenitor cells, contributing further to erythropoietin resistance (Dallalio *et al.* 2006). CKD and hemodialysis patients have elevated hepcidin levels (Ganz *et al.* 2008; Tomosugi *et al.* 2006; Zaritsky *et al.* 2009). However, it is not clear why ESA treatment can increase morbidity and mortality. It has been suggested that an increased tendency to thrombosis or elevated blood pressure may make serious cardiovascular events more likely, but deregulated production of vasoactive factors and abnormal responses to them could also be implicated. Moreover, it has not been established whether the increased mortality is attributable to the increased hemoglobin level or to a direct effect of the ESA (or erythropoietin) itself (Singh 2010; Szczech *et al.* 2008).

The question of how anemia in CKD patients should be treated has therefore become moot, and it extends to a more general question. As Goldsmith (2010) phrased it: *'We are now very much at a "crossroads," where mature reflection is required, because with the latest trials and meta-analyses, these therapies seem not only expensive but also very much a clinical tradeoff (increased risk of adverse effects versus a small gain in fatigue scores). How we arrived at this crossroads is a useful illustration of how easy it is, without properly designed randomized, controlled trials, to assume that clinical benefit must follow therapeutic interventions.'*

Reflections on the CKD-Anemia Controversy

The last sentence in this quotation from Goldsmith suggests that the use of ESAs to normalize hemoglobin levels in anemic CKD patients reflects the pervading influence of Newtonian ideology: thinking in linear cause-effect terms. According to this perspective, loss of function in the kidney parenchyma cells results in abnormally low circulating levels of erythropoietin, and in consequence a hypoplastic anemia; therefore, agents that stimulate erythropoietin production should restore normal erythrocyte production and normal hemoglobin levels. As a hypothesis, this is not inherently implausible; but if it is considered in terms of the 'paradigm of homeostasis' it is clear that it should be viewed with caution. For instance, erythropoietin receptors are not confined to the bone marrow; they are also expressed, for example, in cardiomyocytes, and erythropoietin improves myocardial function in animal models of heart failure (Smith *et al.* 2009). Uremic sera contain hemolytic and anti-erythropoietic factors (Bonomini and Sirolli 2003), so the uremia inevitable in CKD patients could contribute directly to the anemia. The hypertension that often accompanies ESA treatment may have many causes: impaired vascular endothelial vasodilatory responses to hypoxia consequent on uremia, diminished nitric oxide production, increased blood viscosity resulting from increased hematocrit, increased blood volume without compensation by hemodialysis, and so on (Eckardt 2001). These observations and others (see previous section) emphasize the need to consider the pathophysiology of CKD-related anemia, and its treatment, in terms of 'causal network' rather than linear cause-effect connections.

Moreover, the 'paradigm of homeostasis' requires us to look beyond a single pathological consequence of a disease to its further implications. The failed kidney can not excrete excess salt and water. Diminished erythropoietin synthesis and the consequent anemia expose the tissues to hypoxemia, leading to metabolic vasodilation. The resultant peripheral pooling of excess fluid partially compensates the failing kidney and volume overload. Thus, the anemia can - from this perspective - be regarded as a 'homeostatic' response to the major pathological effects of CKD. Such reasoning predicts that normalizing the hematocrit in CKD patients may be detrimental, which is in line with observation.

However, another factor could have aggravated the persistent tendency towards. Newtonian cause-effect reasoning in this context. ESAs are products of biotechnology, so their manufacture, sale and therapeutic use are not only clinically exciting, but they also have economic (and *a fortiori* political) implications. It is well known that medical practice is strongly influenced by the pharmaceutical industries (including, in this case, biotechnology), which conduct or at least finance a large percentage of drug trials. The concept underlying all drug production is that the new drug will have a specific effect, which gives it therapeutic value. In essence, this concept is based on Newtonian ideology.

Conclusion

Such conflicting and controversial issues are not uncommon in routine clinical practice; they are often regarded as "usual". The question arises: do we need a new paradigm, perhaps an elaboration of the 'paradigm of homeostasis', to enable us to understand these issues in a more logical and practically useful way? Most of the publications we have cited in relation to the CKD-anemia example are authoritative review articles, and they point to various aspects of the 'causal network' we have discussed. What this literature lacks - and all similar bodies of literature in medicine lack - is an *a priori* perspective that can immediately assimilate the complexities of relevant 'causal networks'. We have a vast, detailed knowledge-base of human physiology and pathology, and parts of this knowledge-base are always used in medical investigations. But our approaches tend to be piecemeal, phenomenological and often haphazard rather than integrated, theory-based and organized.

The form of the desired paradigm is a matter on which philosophers may be able to advise, in collaboration with physicians who are open-minded about their input, and possibly with systems biologists and others versed in the techniques of modeling. As far as we can anticipate, the hoped-for paradigm will involve the understanding of 'function' and 'effect' that we outlined earlier in this article, and a more precise delineation of the notion of 'causal networks' (a matter on which some systems biologists could certainly advise). It will enable the realities of observation and the mechanistic explanations of 'how' to be integrated with the 'why' of teleonomy, extended to pathological sequelae of the conditions under consideration.

References

Agutter, P.S. and Wheatley, D.N. (1999) On the "problem of purpose" in biology and our acceptance of the Darwinian theory of natural selection. *Foundations of Science*, 4, pp. 3-23.

Agutter, P.S. and Wheatley, D.N. (2008) *Thinking about Life: the History and Philosophy of Biology and Other Sciences*. Dordrecht: Springer.

Bakar, O. (1999) *History and Philosophy of Islamic Science*. Cambridge: Islamic Texts.

Bichat, X. (1801) *Anatomie Générale Appliquée à la Physiologie et à la Médecine*. Paris: Brosson, Gabon et Cie.

Bonomini, M. and Sirolli, V. (2003) Uremic toxicity and anemia. *Journal of Nephrology*, 16, pp. 21-28.

Brosnahan, G. and Fraer, M. (2010) Management of chronic kidney disease: what is the evidence? *Southern Medical Journal*, 103, pp. 222-230.

Buchwald, J.Z. and *BERNARD*, I. (2001) *Isaac Newton's Natural Philosophy*. Cambridge, MA: MIT Press.

Dallalio, G. *et al.* (2006) Hepcidin inhibits in vitro erythroid colony formation at reduced erythropoietin concentrations. *Blood*, 107, pp. 2702-2704.

Del Vecchio, L. *et al.* (2010) Chronic kidney disease-associated anemia: new remedies. *Current Opinion in Investigational Drugs*, 11, pp. 1030-1038.

Domazet-Lošo, T. and Tautz, D. (2008) An ancient evolutionary origin of genes associated with human genetic diseases. *Molecular Biology and Evolution*, 25, pp. 2699-2707.

Dowling, T.C. (2007) Prevalence, etiology, and consequences of anemia and clinical and economic benefits of anemia correction in patients with chronic kidney disease: an overview. *American Journal of Health-System Pharmacy*, 6413[Suppl 8], pp. 3-7.

Drüeke, T.B. *et al.* (2006) Normalization of hemoglobin level in patients with chronic kidney disease and anemia. *The New England Journal of Medicine*, 355, pp. 2071-2084.

Eckardt, K.U. (2001) Anaemia in end-stage renal disease: pathophysiological considerations. *Nephrology, Dialysis, Transplantation*, 16[Suppl 7], pp. 2-8.

Fransella, F. and Bannister, D. (1986) *Inquiring Man: the Theory of Personal Constructs*. 2nd edition. London: Routledge.

Ganz, T. *et al.* (2008) Immunoassay for human serum hepcidin. *Blood*, 112, pp. 4292-4297.

Gillespie, B.S. *et al.* (2007) Anemia management in chronic kidney disease. *Hemodialysis International*, 11, pp. 15-20.

Goldsmith, D. (2010): 2009: a requiem for rHuEPOs - but should we nail down the coffin in 2010? *Clinical Journal of The American Society of Nephrology*, 5, pp. 929-935.

Grant, E. (1996) *The Foundations of Modern Science in the Middle Ages: their Religious, Institutional and Intellectual Contexts*. Cambridge: Cambridge University Press.

Guyer, P. (1987) *Kant and the Claims of Knowledge*. New York: Cambridge University Press.

Henry, J. (2002) *Knowledge is Power: Francis Bacon and the Method of Science*. Cambridge: Icon Books.

Kanbay, M. *et al.* (2010) Erythropoiesis stimulatory agent-resistant anemia in dialysis patients: review of causes and management. *Blood Purification*, 29, pp. 1-12.

Koury, M.J. and Ponka, P. (2004) New insights into erythropoiesis: the roles of folate, vitamin B12, and iron. *Annual Review of Nutrition*, 24, pp. 105-131.

Kuhn, T.S. (1970) *The Structure of Scientific Revolutions*. 2nd edition. Chicago: University of Chicago Press.

Lappe, M. (1994) *Evolutionary Medicine: Rethinking the Origins of Disease*. New York: Random House, Inc.

Lloyd, G.E.R. (1991) *Methods and Problems in Greek Science*. Cambridge: Cambridge University Press.

Lister, J.L. (1863) Croonian lecture: On the coagulation of the blood. *Proceedings of the Royal Society of Medicine (London)*, 13, pp. 355-364.

Locatelli, F. *et al.* (2010) Target haemoglobin to aim for with erythropoiesis-stimulating agents: a position statement by ERBP following publication of the Trial to reduce cardiovascular events with Aranesp therapy (TREAT) study. *Nephrology, Dialysis and Transplantation*, 9, pp. 2846-2850.

Malyszko, J. and Mysliwiec, M. (2007) Hepcidin in anemia and inflammation in chronic kidney disease. *Kidney and Blood Pressure Research*, 30, pp. 15-30.

Mayr, E. (1972) *The Growth of Biological Thought: Diversity, Evolution and Inheritance*. Cambridge, MA: Harvard University Press.

Monod, J. (1970) *Chance and Necessity*. New York: Random House.

Nagel, E. (1979) *Teleology Revisited, and Other Essays in the Philosophy and History of Science*. New York: Columbia University Press.

Nemeth, E. *et al.* (2004) IL-6 mediates hypoferremia of inflammation by inducing the synthesis of the iron regulatory hormone hepcidin. *Journal of Clinical Investigation*, 113, pp. 1271-1276.

Nesse, R.M. and Williams, G.C. (1994) *Why we get Sick: the New Science of Darwinian Medicine*. New York: Times Books.

Pitt, J.C. (1997) *Galileo, Human Knowledge and the Book of Nature: Method Replaces Metaphysics*. Dordrecht: Kluwer

Popper, K.R. (1959) *The Logic of Scientific Discovery*. London: Hutchinson.

Ritz, E. *et al.* (2007) Target level for hemoglobin correction in patients with diabetes and CKD: primary results of the Anemia Correction in Diabetes ACORD Study. *American Journal of Kidney Diseases*, 49, pp. 194-207.

Roger, S.D. and Levin, A. (2007) Epoetin trials: randomised controlled trials don't always mimic observational data. *Nephrology, Dialysis and Transplantation*, 22, pp. 684-686.

Scott, J.F. (1979) *The Scientific Writings of René Descartes*. London: Taylor & Francis.

Singh, A.K. *et al.* (2006) Correction of anemia with epoetin alfa in chronic kidney disease. *The New England Journal of Medicine*, 355, pp. 2085-2098.

Singh, A.K. (2010) Diabetes, anemia and CKD: Why TREAT? *Current Diabetes Reports*, 10, pp. 291-296.

Singh, A.K. (2010) What is causing the mortality in treating the anemia of chronic kidney disease: erythropoietin dose or hemoglobin level? *Current Opinion* in *Nephrology* and *Hypertension*, 19:420-424.

Smith, K. *et al.* (2009) Cellular basis of uraemic cardiomyopathy: a role for erythropoietin? *European Journal of Heart Failure*, 11, 732-738.

Szczech, L.A. *et al.* (2008) Secondary analysis of the CHOIR trial epoetinalpha dose and achieved hemoglobin outcomes. *Kidney International*, 74, pp. 791-798.

Tomosugi, N. *et al.* (2006) Detection of serum hepcidin in renal failure and inflammation by using ProteinChip System. *Blood*, 108, pp. 1381-1387.

Van Der Putten, K. *et al.* (2008) Mechanisms of Disease: erythropoietin resistance in patients with both heart and kidney failure. *Nature Clinical Practice - Nephrology*, 4, pp. 47-57.

Weiner, D.E. *et al.* (2005) Effects of anemia and left ventricular hypertrophy on cardiovascular disease in patients with chronic kidney disease. *Journal of the American Society of Nephrology*, 16, pp. 1803-1810.

Zaritsky, J. *et al.* (2009) Hepcidin – a potential novel biomarker for iron status in chronic kidney disease. *Clinical Journal of the American Society of Nephrology*, 4, pp. 1051-1056.

In: Hypotheses in Clinical Medicine
Editors: M.M. Shoja, P.S. Agutter et al.
ISBN: 978-1-62257-276-2

Chapter 3

Data Management Using Computational Methods to Put the Pieces Together: Time to Move from Theory to Practice

Virginia A. Folcik[1,2,*], *Rubina Kapil*[1], *Keith Warren*[2,3], *and William T. Coleman*[1]
[1]College of Medicine, Department of Internal Medicine, The Ohio State University Wexner Medical Center, Columbus, Ohio, US
[2]The Complexity in Human, Natural, and Engineered Systems Innovation Group, The Ohio State University, Columbus, Ohio, US
[3]College of Social Work, The Ohio State University, Columbus, Ohio, US

Abstract

Graduate education in medicine and biomedical research should include opportunities to study computational methods in addition to requirements for the study of mathematics and biostatistics, as the understanding of computational analysis of data is already a necessity to keep up with scientific progress. In the present chapter, this practical recommendation is considered, and it is emphasized that the pieces of knowledge consisted of the accumulated data generated by medical researchers for more than a century need to be assembled to achieve the excellence in practice. A glimpse on the computational methods of interest is provided.

Hypothesis

Graduate education in medicine and biomedical research should include opportunities to study computational methods in addition to requirements for the study of mathematics and biostatistics. This curriculum expansion is necessary for communication across disciplines,

* E-mail: Nivar.1@osu.edu.

and for new analytical approaches to be instilled in the biomedical community. Those actively conducting biomedical research will benefit from learning about the variety of computational methods available. This idea is not new (Lazebnik, 2002), but it remains to be incorporated into the medical and biomedical research curricula. Cross-disciplinary communication is the key to putting the pieces of data together and solving the *puzzle of health and disease* in the 21st century.

What Are the Pieces?

The pieces that need to be assembled consist of all the accumulated data generated by medical researchers for more than a century. Laboratory experiments probing cell behavior fill the scientific literature with pieces of the puzzle. Cell behavior includes the production and release of proteins or lipid mediators, the translation of messenger RNA (mRNA) into proteins and enzymes, and the transcription of genes from DNA into RNA. The earliest discoveries, such as the identification of cell types and the development of vaccines, are important (Bibel, 1988). However, we have entered a new era of biomedical research. The variety of methods available for data generation and analysis continues to increase. In fact, an entire volume of the journal *Nucleic Acids Research* (January 2004) was dedicated to describing databases of nucleic acids and proteins. The issue of generating too much data was recognized more than a decade ago (Roos, 2001). Gathering lists of data is not enough to answer questions and to solve the puzzles of biology (Fahrer et al., 2001, Ehrenberg et al., 2003). It is the network connections between the data that matter.

Data generation and collection is accelerated by the microarray methods capable of detecting thousands of molecules at once from small samples (Lockhart et al., 1996). High-throughput assays for molecules such as mRNAs, and the serendipitously discovered micro-RNAs [miRs; (Lee et al., 2004)], add volumes to existing data for cellular protein expression from *in vitro* experiments. This wealth of microarray data exists in addition to the complete sequence of the human genome (Consortium, 2001, J. Craig Venter, 2001), as well as the genomes of many other organisms. These data led to "Genome Wide Association Studies" (Couzin and Kaiser, 2007), to identify the functions associated with genes, and the potentially defective genes causing disease. Besides genomes, there are databases of networks of molecules, including transcriptomes (Caron et al., 2001, Su et al., 2004, Hah et al., 2011), cistromes (Tavazoie et al., 1999) and epigenomes (Prokesch and Lazar, 2011), proteomes (Consortium, 2001, Calvo et al., 2006), complexomes (Malovannaya et al., 2011), metabolomes (vanderGreef and Smilde, 2005), inflammasomes (Ogura et al., 2006), and diseaseomes (Goh et al., 2007). In the "ome" vocabulary, a transcriptome is a collection of genes transcribed under steady-state conditions, and cistromes are cis-acting elements in the genome upstream of places where RNA polymerases bind; for example, estrogen receptors (with estrogen) bind cistromes to enhance transcription (Hah et al., 2011). Epigenomes are biochemical mechanisms controlling the differential expression of genes, thus affecting the transcriptome. A proteome is a set of all the proteins expressed under a specified condition.

Data collection necessitates the use of network graphs to make pictorial sense of it all (Barabasi and Oltvai, 2004, Aderem and Smith, 2004). This is made possible by computational methods. Systems Biology, the science of systematically analyzing the "omic" data to find patterns of interactions in biological systems, which includes understanding the regulation and organization of networks associated with biological functions, which has been developed out of necessity (vanderGreef et al., 2007).

Table 1. Free Software

Curator/Name	Function	URL
Michael Eisen's Lab	Clustering and visualization	http://rana.lbl.gov/EisenSoftware.htm
Broad Institute/ GeneCluster 2	Clustering, SOM	http://www.broadinstitute.org/cancer/ software/genecluster2/gc2.html
Swarm Development Group	Agent-based modeling, programming skills required	http://www.swarm.org/index.php/ Swarm_main_page
Duke University Fuqua School of Business, Free Software Downloads	Software add-ons to Excel®	http://faculty.fuqua.duke.edu/~kamakura/ bio/WagnerKamakuraDownloads.htm
NetLogo	Agent-based modeling	http://ccl.northwestern.edu/netlogo/
MASON, George Mason University's Evolutionary Computation Laboratory and the GMU Center for Social Complexity	Agent-based modeling, programming skills required	http://cs.gmu.edu/~eclab/projects/ mason/
Repast3 Argonne National Labs	Agent-based modeling, programming skills required	http://repast.sourceforge.net/ repast_3/index.html
Repast Simphony Argonne National Labs	Agent-based modeling	http://repast.sourceforge.net/ repast_simphony.html
Philip Crooke, John Hotchkiss	Simulator for the Spread of Infections in the ICU	http://www.math.vanderbilt.edu/ ~pscrooke/CCM/Instructions.html

What Are Computational Methods?

Computational methods involve the use of simple mathematics, with iterative and repetitive algorithms, thus requiring the use of a computer. Many computational methods are available for data analysis. The key to optimizing results is knowing which methods extract the most valuable information from the available pieces of data. In general, the scale(s) of the biological system under study dictates the types of computational analysis that yield the most useful, integrated, and translational information. Scale refers to the level of biological detail, from microscopic to macroscopic, including intracellular molecules, organelles, cells, tissues, organs, organisms, and populations. The integration of information from different scales, and the clinical applicability of the results of data analyses, need to be considered the highest priorities in biomedical research (An et al., 2008).

At the Molecular Scale

Computational and statistical algorithms created decades ago (Everitt et al., 2001) are now commonly being applied to analyze molecular biology data. These systematic analyses of large biological data sets, or systems biology methods, have become indispensable tools in molecular biology. The good news is that free software is available for most of the algorithms described, and Table 1 lists some current information (07/2011) for obtaining the software. A Google® search can usually find free software, and the user can examine the credentials of the website. Many statistical methods are available with Microsoft Excel® and free add-ons.

Clustering Algorithms

Clustering algorithms are the basis of many computational methods used to analyze molecular biology data (Eisen et al., 1998). They are used for grouping or ranking data that describes the expression of biomolecules. These algorithms combine statistical methods with computational methods. Gene expression data (mRNAs or miRs) are frequently represented as heatmaps, with colored boxes representing the changes in expression levels of genes of interest under various conditions. Red usually indicates an increase in expression; green represents a decrease. These colored maps are often accompanied by dendrograms, or trees, whose leaves point to genes ordered by patterns of similarity in expression. When dendrograms are included, the clustering is hierarchical, or ordered in some predetermined way with multiple levels of organization. In a standard example (Eisen et al., 1998), all of the individual data points (a treatment condition applied over time; a vector of values) for each gene expression measurement is normalized using the mean of the values. Then, a Pearson correlation coefficient is calculated between all of the vector pairs; the higher the absolute value, the better the correlation. The vector pairs are then ordered by the Pearson correlation coefficient, the initial order (eg. lowest to highest vs. highest to lowest) is arbitrary. The order within pairs involves a choice, a weight based on some overall property of the genes such as average raw expression values. The elements within the pairs should be ordered by weight as the pairs were. The next hierarchical level may be determined by averaging the values in the paired vectors (creating nodes), then repeating the correlation analysis for similarity between nodes, to join new node/pairs at the next level. This is repeated as many times as there are treatment groups minus one. There are other ways to continue the grouping, depending upon the desired output. This algorithm is agglomerative, starting with clusters containing one gene data vector each and joining them until all genes are joined by the hierarchical tree. The result of this procedure is a representation of the data that is visually interpretable and tends to group genes by their functions. This algorithm is also suited to experimental conditions that have a stepwise order or hierarchy, such as the application of a treatment condition over time, or the changes in DNA sequences for genes during the evolution of organisms.

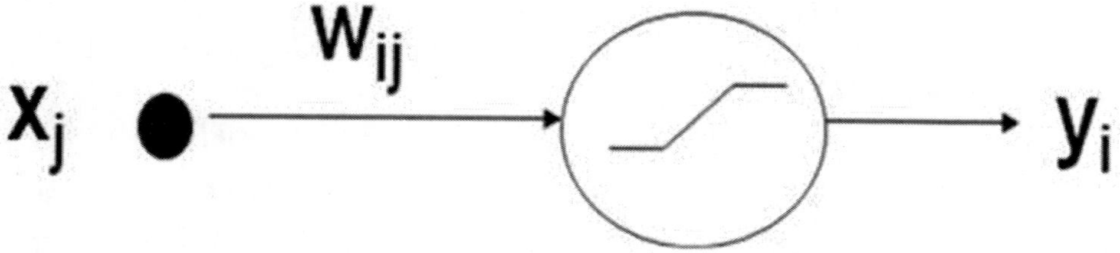

Figure 3.1. McCulloch-Pitts Processing Element (PE). A processing element consists of an input (x), a weight on the input (w), and an activation function (oval; referred to as a node in an SOM) that determines the output (y) for a given input and weight (McCulloch and Pitts, 1943).

K-Means Clustering

Sometimes one knows how many clusters there are, and data (vectors) need to be grouped by similarity into that pre-determined number of clusters, with the number of clusters designated as 'K'. This algorithm begins with random assignment of all data into K groups. The means or centroids of each group are determined (as appropriate to the data vector), and each of the elements is compared to the means/centroids of each group and placed in the group whose mean is closest. The means/centroids of the groups are then re-calculated, and the process is repeated until the composition of the groups no longer changes. This method is useful when there is prior knowledge of the number of groups within the data, but no pre-supposed hierarchical order to the data.

Self-organizing Maps (SOMs)

SOMs are more complicated than K-means clustering, because they contain "processing elements" (Figure 3.1) that allow them to learn by extracting information from input patterns and arranging it into output patterns. They do so without a prior notion of what the output pattern (clustering arrangement) will be. When the output pattern for a learning algorithm is unknown, the learning is termed "unsupervised". SOMs also process datasets that are large and not normally distributed (Tamayo et al., 1999). SOMs cluster inputs in a divisive manner (the opposite of agglomerative), because the data begin as one group and are divided into clusters by the self-organizing algorithm. SOMs were created by Teuvo Kohonen (Kohonen, 1990) as a variation of artificial neural networks. Figure 3.2 shows an arrangement for a SOM network. The input data vectors start out un-clustered, and the output space consists of neighborhoods (often depicted in two dimensions), like a map or a drawer with compartments for arranging items.

The compartments/neighborhoods are represented by the nodes (ovals). The inputs are applied one at a time, and they join the neighborhood (node) that they most closely match. When an input joins a node it alters the vector of values within the node, making it more like the input, and this increases the weight on the node (Figure 3.2, +++, x_7 -> y_3). The nodes with the next closest values have their weights increased (Figure 3.2, ++, x_7 -> y_2) and the next ones have their weights decreased (Figure 3.2, -, x_7 -> y_1). Nodes farther away are unaffected (y_m) and remain unchanged. Each input in a data set is applied, then the process is repeated a predetermined number of times. The end result is the formation of clusters of similar data vectors in an unsupervised manner, i.e., without using prior knowledge of the patterns inherent in the data.

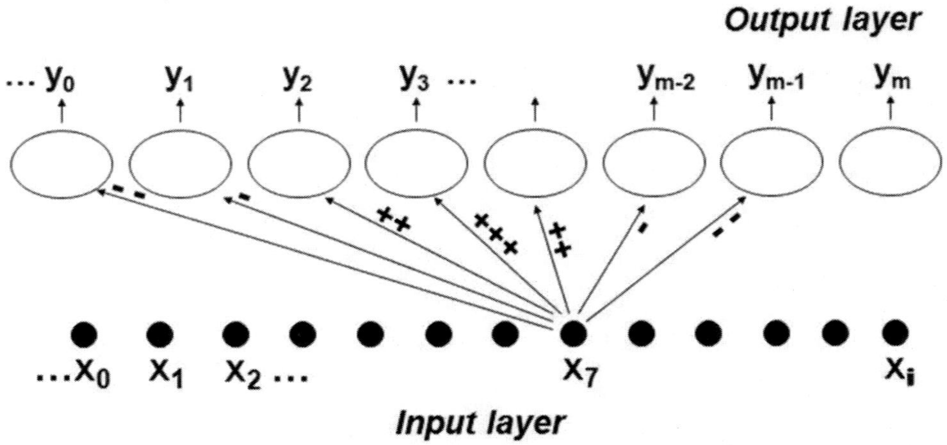

Figure 3.2. Arrangement of a self-organizing map network.

An example of an analysis using SOM demonstrates how the algorithm found patterns of gene expression in four cell lines of hematopoietic origin (Tamayo et al., 1999). Tamayo *et al.* (1999) treated the cell lines (all leukemic) with compounds commonly used *in vitro* to induce differentiation, and the expression patterns of approximately 6,000 genes were assayed. The SOM algorithm was appropriate because no such large-scale analysis had previously been done for gene expression under the given conditions, and discovery of new patterns was the goal. The exploratory analysis produced some results expected from the cell lines, including the expression of differentiation and pro-inflammatory genes by HL-60 cells in response to a stimulus (phorbol 12-myristate 13-acetate) known to produce these responses. Eight unexpected genes were also found in the same cluster. In the NB4 cell line, a cluster was formed by genes involved in differentiation in response to all-trans retinoic acid, a compound used to differentiate these cells and treat leukemia. Some of the genes in the cluster were known, but others that co-expressed were unexpected and provided insight into the mechanism of differentiation. SOM allowed sense to be made of a large data set by identifying patterns of gene expression, and stimulating further experiments.

Artificial Neural Networks - Multiple Scales

The methods discussed above were used to arrange data sets into clusters and identify patterns of gene expression. A more powerful artificial intelligence method, the artificial neural network (ANN), learns to classify data [reviewed by (Wang, 1993)]. The difference between clustering and classification is that clustering puts data into groups (the output is grouped data), and classification is the assignment of a previously unseen input vector to a group or category (the output is a prediction). Once an ANN is trained on a set of inputs and outputs, the ANN can predict the output from an input pattern. An ANN can also provide information about the contribution of the individual data values that constitute the inputs to the various outputs of interest.

The basic element of an ANN is the processing element [PE; Figure 3.1; (McCulloch and Pitts, 1943)], and an ANN is a perceptron (Rosenblatt, 1958). Just as in the SOM, the PEs receive input (x) and produce output (y). Unlike the SOM, which performs clustering in an unsupervised manner, the learning by the PEs in an ANN is supervised. This means that the (final) desired output is known, so the output y (an activation function of the input and weight) is compared to the desired output, and the difference, or error, is used to adjust the weight. Adjustment of the weights on the PEs is how learning is accomplished. Figure 3.1 shows one PE with one input (x_j). A PE may have more than one input, and each input has a weight. The value of the output (y_i) in that case would be a function of the sum of the weighted inputs. The arrangement of the PEs depends upon the input data and the nature of the classification problem. For a more complicated pattern to be recognized, more layers of PEs are needed (Figure 3.3).

Figure 3.3 shows how many PEs may be arranged to create a "multi-layer perceptron", a descriptive name for this type of ANN. As the name suggests, there is more than one layer. Sometimes the input layer is counted, but usually only the hidden layer(s) and the output layer are counted, making this an example of an ANN with two layers. More complicated pattern-recognition problems, such as those that arise in medical applications, require at least two layers. ANNs can take multiple types of data as input, because all of the input-output vector values are scaled to be numbers between -1 and 1, or 0 and 1. The weights are initialized with small random values (Basheer and Hajmeer, 2000). The algorithm used to update the weights on the middle layer is called back-propagation [reviewed in (Rumelhart et al., 1985)]. It takes into account that the desired value of the hidden layer outputs are unknown, and it "back propagates" the error from the final layer (y_1 - y_i) to adjust the weights on the hidden layer.

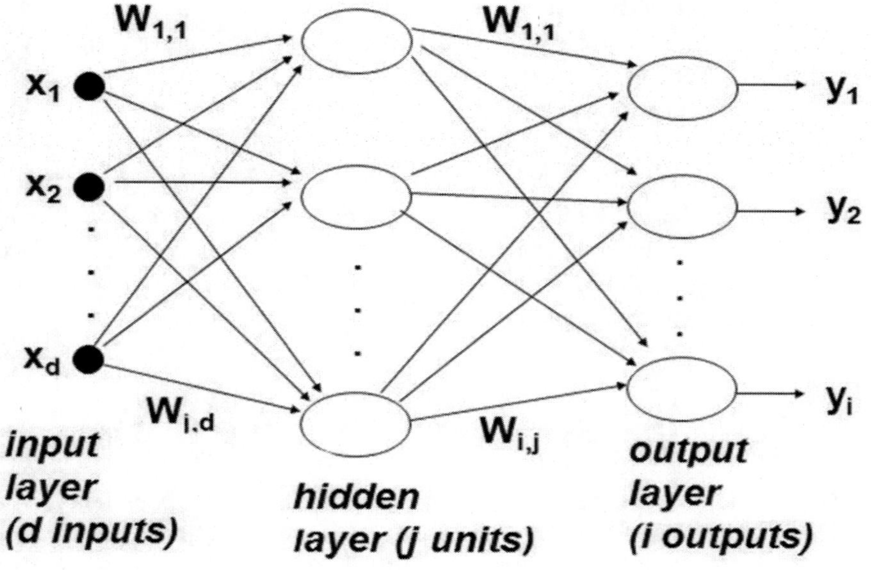

Figure 3.3. Structure of a multi-layer perceptron.

ANNs are trained by repeatedly passing through the training set. Training is complete when the weights change less than a small, pre-determined quantity. The general procedure is to take a data set of inputs and outputs, and randomly choose part of the dataset to leave out. The entire data set is applied to the input layer one input-output vector at a time, with the weights adjusted using the output error as described above. This is called one epoch, or an iteration. Then, the order of input-output vectors in the training set is shuffled, and another epoch is performed. This continues until all of the weights change by a very small amount; there are multiple ways to determine this stopping point. Once training is finished, the ANN can be used to predict the output from the inputs that were left out. The predicted values are compared to the actual values, and the ANN may be adjusted in various ways to optimize the predictive capacity (Basheer and Hajmeer, 2000). Another way that ANNs can be used is to determine the contribution of each input to the final output, by analyzing the final weights of a trained ANN.

There are many examples of the use of ANNs to predict medical outcomes in the literature (Ahmed, 2005). In one example, ANNs were applied to predict long-term survival for patients with diffuse large B-cell lymphoma, using microarray data for gene expression in the blood (O'Neill and Song, 2003). This study used the ANN to distinguish (classify) patients with large B-cell lymphoma from patients with other types of lymphoma, and found that 34 of the originally identified 4,026 genes could predict the specific diagnosis. Another study used ANNs to successfully diagnose and predict survival for patients with colon cancer (Ahmed, 2005). Microarray gene expression data from colon cancer biopsy tissue was used to train the ANN along with survival records from the patients.

ANNs have also been used for other medical issues. For example, patients with the genetic disorder thalassemia have defective hemoglobin, and may be cured by a hematopoietic stem cell transplant from a sibling with matching human leukocyte antigens. Patients do not always have such a sibling, and must look for an unrelated donor if transplant is an option. ANNs have been used to predict the possibility of graft-versus-host disease, a significant barrier to hematopoietic stem cell transplants. Using relevant input variables, a positive prediction rate of 83% was achieved (Caocci et al., 2010).

ANNs can be created with the Neural Network Toolbox® of Matlab® software, or with other commercially available software. Because the algorithms are known, they are not terribly difficult to program, if one has sufficient experience with a programming language. They should, however, be used with full understanding of the algorithm and the use of the optimizing parameters. In general, a few hundred input-output examples are needed to train an ANN. The ANN is trained and run multiple times, using a mean or other measure of centrality on the output(s) for the predicted answer.

Complex Systems - Multiple Scales

One type of system that is well known and has special network properties is a "Complex System" (Barabasi and Bonabeau, 2003). The properties of most biological systems (above the atomic scale) fit the definition of a complex system (Holland, 1995). These systems have different types of elements, and the elements interact with each other according to internal rules. Although the roles of the different types of elements are distinct, they may have some redundancy in function. The redundancy gives a complex system resilience. The individual elements are replaced when they expire, and when taken together, the behavior of the system that is composed of the individual elements is surprisingly complex.

Many interesting books have been written about complex systems. A series of books have been published by the Santa Fe Institute (Santa Fe, New Mexico): *Studies in the Sciences of Complexity*. The key word in the series title is *Sciences*. The first volume describes examples of complex systems, including social insect colonies (anthills, beehives, and wasp nests), in eloquent mathematical and logical detail (Bonabeau et al., 1999). The insects that make up these complex systems solve complex problems using simple behavioral rules that require pattern recognition. Insects of the same species share the behavioral rules and responses to pattern recognition. This is why insect species can be distinguished by the nests or hives that they build. The patterns they recognize, and their responses to these patterns, are hereditary and control the nest-building behavior. Complex systems are abundant among living organisms, constituting a recurrent, intriguing motif among living systems (Holland, 1995).

Network Analysis - Multiple Scales

Graphical networks have become popular tools for visualizing the results obtained from high throughput analysis of biological samples. Network theory has established itself in the biomedical literature (Albert, 2005), and graphs are popular in systems biology (Lander, 2010). The network nature of complex systems has been well-described in layman's terms (Barabasi, 2002). Networks are constructed of elements called nodes, and the connections between the nodes are called edges, or links. One can arbitrarily assign the content of the nodes and the links that connect them, creating endless possibilities for analyses of systems on various scales.

Scale-free Networks

One of the many interesting properties of complex systems is that network analyses of their interacting entities can produce scale-free networks, or networks with a distribution of connections that spans many (numerical) scales of magnitude (Barabasi et al., 2000). The distribution of connections between the nodes in a scale-free network follows a power-law distribution. From a biomedical perspective, there are aspects of these networks that may be exploited (Barabasi, 2007). For instance, because a few of the nodes in a scale-free network may have thousands of edges or connections, they are referred to as hubs in the network (Jeong et al., 2001). These nodes make the network susceptible to a targeted attack, because they connect with many of the other nodes (Albert et al., 2000). The interactions between molecules in a biological system have been analyzed as networks, and the information is being used to find drug targets for intervention in disease (Yildirim et al., 2007).

However, network analyses of biological systems have found features that differ from those networks that are man-made, like the internet. Different kinds of hubs have been identified in human protein-protein interaction networks (Liang and Li, 2007). Proteins forming modules that are highly connected (interactive; intra-modular hubs) have less epigenetic regulation of their expression by miRs than proteins that connect the modules together (inter-modular hubs). The genes for hub proteins connecting modules have more miR binding sites, corresponding to switches on the connections between the modules. These properties suggest that proteins that interact and work together at the same time need less epigenetic regulation than proteins that connect modules and control their activity. Genes for proteins involved in regulatory or developmental processes (inter-modular) also have more miR binding sites than genes involved in intra-modular biosynthetic processes (Stark et al., 2005). This arrangement provides robustness to epigenetic regulatory processes.

Network Analysis - Immune System

One of the most commonly named examples of a complex system is the immune system (Orosz, 2001). The immune system cannot be studied directly as a network, because the immune systems' cells are distributed throughout the body of an organism. They can be isolated from an organism and studied *in vitro* (a Google search of "immune system, *in vitro*" retrieves over 22 million results), but this does not necessarily allow quantification of interactions, whether they be direct (cell-to-cell) or indirect (cell-to-cytokine-to-cell). Some of the network properties of the immune system have been analyzed using agent-based modeling (described below) as a tool (Folcik et al., 2011). The empirical data for immune cell behavior were incorporated into an agent-based model, and the model counted the direct interactions between the immune cells during an inflammatory response. Not surprisingly, immune cells known as dendritic cells were identified as hubs. These cells function in tissue surveillance. Dendritic cells carry information from sites of inflammation to the lymph nodes, where they present the information to the lymphocytes in events requiring cell-to-cell interactions. The unexpected result was that, in simulation runs with a successful immune response that cleared a virus from the virtual tissue, there were far fewer interactions than in the simulation runs that exhibited an unsuccessful response, in which the tissue was destroyed by the viral infection. Swollen virtual lymphoid tissue was also part of the unsuccessful immune response; this occurs in strong inflammatory responses. Studying the immune system as a complex system reveals the connections between cellular behavioral rules and immune system behavior, an example of putting the pieces together.

Network Analysis - Genes and Diseases

Other network characteristics of human biology have been studied, and the nodes and edges have been defined in some very insightful ways, revealing some interesting properties of human susceptibility to disease (Goh et al., 2007). Goh *et al.* (2007) constructed networks that consisted of nodes representing diseases known to involve genetic defects, with edges between them representing the defective genes (the Human Disease Network). They also constructed a network of genes known to cause diseases when they contained defects, and these were connected by edges that represented disorders (the Disease Gene Network). These investigators found that genes widely expressed in tissues and essential for survival (encoding proteins that have many known interactions, i.e. hub proteins) are unlikely to be connected to inherited disease. Defects in such genes are incompatible with survival to birth. On the other hand, genes whose defects cause disease are less abundantly expressed, and not essential to survival past the age of reproduction. Diseases such as cancer, caused by genes disrupted by somatic mutation (after birth), are not limited to peripheral expression, but could be genes encoding hub proteins. These results define heuristics for identifying unknown genetic defects in idiopathic diseases. Work is also underway to find the means to correct any genetic defects by identifying alternative metabolic pathways that can be manipulated into activity to replace defective pathways (Motter et al., 2008). While this effort is in its infancy, it is a manner of creative thinking that may, ultimately, find cures for metabolic diseases.

Agent/Individual-based Modeling – The Individual Scale

At the cellular, tissue/organ, and organismal scale, agent- or individual-based modeling is a useful tool for studying complex systems and conducting virtual experiments (Bonabeau, 2002, Grimm et al., 2005). Agents are the interacting entities, and when they represent whole organisms the method is often called individual-based modeling (Grimm and Railsback, 2005). Most agent-based modeling platforms provide programming elements for signals between agents, so extracellular molecules and characteristics of the environment can be explicitly represented. The role of the environment is an important factor in agent-based models (ABMs), and this type of modeling is uniquely suited for studying agent-environment interactions.

Although agent-based modeling has been around for decades (Gardner, 1970, Reynolds, 1987), the first textbook on how to construct a model is just now being published (Railsback and Grimm, 2012). Railsback and Grimm describe the basic steps in creating an ABM, drawing from their experience and the experience of others who have created the freely available software packages for agent-based modeling (Table 1). The choice of which software to use to create a model often depends on whether one has computer programming skills. Currently, the most popular choice for non-programmers is NetLogo (Table 1). NetLogo is an extension of the software called StarLogo, which was created to be used as a teaching tool at the grade school level (Wilensky and Resnick, 1999).

The modeling process usually begins with a question about a system, such as how it is able to accomplish some task, or what would happen if it were perturbed in some way. ABMs have the unique ability to answer questions of "how" and "why", at least to the extent of predicting the probability of certain hypothesized answers *in silico*. Some regard ABMs as theory building tools, because the answers to questions obtained *in silico* must be validated in the real world. Once the question is posed, one must decide what is represented by the agents, and what is included in their virtual environment. Empirical information about the system is used to build a model. The details should be kept to the minimum necessary to answer the question about the system. Too much as well as too little detail is undesirable (Grimm et al., 2005). Agents' behavior is described using logical statements. The easiest way to think of the rules for behavior for an agent is to imagine being the agent. Then, an agent's behavior can be described in the vocabulary of the system.

Once one decides what details to include, the model should be described in writing (Grimm et al., 2010). The model can then be created, using the preferred type of software. An ABM must also be checked for correct implementation, or verified, to make sure the code is written and executing correctly. There is a paucity in standardized instructions for this step outside of the computer science realm for traditional programming (Ekbote et al., 2010). There are instructions for verification in the new textbook (Railsback and Grimm, 2012). After verification, the ABM can be used to conduct virtual experiments. Often there are some surprises or unexpected behaviors that appear. These may be due to unforeseen logical loopholes in the code, or they may be emergent behaviors of the virtual system. The results of the virtual experiments or simulation runs are compared to what happens in the real world. The virtual system should emulate the behavior of the actual system. The comparison of system behavior to empirical data is called validation. One method for validation is to apply a perturbation to the virtual system that has a known effect in the real system, and compare the outcomes. If the ABM exhibits outcomes that occur in the real system, it is validated. Even so, an ABM that is functional and validated is often a continual work in progress. Revisions may be made, and the cycle of development is repeated (Grimm and Railsback, 2005).

Examples of agent-based models used to answer medically relevant questions include some that are simple, and some that are actually hybrid mathematical models with differential equations. Starting with ABMs that model cells as agents, a few purely logical ABMs exist. One of them is the Basic Immune Simulator (Folcik et al., 2007), and its updated version, the Basic Immune Simulator 2010 (Folcik et al., 2011). Both versions were created using Repast agent-based modeling software (North et al., 2006). This software is for modelers with programming experience. The Basic Immune Simulator has three environments; one representing a functional tissue, one representing lymphoid tissue, and one representing the blood. The agents representing cells move between the environments, just as the cells of the immune system travel through the body. Perturbations to the numbers of agents representing dendritic cells, the sentinels of the immune system, lead to virtual hypersensitivity-reactions in the ABM (Folcik et al., 2007). The Basic Immune Simulator exhibits emergent properties at the system level due to the rules for normal immune cell behavior programmed into the agents. This model continues to be developed to study fibrotic lung disease (Folcik et al., 2009), and will be used to virtually test hypotheses regarding the cellular behavior that leads to idiopathic pulmonary fibrosis.

Others have built hybrid ABMs modeling the immune response using NetLogo (Table 1) and Matlab® software. One ABM has been constructed to study the homing of monocytes to areas of inflammation, including flow dynamics in the microvasculature (Bailey et al., 2007). Their approach was to study blood flow in murine muscle with video cameras peering through miniature windows, focused on microvessels. They analyzed the video to obtain flow dynamics information, and used it, together with empirical information about chemoattraction of cell types into inflammatory tissue areas, to create their model. The role of adhesion molecules expressed by the vessel endothelium to promote the adherence of the monocytes to the vessel wall was also included. Besides the quality of the modeling, what makes this group's studies unique is the creative use of microscopes with cameras to film events taking place *in vivo* in live, anaesthetized animals. Such data are extremely difficult to obtain. Their work fills an information gap, and at the same time puts the information to use in a virtual environment.

The last example is an elegantly simple, but informative, ABM representing caregivers and patients as agents in the medical setting of an Intensive Care Unit (ICU) (Hotchkiss et al., 2005). The model was created using Mathematica® (Table 1). The model addresses the problem of nosocomial (hospital acquired) infection, and how the behavior of the caregivers, the transmissibility of the virtual bacteria, and the configuration of the virtual environment (caregiver traffic flow) affect the numbers of patients infected. The virtual bacteria were chosen to represent those requiring direct caregiver-patient contact for onward transmission. The results demonstrate that increased transmissibility of the virtual bacteria, duration of the caregiver/agent contamination, and number of patients contacted per caregiver, all have a positive correlation with increased patient infection incidence in the model. The behavioral factors most important for containment were rapid detection, and isolation of infected patients. Minimal overlap of caregiver/agent domains (location of the subset of patients per caregiver) prevented mass spread of infection. The model reveals what needs to be modified in the ICU environment, aside from the obvious necessity for adherence to best practices in blood and body fluid precautions. Minimizing the overlap area covered by caregivers can be optimized using the model. The solutions to the problem are changes in the rules for behavior in the ICU.

All of the examples above are a glimpse of the potential for computational methods to advance medical care. The examples provided in this chapter include investigators who learned to think in a way that solves problems, and/or collaborations between individuals with different areas of expertise. A hindrance to this process is the difficulty in communication between the disciplines of biology, biostatistics, bioinformatics, mathematics, and computer science. Cross-disciplinary education is one way that solving the puzzles associated with disease can be accelerated in the coming decades.

What Computational Skills Do Medical Schools Require?

Cross-pollination between disciplines needs to occur, and some overlap in the curriculum at the undergraduate or graduate level would be beneficial. Medical schools and graduate schools vary in their admission requirements for coursework in mathematics, statistics, and computer science. Graduate schools are numerous, and can be flexible in coursework requirements, while medical schools have established curricula and prerequisites. According to the book *Princeton Review: The Best 168 Medical Schools* (Braswell, 2011), 98 of the 168 schools have no requirements or recommendations for mathematics. There are 54 schools that have designated mathematical requirements, and 19 schools with recommended coursework.

Of the 54 schools requiring mathematics in undergraduate coursework, 30 schools ask for "college-level mathematics" coursework, but do not further specify. There are 24 schools, including Duke Medical School and John Hopkins Medical School, requiring calculus and/or statistics classes. There are five schools which require mathematics coursework through Algebra and Trigonometry; this is typically completed as a requirement for all high school graduates. No schools, however, require a computer science background.

Of the 19 schools recommending mathematics in undergraduate coursework, there are five schools that recommend taking both calculus and statistics courses, and five schools that recommend taking either calculus or statistics. There are also another seven schools that recommend taking mathematics courses, but do not specify which courses. Georgetown School of Medicine, Tufts School of Medicine, and the University of Missouri - Kansas City, School of Medicine recommend taking at least one course in computer science. Tufts School of Medicine is unique in recommending both computer science courses, as well as calculus and/or statistics courses. This is a very practical recommendation, given all of the technology that medical students and physicians need to use in daily practice. This should be the norm for the medical schools and for graduate schools in the biomedical sciences, as the understanding of computational analysis of data is already a necessity to keep up with scientific progress.

Acknowledgments

The work was supported by award number R21HL093675 (VAF) from the National Heart, Lung, and Blood Institute of the National Institutes of Health. The content is solely the responsibility of the authors and does not necessarily represent the official views of the National Heart, Lung, and Blood Institute or the National Institutes of Health.

References

Aderem, A. and Smith, K. D. (2004) A systems approach to dissecting immunity and inflammation. *Seminars in Immunology*, 16, pp. 55-67.

Ahmed, F. E. (2005) Artificial neural networks for diagnosis and survival prediction in colon cancer. *Molecular Cancer*, 4, pp. 29-40.

Albert, R. 2005. Scale-free networks in cell biology. *Journal of Cell Science*, 118, pp. 4947-4957.

Albert, R. et al. (2000) Error and attack tolerance of complex networks. *Nature*, 406, pp. 378-382.

An, G. et al. (2008) Translational systems biology: Introduction of an engineering approach to the pathophysiology of the burn patient. *Journal of Burn Care Research*, 29, pp. 277-285.

Bailey, A. M. et al. (2007) Multi-cell agent-based simulation of the microvasculature to study the dynamics of circulating inflammatory cell trafficking. *Annals of Biomedical Engineering*, 35, pp. 916-936.

Barabasi, A. L. (2002) *Linked*. New York, New York: Penguin Group.

Barabasi, A. L. (2007) Network medicine--from obesity to the "diseasome". *The New England Journal of Medicine*, 357, pp. 404-407.

Barabasi, A. L. et al. (2000) Scale-free characteristics of random networks: the topology of the world-wide web. *Physica A*, 281, pp. 69-77.

Barabasi, A. L. and Bonabeau, E. (2003) Scale-Free Networks. *Scientific American*, 288, pp. 60-69.

Barabasi, A. L. and Oltvai, Z. N. (2004) *Network biology: Understanding the cell's functional organization*. Nature Reviews Genetics, 5, pp. 101-113.

Basheer, I. A. and Hajmeer, M. (2000) Artificial neural networks: fundamentals, computing, design, and application. *Journal of Microbiological Methods*, 43, pp. 3-31.

Bibel, D. J. (1988) *Milestones in Immunology: A Historical Exploration*. Madison, Wisconsin: Science Tech Publishers.

Bonabeau, E. (2002) Agent-based modeling: Methods and techniques for simulating human systems. *Proceedings of the National Academy of Sciences of the United States of America*, 99, pp. 7280-7287.

Bonabeau, E. et al. (1999) *Swarm Intelligence: From Natural to Artificial Systems*. New York, New York: Oxford University Press.

Braswell, L. (ed.) (2011) *The Best 168 Medical Schools, 2011 Edition*. Framingham: Random House, Inc.

Calvo, S. et al. (2006) Systematic identification of human mitochondrial disease genes through integrative genomics. *Nature Genetics*, 38, pp. 576-582.

Caocci, G. et al. (2010) Comparison between an artificial neural network and logistic regression in predicting acute graft-vs-host disease after unrelated donor hematopoietic stem cell transplantation in thalassemia patients. *Experimental Hematology*, 38, pp. 426-433.

Caron, H. et al. (2001) The human transcriptome map: Clustering of highly expressed genes in chromosomal domains. *Science*, 291, pp. 1289-1292.

International Human Genome Sequencing Consortium 2001. Initial sequencing and analysis of the human genome. *Nature*, 409, pp. 860-927.

Couzin, J. And Kaiser, J. (2007) Closing the net on common disease genes. *Science*, 316, pp. 820-822.

Ehrenberg, M. et al. (2003) Systems biology is taking off. *Genome Research*, 13, pp. 2377-2380.

Eisen, M. B. et al. (1998) Cluster analysis and display of genome-wide expression patterns. *Proceedings of the National Academy of Sciences*, 95, pp. 14863-14868.

Ekbote, C. et al. (2010) *Verification of an agent-based model: Meeting the challenge of verifying object-oriented code that executes stochastically*. Available from: http://www.swarm.org [Accessed 22/1/2012].

Everitt, B. S. et al. (2001) *Cluster Analysis*. New York: Oxford University Press, Inc.

Fahrer, A. M. et al. (2001) *A genomic view of immunology*. Nature, 409, pp. 836-838.

Folcik, V. A. et al. (2007) The Basic Immune Simulator: An Agent-Based Model to study the interactions between innate and adaptive immunity. *Theoretical Biology and Medical Modelling*, 4, pp. 39.

Folcik, V. A. et al. (2011) Using an agent-based model to analyze the dynamic communication network of the immune response. *Theoretical Biology and Medical Modelling*, 8, pp. 1.

Folcik, V. A. et al. (2009) *Using Agent-Based Modeling to Study Interstitial Lung Disease*. Available from: http://www.swarm.org [Accessed 22/1/2012].

Gardner, M. (1970) Mathematical Games: The fantastc combinations of John Conway's new solitaire game "Life". *Scientific American*, 223, pp. 120-123.

Goh, K. I. et al. (2007) The human disease network. *Proceedings of the National Academy of Sciences*, 104, pp. 8685-8690.

Grimm, V. et al. (2010) The ODD protocol: A review and first update. *Ecological Modelling*, 221, pp. 2760-2768.

Grimm, V. and Railsback, S. F. (2005) *Individual-based Modeling and Ecology*. Princeton, New Jersey: Princeton University Press.

Grimm, V. et al. (2005) Pattern-oriented modeling of agent-based complex systems: Lessons from ecology. *Science*, 310, pp. 987-991.

Hah, N. et al. (2011) A rapid, extensive, and transient transcriptional response to estrogen signaling in breast cancer cells. *Cell*, 145, pp. 622-634.

Holland, J. H. (1995) *Hidden Order: How Adaptation Builds Complexity*. Perseus Books.

Hotchkiss, J. R. et al. (2005) An agent-based and spatially explicit model of pathogen dissemination in the intensive care unit. *Critical Care Medicine*, 33, pp. 168-176.

Jeong, H. et al. (2001) Lethality and centrality in protein networks. *Nature*, 411, pp. 41-42.

Kohonen, T. (1990) The self-organizing map. *Proceedings of the IEEE*, 78, pp. 1464-1480.

Lander, A. D. (2010) The edges of understanding. *BMC Biology*, 8, pp. 40.

Lazebnik, Y. (2002) Can a biologist fix a radio? Or, what I learned while studying apoptosis. *Cancer Cell*, 2, pp. 179-182.

Lee, R. et al (2004) A short history of a short RNA. *Cell*, S116, pp. 89-92.

Liang, H. and Li, W. H. (2007) MicroRNA regulation of human protein-protein interaction network. *RNA*, 13, pp. 1402-1408.

Lockhart, D. J. et al. (1996) Expression monitoring by hybridization to high-density oligonucleotide arrays. *Nature Biotechnology*, 14, pp. 1675-1680.

Malovannaya, A. et al. (2011) Analysis of the human endogenous coregulator complexome. *Cell*, 145, pp. 787-799.

Mcculloch, W. S. and Pitts, W. (1943) A logical calculus of the ideas imminent in nervous activity. *Bulletin of Mathematics and Biophysics*, 5, pp. 115-133.

Motter, A. E. et al. (2008) Predicting synthetic rescues in metabolic networks. *Molecular Systems Biology*, 4, pp. 168.

North, M. J. et al. (2006) Experiences Creating Three Implementations of the Repast Agent Modeling Toolkit. *ACM Transactions on Modeling and Computer Simulation*, 16, pp. 1-25.

O'Neill, M. C. and Song, L. (2003) Neural network analysis of lymphoma microarray data: prognosis and diagnosis near-perfect. *BMC Bioinformatics*, 4, pp. 13-24.

Ogura, Y. et al. (2006) The inflammasome: First line of the immune response to cell stress. *Cell*, 126, pp. 659-662.

Orosz, C. G. (2001) Immunity as a swarm function. *Graft*, 5, 369, pp. 373-375.

Prokesch, A. and Lazar, M. A. (2011) A hormone sends instant messages to the genome. *Cell*, 145, pp. 499-501.

Railsback, S. F. and Grimm, V. (2012) *Agent-Based and Individual-Based Modeling: A Practical Introduction*. Princeton, New Jersey: Princeton University Press.

Reynolds, C. W. (1987) Flocks, herds, and schools: A distributed behavioral model. *Computer Graphics*, 21, pp. 25-34.

Roos, D. S. (2001) Bioinformatics - Trying to swim in a sea od data. *Science*, 291, pp. 1260-1261.

Rosenblatt, F. (1958) The Perceptron: A probabilistic model for information storage and organization in the brain. *Psychological Review*, 65, pp. 386-408.

Rumelhart, D. E. et al. (eds.) (1985) *Learning Internal Representations by Error Propagation*. Cambridge, MA: MIT Press.

Stark, A. et al. (2005) Animal microRNAs confer robustness to gene expression and have a significant impact on 3'UTR evolution. *Cell*, 123, pp. 1133-1146.

Su, A. I. et al. (2004) A gene atlas of the mouse and human protein-encoding transcriptomes. *Proceedings of the National Academy of Sciences*, 101, pp. 6062-6067.

Tamayo, P. et al. (1999) Interpreting patterns of gene expression with self-organizing maps: Methods and application to hematopoietic differentiation. *Proceedings of the National Academy of Sciences*, 96, pp. 2907-2912.

Tavazoie, S. et al. (1999) Systematic determination of genetic network architecture. *Nature Genetics*, 22, pp. 281-285.

van der Greef, J. et al. (2007) The art and practice of systems biology in medicine: Mapping patterns of relationships. *Journal of Proteome Research*, 6, pp. 1540-1559.

van der Greef, J. and Smilde, A. K. (2005) Symbiosis of chemometrics and metabolomics: past, present, and future. *Journal of Chemometrics*, 19, pp. 376-386.

Venter, C. J. et al. (2001). The sequence of the human genome. *Science*, 291, pp. 1304-1351.

Wang, D. (1993) Pattern recognition: Neural networks in perspective. *IEEE Expert*, 8, pp. 52-60.

Wilensky, U. and Resnick, M. (1999) Thinking in levels: A dynamic systems approach to making sense of the world. *Journal of Science Education and Technology*, 8, pp. 1-17.

Yildirim, M. A. et al. (2007) Drug-target network. *Nature Biotechnology*, 25, pp. 1119-1126.

In: Hypotheses in Clinical Medicine
Editors: M.M. Shoja, P.S. Agutter et al.

ISBN: 978-1-62257-276-2

Chapter 4

Could Cytomegalovirus Be Causing Widespread Outbreaks of Chronic Poor Health?

Rodney P. Jones*
Statistical Advisor, Healthcare Analysis & Forecasting
Camberley, UK

Abstract

Evidence is presented for synchronous and recurring increases in medical admissions at between three and eight (most commonly five or six) year intervals. These lead to a typical 10% step-like increase in medical admissions (with other admissions totally unaffected). Such medical admissions are the tip of the iceberg for wider primary care cost increases. A range of non-specific signs and symptoms and specific diagnoses are associated with each step-like increase, whose magnitude increases with age and has a degree of female specificity. Here, the possibility is explored that the ubiquitous herpes virus, cytomegalovirus (CMV), may be behind this international behavior. It is proposed that CMV takes advantage of the wide range of permanent and temporary immune impairments, which exist in what has traditionally been termed 'immune competent' individuals, to exert a wide range of sub-clinical to clinical effects against general population health. Common themes regarding the elderly, signs and symptoms, depression, infection, and inflammation emerge. Indeed, many general practitioner contacts with patients of a vague or syndromic nature may be arising out of the direct and indirect effects of CMV against immune function. Specific research projects needed to test this hypothesis are outlined.

Introduction

The unusually high growth in medical admissions has been an enduring international enigma over the past four to five decades (Hobbs 1995; Kendrick 1995; Capewell 1996;

* E-mail: hcaf_rod@yahoo.co.uk.

Parker *et al.* 1997; Hilder *et al.* 1998; Hilder *et al.* 2000; Morgan *et al.* 1996; Lung and Asthma Information Agency 2001; Kendrick and Conway 2003a-c; NSW Health 2007; MacDonald *et al.* 2008; Roberts *et al.* 2008; Pallin *et al.* 2008; Jones 2009a-i; 2010a-n; 2011a-k; Blunt *et al.* 2010; Gillam 2010). Up to the present, this trend has been largely attributed to factors such as the aging population, health care consumerism, more conservative general practitioners (GP), hospital consultant behavior, and failings in the processes and organization of health and social care. No one seems to have asked the obvious question: could it be that there is a general trend of increasing poor health? Indeed, why have illnesses such as diabetes, allergies, asthma and other immune syndromes apparently increased in parallel with the increase in medical emergency admissions? (Khot *et al.* 1984; Hyams 1998; Anderson *et al.* 2007; Moorman *et al.* 2007; Gonzalez *et al.* 2009; Keil *et al.* 2006).

The author's involvement in this area of research began in 1993 whilst Assistant Director of Information at the Royal Berkshire Hospital (Reading, Berkshire, UK). In the middle of March 1993, the hospital experienced a sudden, unexpected, and permanent increase in medical admissions (Jones 1996a; Jones 1997). Intriguingly, this same event appeared to sweep across the whole of the UK, and a number of studies have sought to explain this behavior (Hobbs 1995; Kendrick 1995; Capewell 1996; Parker *et al.* 1997; Morgan *et al.* 1996). In retrospect, a similar event appeared to occur in New Zealand (Hilder *et al.* 1998). In the USA, an unusual and permanent increase in emergency department attendances also commenced in 1993 (Roberts *et al.* 2008).

My own investigation into this event led to the conclusion that there was some form of infectious outbreak; however, it was not until late 2008 that definitive evidence began to emerge that this was a recurring phenomenon. At this time, I was simultaneously contacted by two large acute hospitals, where managers could not understand why medical beds had suddenly experienced an unexplained influx of patients, and by a Strategic Health Authority seeking to understand why the budgets at Primary Care Organizations (PCO) were suddenly over-spent. Subsequently, I began to search for wider international evidence and explanations in the fields of immunology and virology (Jones 2009a-i; 2010 a-j; 2011a-l).

Since that time, I have also had the unique opportunity of being involved in detailed reviews of emergency medical admissions covering one regional and three PCO geographies in England, and in a review of bed requirements for a large tertiary hospital in Australia (Jones 2011k). All of these reviews were necessitated by the financial and acute bed pressures emanating out of the 2007 outbreak. Most of this work remains unpublished, but only confirms the author's hypothesis regarding an international infectious outbreak. Indeed, when a step change emerges across multiple systems covering a roughly similar set of diagnoses and all clustered around a common initiation date, but with timing differences consistent with something possessing a relatively slow spread (and thereby implying person to person contact), then the possibility of a common infectious cause is highly likely.

The characterization of the unique changes in hospital admission and bed occupancy leading to the analysis of shifts in diagnosis associated with each 'outbreak' was greatly facilitated by the unusually low incidence of influenza over the period January 2000 to August 2009. Such gaps are very rare; the last extended period of very low incidence of influenza occurred between 1879 and 1889 (Thacker 1986). Hence, the analysis of hospital admissions surrounding the 2002 and 2007 outbreaks could be conducted in the absence of the potentially confounding effects of influenza. It is highly likely that the dominating effect of influenza outbreaks upon emergency admissions prior to 2000 acted to obscure the effects of these 'outbreaks', especially since so many studies use annual totals rather than the daily and monthly time series that the author has used to study the detail of these outbreaks.

In the above context, the re-examination of the long-term trends in medical admissions in the four countries of the UK, USA, Canada and Australia (Jones 1996a; Jones 1997; Jones 2009a-i; 2010a-j; 2011a-k), together with Austria, Estonia and Switzerland (author's unpublished analysis), has revealed curious cyclic patterns, which are reminiscent of the behavior that would characterize an infectious disease outbreak. An excellent example of such cyclic behavior is the observation that the incidence of syphilis (which has an element of acquired immunity) follows an approximate nine year cycle, while that for gonorrhea (no acquired immunity) does not exhibit cyclic behavior (Grassley *et al.* 2005). Every infectious disease involving acquired immunity has its own unique time cycle, which is altered by immunization programmes (Andersen *et al.* 1984; Flemming *et al.* 1991; Dushoff 1996; Dowell 2001; Koelle and Pascual 2004; Grassley and Fraser 2006).

In the UK, the pattern of NHS surplus and deficit, emergency department attendance, bed occupancy, and the size of the inpatient elective waiting list (a knock-on effect from bed occupancy and the availability of funds as a result of the cycle in surplus and deficit) also conform to such a cyclic pattern (Jones 2010f; Jones 2011a,c,h). In the USA, a similar pattern in health care expenditure is known as the 'health insurance underwriting cycle' and leads to a cycle of profit and loss in the health insurance industry (Gabel *et al.* 1991; Kipp. *et al.* 2003; Born and Santerre 2008; Jones 2010c,f).

This chapter will examine the evidence for patterns in acute admissions, bed occupancy and wider health care costs, which cannot be explained by demographic changes, funding, or wider differences in health care organization, policy or implementation. A hypothesis will be explored to investigate if the ubiquitous herpes virus, cytomegalovirus, could be responsible for the range of diagnoses observed that accompany each outbreak.

Upward Trend or a Series of Step-like Changes?

A step change in the rate of admissions or incidence of a disease is an unexpected increase that occurs over a very short time, leading to the establishment of a new, but higher, rate or incidence. This is illustrated in Figure 4.1, using admissions from England over the decade 1998/99 to 2008/09, where two step changes can be seen to occur in the latter part of the financial years 2002/03 and 2007/08, leading to a jump in admissions in the next financial year (April to March). The particular cluster of diagnoses used in Figure 4.1 experience this step change, while other diagnoses follow more usual time trends (Jones 2009i; Jones 2010k-m,i).

This step-like behavior is particular to certain medical specialties (Jones 2009f,i; Jones 2010a,e) and diagnoses (Jones 2009d,i; 2010b,l; 2011c), and is mainly related to emergency or unscheduled admissions (Jones 2009a-e). The unique association of these diagnoses with medical admissions is further illustrated in Figure 4.2. This behavior can be discerned in the four countries of the UK (England, Northern Ireland, Scotland and Wales), Australia, Canada, New Zealand and the USA (Jones 2010f,j-m). Such behavior can also be seen in Austria, Estonia and Switzerland (author's unpublished analysis), and can be inferred from studies noting an unexplained 10% increase in medical emergency admissions and costs per bed day in Dublin (Ireland) in late 2002, with a specific increase in syncope and chest pain, administration of intravenous antibiotics, and diagnostic ultrasound of heart, abdomen and vessels (Moloney *et al.* 2005). Total admissions in Athens (Greece) also show a step increase in 2002, along with an increase in the variability associated with admissions (Boutsioli 2009). Similar increases in the variation associated with emergency admissions and bed occupancy immediately after each step change have also been noted in the UK and Australia (Jones 2010m; Jones 2011h,m). All the observed step increases appear to initiate around or slightly after the years 2002 or 2007, as seen in Figures 4.1 and 4.2, with evidence for additional step changes in the years prior to 2002 in the USA and UK.

Additional studies have revealed that the step-like changes are also age- and gender-related (Jones 2010f-g,j; Jones 2011c,i), appear to show spatial spread over time (Jones 1996a; Jones 2011a), and involve the totality of health care costs and not just emergency hospital admissions (Jones 2010f,i). The author's own unpublished work suggests that the relationship with age appears to involve some degree of behavior relating to age at the previous 'outbreak', which would be consistent with the phenomenon known as 'antigenic original sin' (Morens *et al.* 2010), where an infectious agent is implicated which invokes an immune response that may or may not be beneficial at the next exposure to this agent. This is consistent with sequential infection by multiple CMV strains (see later).

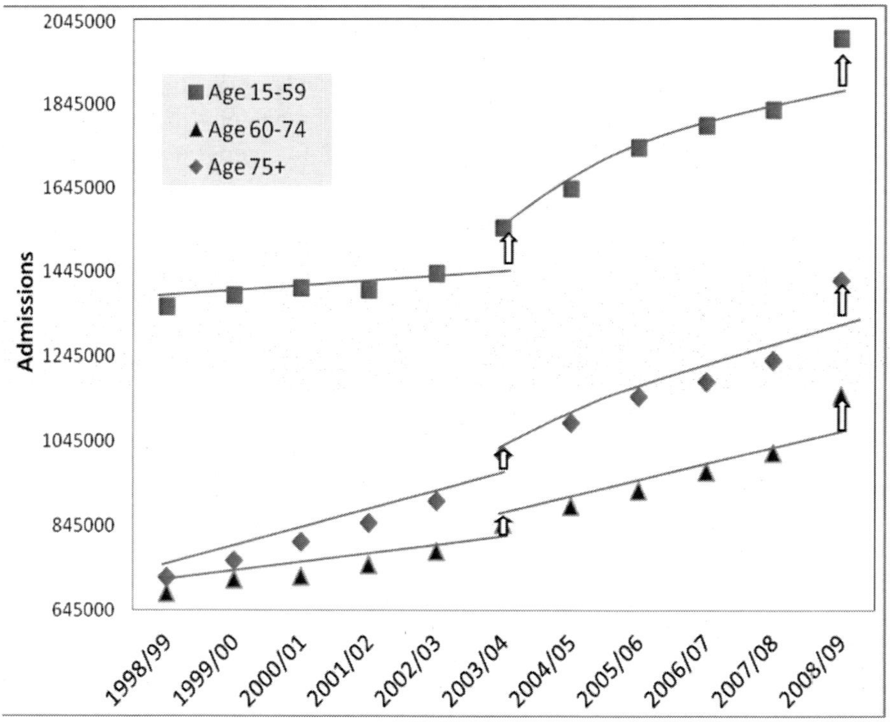

Figure 4.1. Step-like increases in admissions for a cluster of diagnoses across England (Adapted from Jones (2010b) – reproduced with permission from British Journal of Healthcare Management).

Table 1
Pattern in total occupied beds for various regions within England

Strategic Health Authority	**2005/06**	**2006/07**	**2007/08**	**2008/09**	**2009/10**	**Max: Min**
North Central London	95.9	93.1	**79.2**	99.8	103.4	131%
West Midlands South	97.8	98.9	**91.1**	109.7	103.8	120%
North West London	95.1	87.8	**84.9**	100.2	101.9	120%
Bedfordshire & Hertfordshire	97.0	92.8	**88.2**	101.3	103.6	118%
Surrey & Sussex	98.7	92.2	**85.1**	99.4	91.7	117%
Shropshire & Staffordshire	97.3	95.9	**88.5**	99.7	102.1	115%
County Durham & Tees Valley	99.7	106.1	**92.4**	101.9	105.3	115%
Hampshire & Isle of Wight	94.9	87.9	**85.8**	98.4	89.2	115%
North East London	95.7	90.8	**83.5**	92.2	93.6	112%
Northumberland, Tyne & Wear	101.0	96.9	**96.0**	106.3	107.0	111%
Thames Valley	97.6	89.9	**95.1**	95.9	98.8	110%
South East London	96.0	101.8	**93.3**	101.2	98.4	109%
Leicester, Northampton, Rutland	99.1	96.5	**91.7**	94.4	99.9	109%
Birmingham & the Black Country	96.4	94.3	**91.0**	98.9	98.9	109%
Dorset & Somerset	98.8	93.3	**92.6**	100.2	97.1	108%
Trent	98.4	95.6	**93.4**	99.2	101.0	108%
South West London	97.8	92.7	**91.5**	98.1	97.0	107%
Kent & Medway	101.6	97.3	**92.8**	95.1	90.9	107%
Avon, Gloucestershire & Wiltshire	97.6	96.2	**91.5**	97.8	97.6	107%
N & E Yorkshire	97.8	93.4	**89.1**	94.1	94.6	106%
Cumbria & Lancashire	91.2	91.7	**90.5**	95.8	92.0	106%
Essex	101.4	98.3	**94.8**	96.8	100.0	105%
South West Peninsula	96.1	**90.0**	93.3	94.5	93.5	105%
South Yorkshire	101.5	97.7	**94.5**	98.0	99.1	105%
West Yorkshire	97.0	**94.9**	96.0	97.6	93.7	104%
Cheshire & Merseyside	95.3	91.4	**89.1**	92.6	91.4	104%
Greater Manchester	101.6	99.0	**96.8**	97.2	99.8	103%
Norfolk, Suffolk & Cambridgeshire	93.5	86.9	**85.5**	87.7	88.0	103%

Data were extracted from the 'Strategic Health Authority of Residence' tables on the Hospital Episode Statistics (HES) Online website (http://www.hesonline.nhs.uk). Total bed occupancy includes maternity and mental health, and is relative to 2004/05 as the reference point (value = 100.0). Same day stay elective is also included, and has been assigned a nominal one day length of stay to adjust for potential differences in day surgery rates although the effect is minimal. The maximum to minimum ratio is for the maximum bed occupancy occurring after the minimum.

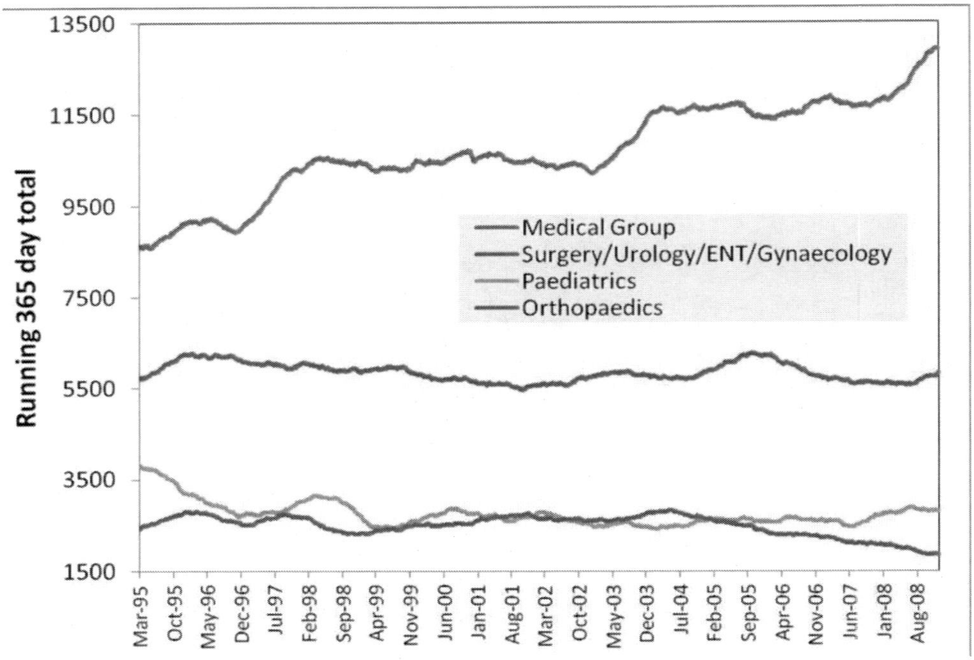

Figure 4.2. Medical and non-medical acute emergency admissions. Data kindly provided by the Royal Berkshire Hospital NHS Foundation Trust. Data exclude zero day stay admissions owing to a potential overlap with emergency department (ED) attendances arising out of the four hour maximum waiting time target. Note that a step change in admission rate will show up as a ramp-like feature in a running 365-day total chart.

Hence, it would seem that large step-like increases in medical admissions and total health care costs are occurring in the major developed countries in a roughly synchronous manner that is suggestive of an infectious outbreak. It would be exceedingly difficult to attribute such changes to any form of common funding, policy, or hospital behavior. A consideration of the diagnoses typically associated with each step change may therefore shed light on the nature of the outbreak or international epidemic; however, before doing this it is useful to investigate the magnitude of the financial and operational implications to international health care.

Financial and Operational Consequences

All health care systems operate within the constraints of financial and operational resources. Throughout the 1980s, the US health insurance industry began to suspect that a cycle of profit and loss may be operating (Kipp *et al.* 2003), and the evidence for this was formally reported in 1991 (Gabel *et al.* 1991). Further research suggested that this cycle appeared to be linked to a curious, sudden, approximately 6% (range 3% to 15%) increase in inflation-adjusted total costs (Born and Santerre 2005; Jones 2010c,f). Such increases will arise from a rapid change in the volume, case-mix and/or complexity of the health care contacts, the sum of which leads to the total cost. The pattern of hospital admissions, occupied bed days and wider costs seen in other countries appears to mirror a cycle very similar, if not identical, to the health insurance underwriting cycle seen in the USA; although the exact shape of the response over time depends on the geography studied, i.e. for large geographic areas such as the USA the response is a composite of spread over time (as demonstrated in Table 1).

An illustration of the sheer magnitude of such a change is given in Table 1 and Figure 4.3, where the trend in occupied beds within England is examined between 2004/05 and 2009/10. It should be noted that the pattern in occupied bed days is slightly different from that of admissions because the average length of stay is reducing over time (Jones 2009g). This tends to generate a more undulating cycle in occupied bed days rather than the more pronounced step-like pattern in admissions (Jones 2009d,f; Jones 2010a). However, as can be seen, there is a downward trend from 2004/05 either to 2006/07 (four regions) or, most often, to 2007/08, and in just one instance (Greater Manchester), to a minimum covering 2007/08 and 2008/09. The key points are that the downward trend is interrupted by a large (and totally unexplained) increase in the following financial year (although the exact change occurs at a point mid-way through the year), and that considerable regional variation is seen in the spread over time. Neither the downward trend nor the resulting sudden increase can be explained by any demographic, policy, or funding change, and the bulk of the trend is from unscheduled admissions (Jones 2009a,i). Each of the larger districts in Table 1 is made up from around five PCOs, and the pattern observed in these smaller locations is roughly the same, but within the larger regions there is greater evidence for geographic spread over time (Jones 2011a).

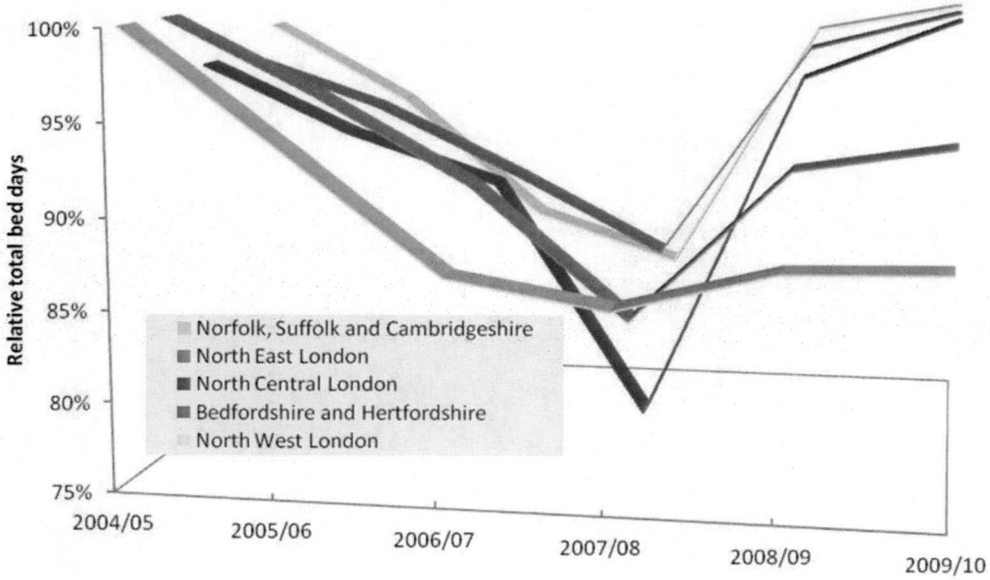

Figure 4.3. Time-based trends for different English regions. Bed demand is relative to the highest year in the time series (value = 100%).

Immediately following this dramatic change, all PCOs across England experienced financial difficulties (Jones 2010a,c,f,i). The varying extent of these financial difficulties can be explained by the different trajectories shown in Table 1, and is further illustrated in Figure 4.3 - North Central London had to cope with a 30% increase in bed-day related costs, while Dorset and Somerset had only to cope with a 7% increase, and Greater Manchester with just a

3% increase. The average increase for England was 7.7%. A 7% step-change in occupied bed-days at a conservative cost of £200 per bed day (Jones 2008) results in a minimum of £680 million ($1,120 million USD) of additional costs, and it is therefore not surprising to note that PCOs in England quickly slid into a deficit similar to that observed in the US health insurance underwriting cycle (Gabel *et al.* 1991; Born and Santerre 2005).

The trend in available beds (as opposed to occupied beds) supports the proposal that the increase in occupied beds was totally unexpected. This then led to the opening of beds that had been previously closed, in order to cope with the additional bed demand (Jones 2009f). While the downward part of the cycle was occurring, the trend showing a reduction in total bed days was widely attributed to 'efficiency' measures acting to reduce the average length of stay, which is partly true (Jones 2009g) but fails to explain the sudden and sustained increase immediately after the minimum point had been reached.

Table 2. List of potential diagnoses which increased after the 2002 and 2007 outbreaks in England

ICD Code	Description	2003/04	2008/09	03/04 step	08/09 step	Category
A01	Typhoid and paratyphoid fevers	247	367	46%	5%	Potential
A03	Shigellosis	68	87	11%	14%	Potential
A07	Other protozoal intestinal diseases	239	212	45%	33%	Potential
A30	Leprosy [Hansen's disease]	21	4	75%	33%	Potential
A38	Scarlet fever	259	421	4%	43%	Potential
A40	Streptococcal septicemia	1,060	1,213	8%	9%	Potential
A43	Nocardiosis	9	8	350%	700%	Potential
A46	Erysipelas	354	281	14%	6%	Potential
A20-A49	**Certain bacterial diseases**			**7%**	**3%**	**Possible**
A50	Congenital syphilis	10	15	43%	88%	Potential
A52	Late syphilis	93	99	29%	8%	Potential
A53	Other and unspecified syphilis	29	26	45%	18%	Potential
A68	Relapsing fevers	6	8	200%	60%	Potential
B05	Measles	108	409	40%	16%	Potential
B09	Viral infection membrane lesions	415	679	11%	19%	Potential
B19	Unspecified viral hepatitis	230	215	28%	10%	Potential
B20	HIV with infectious parasitic	1,040	1,627	8%	11%	Potential
B20-B24	**HIV disease**			**2%**	**4%**	**Possible**
B26	Mumps	143	281	49%	42%	Potential
B33	Other viral diseases, NEC	182	117	60%	19%	Potential
B34	Viral infection of unspecified site	39,911	48,619	4%	12%	Possible
B25-B34	**Other viral diseases**			**4%**	**11%**	**Strong**
B36	Other superficial mycoses	44	65	26%	76%	Potential
B37	Candidiasis	1,489	1,745	11%	3%	Potential
B43	Chromo- & pheomycotic abscess	3	10	200%	150%	Potential

ICD Code	Description	2003/04	2008/09	03/04 step	08/09 step	Category
B35-B49	**Mycoses**			**8%**	**5%**	**Strong**
B56	African trypanosomiasis	9	12	800%	33%	Potential
B76	Hookworm diseases	12	7	71%	250%	Potential
B87	Myiasis	6	15	50%	36%	Potential
B95	Streptococcus and staphylococcus	68	26	10%	136%	Potential
C48	Neoplasm of retro- & peritoneum	1,157	1,526	24%	15%	Strong
D22	Melanocytic naevi	1,464	1,462	15%	22%	Strong
E11	Non-insulin-dependent diabetes	13,669	17,615	7%	8%	Possible
E16	Disorders of pancreatic secretion	7,596	12,900	6%	12%	Possible
E66	Obesity	1,212	5,287	29%	47%	Possible
E87	Electrolyte and acid-base balance	8,521	15,614	19%	15%	Possible
E15-E90	**Endocrine metabolic diseases**			**10%**	**12%**	**Strong**
F10	Mental disorders due to alcohol	31,565	42,995	10%	3%	Possible
F10-F19	**Due to psychoactive substances**			**7%**	**1%**	**Possible**
G00-G09	**CNS inflammations**			**99%**	**107%**	**Strong**
G10-G13	**CNS degenerative diseases**			**96%**	**97%**	**Strong**
G20-G26	**Movement disorders**			**98%**	**105%**	**Strong**
G43	Migraine	6,954	11,282	7%	16%	Strong
G44	Other headache syndromes	2,260	3,178	9%	10%	Possible
G45	Transient ischemic attacks	16,633	21,185	6%	13%	Strong
G40-G47	**Epilepsy, migraine, etc**			**3%**	**23%**	**Strong**
G51	Facial nerve disorders	2,478	3,993	7%	13%	Possible
G97	Postprocedural nervous system	445	797	21%	29%	Strong
H10-H13	**Disorders of conjunctiva**			**9%**	**-**	**Strong**
H35	Other retinal disorders	3,064	4,113	12%	11%	Possible
H47	Disorders of optic [2nd] nerve	448	581	23%	18%	Strong
H53	Visual disturbances	2,641	4,275	11%	16%	Possible
H66	Suppurative otitis media	6,957	6,627	7%	7%	Strong
I00-I09	**Rheumatic heart disease**			**-**	**15%**	**Possible**
I10-I15	**Hypertensive diseases**			**1%**	**10%**	**Possible**
I26-I28	**Pulmonary heart & circulation**			**2%**	**10%**	**Possible**
I34	Nonrheumatic mitral valve	2,553	2,908	10%	6%	Strong
I42	Cardiomyopathy	3,445	3,988	8%	8%	Strong
I48	Atrial fibrillation and flutter	55,910	68,088	6%	2%	Possible
I51	Descriptions of heart disease	1,547	2,331	14%	40%	Strong
I63	Cerebral infarction	35,770	44,354	2%	6%	Strong
I95	Hypotension	8,387	13,635	13%	10%	Possible
I95-I99	**Other circulatory disorders**			**10%**	**9%**	**Strong**
J00	Acute nasopharyngitis	773	1,628	13%	29%	Possible

Table 2. (Continued)

ICD Code	Description	2003/04	2008/09	03/04 step	08/09 step	Category
J00-J06	**Acute upper RT infections**			**114%**	**101%**	**Strong**
J06	Acute upper RT of multiple sites	45,411	50,348	13%	12%	Strong
J10	Influenza identified virus	322	314	201%	140%	Strong
J11	Influenza virus not identified	950	673	42%	28%	Strong
J18	Pneumonia organism unspecified	88,038	125,601	9%	15%	Strong
J10-J18	**Influenza & pneumonia**			**9%**	**15%**	**Strong**
J22	Unspecified acute LRT infection	77,965	91,245	8%	13%	Strong
J20-J22	**Other acute LRT infections**			**8%**	**12%**	**Strong**
J40	Bronchitis not specified	1,265	1,671	14%	11%	Strong
J44	Other chronic OPD	103,917	109,977	13%	10%	Strong
J45	Asthma	55,875	61,048	10%	11%	Strong
J47	Bronchiectasis	5,203	6,430	11%	7%	Possible
J40-J47	**Chronic LRT diseases**			**10%**	**10%**	**Strong**
ICD Code	**Description**	**2003/04**	**2008/09**	**03/04 step**	**08/09 step**	**Category**
J60-J70	**Lung diseases external agents**			**20%**	**5%**	**Strong**
J84	Interstitial pulmonary diseases	4,960	5,854	11%	6%	Strong
J86	Pyothorax	1,910	2,573	11%	11%	Strong
J98	Other respiratory disorders	4,621	5,500	6%	11%	Possible
J80-J99	**Other respiratory diseases**			**4%**	**6%**	**Strong**
K04	Diseases of pulp and periapical	3,974	5,278	8%	5%	Possible
K57	Diverticular disease of intestine	20,702	22,161	3%	3%	Possible
K59	Functional intestinal disorders	34,006	40,602	6%	6%	Strong
K70-K77	**Diseases of liver**			**3%**	**1%**	**Possible**
K85	Acute pancreatitis	13,879	17,160	6%	5%	Possible
K92	Diseases of digestive system	35,839	42,534	3%	6%	Possible
K90-K93	**Other digestive system**			**2%**	**6%**	**Possible**
L02	Cutaneous abscess, furuncle, etc	23,199	28,571	9%	6%	Possible
L03	Cellulitis	48,889	56,232	10%	4%	Possible
L00-L14	**Infections/disorders of skin**			**6%**	**3%**	**Strong**
M15	Polyarthrosis	2,772	7,215	19%	36%	Possible
M25	Other joint disorders	30,681	50,866	6%	21%	Possible
M54	Dorsalgia	33,679	48,031	10%	8%	Strong
M40-M54	**Dorsopathies**			**8%**	**10%**	**Strong**
M62	Other disorders of muscle	2,172	2,520	10%	16%	Strong
M79	Other soft tissue disorders	46,936	66,176	4%	10%	Possible
M60-M79	**Soft tissue disorders**			**6%**	**7%**	**Strong**
N00-N08	**Diseases of the kidney**			**5%**	**8%**	**Strong**
N12	Tubulo-interstitial nephritis	6,405	10,045	11%	14%	Possible

ICD Code	Description	2003/04	2008/09	03/04 step	08/09 step	Category
N17-N19	**Renal failure**			**23%**	**3%**	**Strong**
N20	Calculus of kidney and ureter	21,890	30,502	11%	8%	Possible
N20-N23	**Urolithiasis**			**11%**	**5%**	**Strong**
N25-N29	**Disorders of kidney & ureter**			**3%**	**8%**	**Strong**
N39	Other disorders of urinary system	82,586	130,444	10%	9%	Strong
N30-N39	**Other diseases urinary system**			**7%**	**8%**	**Strong**
N99	Other disorders genitourinary			107%	102%	Strong
O90	Complications of the puerperium	3,961	6,323	16%	5%	Possible
O91	Infections of breast childbirth	509	835	22%	16%	Strong
P08	Disorders gestation & birth weight	5,332	8,827	6%	10%	Strong
P20	Intrauterine hypoxia	23,144	25,084	6%	3%	Possible
P28	Perinatal respiratory conditions	6,612	8,845	8%	9%	Strong
P36	Bacterial sepsis of newborn	1,010	2,310	15%	31%	Strong
P92	Feeding problems of newborn	7,387	12,478	7%	10%	Possible
R00	Abnormalities of heart beat	15,496	21,927	13%	8%	Strong
R06	Abnormalities of breathing	53,006	76,785	8%	14%	Strong
R07	Pain in throat and chest	181,967	252,091	9%	6%	Strong
R00-R09	**Circulatory/respiratory**			**8%**	**7%**	**Strong**
R10	Abdominal and pelvic pain	181,762	227,143	6%	3%	Possible
R18	Ascites	4,854	8,403	13%	9%	Possible
R20	Disturbances of skin sensation	3,621	6,603	10%	17%	Possible
R20-R23	**Skin & subcutaneous tissue**			**2%**	**6%**	**Possible**
R25	Abnormal involuntary movements	2,873	4,125	8%	8%	Possible
R26	Abnormalities of gait and mobility	7,198	6,954	5%	10%	Possible
R25-R29	**Nervous & musculoskeletal**			**5%**	**11%**	**Strong**
R31	Unspecified hematuria	15,736	20,379	6%	6%	Possible
R33	Retention of urine	25,113	27,183	3%	4%	Strong
R41	Cognitive function & awareness	18,341	27,112	12%	13%	Possible
R42	Dizziness and giddiness	12,787	19,252	12%	11%	Strong
R40-R46	**Cognition, perception, etc**			**12%**	**13%**	**Strong**
R47	Speech disturbances,	2,357	5,191	11%	24%	Possible
R50	Fever of unknown origin	15,134	22,455	13%	5%	Strong
R51	Headache	32,540	50,753	9%	9%	Possible
R53	Malaise and fatigue	10,415	14,632	11%	13%	Strong
R54	Senility	27,665	42,175	8%	16%	Possible
R55	Syncope and collapse	64,032	91,643	10%	9%	Strong
R56	Convulsions	35,375	41,528	9%	5%	Strong
R68	Other general symptoms	3,023	5,559	13%	65%	Strong
R50-R68	**General symptoms & signs**			**9%**	**10%**	**Strong**
R69	Unknown causes of morbidity	229,695	116,827	19%	10%	Strong

Table 2. (Continued)

ICD Code	Description	2003/04	2008/09	03/04 step	08/09 step	Category
R79	Abnormal findings of blood	1,710	5,460	25%	15%	Possible
T40	Poisoning by narcotics	6,545	9,954	12%	4%	Possible
T42	Poisoning by antiepileptic, etc	12,608	15,435	11%	5%	Strong
T36-T50	**Poisonings by drugs**			**12%**	**1%**	**Strong**
T66-T78	**Other external causes**			**14%**	**4%**	**Strong**
T83	**Complications GU devices**	**6,825**	**11,279**	**5%**	**13%**	**Possible**
T80-T88	**Surgical & medical care**			**7%**	**5%**	**Strong**
T90-T98	**Sequelae of injuries**			**-**	**25%**	**Possible**
Z04	Examination and observation	10,334	15,273	41%	57%	Strong
Z00-Z13	**Examination and investigation**			**2%**	**14%**	**Strong**
Z27	Immunization	646	333	24%	24%	Possible
Z45	Adjustment of implanted device	6,765	8,467	5%	9%	Possible

Material in this table has been adapted from Jones (2010k,l). The first study used ICD chapter sub-groups, i.e. J02-J22 (Other acute lower respiratory tract infections) in order to gain the benefit of larger numbers (Jones 2010k) while the second study (Jones 2010l) used ICD three digit diagnoses with larger numbers of admissions to investigate in more detail. The 'Category' column gives an assessment of which diagnoses have the strongest evidence for a step change: Strong – good evidence, Possible – possible role for other factors or a knock-on effect, Potential – mainly small number diagnoses.

In conclusion, the financial and operational impact of each outbreak is very large, and leads to significant disruption in the operation of the health care system. How do we go about explaining this cycle of events?

An Infectious Outbreak?

As discussed, the increase in emergency admissions (especially of a medical nature) and emergency department attendances is not a new phenomenon, but goes back at least four decades. However, the point of interest is that this increase occurs at certain points in time rather than as a continuous long-term trend, and that this increase appears to be roughly synchronous among countries.

In this respect, it is well known that all infectious diseases with an acquired immune response exhibit unique time cycles specific to the type of infection (Anderson *et al.* 1984; Flemming *et al.* 1991; Dushoff 1996; Dowell 2001; Koelle and Pascual 2004; Grassly *et al.* 2005; Grassly and Fraser 2005). It has been proposed that the spectrum of diagnoses that commonly increase with each 'outbreak' appear to be associated with some form of immune system disturbance, meaning that admissions for infection and inflammation (in its widest sense) all appear to increase – see Table 2 (Jones 2010k-m).

The evidence that this could be the work of a previously unrecognized infectious agent is as follows (Jones 2006a; Jones 2009a-c,i; Jones 2010k-m; Jones 2011a,d,h):

1. The unique behavior has been consistent over a very long time frame (back to the 1960s).
2. The 'outbreak' results in a step increase specific to medical admissions as opposed to wider surgical, trauma or pediatric, so it is not due to some generalized factor affecting all admissions.
3. Within a very short time (six to eight weeks), the admission rate steps up to a new and higher rate.
4. Regional variability in the timing and extent of the step increase is consistent with an infectious outbreak.
5. The 'outbreak' is characterized by an increase in excess deaths, which lasts for around six to eight weeks.
6. The increase in emergency admissions is accompanied by a permanent and parallel increase in occupied beds.
7. A range of vague and non-specific signs and symptoms plus more specific diagnoses appear to increase during the 'outbreak'.
8. The outbreak appears to coincide with a non-specific increase in GP referral for an outpatient appointment, and this could be interpreted as an increase in general poor health that appears to accompany the outbreak.
9. There is no apparent seasonality, in that similar onsets for each outbreak are observed across northern and southern hemispheres (see later discussion regarding lack of seasonality in CMV reactivation).
10. In the UK there is evidence to suggest that each outbreak initiates earliest in Scotland, and that there is some degree of north to south spread (see later discussion regarding a possible role for vitamin D sufficiency).
11. The author has noted a spatial spread over time among a population admitted to a single hospital by virtue of natural boundaries to movement such as the ocean, rivers or road network, thus a shift in acute thresholds for admission can be ruled out as the cause of this behavior (unpublished analysis).

It is important to note that the increase affecting the greatest number of admissions was for diagnoses of a non-specific nature, i.e. signs and symptoms, and it is the author's opinion that a genuine but subtle step-change in the overall health of the population has occurred. The differential response of the combined acute, primary care and social care system to each outbreak then determines the resulting cost pressures. A poorly integrated system is likely to 'over react', and thereby create additional cost and acute bed pressures. In a poorly integrated system, a large increase in symptoms of poor health, especially among the elderly (where definitive diagnosis is difficult), overwhelms primary and social care and acute admission becomes the default, although it would seem that acute doctors cannot quite explain what exactly is wrong with the additional patients. This additional influx of patients also overwhelms the coding processes within hospitals, leading to an additional increase in default coding (Jones 1996b, Jones 2009h). Factors such as high bed occupancy, leading to hospital acquired infection and allocation of patients into the incorrect specialty bed pool for optimum care (Jones 2009h; Jones 2011f-g,l), act to exacerbate the situation further, and the stretched resources in health and social care can lead to further blockages to discharge (Jones 2011j). These knock-on effects probably explain the very high increase in occupied beds seen in the health care systems toward the top of Table 1, especially in London (Jones 2011i).

It is postulated that the infectious agent is viral. Certain viruses maintain a state of permanent or persistent infection in the host, and this could account for the step-like change in emergency admission rates, which will arise from the pool of infected persons who could be experiencing some form of impaired or altered immunity. Hence, if the hypothesis of repeating international outbreaks is correct, then we must, of necessity, be looking for a ubiquitous virus known to establish a persistent infection, but that must additionally possess powerful immune-modulating properties. In this respect, the ubiquitous herpes virus, cytomegalovirus (CMV), could be implicated (Jones 2011d), although until recent years this virus has been largely regarded as only posing a risk either to the developing fetus, where it is responsible for 40% of all congenital malformations (Bate *et al.* 2010), or the severely immunocompromised, such as HIV/AIDS and transplant recipients.

Cytomegalovirus

Cytomegalovirus (CMV) is a member of the herpes group of DNA viruses. Varying between countries, 20% to 100% of the population is infected, depending upon the age, gender, region and risk factors (Cannon *et al.* 2010; Hyde *et al.* 2010). It causes a persistent infection with reactivation (via a range of mechanisms) to cause observable clinical symptoms, which include a lupus- or influenza-like illness with fatigue, headache, fever and occasional respiratory infection. These symptoms match some of the more non-specific diagnoses that accompany each outbreak. Indeed, an increase in influenza-like symptoms was noted in primary care during the 1993 outbreak (Jones 1996a). Infection of varying severity can occur in almost any body organ or cell type, and is often resolved with specific anti-viral therapy (Soderberger-Naucler 2006; Varani *et al.* 2009; Varani *et al.* 2010).

Of all the herpes viruses, CMV has the greatest number of genes committed to a formidable arsenal of immune evasive and disruptive strategies directed against the innate and adaptive immune responses of the host (Miller-Kittrell and Sparer 2009; van de Berg *et al.* 2010; Derhovanessian *et al.* 2009), leading to active immune suppression, amplification of inflammation, and autoimmune phenomena (Miller-Kittrell and Sparer 2009; Varani *et al.* 2010; Varani and Landini 2011). CMV also appears to be unique among DNA viruses in that the viron contains four species of mRNA with unknown function (Huang and Johnson 2000).

CMV is curious in that it has no recognized serotypes (in contrast to the influenza virus), but instead has a wide range of strains with high genetic diversity (Stanton *et al.* 2010). Different strains appear to prefer specific organs/tissues, and individuals can be simultaneously or sequentially infected with distinct strains (Ver Braak *et al.* 1998; Stanton *et al.* 2010).

Transmission is via body fluids (blood, breast milk, mucus, saliva, semen, urine and vaginal secretions), and requires a degree of direct contact (Cannon *et al.* 2011). This mode of transmission concurs with the rather slow further spread following the initial outbreak(s). Sexual transmission is one of the more significant risk factors (Robain *et al.* 1998; Cannon *et al.* 2011) The virus can cross the species boundary with primates (Swinkels *et al.* 1984), and fairly rapid mutation is observed when the virus is subject to serial culture *in vitro* (Stanton *et al.* 2010). Hence, a significant *in vivo* mutation (which is slower than *in vitro*) in a particular strain could be rapidly carried by high volume air, rail, road and sea transport (Hollingsworth *et al.* 2007) from the initial locus to create an international 'epidemic' of poor health. Evidence that CMV seroprevalence is higher in particular years, and the curious gender differences, will be discussed later. It should also be noted that the apparent lack of seasonality with regard to the proposed outbreaks is consistent with direct person to person transmission, and also with the lack of seasonality in CMV re-activation (Ling *et al.* 2003).

Recent research has suggested that a range of sub-clinical effects can also occur, which lead to the virus being a risk factor in a diverse range of clinical situations. These include inflammatory and autoimmune diseases (Varani *et al.* 2009; Varani *et al.* 2010), survival in the intensive care unit (Andre *et al.* 2009), diverse expressions of poor health especially in the elderly (Pawalec *et al.* 2005; Pawalec *et al.* 2009; Vescovini *et al.* 2010; Wang *et al.* 2010), a trigger for breast cancer (Cox *et al.* 2010; Harkinns *et al.* 2010), a trigger for depression (Phillips *et al.* 2008), and as a risk factor in cardiovascular disease (CVD) where CMV seropositive individuals with high C-reactive protein (a marker of inflammation) have a 30% higher risk of death from CVD (Simanek *et al.* 2011). Chronic inflammation in endothelial cells (as in vascular disease) can be induced by the induction of fractalkine when the frequency of CMV-specific T cells is high (Bolovan-Fritts and Spector 2011). Research has shown that CMV is present in 97% of breast ductal carcinoma cases compared to 63% of normal breast glandular epithelium (Harkins *et al.* 2010), and that the elevation of CMV antibodies precedes the development of breast cancer in some women (Cox *et al.* 2010).

A range of studies have shown that the healthy elderly are either not infected with CMV or have very low levels of antibody titer, suggesting that the virus is maintained in a latent state. The frail or unwell elderly are characterized by increasingly high antibody titers (Derhovanessian *et al.* 2010; Vescovini *et al.* 2010; Wang *et al.* 2010), which in one study was linked to associated increases in diabetes, cardiovascular disease, frailty and mortality (Wang *et al.* 2010), and what is known as the immune risk profile (IRP) (Derhovanessian *et al.* 2009; Pawelec *et al.* 2009). The IRP is a cluster of immune changes that appear to mark the onset of the transition ultimately to death. It is characterized by poor T-cell proliferation and response to mitogens, low numbers of B-cells, and an inverted CD4/CD8 ratio caused by the proliferation of CD8 cells and (in most instances) by CMV seropositivity (Pawelec *et al.* 2005; Pawalec *et al.* 2009). CMV also leads to the equivalent of premature aging in T cells, which is linked to diseases such as atherosclerosis (van de Berg *et al.* 2010). Shedding of CMV, which is largely absent in mid-life, is frequently observed in the elderly, along with dual reactivation of both EBV and CMV (Stowe *et al.* 2007). For a large proportion of the elderly the infection has, therefore, switched from latent (or persistent low grade virus replication) to chronic (with active shedding). In this respect the mechanisms distinguishing true latency from persistent, low grade infection are not yet known.

CMV Strain Diversity

As mentioned above, CMV exists as a large and genetically diverse number of strains (Puchhamer-Stockl *et al.* 2011). This is reflected in the glycoprotein diversity of the envelope

(Novak *et al.* 2009), which acts to hamper vaccine development. Multiple strain infections are commonly observed, and up to six strains can simultaneously hyper-infect an individual, with the ratio between these strains changing over time (Gorzer *et al.* 2010). Some 16% of congenitally infected infants have multiple strains (Ross *et al.* 2010), and in a study of healthy young women who had only recently become seropositive to CMV, some 25% had an identical strain, 71% harbored unique strains, and 4% had two strains (Murthy *et al.* 2011). In another study, multiple clusters of strains were detected among children at six day care centers in two cities in the USA (Bale *et al.* 1999). Since CMV is uniquely characterized by such an enormous variety of strains, why is such diversity needed? It is proposed that strain diversity is the unique answer to optimum infection in humans exhibiting a similarly diverse range of immune impairments. Such differences may also enable each strain to exhibit a degree of organ specificity (Woo *et al.* 1997). It is proposed that descriptions such as 'immune competent' or 'healthy' have failed to indicate the correct situation, and that the issue of immune impairment needs to be more widely appreciated.

Immune Competent?

The classic textbook description of CMV infection is that it is largely dormant and without observable clinical symptoms in most immune competent hosts, and that only the immune compromised host is at risk of serious clinical infection. However, such a clear cut distinction may have acted to deflect clinical and research interest away from the more subtle effects of this virus.

Indeed, to understand the maximum potential for this virus to act, we need to understand the much wider range of permanent and temporary immune impairments that characterize the supposedly 'immune competent' or 'healthy' host. All individuals have the potential for some degree of temporary or permanent immune impairment due to a wide variety of factors such as: ageing (Lustgarten 2009; Mayor 2009; Deeks and Phillips 2010), gender, especially around puberty (Tanriverdi *et al.* 2003; Fairweather and Rose 2004; Jaspan *et al.* 2006; Lamason *et al.* 2006; Libert *et al.* 2010), the developing fetus and very young children (West 2002; Tu *et al.* 2004), pregnancy (Jamieson *et al.* 2006; Westman 2010; Kastelan *et al.* 2010), circadian cycles in immune components and sleep disruption (Born *et al.* 1997), strenuous physical activity (Gleeson *et al.* 2004), chronic stress and anxiety (Kiecolt-Glaser *et al.* 1987; Kiecolt-Glasser and Glasser 2002; Prasch *et al.* 2000; Davidson *et al.* 2003; Reiche *et al.* 2004), war, natural disasters and trauma (Hyams *et al.* 1996; Ironson *et al.* 1997; Vojdani and Thrasher 2004; Whistler *et al.* 2009), depression (Kiecolt-Glaser and Glaser 2002; Dantzer *et al.* 2008), exposure to environmental toxins, including the resulting DNA damage (Hyams 1998; Kawanishi *et al.* 2006; Ohshima and Bartsch H 1994), poor nutrition (Linder 1987; Azad *et al.* 1999; Savino 2002; Gleeson *et al.* 2004; Evans 2005; Haase and Rink 2009), deficiency in iron, zinc and selenium (Broome *et al.* 2004; Hurwitz *et al.* 2007; Wardwell *et al.* 2008; Mocchegiani *et al.* 2009; Haase and Rink 2009; Papp *et al.* 2010), acid/base imbalance (Lardner 2001), season of the year, altitude and latitude, including magnitude of exposure to ultraviolet radiation and vitamin D levels (Dowel 2001; van der Mei *et al.* 2001; Altizer *et al.* 2006; DeLappe *et al.* 2006; Grassley and Fraser 2006; Zittermann *et al.* 2009; Hayes 2010), existing autoimmune disease(s) (Gottleib *et al.* 1979), variation in thymic T-cell production (Lorenzi *et al.* 2008; Lorenzi *et al.* 2009), genetic factors, including specific gene mutations (leading to what are known as primary immunodeficiencies) and epigenetic factors such as environment-induced DNA methylation (Casanova *et al.* 2008; Thomas *et al.* 2009; Hamza *et al.* 2010; Bousfiha *et al.* 2010; Mathers *et al.* 2010), which may explain the unique patterns in immune response that render some individuals resistant to HIV infection (Suy *et al.* 2007), type 1 or type 2 diabetes (Muller *et al.* 2005; Danquah *et al.* 2010), diseases such as cirrhosis of the liver (Varani *et al.* 2000), or the presence of persistent viral infection (Bonhoeffer and Nowak 1994; Worobey and Holmes 1999; Goulding *et al.* 2001; Wills *et al.* 2002; Wherry *et al.* 2003; Garcia-Pineres *et al.* 2006; Freeman *et al.* 2006; De Martel *et al.* 2008; Voisset *et al.* 2008; Zuniga *et al.* 2008; Deeks and Phillips 2010).

Given the complexity of the immune system, and the fact that new classes of immune cells are regularly being discovered (Miossec *et al.* 2009), such observations are not surprising and suggest that the supposedly 'immune competent' population has a wide variety of exploitable immune impairments. If we accept the proposal that the multiplicity of CMV strains is central to the biological success of this virus, we then have a basis for understanding how the seemingly immunocompetent population could experience a wide range of sub-acute, acute and chronic CMV infections. Indeed, the whole issue of immune impairments may be central to the explanation of *in vivo* CMV biology, and the very use of averages and tests for statistical significance are based on the assumption that individuals react to infection and disease in a unique way.

We now need to reconcile the observed characteristics of the outbreaks of poor health against the known and potential effects of CMV, and the following sections will investigate several of the key areas.

The Elderly

In England, 50% of all admissions (including elective/planned) are for those aged over 60, and this proportion reaches 65% for the medical group of specialties. In the elderly, infection often manifests as changes in cognitive function (including depression) and physical function, rather than the classical signs of infection seen in the young (High *et al.* 2005). Chronic inflammatory conditions associated with high levels of circulating cytokines lead to muscle wastage and disability (irrespective of age), although in the elderly the natural innate inflammatory responses are enhanced and prolonged (High *et al.* 2005, Stout-Delgado *et al.* 2009). Assessment scores for both cognitive and physical function are therefore good predictors of emergency department attendance (Walker *et al.* 2005) as well as infection and/or inflammation, and can often continue to decline after the immediately apparent cause of the 'infection' (urinary tract infection, pneumonia, etc) has been treated (High *et al.* 2005). In elderly Latinos, functional impairment has been shown to be clearly linked to levels of C-reactive protein (CRP), which is a marker for inflammation, and CMV has also been implicated (Aiello *et al.* 2008a). The role of CMV inflammation is discussed in more detail in a later section.

Several studies have noted that specific and unexplained increase in admissions, as described in Chapter R of the International Classification of Disease (ICD) 'signs and symptoms', is associated with an increase in medical emergency admissions for the elderly

(Walsh *et al.* 2008, Kendrick and Conway 2003a-c, NHS Scotland, 2005), especially R00-09 (circulatory and respiratory) and R50-68 (general signs and symptoms) (Blunt *et al.* 2010). Re-analysis of the same data has demonstrated that particular signs and symptoms exhibited a characteristic step-like increase immediately after the 2002 and 2007 'outbreaks' seen in the UK (Jones 2009i; Jones 2010k-m) and a similar 'outbreak' seen in Australia (Jones 2011k). In the USA, a specific increase in emergency department attendances for 'other and undefined diagnoses' has been observed since 1993, and this translated into peaks in admission via the emergency department around 1993, 1997 and 2003. The highest increase was noted in those aged over 65, of African descent, and requiring three or more medications (Roberts *et al.* 2008). Hence, the general difficulty in assigning a definitive diagnosis in the elderly is consistent with the specific step increase in admissions for signs and symptoms, and this may have masked the true underlying etiology.

In addition to the more general 'signs and symptoms', there is an additional set of more specific diagnoses that appear to be implicated, and these are listed in Table 2. While the list in Table 2 may appear somewhat extended, it should be noted that it represents a very small subset of the 1,655 ICD diagnoses used across England (of which the top 200 account for 75% of all admissions). However, in its widest sense all diagnoses have a common link with infection or inflammation, with the inflammatory immune responses and the consequences of these.

Additional research into this list is required, as some have a 'confirmed' step increase while others are possible diagnoses requiring further validation. Indeed, it is possible that some are direct effects of the outbreak while others are indirect or knock-on effects. Diagnoses relating to cancers, neonates and congenital conditions are largely unstudied. It is also possible that some of the diagnoses noted in Table 2 may be 'nearest fit' diagnoses. The issue regarding the accuracy of diagnosis is discussed later. If we accept that we are dealing with a relatively slow moving infectious outbreak leading to a cascade of diagnoses, some of which may involve time lags, then complex spatial analysis is required to match up the point of onset in each location to magnify the resulting diagnostic changes over time. This approach will then allow greater clarity as to which diagnoses are genuinely associated with the outbreak, and the degree of time lag for other diagnoses that may also be gender related (Jones 2011c).

Gender

While the two genders appear to have identical immune systems, evidence is emerging for gender-specific immune functional differences. Each autoimmune disease exhibits a unique gender ratio regarding incidence (Libert *et al.* 2010), and only women are capable of the unique immune changes required during pregnancy (Westman 2010). One of the characteristics of the curious step-increase in medical admissions is an apparently greater effect against females, or gender- and time-related effects in particular diagnoses (Jones 2009i; Jones 2010f,g,j; Jones 2011c,i). In this respect, CMV seropositivity is more prevalent in females and generally occurs at an earlier age (Matos *et al.* 2010), and this has been attributed to greater exposure to young children who can shed CMV for up to 29 months post infection (Tu *et al.* 2004). CMV antibody levels are usually higher in women (Matos *et al.*

2010), and women show a higher release of interferon-γ and interleukin-2 than men in response to active CMV infection (Villacres *et al.* 2004).

Role of the Thymus

The correct function of the thymus in attracting and converting bone marrow-derived precursor cells is vital for the production of T lymphocytes (see review by Boyd *et al.* 2008) and dis-regulation of this process leads to autoimmunity (Baldwin *et al.* 2004). CMV is now strongly implicated in a range of autoimmune diseases (Varani *et al.* 2009; Varani *et al.* 2010; Varani and Landini 2011). Measles, HIV, varicella-zoster, coxsackievirus-B4, echovirus type 6 and CMV are all capable of infecting the thymus (Numazaki *et al.* 1989; Valsamakis *et al.* 1998; Ventura *et al.* 2001; de la Rossa and Leal 2003), leading to various impairments in T-cell production, the production of virus-infected T-cells (such as with HIV), and reduced secretion of interleukin-1-like activity (Wainberg *et al.* 1988; King *et al.* 1992; Brilot *et al.* 2004). The thymus is also a specific target in malnutrition (Linder 1987; Savino 2002), suggesting that the malnourished elderly, who are over-represented in acute medical admissions (Azad *et al.* 1999; Evans 2005; Haase and Rink 2009), could be a specific target for CMV. In some instances the virus can be eliminated from the thymus by the addition of donor T-cells containing virus-specific cytotoxic T lymphocytes (King *et al.* 1992), and this may explain the beneficial effects of thymus extracts in treating instances of chronic respiratory tract and other infections (Wilson 1999).

The production of T-cells by the thymus can be accurately determined using T cell receptor excision circle (TREC) studies. TRECs are episomal DNA by-products of T cell receptor rearrangements that are only expressed by T cells of thymic origin, with each cell containing a single copy of TREC. In 'healthy' individuals the TREC count declines in a logarithmic manner with age, from around 1.1 x 10^9 cells per day at age 1 to around 1 x 10^7 at age 80, and this is also associated with a change in the ratio of CD4+/CD8+ and CD8_TREC/CD8+ (Ye and Kirschener 2002; McFarland *et al.* 2000). However, for individuals of the same age, thymic T-cell production can vary by at least 10-fold, with the extent of this variation appearing to be least between 15 and 35 years, then significantly increasing above age 35 (Lorenzi *et al.* 2008). Production of T-cells is typically higher in females (Lorenzi *et al.* 2008; Lorenzi *et al.* 2009). Aberrations in thymic morphology and reduced T-cell production are known to be associated with auto-immune, infectious, and allergic diseases (Zairat'iants 1991) such as myasthenia gravis (Vakilian *et al.* 2006), systemic lupus erythematosus (Gottlieb *et al.* 1979; Kayser *et al.* 2004), rheumatic heart disease (Henry 1968) and inflammatory skin diseases such as atopic dermatitis (AD) and psoriasis (Just 2006). Interestingly, patients with AD exhibit a high variation in TREC over time (Just 2006), which appears to be a similar phenomenon to the symptom flare cycles observed with Lyme disease, and may arise from oscillatory cycles in cytokine levels triggering an autoimmune response (Gruber 2010).

The vital role of the thymus in maintaining immune function following CMV infection has been demonstrated in a study investigating patients whose thymus was removed during early childhood. In this study, CMV-infected thymectomized patients who had reached the age of 22 exhibited an altered T cell profile characteristic of those aged over 75, which was similar to the IRP. The strongest alteration in this profile was associated with a group of patients who were 86% CMV seropositive, in contrast to other thymectomized patients who were only 36% CMV seropositive (Sauce *et al.* 2009). In AIDS, it has also been noted that restoration of thymic mass by growth hormones acts to restore T cell production (Taub *et al.* 2010).

In one study using human thymic tissue grafted into SCID-hu mice, human CMV (HCMV) was concentrated in the medulla of the thymus, with the epithelial cells being the primary target rather than the hematopoietic cell population (Mocarski *et al.* 1993). Similar damage to the thymic epithelial cells occurs in severe malnutrition due to expansion of cytotoxic suppressor (CD8) lymphocytes, which has been proposed to lead to immune dysfunction (Linder 1987). In guinea pigs with CMV-induced mononucleosis, the virus was cleared from the blood and bone marrow within one month; however, it remained resident in thymic and lymph tissue (Griffith *et al.* 1981) with unknown long-term effects. In BALB/c mice infected with a sublethal dose of murine CMV (MCMV), the thymocytes exhibited extensive apoptosis due to aberrant Ca^{2+} mobilization, although MCMV DNA could only be found in the thymic stromal cells and not in the thymocytes (Koga *et al.* 1994). It is clear that CMV can establish long-term infection in the thymus, leading to the production of defective (but not infected) thymocytes. Such resident CMV infection could also hasten the decline in thymic function with age, as evident by the wide range in TREC production observed in humans of the same age (Gress and Deeks 2009). Lastly, in patients with hematological malignancies, naïve CD8 cells from umbilical blood failed to clear CMV viremia, but required T cell neogenesis (as $CD4^+CD45RA^+$) via the thymus to be effective (Braun *et al.* 2010). It is widely recognized that, in some individuals, up to 30% of the circulating $CD4^+$ and $CD8^+$ memory cell population is committed to controlling CMV (Sylwester *et al.* 2005, Naeger *et al.* 2010), and this compromises the patient's ability to respond to new infections, thus leading to the observed increase in susceptibility to infection during each outbreak. Under these circumstances it is only those individuals with an active thymus who will have the reserve capacity to continue producing non-CMV committed T-cells.

There appear to be no studies regarding the possible role of CMV infection of the thymus in the progression of immunosenescence, various system diseases, or premature death. In this respect, testing for CMV infection during autopsies of those dying from different diseases or at different ages may shed further light on this topic.

Vitamin D

In the UK each outbreak appears to commence slightly earlier in Scotland, and shows some degree of north-south movement (Jones 1996a; Jones 2010i). It has been suggested that vitamin D sufficiency/insufficiency may explain this observation (Jones 2010i). Vitamin D is known to be involved in both innate and adaptive immunity, and hence, autoimmune disease, various diseases including some cancers, resistance to infection, the production of antimicrobial peptides called defensins, and depression (Adams and Hewison 2008; Yamschchikov *et al.* 2009; Zitterman *et al.* 2009; Ganji *et al.* 2010; Sabetta *et al.* 2010).

It is of interest to note that 1,25 $(OH)_2$-vitamin D3 is concentrated in the nuclei of reticular cells of the medulla and cortex of the thymus (Stumpf and O'Brien 1987), but not in the nuclei of lymphocytes. However, vitamin D receptor (VDR), a member of the nuclear receptor family of transcription factors, is found in significant concentrations in the immature cells of the thymus and in mature CD8 T lymphocytes (Deluca and Cantorna 2001). Hence, vitamin D levels could also play an important part in regulating thymic function (discussed above), along with wider infection/inflammation issues.

There is only one study to date regarding vitamin D levels and CMV, dealing with pediatric onset multiple sclerosis (MS). The MS group, rather surprisingly, had lower CMV antibody levels associated with vitamin D insufficiency and, conversely, vitamin D sufficiency was associated with higher CMV antibody levels, while in the control group, vitamin D sufficiency was associated with lower CMV antibody levels (Mowry *et al.* 2011). It would appear that, in the absence of MS, vitamin D sufficiency is implicated in avoiding the deleterious effects of CMV, with low CMV antibody levels suggesting controlled infection, but may interact with particular immune impairments in unexpected ways. See the next section for a similar dichotomous response to CMV inflammation in the presence of a specific gene mutation.

More research regarding the role of vitamin D sufficiency/insufficiency in association with CMV infection is required, especially for the elderly where diminishing renal function leads to hyperthyroidism, requiring a higher intake of vitamin D to counteract this effect (Vieth *et al.* 2003), and in pregnancy where vitamin D deficiency is implicated in impaired maternal and fetal outcomes (Lapillonne, 2010) – could this be a hidden interaction with CMV infection?

Inflammation

The observed cluster of inflammation-related diagnoses is an important clinical benchmark, and CMV-seropositive individuals with elevated CRP have a 30% increase in all-cause mortality (Simanek *et al.* 2011), indicating wide-reaching effects promoting disease in its widest sense. This has been termed mosaic aging, where the weakest organ/system fails first (Walker and Herndon 2010), and CMV may be the 'stress factor' in particular cases.

In elderly Latinos, functional impairment has been shown to be clearly linked to levels of C-reactive protein (CRP), which is a marker for inflammation, in which CMV was also implicated (Aiello *et al.* 2008a). However, the linkage with CMV becomes clearer when it is realized that the APOE-epsilon 4 genotype leads to alternative CRP responses (Aiello *et al.* 2008b). Those possessing this particular genotype have lower levels of CRP and exhibit higher levels of CMV antibodies. This disparity in the role of CRP explains why the role of CMV was difficult to discern in the study using just CRP levels as an inflammatory marker (Aiello *et al.* 2008a), as specific immune impairments lead to particular pathways of CMV attack. The APOE-epsilon 4 genotype response was noted to be specific to CMV, not to HSV-1 (Aiello *et al.* 2008b).

Dendritic cells (DC) are highly specialized cells that determine the quality and magnitude of immune reactions against foreign- or self-antigens, and exposure to exogenous or endogenous interleukin-10 (IL-10), an anti-inflammatory cytokine, is critical to their maturation, effectiveness and longevity (Chang *et al.* 2007). CMV contains genetic material encoding a specific IL-10 homolog (an IL-10 impostor), which is highly effective at inhibiting the maturation and functionality of DC at all stages of DC activation (Chang *et al.* 2004), and also suppresses type 1 interferon production by DC (Chang *et al.* 2009). These two factors initiate a cascade of long-term deficits in both innate and adaptive immune and inflammatory responses (Slobedman *et al.* 2009, Chang and Barry 2010), which can be used to explain why both active and apparently 'inactive' CMV infection can lead to increased sensitivity to infection and inflammation. During productive infection, CMV is also known to produce at least five other less abundant IL-10 like variants (Slobedman *et al.* 2009).

In addition to the above, CMV infection increases the expression of 5-lipoxygenase (leading to leukotriene B4 production) and COX 2 (and therefore prostaglandin release), which are crucial in inflammation (Qiu *et al.* 2008), along with other inflammatory cascades (Varani and Landini 2011). Lymphocytes in the elderly are known to be more sensitive to the inhibitory effects of prostaglandin E2 (Goodwin 1979).

Hence, it would seem that specific mechanisms do indeed exist for CMV to initiate an increased susceptibility to infection and an increase in inflammatory-related conditions, as observed in the outbreaks of acute hospital admissions.

Chronic Disease

There are several additional intriguing possibilities for the role of CMV in chronic diseases. The first comes from the observation that the expression of CMV genes in infected cells leads to mutations in the host DNA, acting to sensitize the host DNA to mutagenic agents (Albrecht *et al.* 1997). It is possible that one of the adverse roles of CMV in the developing fetus is to cause gene mutation (Cheeran *et al.* 2009). The second possibility comes from the encyclopedic study of Hanan Polanski (2003) into the role of micro-competition between foreign DNA and host DNA in the regulation of gene expression. Microcompetition in effect leads to gene expression, which acts as if the gene were mutated, and this then leads to the initiation of a variety of chronic disease processes. This mechanism is especially relevant to the range of cell types (such as microglia) where CMV enters the cell, releases its DNA, but does not progress to productive infection (Cheeran *et al.* 2009).

Lastly, poor psychological well-being and chronic heart failure have both been observed to be associated with shorter leukocyte telomere length (Huzen *et al.* 2010), and the same effect on both leukocytes (differentiated T-cells) and lymphocytes has been noted in active CMV infection (van de Berg *et al.* 2010). Shortened telomere length in circulating leukocytes has been proposed to be associated with age-related diseases such as atherosclerosis (Huzen *et al.* 2010). All of the above are plausible but largely unstudied areas for potential roles for CMV in the accelerated aging of the immune system and disruption of DNA expression, leading to chronic disease.

Under-Diagnosis in the Primary Care

In general practice, fewer than 20% of the most frequent diagnoses account for 80% of consultations, hence, just 20% of consultations relate to the 80% of less frequent diagnoses. In general, 50% of diagnoses remain a description of symptoms, 40% are named syndromes, and only 10% are confirmed diagnoses (Fink *et al.* 2009). Since CMV is only considered to be a danger to the developing fetus (Revello and Gerna 2002) and in the seriously immunocompromised (Boeckh and Geballe 2011), the majority of GPs will not even consider CMV as a possibility behind non-specific symptoms. However, although it is thought largely to lie latent, CMV can be isolated from 61% of saliva samples, 37% of urine samples and 10% of uterine secretions, suggesting that 'sub-clinical' active infection is fairly frequent (Gautheret *et al.* 1997), and one of the key observations of a recent review is that "seroconverting adults shed for many months rather than weeks" (Cannon *et al.* 2011). Of particular interest is the fact that detection in urine depends on the degree of immune deficiency; it is more common in those with HIV (Gautheret *et al.* 1997) and is specifically related to the level of CD4 cells (Clarke *et al.* 1993). In this respect, it is of interest to note that the review of Cannon *et al.* (2011) on CMV shedding appears to show that in children there is a disposition to shedding in the urine compared to saliva, and this might be linked to the observation that children appear to have a specific CD4-based immune weakness specific to CMV (Tu *et al.* 2004). The comments above regarding the range of immune impairments are apposite, and the ratio of saliva/urine positive samples may well prove to be an indicator of particular types of CMV-specific immune impairments.

Especially relevant to the primary care context is the association between active CMV infection and depression (Phillips *et al.* 2008), an effect that is also common in other immune impairing diseases such as HIV infection (Evans *et al.* 2002), Lyme disease (Rissenberg and Chambers 1998) and hepatitis C infection (Goulding *et al.* 2001). It is of interest to note that primary care costs associated with markers of depression and mental health increased by over 20% following the 2007 outbreak in England (substance misuse +31%, organic mental disorders + 24%, psychotic disorders +43%, chronic pain +20%, poisoning +39%) (Jones 2010i). The links between inflammation and depression are being increasingly recognized (Dantzer *et al.* 2008), but could these be the tip of the iceberg for primary care?

Studies investigating the prevalence of high levels of CMV antibodies are likewise needed in a primary care setting, especially for patients exhibiting unexplained physical and apparent psychological/neurological symptoms. For example, young mothers who have just become CMV seropositive via contact with their own children show prolonged CMV shedding for up to six months, but in some individuals this can last up to 15 months (Tu *et al.* 2004). Do these represent a particular risk group for secondary infections and depression? Out of interest, the author asked a GP for a list of common consultations regarding health issues in young mothers, and the following were identified: menstrual pains, headache, abdominal bloating, depression and tiredness (Dr Clare Gerada, personal communication). These are non-specific syndromes, which will require further investigation to see if they correlate with active CMV infection, especially since sleep disruption is common in young mothers and is a known cause of immune impairment (Born *et al.* 1997). Indeed, a wider study investigating levels of CMV antibodies (or CMV seropositivity plus indicators of inflammation and/or low grade infection) in patients consulting their GP regarding symptoms of tiredness and lethargy is probably needed.

Under-diagnosis in Hospital Care

In recent times, clinicians have increasingly recognized a variety of CMV-induced diseases (or disease mimicry) in 'immunocompetent' patients, which resolve with anti-viral treatment (Varani *et al.* 2000; Varani *et al.* 2009; Varani *et al.* 2010; Varani and Landini, 2011). For example, one previously healthy young patient developed life-threatening fulminant pneumonia due to co-infection with *Mycoplasma pneumoniae* (Jacobi *et al.* 2010). Given that the lung is a major organ for CMV infection, it is not surprising to note that interstitial pneumonia is a frequent manifestation of CMV re-activation or re-infection (Balthesen *et al.* 1993). Some 92% of young children with pneumonia in Papua New Guinea had CMV antibodies, although only 1% had a 4-fold rise in antibody levels (Shann *et al.* 1986). Indeed, the range of lung infections (and possible misdiagnoses) increased after the 2002 and 2007 outbreaks in England, including upper and lower respiratory tract infections, unspecified pneumonia, presumed influenza, unspecified bronchitis, bronchiectasis, unspecified COPD, and other interstitial pulmonary diseases and respiratory disorders (Jones 2010k-m). In both adults and children viral infection is one of the most common reasons for re-admission to hospital for asthma (Kuo *et al.* 2001) and, given the increased susceptibility to infection surrounding each outbreak, the possibility of CMV active infection as an underlying risk factor should be investigated.

Neuropathogenesis resulting from CMV infection of the developing fetus is well recognized (Cheeran *et al.* 2009). However, a range of neuro-inflammatory symptoms have also been observed to increase in emergency hospital admission for adults following the 2002 and 2007 outbreaks in England, including migraine and headache syndromes, post-procedural nervous system disorders, disorders of the optic and facial nerve, unspecified convulsions, abnormal involuntary movements, CNS degenerative and movement disorders. The study of neuro-inflammation is a developing area (Majde 2010). Immune function in the CNS is largely regulated by the microglia, which are responsible for phagocytosis, non-specific inflammation and adaptive immune responses, and dis-regulation of microglia is presumed to lead to the neurological disorders (Aloisi 2001). CMV is known to enter microglia, but does not progress to a productive infection (Cheeran *et al.* 2009). The gene expression implied by the multiple and adaptive roles of the microglia could render these cells open to DNA microcompetition, leading to defective gene expression (Polanski 2004). Disorders arising from direct infection of astrocytes, in which CMV establishes a productive infection, are also possible (van der Pol *et al.* 1999; Cheeran *et al.* 2009). All other CNS cells exhibit a similar range from the potential for DNA-based microcompetition through to active infection. Another route to neuroinflammation comes from the observation that neural precursor cells are produced in the hippocampus even in adults. In adult mice the induction of an adaptive immune response with T-cell activation leads to a transient increase in the proliferation and neogenesis of these neural precursor cells (Wolf *et al.* 2009). Human CMV is known to inhibit differentiation of neural precursor cells into astrocytes and to induce their apoptosis (Odeberg *et al.* 2006; Odeberg *et al.* 2007).

While it has been observed that pediatric (children up to the age of 16) admissions do not generally follow the step-changes observed in adults (Jones 2009i), the CMV hypothesis should not preclude an increase in admissions associated with the primary or secondary effects of CMV infection in very young patients. Evidence that this may be occurring is presented in Figure 4.4, where a time trend from Northern Ireland for infants under the age of one year shows a large spike in admissions for any diagnosis associated with an infection, such as tonsillitis, respiratory tract infections, and viral infections, in the year immediately following the mid-2002/03 and mid-2007/08 outbreaks seen in Northern Ireland (Jones 2010m). This observation is consistent with the observation that CMV infection in the very young remains active for around 8 to 29 months post infection, and that this is due to a selective deficiency in the $CD4^+$ T-cell response to CMV in children (Tu *et al.* 2004). It would appear that further study is warranted to determine whether these admissions are for neonates conceived during the outbreak, or are secondary infections in infants arising from primary CMV infection during the outbreak. In Northern Ireland, the outbreak was noted to occur in October of 2002 and 2007 (Jones 2010m) and hence, conceptions around that point would appear in the 2003/04 and 2008/09 financial year data.

Does the Incidence of CMV Fluctuate over Time?

If the CMV hypothesis is correct, it should be possible to detect fluctuations in the proportion of CMV seropositive individuals. Given the generally observed 10% increase in medical admissions associated with each outbreak, it is possible to estimate the degree of change in CMV-infected individuals. In England, there are around 4.2 million emergency medical admissions per annum, so a 10% step-change would involve some 420,000 extra admissions (persons). The adult population of England is in excess of 42 million so we have an implied 1% (minimum initial) increment in the level of infected adults. If the outbreak is due to the emergence of a new strain, the level of CMV seropositive individuals may not necessarily increase by 1% since infection with multiple strains is possible and the common tests for CMV seropositivity are not strain specific. A 1% seroconversion rate is at the lower end of most published studies (Hyde *et al.* 2010), although one study over an 11-year period in Germany covering healthy blood donors had an average rate of 0.46% with maximum of 1.33% in the 30-35 age group (Hecker *et al.* 2004). The proposed 1% rate is therefore feasible for the emergence of a new strain, as the known seroconversion rate is sufficient to spread a new strain to the required numbers of individuals, especially as children are known carriers of viral and other infections to their elderly relatives (Braunstein and Mandal 2008).

The first piece of evidence comes from a study conducted in Spain, which occurred around the time of the 1993 outbreak. Samples were collected between October 1993 and February 1994, immediately after the March 1993 outbreak observed in the UK, and again six years later between September 1999 and May 2000. CMV seroprevalence was lower in all age groups in 1999/00 compared to 1993/94, especially in the 6-10 and 31-40 age groups, and least in the 2-5 year age group (de Ory *et al.* 2004). This appears consistent with the hypothesis of a CMV outbreak in early 1993 and not immediately prior to or during September 1999 to May 2000. Unfortunately, we have no retrospective hospital admission data against which to test the effect on medical admissions.

Another study conducted in England concluded that, in the interval 1991 to 2002, CMV seropositivity was highest in children born between 1985 and 1989 (Vyse *et al.* 2009). This appears to link back to a suspected outbreak around 1986, observed in Scotland as a step change in the emergency admissions (Kendrick and Conway 2003a-c), in accident and emergency attendances in early 1987 in England (Jones 2010h), and in total health care costs around 1986 in the USA (Jones 2010f). The somewhat wide time bands employed in this study prevent more detailed conclusions, but expectant mothers are a known high risk group for either primary CMV infection or secondary infection with a new strain (Schoenfisch *et al.* 2011).

A further study in the USA using broad seven-year time intervals of 1988-1994 and 1999-2004 showed generally higher seroprevalence in 1988-1994 for 15 out of 25 demographic types, with age 40-49 being the only group to reach statistical significance (Bate *et al.* 2010). Since both time intervals overlap periods where a number of unexpected step-like shifts in the cost of health care occurred in the USA (Jones 2010f), it is not possible to reach any concrete conclusion; this publicly available dataset should be subject to re-analysis using single-year increments as part of the process of validating this hypothesis.

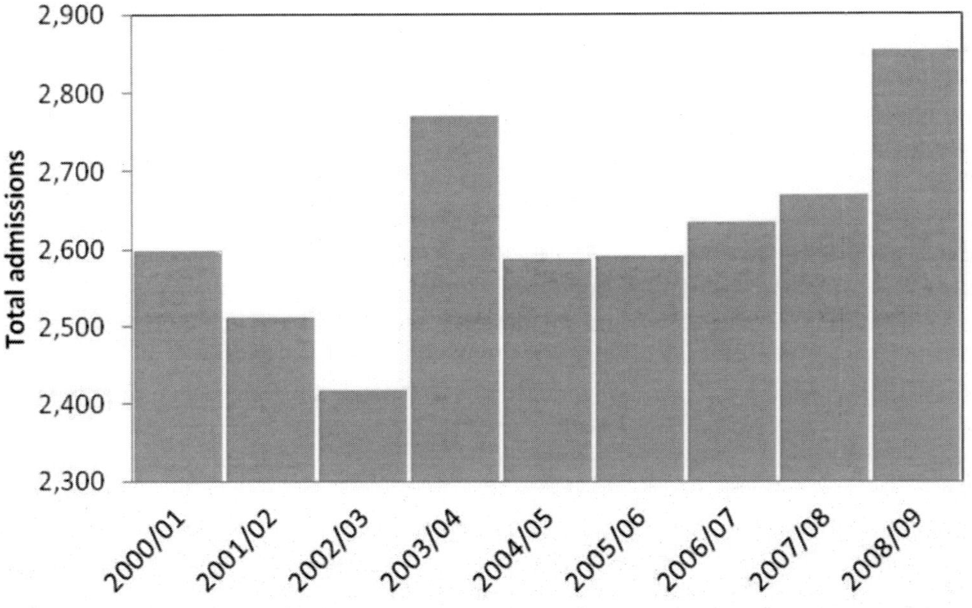

Figure 4.4. Admissions for young children aged less than 1 in Northern Ireland. Data for Northern Ireland were kindly provided by the Information and Analysis Directorate of the Department of Health, Social Services and Public Safety (DHSSPS). Admissions are for any diagnosis in which infection is implicated. Based on Poisson statistics, the 2003/04 spike represents a 5.2 standard deviation difference over the average of the previous three years, and 2008/09 represents a 4.5 standard deviation difference over the average of the previous four years. In both instances the spike represents an approximate 10% increase.

Lastly, a comprehensive review of seroconversion rates among similar risk groups by Hyde *et al.* (2010) shows sufficient variation in conversion rates, owing to the studies being conducted throughout a 40-year time period with a variety of shorter and longer sample periods, to suggest that time-based variation is a real possibility. Populations starting at a similar proportion of seropositivity showed at least a 7% range in conversion rates, which is well above the level of a 1% change needed to initiate the required increase in hospital admissions.

Establishing the validity of the hypothesis will therefore require the collection of statistically significant numbers of samples across multiple age groups at intervals of around one year, particularly in the older age groups (age > 60 years) where the bulk of the increase in emergency admissions occurs. Sampling from those with or without emergency hospital admission will also be required, and levels of CMV antibodies and/or other quantitative measures for active or low level multiplication would be useful additional information.

Synergistic Infections

While the bulk of our understanding of the immunological effects of CMV have come from *in vitro* studies (Boeckh and Geballe 2011), it is important to realize that infection with multiple persistent viruses (CMV, EBV, HSV, etc), bacteria and fungi is common among the population, where multiple and additive immune impairments from the persistent flora interact with the existing immune impairments in the host. In addition to this are the immunological challenges posed by common recurrent infections (influenza, rhinovirus, RSV, etc) and subsequent opportunistic bacterial infections (Baranek and Dalod 2008). For these reasons, it has been an enduring challenge to separate out the role of CMV as the direct agent, risk factor or opportunist. However, it is hoped that, by viewing the totality of immune impairments, the role of CMV can be seen in the wider context as a direct agent of disease (under a wider variety of circumstances than has been formerly appreciated), and as a general immune eroding force with effects that are cumulative with age.

Re-evaluation of Published Time Series

The re-evaluation of published time series for specific diseases may give further confirmation, especially where immune function is implicated in the ultimate expression of the disease. For example, admission for anaphylactic shock in England showed a distinct step change in 1993/94 (at the point surrounding the March 1993 outbreak) compared to the 1992/93 financial year (Sheikh and Alves 2000). A study on the use of ambulance services from 1988 to 1996 showed evidence for a step change around 1993, which appeared to be specific to medical conditions (Wrigley *et al.* 2002). A distinct cyclic pattern can also be observed in the trends for asthma (Anderson *et al.* 2007). Such re-evaluation is required simply because researchers were not aware of the possibility of step changes in the time series and tended to employ linear trends in the analysis of 'growth'. Indeed, ignoring this very possibility led Blunt *et al.* (2010) to reach the incorrect conclusion that the increase in emergency admissions in England between 2004/05 and 2009/10 was simply due to acute hospitals reducing their threshold to admission – which fails to explain the trends in occupied bed days shown in Table 1 and the wider international synchrony between outbreaks.

Conclusion

Advances in medicine are via observation and the formulation of a plausible clinical hypothesis. The hypothesis presented here requires further research to establish the exact role(s) for CMV, and to consider appropriate public health measures as the solution to the real root cause. This will require longitudinal studies of the levels of inflammatory cytokines in the hospitalized and non-hospitalized cohorts, and corresponding levels of CMV-specific antibodies, with a particular focus on elderly age groups and possibly different racial groups and/or groups with specific gene mutations. Measurement of antibody levels should also be associated with other tests capable of detecting low grade virus replication in different sites (quantitative detection of viral DNA in urine, saliva and other body fluids and/or quantitative detection of viral antigens/DNA/RNA in tissues when biopsies are available). The curious dichotomous immune response to CMV in the presence of particular immune impairments (MS and the APOE epsilon-4 genotype) needs to be more widely recognized as a potential confounding factor.

While many of the studies on the rise in emergency admissions have sought to implicate social trends such as the breakdown of the family unit and the elderly living alone as the primary cause, it is perhaps better to suggest that they are contributory rather than causative factors, and might have only acted to amplify the effect on the medical emergency admissions. This amplification, along with the low levels of influenza over the nine years from 2000 onward, has probably helped to bring the basic root cause to light.

The possibility that age at previous exposure(s) may be important implies that the traditional use of age standardization (usually with five-year age bands) may be acting to obscure what are effectively cohorts of patients moving forward in time, and researchers need to be alert to this possibility.

The possibility of new strains emerging is very real. For example, the emergence of a new strain of the West Nile Virus (WNV) in the USA in 1992 has been implicated in the rapid spread of WNV throughout the North American continent subsequent to that date (Lindsey *et al.* 2010: McMullen *et al.* 2011). If at all possible, the proposed emergence of a significant new strain of CMV in the early 1960s needs to be confirmed (Jones 2010f).

Whatever the cause, the agent is 'highly infectious' in the sense that the local medical admission rate moves rapidly from a lower to a permanently higher rate in a matter of weeks, and has enormous implications on the financial pressures faced by health services around the world. If the above association with CMV is correct, then the search for an effective vaccine against CMV needs to be accelerated, as this virus may be responsible for billions of dollars of international healthcare expenditure. The trends in healthcare costs, bed demand and admissions are certainly not acting in the way they are 'supposed' to behave and, at the present, the CMV hypothesis is the best starting point for further investigation. In order to have the necessary research programmes in place to track the outbreak and its causes, all concerned need to be alert to the fact that the next outbreak is likely to occur in the interval 2012 to 2016.

Acknowledgments

The valuable comments of Dr Stefania Varani are acknowledged.

References

Adams, J. and Hewison, M. (2008) Unexpected actions of vitamin D: new perspectives on the regulation of innate and adaptive immunity. *Nature Clinical Practice: Endocrinology and Metabolism*, 42 pp. 80-90.

Aiello, A. (2008a) Persistent infection, inflammation, and functional impairment in older Latinos. *Journal of Gerontology A: Biological Science and Medical Science*, 63, pp. 610-618.

Aiello, A. *et al* (2008b) C-reactive protein mediates the effect of apolipoprotein E on cytomegalovirus infection. *Journal of Infectious Diseases*, 197, pp. 34-41.

Albrecht, T. *et al* (1997) Increased frequency of specific locus mutation following human cytomegalovirus infection. *Virology*, 230, pp. 48-61.

Aloisi, F. (2001) Immune function of microglia. *Glia*, 36, pp. 165-179.

Altizer, S. *et al.* (2006) Seasonality and the dynamics of infectious diseases. *Ecology Letters*, 9, pp. 467-484.

Anderson, H. *et al* (2007) 50 years of asthma: UK trends from 1955 to 2004. *Thorax*, 62, pp. 85-90.

Anderson, R. *et al* (1984) Oscillatory fluctuations in the incidence of infectious disease and the impact of vaccination: time series analysis. *Journal of Hygiene*, 93, pp. 587-608.

Andre, K. and Florescu, D. (2009) Prevalence and mortality associated with cytomegalovirus infection in nonimmunosuppressed patients in the intensive care unit. *Critical Care Medicine*, 37, pp. 2350-2358.

Azad, N. *et al* (1999) Nutrition survey in an elderly population following admissions to a tertiary hospital. *Canadian Medical Association Journal*, 161, pp. 511-515.

Baldwin, T. *et al* (2004) The Fourth Way? Harnessing aggressive tendencies in the thymus. *The Journal of Immunology*, 173, pp. 6515-6520.

Bale, J. *et al.* (1999) Circulation of cytomegalovirus strains among child care centers. Paediatric Research, 45, p. 100A

Balthesen, M. *et al.* (1993) Lungs are a major organ site of cytomegalovirus latency and recurrence. *Journal of Virology*, 67, pp. 5360-5369.

Baranek, T. and Dalod, M. (2008) How opportunistic agents benefit from viral infections: the plasmactoid dendritic cell connection. *Cell Host and Microbe*, 4, pp. 305-307.

Bate, S. *et al.* (2010) Cytomegalovirus seroprevalence in the United States: The national health and nutrition examination surveys. 1988-2004. *Clinical Infectious Diseases*, 50, pp. 1439-1447.

Blunt, I. *et al.* (2010) *Trends in Emergency admissions in England 2004-2009.* [www] London, The Nuffield Trust. Available from: .http://www.nuffieldtrust.org.uk/sites/files /nuffield/Trends_in_emergency_admissions_report.pdf.

Boeckh, M. and Geballe, A. (2011) Cytomegalovirus: pathogen, paradigm, and puzzle. *The Journal of Clinical Investigation*, 121, pp. 1673-1680.

Bolovan-Fritts, C. and Spector, S. (2011) Endothelial damage from cytomegalovirus-specific host immune response can be prevented by targeted disruption of fractalkine-CX3 CR1 interaction. *Blood*, 111, pp.175-182.

Bonhoeffer, S. and Nowark, M. (1994) Intra-host versus inter-host selection: Viral strategies of immune function impairment. *Proceedings of the National Academy of Science USA*, 91, pp. 8062-8066.

Born, J. *et al.* (1997) Effects of sleep and circadian rhythm on human circulating immune cells. *Journal of Immunology*, 158, pp. 4454-4464.

Born, P. and Santerre, R. (2008) Unravelling the health insurance underwriting cycle. *Journal of Insurance Regulation*, 26, pp. 65-84.

Bousfiha, A. *et al.* (2010) Primary immunodeficiencies of protective immunity to primary infections. *Clinical Immunology*, 135, pp. 204-209.

Boutsioli, Z. (2009) Measuring unexpected hospital demand: The application of a univariate model to public hospitals in Greece. *Hospital Topics*, 87, pp. 14-21.

Boyd, R. *et al.* (2008) Disease prevention and vaccination prior to thymic reactivation. [www] Patent Application IPC8 Class:AA61K 3820FI, Northwood Immunology, Ltd. Available from: ttp://www.faqs.org/patents /app/20080279812 [Accessed 28/8/11].

Braun, J. *et al.* (2010) Clearance of CMV Viremia and survival after double umbilical cord blood transplantation in adults, depends on reconstitution of thymopoiesis. *Blood*, 115, pp. 4111-4119.

Braunstein, J. and Mandal, K. (2008) Pediatric population size is associated with geographic patterns of acute respiratory infections among adults. *Annals of Emergency Medicine*, 52, pp. 63-68.

Brilot, F. *et al.* (2004) Coxsackievirus B4 infection of human fetal thymus cells. *Journal of Virology*, 78, pp. 9854-9861.

Broome, C. *et al.* (2004) An increase in selenium intake improves immune function and poliovirus handling in adults with marginal selenium status. *American Journal Clinical Nutrition*, 80, pp. 154-162.

Cannon, M. (2010) Review of cytomegalovirus seroprevalence and demographic characteristics associated with infection. *Reviews in Medical Virology*, 20, pp. 202-213.

Cannon, M. *et al.* (2011) Review of cytomegalovirus shedding in body fluids. and relevance to congenital cytomegalovirus infection. *Reviews in Medical Virology*, 21, pp. 240-255.

Capewelll, S. (1996) The continuing rise in emergency admissions. *British Medical Journal*, 312, pp. 991-992.

Casanova, J. *et al.* (2008) Revisiting human primary immunodeficiencies. *Journal of Internal Medicine*, 264, pp. 115-127.

Chang, W. and Barry, P. (2010) Attenuation of innate immunity by cytomegalovirus IL-10 establishes a long-term deficit of adaptive antiviral immunity. *Proceedings of the National Academy of Science USA*, 107, pp. 22647-22652.

Chang, W. *et al.* (2009) Human cytomegalovirus suppresses type 1 interferon secretion by plasmacytoid dendritic cells through its interleukin 10 homolog. *Virology*, 390, pp. 330-337.

Chang, W. *et al.* (2007) Exposure of myeloid dendritic cells to exogenous or endogenous IL-10 during their maturation determines their longevity. *Journal of Immunology*, 178, pp. 7794-7804.

Chang, W. *et al.* (2004) Human cytomegalovirus-encoded interleukin-10 homolog inhibits maturation of dendritic cells and alters their functionality. *Journal of Virology*, 78, pp. 8720-8731.

Cheeran, M. *et al.* (2009) Neuropathogenesis of congenital cytomegalovirus infection: Disease mechanisms and prospects for intervention. *Clinical Microbiology Reviews*, 22, pp. 99-126.

Clarke, L. *et al.* (1993) Epidemiology and natural history of cytomegalovirus (CMV) infection on HIV-1 seropositive women. *Abstracts of the 93rd General Meeting of the American Society for Microbiology*, 93, p. 494.

Cox, B. *et al.* (2010) Breast cancer. cytomegalovirus and Epstein Barr virus: a nested case-control study. *British Journal of Cancer*, 102, pp. 1665-1669.

Dananquah, L. *et al.* (2010) Type 2 diabetes mellitus and increased risk of malaria infection. *Emerging Infectious Diseases*, 16, pp. 1601-1604.

Dantzer, R. *et al.* (2008) From inflammation to sickness and depression: when the immune system subjugates the brain. *Nature Reviews in Neuroscience*, 9, 46-57.

Davidson, R. *et al.* (2003) Alterations in brain and immune function produced by mindfulness meditation. *Psychosomatic Medicine*, 65, pp. 564-570.

Deeks, S. and Phillips, N. (2010) HIV infection. antiretroviral treatment. ageing. and non-AIDS related morbidity. *British Medical Journal*, 338, pp. 288-292.

De Lappe, E. *et al.* (2006) Vitamin D insuffiency in older female community-dwelling acute hospital admissions and the response to supplementation. *European Journal of Clinical Nutrition*, 60, pp. 1009-1015.

De La Rosa, R. and Leal, M. (2003) Thymic involvement in recovery of immunity among HIV-infected adults on highly active anti retroviral therapy. *Journal of Antimicrobiol Chemotherapy*, 52, pp. 155-158.

Deluca, H. and Cantorna, M. (2001) Vitamin D: its role and uses in immunology. *The FASEB Journal*, 15, pp. 2579-2585.

Derhovanessian, E. *et al.* (2009) Biomarkers of human immunoscenescence: impact of cytomegalovirus infection. *Current Opinion in Immunology*, 21, pp. 1-6.

Derhovanessian, E. *et al.* (2010) Hallmark features of immunosenescence are absent in familial longevity. *Journal of Immunology*, 185, pp. 4618-4624.

De Martel, and C. Franceschi, S. (2008) Infections and cancer: established associations and new hypotheses. *Critical Reviews in Oncology and Haematology*, 70, pp. 183-194.

Deory, F. *et al.* (2004) Is there a change in cytomegalovirus seroepidemiology in Spain? *European Journal of Epidemiology*, 19, pp. 85-89.

Dowell, S. (2001) Seasonal variation in host susceptibility and cycles of certain infectious diseases. *Emerging Infectious Diseases*, 7, pp. 369-374.

Dushoff, J. (1996) Incorporating immunological ideas in epidemiological models. *Journal of Theoretical Biology*, 180, pp. 181-187.

Evans, C. (2005) Malnutrition in the elderly. A multifactorial failure to thrive. *The Permanente Journal*, 9, pp. 38-41.

Evans, D. *et al.* (2002) Association of depression with viral load. CD8 T lymphocytes. and natural killer cells in women with HIV infection. *American Journal of Psychiatry*, 159, pp. 1752-1759.

Fairweather, D. and Rose, N. (2004) Women and autoimmune diseases. *Emerging Infectious Diseases*, 10, pp. 2005-2011.

Fink, W. *et al.* (2009) Diagnoses by General Practitioners: accuracy and reliability. *International Journal of Forecasting*. 25, pp. 784-793.

Fleming, D. *et al.* (1991) *Annual and Seasonal Variation in the Incidence of Common Diseases*. London: The Royal College of General Practitioners.

Freeman, E. *et al.* (2006) Herpes simplex virus 2 infection increases HIV acquisition in men and women: systematic review and meta-analysis of longitudinal studies. *AIDS*, 20, pp. 73-83.

Gabel, J. *et al.* (1991) Tracing the cycle of health insurance. *Health Affairs*, 10, pp. 48-61.

Ganji, V. *et al.* (2010) Serum vitamin D concentrations are related to depression in young adult US population: the third National health and Nutrition Examination Survey. *International Archives of Medicine*, 3, 29, doi: 10.1186/1755-7682-3-29.

Garcia-Pineres, A. *et al.* (2006) Persistent human human papillomavirus infection is associated with generalised decrease in immune responsiveness in older women. *Cancer Research*, 66, pp. 11070-11076.

Gautheret, A. *et al.* (1997) Retention of human beta herpes virinae in saliva and urine form immunocompromised and immunocompetent subjects. *Journal of Clinical Microbiology*, 35, pp. 1600-1603.

Gillam, S. (2010) Rising hospital admissions. *British Medical Journal*, 340 (7741), pp. 275-276.

Gleeson, M. *et al.* (2004) Exercise, nutrition and immune function. *Journal of Sports Sciences*, 22, pp. 115-125.

Glezen, W. (1982) Serious morbidity and mortality associated with influenza epidemics. *Epidemiologic Reviews*, 4, pp. 26-44.

Gonzalez, E. *et al.* (2009) Trends in the prevalence and incidence of diabetes in the UK:1996-2005. *Journal of Epidemiology and Community Health*, 63, pp. 332-336.

Goodwin, J. (1979) Increased sensitivity of prostaglandin E2 in old people. *Prostaglandins in Medicine*, 3, pp. 395-340.

Gorzer, I. *et al.* (2010). Deep sequencing reveals highly complex dynamics of human cytomegalovirus genotypes in transplant patients over time. *Journal of Virology*, 84, pp. 7195-203.

Gottlieb A. *et al.* (1979) Immune function in systemic lupus erythematosus. Impairment of *in vitro* T-cell proliferation and *in vivo* antibody response to exogenous antigen. *Journal of Clinical Investigation*, 63, pp. 885-892.

Goulding, C. *et al.* (2001) Prevalence of fibromyalgia. anxiety and depression in chronic hepatitis C virus infection: relationship to RT-PCR status and mode of acquisition. European *Journal of Gastroenterology and Hepatology*, 13, pp. 507-511.

Grassly, N. and Fraser, C. (2006) Seasonal infectious disease epidemiology. *Proceedings of the Royal Society: Biological Sciences*, 273, pp. 2541-2550.

Grassly, N. *et al.* (2005) Host immunity and synchronised epidemics of syphilis across the United States. *Nature*, 433, pp. 417-421.

Gruber, J. (2010) *Lyme disease: stastical evaluation of a symptom log and an empirical theory of flare cycles*. [www] Lymenet.de Available from: www.lymenet.de/symptoms/cycles/statistics.htm [Accessed 19/08/11].

Garcia-Pineres, A. *et al.* (2006) Persistant human papillomavirus infection is associated with generalised disease and immune resposiveness in older women. *Cancer Research*, 66, pp.11010-11076.

Gress, R. and Deeks, S. (2009) Reduced thymus activity and infection prematurely age the immune system. *Journal of Clinical Investigation*, 119, pp. 2884-2887.

Griffith, B. *et al.* (1981) Cytomegalovirus and induced mononucleosis in guinea pigs. *Infection and Immunity*, 32, pp. 857-863.

Haase, H. and Rink, L. (2009) The immune system and the impact of zinc during aging. *Immunity and Aging*, 6, doi 10.1186/1742-4933-6-9.

Hamza, T. *et al.* (2010).Common genetic variation in the HLA region is associated with late onset Parkinsons disease. *Nature Genetics*, 42, pp. 781-785.

Harkins, L. *et al.* (2010) Detection of human cytomegalovirus in normal and neoplastic breast epithelium. *Herpesviridae*, 1, doi: 10.1186/2042-4280-1-8.

Hayes, D. (2010) Cancer protection related to solar ultraviolet radiation. altitude and Vitamin D. *Medical Hypotheses*, 75, pp. 378-382.

Hecker, M. *et al.* (2004) Continuous cytomegalovirus seroconversion in a large group of healthy blood donors. *Vox Sanguinis*, 86, pp. 41-44.

Henry, K. (1968) The thymus in rheumatic heart disease. *Clinical and Experimental Immunology*, 3, pp. 509-523.

High, K. *et al.* (2005) A New Paradigm for clinical investigation of infectious syndromes in older adults: Assessing functional status as a risk factor. *Journal of the American Geriatric Society*, 53, pp. 528-535.

Hilder, P. *et al.* (1998) *Acute medical admissions: A critical appraisal of the literature.* NZHTA Report 6. Available from www.nzhta.chmeds.ac. nz/publications/nzhta6.pdf [Accessed 28/8/11].

Hilder, P. *et al.* (2000) The rise in medical admissions. *Australian and New Zealand Journal of Medicine*, 30, pp. 252-260.

Hobbs, R. (1995) Rising emergency admissions. *British Medical Journal*, 310, pp. 207-208.

Hollingsworth, T. *et al.* (2007) Frequent travellers and rate of spread of epidemics. *Emerging Infectious Diseases*, 13, pp. 1288-1294.

Huang, E-S. and Johnson, R. (2000) Human cytomegalovirus - no longer just a DNA virus. *Nature Medicine*, 6, pp. 863-864.

Hurwitz, B. *et al.* (2007) Suppression of human immunodeficiency virus type 1 viral load with selenium supplementation. *Archives of Internal Medicine*, 167, pp. 148-154.

Huzen, J. *et al.* (2010) Telomere length and psychological well-being in patients with chronic heart failure. *Age and Aging*, 39, pp. 223-227.

Hyams, K. (1998) Developing case definitions for symptom-based conditions: the problem of specificity. *Epidemiologic Reviews*, 20, pp. 148-156.

Hyams, K. *et al.* (1996) War syndromes and their evaluation: from the US Civil War to the Persian Gulf War. *Annals of Internal Medicine*. 125, pp. 398-405.

Hyde, T. *et al.* (2010) Cytomegalovirus seroconversion rates and risk factors: implications for congenital CMV. *Reviews in Medical Virology*, 20, pp. 311-326.

Ironson, G. *et al.* (1997) Posttraumatic stress symptoms, intrusive thoughts, loss and immune function after Hurricane Andrew. *Psychosomatic Medicine*, 59, pp. 128-141.

Jacobi, C. *et al.* (2010) Life threatening pneumonia caused by human cytomegalovirus and mycoplasma pneumonia coinfection in a young immunocompetent patient. *Journal of Medical Microbiology*, 59, pp. 980-983.

Jamieson, D. *et al.* (2006) *Emerging infections and pregnancy.* Emerging Infectious Diseases 12 (11) www.cdc.gov/ncidod/eid/vol12no11/06-0152.htm

Jaspan, H. *et al.* (2006) *The maturing immune system: Adolescent immunity.* [www] Medscape Today. Available from: www.medscape.com/ viewarticle/524225_4 [Accessed 28/8/11].

Jones, R. (1996a) *Emergency admissions in the United Kingdom: Trend upward or fundamental shift?.*[www] Healthcare Analysis and Forecasting, Camberley, UK. Available from: http://www.docstoc.com/ docs/9258083/Increase-in-emergency-admissions---trend-or-step-change [Accessed 28/8/11].

Jones, R. (1996b) *Getting the best from hospital patient information.* [www] Healthcare Analysis and Forecasting. Available from: http://www.hcaf. biz/Recent/Handbook.pdf [Accessed 28/8/11].

Jones, R. (1997) Admissions of difficulty. *Health Service Journal*, 107, pp. 28-31.

Jones, R. (2008) Limitations of the HRG tariff excess bed days. Br*itish Journal of Healthcare Management*, 14, pp. 354-355.

Jones, R. (2009a) Trends in emergency admissions. *British Journal of Healthcare Management*, 15, pp. 188-196.

Jones, R. (2009b) Cycles in emergency admissions. *British Journal of Healthcare Management*, 15, pp. 239-246.

Jones, R. (2009c) *Cycles in emergency admissions* - supplement. [www] Healthcare Analysis and Forecasting. Available from: http://www.hcaf.biz/Emergency%20Admissions /Cycles_in_emergency_admissions_Supplement.pdf [Accessed 26/10/11].

Jones, R. (2009d) Emergency admissions and hospital beds. *British Journal of Healthcare Management*, 15, pp. 289-296.

Jones, R. (2009e) Emergency admissions and financial risk. *British Journal of Healthcare Management*, 15, pp. 344-350.

Jones, R. (2009f) Building smaller hospitals. *British Journal of Healthcare Management*, 15, pp. 511-512.

Jones, R. (2009g) Length of stay efficiency. *British Journal of Healthcare Management*, 15, pp. 563-564.

Jones, R. (2009h) Crafting efficient bed pools. *British Journal of Healthcare Management*, 15, pp. 614-616.

Jones, R. (2009i) *Additional studies on the three to six year pattern in medical emergency admissions.* [www] Healthcare Analysis and Forecasting. Available from: http : //www.hcaf.biz/Recent/Additional_Studies.pdf [Accessed 28/8/11].

Jones, R. (2010a) Cyclic factors behind NHS deficits and surpluses. *British Journal of Healthcare Management*, 16, pp. 48-49.

Jones, R. (2010b) Emergency preparedness. *British Journal of Healthcare Management*, 16, pp. 94-95.

Jones, R. (2010c) Do NHS cost pressures follow long-term patterns? *British Journal of Healthcare Management*, 16, pp. 192-194.

Jones, R. (2010d) Benchmarking length of stay. *British Journal of Healthcare Management*, 16, pp. 248-250.

Jones, R. (2010e) Forecasting demand. *British Journal of Healthcare Management*, 16, pp. 392-393.

Jones, R. (2010f) Nature of health care costs and financial risk in commissioning. *British Journal of Healthcare Management*, 16, pp. 424-430.

Jones, R. (2010g) Nature of health care costs and the HRG tariff. *British Journal of Healthcare Management*, 16, pp. 451-452.

Jones, R. (2010h) Forecasting emergency department attendances. *British Journal of Healthcare Management*, 16, pp. 495-496.

Jones, R. (2010i) Trends in programme budget expenditure. *British Journal of Healthcare Management*, 16, pp. 518-526.

Jones, R. (2010j) Gender ratio and hospital admissions. *British Journal of Healthcare Management*, 16, p. 541.

Jones, R. (2010k) Unexpected, periodic and permanent increase in medical inpatient care: man-made or new disease. *Medical Hypotheses*, 74, pp. 978-983.

Jones, R. (2010l) Can time-related patterns in diagnosis for hospital admission help identify common root causes for disease expression. *Medical Hypotheses* 75, pp. 148-154.

Jones, R. (2010m) The case for recurring outbreaks of a new type of infectious disease across all parts of the United Kingdom. *Medical Hypotheses*, 75, pp. 452-457.

Jones, R. (2010n) Myths of ideal hospital size. *Medical Journal of Australia*, 193, pp. 298-300.

Jones, R. (2011a) Infectious outbreaks and the capitation formula. *British Journal of Healthcare Management*, 17, pp. 36-38.

Jones, R. (2011b) Cycles in inpatient waiting time. *British Journal of Healthcare Management*, 17, pp. 80-81.

Jones, R. (2011c) Cycles in gender-related costs for long-term conditions. *British Journal of Healthcare Management*, 17, pp. 124-125.

Jones, R. (2011d) CMV and health care costs. *British Journal of Healthcare Management*, 17, pp. 168-169.

Jones, R. (2011e) Is demand for beds about death or demography. *British Journal of Healthcare Management*, 17, pp190-197.

Jones, R. (2011f). Hospital bed occupancy demystified. *British Journal of Healthcare Management*, 17, pp. 242-248.

Jones, R. (2011g). A&E performance and inpatient bed occupancy. *British Journal of Healthcare Management*, 17, pp. 256-257.

Jones, R. (2011h) Bed occupancy: the impact on hospital planning. *British Journal of Healthcare Management.* 17, pp. 307-313.

Jones, R. (2011i) The need for single room hospital accommodation. *British Journal of Healthcare Management*, 17, pp. 316-317.

Jones, R. (2011i) Demand for hospital beds in primary care organisations. *British Journal of Healthcare Management*, 17, pp. 360-367.

Jones, R. (2011k) *A Review of Bed Requirements at the Royal North Shore Hospital*. [www] Healthcare Analysis and Forecasting, Camberley, UK. Available from: http://www.hcaf.biz [Accessed 28/8/11].

Jones, R. (2011l) A paradigm shift for bed occupancy. *British Journal of Healthcare Management*, 17, pp. 376-377.

Jones, R. (2011m) Volatility in bed occupancy for emergency admissions. *British Journal of Healthcare Management*, 17, pp. 424-430.

Just, H. (2006) *Thymus function in inflammatory skin diseases*. PhD thesis, Faculty of Health Sciences, University of Aarhus, Sweden.

Kasastelan, S. *et al.* (2010) Maternal immune system adaption to pregnancy - a potential influence on the course of diabetic retinopathy. *Reproductive Biology and Endocrinology*, 8, doi: 10.1186/1477-7827-8-124.

Kawanishi, S. *et al.* (2006) Oxidative and nitrative DNA damage in animals and patients with inflammatory diseases in relation to inflammation-related carcinogenesis. *Biological Chemistry*, 387, pp. 365-372.

Kayser, C. *et al.* (2004) Decreased number of T cells bearing TCR rearrangement excision circles (TREC) in active recent onset systematic lupus erythematosus. *Lupus*, 13, pp. 906-911.

Keil, T. *et al.* (2006) European cohort studies on asthma and atopic diseases: 1. Comparison of study designs - a GA2LEN initiative. *Allergy*, 61, pp. 221-228.

Kendrick, S (1995) Emergency admissions: what is driving the increase? *Health Service Journal*, 105, pp. 26-28.

Kendrick, S. and Conway, M. (2003a) *Increasing emergency admissions among older people in Scotland: a whole system audit.* [www] Information and Statistics Division, Common Services Agency, NHS Scotland. Available from: http://www. isdscotland.org/isd/files/ Whole_ System%20_WP1_text.pdf [Accessed 28/8/11].

Kendrick, S. and Conway, M. (2003b) *Increasing emergency admissions among older people in Scotland: a whole system account – Trends 1981-2001.* Whole System Project Working Paper 1. [www] Information and Statistics Division, Common Services Agency, NHS Scotland. Available from: www.isdscotland.org/isd/files/Whole _System_WP1_figures.pdf [Accessed 28/8/11].

Kendrick, S. and Conway, M. (2003c) *Increasing emergency admissions among older people in Scotland: A whole system account.* [www] Information and Statistics Division NHS Scotland. Available from: http://www.isdscotland. org/isd/servlet/FileBuffer ? namedFile =Whole_System+_WP1_text.pdfandpContentDispositionType=inline [Accessed 28/8/ 11].

Khot, A. *et al* (1984) Seasonal variation and time trends in childhood asthma in England and Wales 1975-81. *British Medical Journal*, 289, pp. 235-237.

Kiecott-Glaser, J. and Glaser, R. (2002) Depression and immune function - central pathways to morbidity and mortality. *Journal of Psychosomatic Research*, 53, pp. 873-876.

Kiecott-Glaser, J. *et al.* (1987) Chronic stress and immunity in family caregivers of Alzeimer's disease victims. *Psychosomatic Medicine*, 49, pp. 523-535.

King, C. *et al.* (1992) Viral infection of the thymus. *Journal of Virology*, 66, pp. 3155-3160.

Kipp, R. *et al.* (2003) *Health insurance underwriting cycle: Effect on health plan premiums and profitability*. [www] Milliman, USA. Available from: ttp://www.aha.org/aha/content /2003/pdf/MillimanReport030410.pdf [Accessed 18/08/11].

Koelle, K. and Pascual, M. (2004) Disentangling extrinsic from intrinsic factors in disease dynamics: A nonlinear time series approach with an application for cholera. *American Naturalist*, 163, pp. 901-913.

Koga, Y. *et al.* (1994) Priming of immature thymocytes to CD3-mediated apoptosis by infection with murine cytomegalovirus. *Journal of Virology*, 68, pp. 4322-4328.

Kuo, A, and Craig, T. (2001) A retrospective study of risk factors for repeat admissions for asthma in a rural/surburban university hospital. *JAOA*, 101, pp. S14-S17.

Lamason, R. *et al.* (2006) Sexual diamorphism in immune response genes as a function of puberty. *BMC Immunology*, 7, doi: 10.1186/1471-2172-7-2.

Lapillonne, A. (2010) Vitamin D deficiency during pregnancy may impair maternal and fetal outcomes. *Medical Hypotheses*, 74, pp. 71-75.

Lardner, A. (2001) The effect of extracellular pH on immune function. *Journal of Leukocyte Biology*, 69, pp. 522-530.

Libert, C. *et al.* (2010) The X chromasome in immune function: when a chromosome makes a difference. *Nature Reviews Immunology*, 10, pp. 594-604.

Linder, J. (1987) The thymus gland in secondary immunodeficiency. *Archives of Pathology and Laboratory Medicine*, 111, pp. 1118-1122.

Lindsey, N. *et al.* (2010) Surveilance for Human West Nile Virus Disease – United States, 1999-2008. *MMWR*, 59, pp. 1-17.

Ling, P. *et al.* (2003) The dynamics of herpesvirus and polyomavirus reactivation and shedding in health adults: a 14-month longitudinal study. *Journal of Infectious Diseases*, 187, pp. 1571-1580.

Lorenzi, A. *et al.* (2009) Thymic function in juvenile idiopathic arthritis. *Annals of the Rheumatic Diseases*, 68, pp. 983-990.

Lorenzi, A. *et al.* (2008) Determination of thymic function directly from peripheral blood:A validated modification of an established method. *Journal of Immunologic Methods*, 339, pp. 185-194.

Lung and Asthma Information Agency. (2001) *Trends in emergency hospital admissions for lung disease*. [www] LAIA Factsheet, 2001/4. Available from: http://www.laia.ac.uk/factsheets/20014.pdf [Accessed 18/08/11].

Lustgarten, J. (2009) Cancer, aging and immunotherapy: lessons learned from animal models. *Cancer, Immunology and Immunotherapy*, 58, pp. 1979-1989.

Majde, J. (2010) Neuroinflammation resulting from covert brain invasion by common viruses – A potential role in local and global neurodegeneration. *Medical Hypotheses*, 75, pp. 204-213.

Mathers, J. *et al.* (2010) Induction of epigenetic alterations by dietary and other environmental factors. *Advances in Genetics*, 71, pp. 3-39.

Matos, S. *et al.* (2010) Seroprevalence of cytomegalovirus infection among healthy blood donors in Bahia state, Brazil. *Revista Brasileria de Hematologia e Hemoterapia*, 32, doi: 10.1590/S1516-84842010005000009.

Mayor, S. (2009) Unravelling the secrets of ageing. *British Medical Journal*, 338, pp. 136-138.

Mcdonald, A. *et al.* (2008) Increasing US emergency department visit rates and subsequent hospital admission for atrial fibrillation from 1993 to 2004. *Annals of Emergency Medicine*, 51, pp. 58-65.

Mcfarland, R. *et al.* (2000) Identification of a human recent thymic emigrant phenotype. *Proceedings of the National Academy of Science USA*, 97, pp. 4215-4220.

Mcmullen, A. *et al.* (2011) Evolution of new genotype of West Nile Virus in North America. *Emerging Infectious Diseases*, 17, pp. 785-793.

Miller-Kittrell, M. and Sparer, T. (2009) Feeling manipulated: cytomegalovirus immune manipulation. *Virology Journal*, 6, doi: 10.1186/ 1743-422X-6-4.

Miossec, P. *et al.* (2009) Mechanisms of disease: Interleukin-17 and Type 17 helper T cells. *The New England Journal of Medicine*, 361, pp. 888-898.

Mocarski, E. *et al.* (1993) Human cytomelalovirus in a SCID-hu mouse:thymic epithelial cells are prominent targets of viral replication. *Proceedings of the National Academy of Science USA*, 90, pp. 104-108.

Mocchegiani, E. *et al.* (2009) Zinc and metallothioneins and longevity: Interrelationships with niacin and selenium. *Current Pharmaceutical Design*, 14, pp. 2719-2732.

Molony, E. *et al.* (2005) Impact of an acute medical admission unit on length of hospital stay, and emergency department 'wait times'. *QJM*, 98, pp. 283-289.

Moorman, J. *et al.* (2007) National surveillance for asthma – United States, 1980-2004. *MMWR*, 56, pp. 1-14; 18-54.

Morens, D. *et al.* (2010) The wages of original antigenic sin. *Emerging Infectious Diseases*, 16, pp. 1023-1024.

Morgan, K. *et al.* (1993) The rise in emergency admissions – crisis or artifact? Temporal analysis of health services data. *British Medical Journal*, 319, pp. 158-159.

Mowry, E. *et al.* (2011) Vitamin D status and antibody levels to common viruses in pediatric-onset multiple sclerosis. *Multiple Sclerosis*, 17, pp. 666-671.

Muller, L. *et al.* (2005) Increased risk of common infections in patients with type 1 and type 2 diabetes mellitus. *Clinical Infectious Diseases*, 41, pp. 281-288.

Murthy, S. *et al.* (2011) Detection of a single identical cytomegalovirus (CMV) strain in recently seroconverted young women. *PLoS ONE*, 6, doi: 10.1371/journal.pone.0015949.

Naeger, D. *et al.* (2010) Cytomegalovirus-specific T cells persist at very high levels during long-term antiretroviral treatment of HIV disease. *PLoS ONE*, 5, doi: 10. 1371/journal. pone.0008886.

Nhs Scotland. (2005). *Building a health service fit for the future. Vol 2: A guide for the NHS.* [www] Available from: http://www.Scotland.gov. uk/Publications/2005/05/23141500/ 15035 [Accessed 19/08/11].

Novak, Z. *et al.* (2009) Enzyme linked immunosorbent assay method for detection of cytomegalovirus strain-specific antibody responses. *Clinical and Vaccine Immunology*, 16, pp. 288-90.

Nsw Health. (2007) *Key drivers of demand in the emergency department. A hypothesis driven approach to analyse demand and supply.* [www] nsw Department of Health, Australia. Available from: www.health.nsw. gov.au/pubs/2007/pdf/booze_allen_report_1-10.pdf [Accessed 28/8/11].

Numazaki, K. *et al.* (1989) Effects of infection by HIV-1, cytomegalovirus and human measles virus on cultured human thymic epithelial cells. *Microbiology and Immunology*, 33, pp. 733-745.

Odeberg, J. *et al.* (2006) Human cytomegalovirus inhibits neuronal differentiation and induces apoptosis in human neural precursor cells. *Journal of Virology*, 80, pp. 8929-8939.

Odeberg, J. *et al.* (2007) Late human cytomegalovirus (HCMV) proteins inhibit differentiation of human neural precursor cells into astrocytes. J*ournal of Neurological Research*, 85, pp. 583-593.

Ohshima, H. and Bartsch, H. (1994) Chronic infections and inflammatory process as cancer risk factors. Possible role of nitric ozide in carcinogenesis. *Mutation Research*, 305, pp. 253-264.

Pallin, D. *et al.* (2008) Increased US emergency department visits for skin and soft tissue infections, and changes in antibiotic choices, during the emergence of community-associated methicillin-resistant Staphylococcus aureus. *Annals of Emergency Medicine*, 51, pp. 291-298.

Papp, L. *et al.* (2010) Selenium and selenoproteins in health and disease. *Antioxidation Redox Signal*, 12, pp. 793-795.

Parker, G. *et al.* (1997) *Emergency referral of elderly people to acute hospital care: a pilot study to examine the roles of clinical and non-clinical factors*. [www] University of Leicester, Nuffield Community Care Studies Unit. Available from: www2.le.ac.uk/ departments/health-sciences/extranet/research-groups/Nuffield/pdf/ TRHA57. pdf [Accessed28/8/11].

Pawelec, G. *et al.* (2005) Human immunoscenescence: is it infectious? *Immunological Reviews*, 205, pp. 257-268.

Pawelec, G. *et al.* (2009) Cytomegalovirus and human immunoscenescence. *Reviews in Medical Virology*, 19, pp. 47-56.

Phillips, A. *et al.* (2008) Cytomegalovirus is associated with depression and anxiety in older adults. *Brain, Behaviour, and Immunity*, 22, pp. 52-55.

Polanski, H. (2003) *Micro competition with foreign DNA and the origin of chronic disease.* [www] Center for the biology of Chronic Disease, Rochester NY. Available from: http://www.cbcd.net/Book%20by %20Hanan%20Polansky%20(Purple%20Book).pdf [Accessed 28/8/11].

Prasch, S. *et al.* (2000) A novel link between stress and human cytomegalovirus (HCMV) infection: sympathetic hyperactivity stimulates HCMV activation. *Virology*, 272, pp. 357-365.

Puchhammer-Stockl, E. and Goorzer, I. (2011) Human cytomegalovirus: an enormous variety of strains and their possible clinical significance. *Future Virology*, 6, pp. 259-71.

Qui, H. *et al.* (2008) Human CMV infection induces 5-lipoxygenase expression and leukotriene B4 production in vascular smooth muscle cells. J*ournal of Experimental Medicine*, 205, pp. 19-24.

Reiche, E. *et al.* (2004) Stress, depression, the immune system and cancer. *The Lancet Oncology*, 5, pp. 617-625.

Revello, M. and Gerna, G. (2002) Diagnosis and management of human cytomegalovirus infection in mother, foetus and newborn infant. *Clinical Microbiology Reviews*, 15, pp. 680-715.

Rissenberg, M. and Chambers, S. (1998) Distinct pattern of cognitive impairment noted in study of Lyme patients. *The Lyme Times*, 20, pp. 29-32.

Robain, M. *et al.* (1998) Incidence and sexual risk factors of cytomegalovirus seroconversion in HIV-infected subjects. *Sexually Transmitted Diseases*, 25, pp. 476-480.

Roberts, D. *et al.* (2008) Increasing rate of emergency department visits for elderly patients in the United States, 1993 to 2003. *Annals of Emergency Medicine*, 51, pp. 769-774.

Ross, S. *et al.* (2010) Cyt*omegalovirus strain diversity in newborns with congenital infection.* [www] 48th Annual meeting of the Infectious Diseases Society of America, Vancouver. Available from: http://idsa. confex.com/idsa/2010/webprogram/Paper4045. html [Accessed 19/08/11].

Sabetta, J. *et al.* (2010) Serum 25-hydroxyvitamin D and the incidence of acute viral respiratory tract infections in healthy adults. *PLoS ONE*, 5, doi: 10.1371/journal.pone. 0011088.

Sauce, D. *et al.* (2009) Evidence of premature immune aging in patients thymectomized during early childhood. *Journal of Clinical Investigation*, 119, pp. 3070-3078.

Savino, W. (2002) The thymus gland is a target in malnutrition. *European Journal of Clinical Nutrition*, 56(Suppl3), pp. S46-S49.

Schoenfisch, A. *et al.* (2011) Cytomegalovirus shedding is highly correlated with matters of immunosupression in CMV-seropositive women. *Journal of Medical Microbiology*, 60, pp. 768-774.

Shann, F. *et al.* (1986) Pneumonia associated with infection with pneumocystis, respiratory synctial virus, chlamydia, mycoplasma and cytomegalovirus in children in Papua New Guinea. *British Medical Journal (Clinical Research Edition)*, pp. 292.

Sheikh, A. and Alves, B. (2000) Hospital admission for acute anaphylaxis: time trend study. *British Medical Journal*, 320, pp. 1441.

Simanek, A. *et al.* (2011) Seropositivity to cytomegalovirus, inflammation, all-cause and cardiovascular disease-related mortality in the United States. *PLoS ONE*, 6, doi: 10.1371/journal.pone.0016103.

Slobedman, B. *et al.* (2009) Virus-encoded homologs of cellular interleukin-10 and their control of host immunity. *Journal of Virology*, 83, pp. 9618-9629.

Soderberg-Naucler, C. (2006) Does cytomegalovirus play a causative role in the development of various inflammatory diseases and cancer? *Journal of Internal Medicine*, 259, pp. 219-246.

Stanton, R. *et al.* (2010) Reconstruction of the complete human cytomegalovirus genome in BAC reveals RL13 to be a potent inhibitor of replication. *The Journal of Clinical Investigation*, 120, pp. 3191-3208.

Stowe, R. *et al.* (2007) Chronic herpesvirus reactivation occurs in aging. *Experimental Gerontology*, 42, pp. 563-570.

Stout-Delgado, H. *et al.* (2009) Aging promotes neutrophil-induced mortality by augmenting 1L-17 production during viral infection. *Cell Host and Microbe*, 6, pp. 446-456.

Stumpf, W. and O'brien, L. (1987) Nuclear receptors for 1,25$(OH)_2$vitaminD3 in thymus reticular cells studied by autoradiography. *Histochemistry*, 87, pp. 367-369.

Suy, A. *et al.* (2007) Immunological profile of heterosexual highly HIV-exposed uninfected individuals: predominant role of CD4 and CD8 T-cell activation. *Journal of Infectious Diseases*, 196, pp. 1191-1201.

Swinkels, B. *et al.* (1984) Initial characterization of four cytomegalovirus strains isolated from chimpanzees. *Archives of Virology*, 82, pp. 125-128.

Sylwester, A. *et al.* (2005) Broadly targeted human cytomegalovirus-specific CD4+ and CD8+ T cells dominate the memory compartment of exposed subjects. *Journal of Experimental Medicine*, 2002, pp. 673-685.

Tanriverdi, F. *et al.* (2003) The hypothalmic-pituitary-gonadal axis: immune function and autoimmunity. *Journal of Endocrinology*, 176, pp. 293-304.

Taub, D. *et al.* (2010) Rejuvination of the aging thymus: growth hormone-mediated and ghrelin-mediated signalling pathways. *Current Opinion in Pharmacology*, 10, pp. 408-424.

Thacker, S. (1986) The persistence of influenza A in human populations. *Epidemiologic Reviews*, 8, pp. 129-142.

Thomas, D. *et al.* (2009) Genetic variation in 1L28B and spontaneous clearance of hepatitis C virus. *Nature*, 461, pp. 798-801.

Tu, W. *et al.* (2004) Persistent and selective deficiency of CD4+T cell immunity to cytomegalovirus in immunocompetent young children. *The Journal of Immunology*, 172, pp. 3260-3267.

Vakilian, A. *et al.* (2006) Clinical manifestations, accompanying disease pathologies in 102 patients with myasthemia gravis. *Journal of Research in Medical Sciences*, 11, pp. 63-66.

Valsamkis, A. *et al.* (1998) Recombinant measles virus with mutations in the C, V and F gene have altered growth phenotypes *in vivo*. *Journal of Virology*, 72, pp. 7754-7761.

van de Berg, P. *et al.* (2010) Cytomegalovirus infection reduces telomere length in circulating T cell pool. *Journal of Immunology*, 184, pp. 3417-3423.

van der Mei, I. *et al.* (2001) Regional variation in multiple sclerosis prevalence in Australia, and its association with ambient ultraviolet radiation. *Neuroepidemiology*, 20, pp. 168-174.

van der Pol, A. *et al.* (1999) Cytomegalovirus cell tropism, replication, and gene transfer in brain. *The Journal of Neuroscience*, 19, pp. 10948-10965.

Varani, S. *et al.* (2000) Laboratory signs of acute or recent cytomegalovirus infection are common in cirrhosis of the liver. *Journal of Medical Virology*, 62, pp. 25-28.

Varani, S. *et al.* (2009) Human cytomegalovirus targets different subsets of antigen-presenting cells with pathological consequences for host immunity: implications for immunosuppression, chronic inflammation and autoimmunity. *Reviews in Medical Virology*, 19, pp. 131-145.

Varani, S. *et al.* (2010) Cytomegalovirus-induced autoimmunity. In: Petrov, M. E. (ed.) *Autoimmune Disorders: Symptoms, Diagnosis and Treatm*ent. New York: Nova Science Publishers, Inc.

Varani, S. and Landini, M. (2011) Cytomegalovirus-induced immunopathology and its clinical consequences. *Herpesviridae*, 2, doi: 10. 1186/2042-4280-2-6.

Ventura, K. *et al.* (2001) Fatal neonatal echovirus and infection: autopsy case report and review of literature. *Modern Pathology*, 14, pp. 85-90.

ver Braak, F. *et al.* (1998) Cytomegalovirus (CMV) strain differences between the eye and blood in AIDS patients with CMV retinitis. *AIDS*, 7, pp. 713-718.

Vescovini, R. *et al.* (2010) Intensive antiextracellular adaptive immune response in very old subjects with impaired health and cognitive and functional status. *Journal of Immunology*, 184, pp. 3242-3249.

Vieth, R. *et al.* (2003) Age-related changes in the 25-hydroxyvitamin D versus parathyroid hormone relationship suggest a different reason why older adults require more vitamin D. *Journal of Clinical Endocrinology and Metabolism*, 28, pp. 185-191.

Villacres, M. *et al.* (2004) Predominant type 1 CMV-specific memory T-helper response in humans: evidence for gender differences in cytokine secretion. *Human Immunology*, 65, pp. 476-485.

Voisset, C. *et al.* (2008) RNA "rumor" viruses: the search for novel human retroviruses in chronic disease. *Microbiology Molecular Biology* Reviews, 72, pp. 157–196.

Vojdani, A. and Thrasher, J. (2004) Cellular and humoral immune abnormalities in gulf war veterans. *Environmental Health Perspectives*, 112, pp. 840-846.

Vyse, A. *et al.* (2009) The burden of infection with cytomegalovirus in England and Wales: How many women are infected in pregnancy. *Epidemiology and Infection*, 137, pp. 526-533.

Wainberg, M. *et al.* (1998) Infection of human thymic epithelial cells by human cytomegalovirus and other viruses: effect on secretion of interlevkin-1-like activity. *Clinical and Experimental Immunology*, 72, pp. 415-421.

Walker, L. *et al.* (2005) The Sherbrooke questionnaire predicts use of emergency services. *Age and Ageing*, 34, pp. 233-237.

Walker, L. and Herndon, J. (2010) Mosaic aging. *Medical Hypotheses*, 74, pp. 1048-1051.

Walsh, B. *et al.* (2008) Trends in hospital inpatient episodes for signs, symptoms and ill-defined conditions: observational study of older people's hospital admissions in England, 1995-2003. *Age and Ageing,* 37, pp. 455-478.

Wang, G. *et al.* (2010) Cytomegalovirus infection and the risk of mortality and frailty in older women: A prospective observational cohort study. *American Journal of Epidemiology*, 171, pp. 1144-1152.

Wardwell, L. *et al.* (2008) Nutrient intake and immune function of elderly subjects. *Journal of the American Dietetic Association*, 108, pp. 2005-2012.

West, L. (2002) Defining critical windows in the development of the human immune system. *Human and Experimental Toxicology*, 21, pp. 499-505.

Westman, A. (2010) Immunity, thyroid function and pregnancy: molecular mechanisms. *Nature Reviews - Endocrinology*, 6, pp. 311-318.

Wherry, E. *et al.* (2003) Viral persistence alters D CD8 T-cell immunoscenescence and tissue distribution and results in distinct stages of functional impairment. *Journal of Virology*, 77, pp. 4911-4927.

Whistler, T. *et al.* (2009) Impaired immune function in Gulf War illness. *BMC Medical Genomics*, 2, doi: 10.1186/1755-8794-2-12.

Wills, M. *et al.* (2002) Vaccines against persistent DNA virus infections. B*ritish Medical Bulletin*, 62, pp. 125-138.

Wilson, J (1999) *Thymus extracts: an international literature review of clinical studies.* [www] Hepatitisfree.com Available from: http// hepatisfree.com/thymus-article.html [Accessed 19/08/11].

Wolf, S. *et al.* (2009) Adaptive peripheral immune response increases proliferation of neural precursor cells in adult hippocampus. *The FASEB Journal*, 23, pp. 3121-3128.

Wrigley, H. *et al.* (2002) Trends in demand for emergency ambulance services in Wiltshire over nine years: observational study. *British Medical Journal*, 324, pp. 646-647.

Woo, P. *et al.* (1997) Distinct genotypic distributions of cytomegalovirus (CMV) envelope glycoprotein in bone marrow and renal transplant recipients with CMV disease. *Clinical and Diagnostic Laboratory Immunology*, 4, pp. 515-518.

Worobey, M. and Holmes, E . (1999) Evolutionary aspects of recombination in RNA viruses. *Journal of General Virology*, 80, pp. 2535-2543.

Wrigley, H. *et al.* (2002) Trends in demand for emergency ambulance services in Wiltshire over nine years: observational study. *British Medical Journal*, 324, pp. 646-647.

Yamschchikov, A. *et al.* (2009) Vitamin D for treatment and prevention of infectious diseases: A systematic review of randomized controlled trials. *Endocrine Practice*, 15, pp. 438-449.

Ye, P. and Kirscener, D. (2002) Re-evaluation of Tcell receptor excision circles as a measure of human recent thymic emigrants. *The Journal of Immunology*, 168, pp. 4968-4979.

Zairat'iants, O. (1991) Thymus hyperplasia: classification, problems of patho- and morphogenesis, importance in human pathology [Russian]. Arkhives Patholgy, 53, pp. 3-12.

Zitterman, A. *et al.* (2009) Vitamin D and the adaptive immune system with special emphasis to allergic reactions and allograft rejection. Infl*ammation and Allergy Drug Targets*, 8, pp.161-168.

Zuniga, E. *et al.* (2008) Persistent virus infection inhibits type I interferon production by plasmacytoid dendritic cells to facilitate opportunistic infections. *Cell Host and Microbe*, 4, pp. 374–386.

In: Hypotheses in Clinical Medicine
Editors: M.M. Shoja, P.S. Agutter et al.
ISBN: 978-1-62257-276-2

Chapter 5

Crohn's Disease and the Cold Chain Hypothesis: An Update

Ulrich Meinzer, Frederick Barreau and Jean-Pierre Hugot*
Institut National de la Santé et de la Recherché Médicale (INSERM), Paris, France
Université Paris-Diderot, Sorbonne Paris-Cité, Paris, France
Service de Gastroentérologie et Nutrition Pédiatriques, Hôpital Robert Debré,
Assistance Publique Hôpitaux de Paris, Paris, France

Abstract

Crohn's Disease (CD) is characterized by chronic or relapsing inflammatory lesions of the digestive tract. CD is frequent in developed countries and seems to be associated with the modern Western way of life. We hypothesize that the development of refrigeration may contribute to CD outbreaks. Indeed, epidemiological data argue for a spatial and temporal relationship between these two parameters. Two case control studies in the United Kingdom and Iran confirmed an association between CD incidence and exposure to food refrigeration in childhood. Among refrigerated foods, meat and fish are most associated with CD. In Japan, outbreaks of CD are correlated with the increased consumption of fish. Two retrospective case control studies, a twin study and a prospective cohort study reported an association between high consumption of meat and fish and CD. Finally, a semi-vegetarian diet seemed to be beneficial for CD patients. *Yersinia* is a psychrotrophic bacterium able to grow at low temperatures especially in meat products. Numerous case reports indicate that CD may occur after *Yersinia* infection. Humoral and cellular immune responses toward *Yersinia* are associated with CD and *Yersinia* has been found more frequently in CD lesions than in control biopsies. CD and yersiniosis share many common clinical findings. They are characterized by inflammatory lesions centered on gut lymphoid formations, especially Peyer's patches. Finally, NOD2, the main CD susceptibility gene, is also associated with gut lymphoid dysfunction and resistance toward oral *Yersinia* infection. Taken together, these data allow a hypothetic causality chain to be built, which may be tested at several levels from the molecule to the population.

* E-mail: jean-pierre.hugot@rdb.aphp.fr.

Introduction

Crohn's disease (CD) and ulcerative colitis (UC), the two main types of inflammatory bowel disease (IBD), are chronic relapsing inflammatory disorders of the gastrointestinal tract. The peak of IBD onset is observed in the third decade of age. Patients typically suffer from frequent and chronically relapsing flares resulting in diarrhea, abdominal pain, rectal bleeding and malnutrition. IBD can be complicated by intestinal obstruction and perforation, anal lesions, intestinal cancer and adverse effects of drugs and surgery (Podolsky 2002). CD generally involves the ileum and colon but it can affect any region of the GI tract, often discontinuously. UC involves the rectum and may affect any part of the colon or the entire colon (pancolitis) in an uninterrupted pattern. The inflammation is often transmural in CD but is typically confined to the mucosa in UC. Intestinal granulomas, strictures, and fistulas are typical findings in CD but are absent in UC. Patients with IBD are at risk for primary sclerosing cholangitis, ankylosing spondylitis, psoriasis, vascular thrombosis, and small bowel and colorectal cancers.

The prevalence of CD in North America ranges from 44 to 201/100,000, and that for UC from 7.5 to 238/100,000. Corresponding figures in Europe are 8 to 214/100,000 for CD prevalence and 21 to 294/100,000 for UC. When these figures are extrapolated to the population of the European Community, it can be estimated that 1 million persons in Europe have CD and 1.4 million have UC. A study based on health insurance data estimated that there were more than 1.3 million IBD patients in the US. Finally, IBDs are emerging diseases in developing countries (Cosnes *et al.* 2011).

The mean annual total expenditure on health care is 1871€/patient-year for IBD in Europe (Odes *et al.* 2006). In addition, IBDs are life-long disabling diseases occurring in the young adult so they entail high indirect costs. The diseases have a major impact on quality of life for affected persons and their families. They can lead to hospitalizations, surgery, complications and death. As a whole, IBDs are thus seen as a public health problem.

IBDs are complex genetic disorders with both genetic and environmental risk factors. Recently, progress in the molecular understanding of these diseases has been achieved by genome-wide association studies. This approach has identified a hundred IBD susceptibility genes (for review see Khor *et al.* 2011). Identification of these genes allowed researchers to focus on key molecular pathways including innate immunity, autophagy, and TH17 lymphocyte differentiation. Among the many CD susceptibility genes, NOD2 exhibits the highest risk (more than 30-fold for people carrying two frame-shift mutations).

Less progress has been achieved in the identification of environmental factors involved in the development of IBD. However, there is strong evidence that living conditions and environmental factors contribute significantly to the risk for these conditions. For example, the dramatic increase in IBD incidence in many countries during recent decades is incompatible with a purely genetic disease (Carbonnel *et al.* 2009; Cosnes *et al.* 2011). Also, data from migration studies indicate that second generation immigrants take on the risk of the new environment (Probert *et al.* 1992). The single CD risk factor established to date is smoking. Tobacco increases the risk of CD occurrence with an odds ratio (OR) of 1.76 (95% confidence interval (95% CI): 1.40-2.22) (Mahid *et al.* 2006). It is also associated with a more severe clinical presentation in diagnosed patients. However, tobacco is usually seen as modulating the phenotype rather than as a causative factor.

In the absence of knowledge about CD risk factors, preventive actions are limited. However, there is an urgent need to develop such actions. First, any preventive action that could (even modestly) reduce the relapse rate and/or the incidence of the disease would have a significant economic impact. Secondly, treatments remain palliative and mainly based on costly anti-inflammatory, immunosuppressant, and biological drugs. These drugs have severe side-effects that limit their use, especially in this context of life-long disorders. Thirdly, there is a strong demand from the patients' community for recommendations that will protect at-risk people against the disease (or protect diagnosed people against relapse) rather than passively bearing it.

Wide exploration of the roles of putative environmental risk factors (called the exposome) has been recently proposed (Rappaport 2011). However, this approach has not yet been developed in CD. Research on the environmental causes of IBD thus remains hypothesis-driven. Among the many working hypotheses proposed to explain CD outbreaks (Korzenik 2005), we have proposed analysis of the role of refrigeration (Hugot *et al.* 2003a).

Refrigeration and CD

CD emerged as a public health problem in North America and Europe during the second part of the twentieth century (Mayberry and Rhodes 1984; Binder 2004). This observation does not seem to be attributable to the improvement of diagnostic procedures alone, so CD is likely to be linked with the modern Western way of life. This opinion is further supported by the fact that CD incidence is now increasing in developing countries in North Africa, South Asia and South America (Cosnes *et al.* 2011). In contrast, in older developed countries, where the modern way of life is widespread, the disease now affects all ethnic and socioeconomic groups and its incidence is relatively stable.

The adoption of the modern Western way of life has affected all aspects of life simultaneously: housing, clothes, pollution, hygiene, drugs, leisure, travels, diet, etc. On the basis of epidemiological data alone, it is therefore difficult to propose any specific candidate risk factor for CD. For this reason, additional information has to be taken into account to define more specific candidate risk factors.

First, CD is probably associated with bacteria present in the digestive tract. Several lines of evidence support this opinion including studies on intestinal diversion and re-instillation of ileal flux into excluded intestinal segments (for review see Janowitz *et al.* 1998). Recently, it has been shown that the gut microbiota is altered in CD patients (Qin *et al.* 2010). Moreover, the most important CD susceptibility genes (e. g. NOD2, IRGM, ATG16L1) are involved in the innate immune response toward bacteria.

Second, CD seems to be associated with dietary components. The best argument is provided by the clinical observation that nutritional treatments are efficient in CD, at least in children or at the beginning of the disease in adults (Smith 2008). The exact mechanism by which enteral nutrition modulates CD lesions is not understood but it is widely recognized by pediatricians that enteral feeding works only when it is exclusive. This finding suggests that the eviction of diet-driven antigens may play a role in CD.

Third, CD is associated with hygiene and home comfort. Several reports have documented an increased risk of CD in people with high domestic hygiene standards often in childhood (Koloski *et al.* 2008; Gent *et al.* 1994; Malekzadeh *et al.* 2009). In contrast, CD is less frequent in populations with less sanitized ways of life such as “travelers” (Karlinger *et al.* 2000; McCormick and Manning 2001). Finally, the report that risk factors shared by siblings during childhood may play a role in CD is also consistent with the idea that hygiene and domestic comfort contribute to the disease (Hugot *et al.* 2003b).

Considering all these findings, we noted that refrigeration links the modern way of life, bacteria, diet and domestic hygiene (Hugot *et al.* 2003a). In Western countries, the starting dates of CD outbreaks are often difficult to define precisely but population-based data suggest that CD increased in the ‘40s or earlier in USA, in the ‘50s or earlier in Sweden, in the ‘60s in the United Kingdom, and later in Southern Europe (Binder 2004).

Domestic chilling has developed since the 19th century when ice was conserved in containers. The first refrigerating machines were built around 1875. During the first part of the 20th century, the USA was more advanced than other countries in terms of refrigeration and the first domestic refrigerator was developed by Kelvinator in 1918 (Thévenot 1978). It is estimated that 49% of American families had a ‘fridge by 1937. This may explain retrospectively why CD was fully recognized in the ‘30s in New York.

In Europe, the refrigerator was present only in rich households during the 1930s and its use became widespread only after World War II, following improvements of the standard of living and electrification (Thévenot 1978). For example, it is estimated that in 1958, only 10% of French and 12% of British families had a refrigerator at home; in Spain, the Union of Soviet Socialist Republics and Japan, the figure was 2%. In Sweden, the incidence of CD was surprisingly higher than in other European (including Scandinavian) countries in the ‘60s. Interestingly, the Swedish company Electrolux successfully developed a ‘fridge as early as 1931. Thus, the percentage of households with refrigerators in 1957 was higher in Sweden (55%) than in the rest of Europe. All these examples reveal a temporal and geographical coincidence between the development of the refrigerator and the outbreak of CD.

To explore the relationship between refrigeration and CD better, exposure to refrigerators was analyzed in case-control studies. Such studies are difficult because of the general exposure to the suspected risk factor in the population. In order to resolve this problem, Forbes and colleagues studied the oldest CD patients from a large population-based cohort (Forbes and Kalantzis 2006). They reported that patients had been exposed to refrigerators during childhood more often than controls.

We also performed a case-control study on CD and ‘fridge exposure. However, instead of working on the first cases reported in Western countries, we explored recently diagnosed CD cases in Iran, a country where CD is an emerging disease (Malekzadeh *et al.* 2009). We also found a limited but significant excess of ‘fridge exposure at birth in CD patients compared to controls.

Two independent case-control studies thus support the cold-chain hypothesis. However, these reported associations do not prove causality. As expected, several other items related to domestic hygiene and comfort were also found to be linked with CD in our study (Malekzadeh *et al.* 2009). Thus, refrigeration may only be a confounding factor statistically associated with CD rather than a causative factor leading to CD. Intervention studies are needed to resolve this question. However, it is obviously impossible to build prospective studies on large cohorts of people avoiding refrigerated food.

Animal Proteins and CD

If the cold chain hypothesis is true, CD should be associated with the consumption of refrigerated food. Fresh meat and fish are among the diet products that are the most dependent on the cold chain for preservation and distribution. They have been associated with IBD in several recent studies.

An observational study of dietary trends in the Japanese population reported a relationship between fish consumption and IBD outbreaks (Sakamoto *et al.* 2005). Two retrospective case-control studies also found an association between meat intake and IBD in Europe (Maconi *et al.* 2010; D'Souza *et al.* 2008). Finally, comparisons of dietary habits between discordant IBD twins also point to high meat consumption as a risk factor associated with IBD (Spehlmann *et al.* 2012). However, the recall biases inherent in the design of retrospective studies limit the impact of their conclusion. Only one recent population-based prospective study is available for CD (Jantchou *et al.* 2010). More than 67,000 healthy French women were prospectively followed for an average period of 10.4 years. Seventy-seven IBD patients were identified. Affected women ate more animal proteins than controls. Regarding the sources of animal proteins, consumption of meat and fish but not of eggs or dairy products was associated with IBD (hazards ratio of the third versus the first tertile was 1.87 (95% CI: 1.00-3.49, *P* value: 0.02). Finally, an open clinical trial recently reported that a traditional Japanese semi-vegetarian diet was effective in preventing CD relapse (Chiba *et al.* 2010). We are aware that all these recent studies have to be further confirmed and/or replicated. However, they all point to high consumption of meat and fish as a putative CD risk factor.

Yersinia and CD

Some bacteria (called psychrotrophic) are able to grow at low temperatures. They have an optimum growth at temperatures higher than 30°C but they are able to grow, at a slower rate, at temperatures between –1°C and +10°C, which are typically observed in refrigerators. It is thus possible that the increased consumption of refrigerated food has increased exposure to these bacteria.

The common psychrotrophic bacteria with pathogenic properties are *Listeria monocytogenes, Yersinia enterocolitica, Clostridium botulinum, Pseudomonas fluorescens* and *Bacillus cereus* (Champagne *et al.* 1994). Antibodies directed against the I2 fragment of *Pseudomonas fluorescens* have been associated with CD (Wei *et al.* 2002). *L. monocytogenes* is a Gram-positive bacillus that induces acute diarrhea. It has been identified in CD lesions by immunohistochemical analysis (Liu *et al.* 1995), but not by PCR (Walmsley *et al.* 1998; Chen *et al.* 2000; Chiba *et al.* 1998; Swidsinski *et al.* 2002). Thus, among the psychrotrophic bacteria, we considered *Yersinia* the best candidates.

Yersinia species are Gram-negative bacteria growing in aero-anaerobic conditions. *Y. enterocolitica* and *Y. pesudotuberculosis* are ubiquitous and they have been detected in the digestive tracts of many wild or domestic animals (Bottone 1999). *Yersinia* species (most often *Y. enterocolitica*-like species) are present in a large variety of refrigerated foods, especially in meat. They are found in up to 50% of pork tongues, 30% of pork samples, 10% of beef products, 50% of chicken samples, 10% of milk products, 50% of prepared salads in restaurants and 4% of sandwiches from supermarkets. These data indicate that exposure to *Yersinia* species is common and mainly related to meat. However, more detailed analyses are required to define better the pathogenicity of the bacterial strains encountered within food and the quantitative exposure to *Yersinia* species in real life.

There are numerous case reports in the literature showing that *Yersinia* infection may inaugurate a disease that will later be classed as CD. Saebo and colleagues interviewed a cohort of Norwegian patients with documented positive/negative serologies against *Y. enterocolitica*, on average 9.5 years after the serological test (Saebo *et al.* 2005). Fifteen percent of IBD incidence cases occurred in serologically positive people ($P < 0.001$). Reactivity against *Yersinia* species is also documented for the cellular immune response. Mucosal T-cells present in the guts of CD patients are specifically reactive against *Yersinia* antigens but not to other bacterial antigens (Ibbotson *et al.* 1992). Altogether, these findings indicate that CD is associated with the capacity of the host to develop strong clinical and/or immunological responses after *Yersinia* exposure.

Two independent groups using specific PCR primers have detected *Yersinia* species in, respectively, 63% (13/19) and 31% (17/54) of people with CD (Kalinowski *et al.* 1998; Lamps *et al.* 2003). Intestinal samples were positive for *Y. enterocolitica*, *Y. pseudotuberculosis*, or both. The clinical and histological features of the *Yersinia*-positive cases were indistinguishable from *Yersinia*-negative cases. Disease misclassification is unlikely, since median follow-up in the two study groups were 9 and 10 years, respectively. These data indicate that *Yersinia* spp. can exist in CD lesions. They are mainly found in lymphoid formations of the digestive tract. This finding may explain some negative studies (Cartun *et al.* 1993; Knösel *et al.* 2009). Finally, it is notable that *Yersinia* spp. are not among the predominant micro-organisms and that CD cannot be considered as an "infection" by *Yersinia* (Swidsinski *et al.* 2002).

In conclusion, there is a documented relationship between *Yersinia* species and CD. However, further work with larger groups of patients is needed to confirm that *Yersinia* may be seen in CD lesions, to define the virulence factors of the identified strains better, and to confirm that CD is associated with an exacerbated immune host response towards these bacteria.

Lymphoid Follicles and CD

Going on with the cold chain hypothesis, we have now to suppose that chronic exposure to low doses of *Yersinia* species may contribute to chronic or relapsing intestinal inflammation. Enteropathogenic *Yersinia* strains, including *Y. pseudotuberculosis* and *Y. enterocolitica*, most often cause self-limited enteritis and mesenteric adenolymphitis in children and young adults. Gut and lymph node lesions can exhibit granuloma formations on histological examination. Like *Helicobacter pylori*, *Yersinia* is able to produce a urease, which is known to be essential in gastritis - a finding that could be related to the focally enhanced gastritis frequently observed in CD (Parente *et al.* 2000). *Yersinia* is also able to produce a heat-shock protein (p60) potentially involved in diarrhea and autoimmune colitis in animal models (Sukegawa *et al.* 2000). Finally, *Yersinia* species may induce reactive arthritis and erythema nodosa. All these clinical findings are common to CD and yersiniosis, explaining why these two disorders have classically to be differentiated during the diagnosis procedure.

Yersinia species are able to produce an invasin, which interacts with integrins containing a β1 chain. The invasin allows the bacteria to penetrate M cells (Isberg and Barnes 2001). This specific tropism for M cells makes *Yersinia* pathogenic to the lymphoid follicles. Histological observation of *Yersinia* infection in mice shows vesicles centered on lymphoid follicles, which are progressively destroyed with micro-abscess formation (Autenrieth and Firsching 1996). In the small bowel, lymphoid follicles are grouped forming Peyer's patches. In infected mice, 30-50% of the Peyer's patches are involved.

CD, like yersiniosis, is characterized by discontinuous inflammation. Several authors have reported that aphtoid ulcerations (which are considered the inaugural CD lesions) are centered on lymphoid follicles (Fujimura *et al.* 1996; Gullberg and Söderholm 2006). CD lesions occur predominantly where there is a high density of lymphoid follicles: in the small bowel where the follicles are grouped forming Peyer's patches, and in the colon where they are isolated. In the small intestine, CD lesions are more frequent in the distal ileum, where Peyer's patches are most abundant. Within the colon, there is also a rough correlation between the frequency of CD lesions and the density of lymphoid follicles. Indeed, the density of lymphoid follicles is 29.2/cm^2 at the recto-anal junction, 25.4/cm^2 in the rectum, 18.4/cm^2 in the cecum and 15/cm^2 elsewhere in the colon (Langman and Rowland 1986, 1992).

In addition to this spatial relationship, a temporal relationship has also been proposed (Van Kruiningen *et al.* 1998). The Peyer's patches develop from birth to 10-15 years of life and then undergo involution. The age-dependent incidence curve for CD is roughly parallel to the number of Peyer's patches, with a peak in the third decade. A delay of 10 years is thus observed between the development of Peyer's patches and peak occurrence of symptoms. Such a delay is compatible with the hypothesis of a chronic inflammation. More interestingly, ileal CD has been shown to be rare in seniors (Polito *et al.* 1996) and in younger children who have fewer Peyer's patches (Meinzer *et al.* 2005). In the colon, the number of lymphoid follicles is less subject to age variations, and colonic CD can be seen in all age groups (Langman and Rowland 1992).

In summary, at the histopathological level, *Yersinia* infection and CD share many resemblances especially with respect to their lymphoid follicle-centered lesions. It is thus possible that CD lesions could be driven by recurrent or chronic exposure to *Yersinia* species.

NOD2 and CD

CD occurs in genetically at-risk people. It is thus expected that the genes predisposing to CD should play a role in Peyer's patch function and in the host response towards *Yersinia*. As the first identified CD susceptibility gene, NOD2 is the best studied. NOD2 mutations are found in up to 50% of CD patients. NOD2-mutated patients usually show involvement of their terminal ileum and increased intestinal permeability (Lesage *et al.* 2002).

Table 1. Summary of the arguments for the cold chain hypothesis

Main links of the "cold chain"	Arguments supporting its relationship with CD
Refrigeration	• Spatial and temporal relationship between domestic cold development and CD outbreak (Thévenot 1978; Binder 2004) • Two case control studies showing an association between 'fridge at home in childhood and CD (Forbes and Kalantzis 2006; Malekzadeh *et al.* 2009).
Animal proteins	• Temporal relationship between IBD and fish consumption in Japan (Sakamoto *et al.* 2005) • Two case-control studies showing an association between meat and fish consumption and IBD (D'Souza *et al.* 2008; Maconi *et al.* 2010) • A twin study showing high meat consumption in affected twins (Spehlmann *et al.* 2012) • A prospective cohort study showing an association between fish and meat and IBD (Jantchou *et al.* 2010) • An interventional study showing a benefit of a semi-vegetarian diet in IBD (Chiba *et al.* 2010)
Yersinia species	• Numerous case reports where CD is consecutive to *Yersinia* infection • A retrospective study showing that CD occurs more frequently after a documented yersiniosis (Saebo *et al.* 2005) • CD mucosal lymphocytes are reactive against *Yersinia* (Ibbotson *et al.* 1992) • *Yersinia* DNA is more frequently found in CD lesions than in control biopsies (Kalinowski *et al.* 1998; Lamps *et al.* 2003; Swidsinski *et al.* 2002)
Lymphoid tissue	• Yersiniosis and CD share numerous clinical features • Yersiniosis and CD are characterized by inflammatory lesions centered on gut-associated lymphoid follicles (Fujimura *et al.* 1996; Gullberg and Söderholm 2006). • There is a spatial and temporal relationship between ileal CD and Peyer's patches (Van Kruiningen *et al.* 1997; Polito *et al.* 1996; Meinzer *et al.* 2005)
NOD2	• NOD2 is associated with CD (Hugot *et al.* 2001; Ogura *et al.* 2001) • Nod2 is involved in Peyer's patch function (Barreau *et al.* 2007, 2010) • NOD2 deficiency is associated with resistance toward oral *Yersinia* infection (Meinzer *et al.* 2008) • YopJ, a *Yersinia* virulence factor, modulates NOD2 function (Meinzer *et al.* in press).

In NOD2 knock-out mice or mice carrying a mutation homologous to the human frame-shift mutation, the Peyer's patches are more numerous and bigger than in control mice. This phenotype appears after bacterial gut colonization and disappears after treatment with oral antibiotics (Barreau *et al.* 2007). Additional data suggest that Peyer's patch dysfunction is driven by the commensal flora via a balance between proinflammatory Toll-like Receptors

(TLR) and NOD2 (Barreau *et al.* 2010). The Peyer's patches of NOD2-deficient mice are characterized by a large number of CD4+ T-cells and high levels of pro-inflammatory cytokines. More interestingly, the permeability of Peyer's patches is increased, as shown by studies performed with markers of bacterial translocation, paracellular and transcellular permeability (Barreau *et al.* 2010).

Indirect findings also argue for a role of NOD2 in the Peyer's patch. NOD2 mutations have been associated with Graft Versus Host Disease (GVHD), which is related to Peyer's patch function as shown by its resistance in mice with defective Peyer's patch development (for a review see Penack *et al.* 2010). Altogether, these data indicate that NOD2 contributes to the homeostasis of PPs.

NOD2 is involved in the recognition of small molecules derived from the peptidoglycans of most bacteria (Franchi *et al.* 2009). Under activation, NOD2 activates several pathways including NF-κB, IL-1β and autophagy. Since NOD2 is intracellular, invasive bacteria defined by their ability to enter the cell or to transfer virulence factors into the cytoplasm can be seen as the best candidates for NOD2 activation. Indeed, the role of NOD2 has been established for several invasive bacteria such as *Mycobacteria*, *Streptococcus*, *Listeria*, anthrax, *Staphylococcus*, etc.

When infected with *Yersinia pseudotuberculosis*, NOD2-deficient mice exhibit a delayed mortality (Meinzer *et al.* 2008). This phenotype is observed only after enteral infection while NOD2 deficiency does not change the host response via the intraperitoneal route. Looking at Peyer's patches, deficient mice are characterized by delayed colonization of the gut-associated lymphoid tissue, increased production of proinflammatory cytokines and a lower dissemination in deep organs such as spleen and liver. As a result, *Yersinia* seems to need NOD2 to achieve its virulence within the gut. However, the price paid for *Yersinia* resistance by NOD2-deficient animals is an excess of inflammation in Peyer's patches.

The virulence factors of *Yersinia* species are mainly carried by a plasmid (pYV) encoding the *Yersinia* outer proteins (Yop), which are injected into the cell via a needle-like structure known as the secretory apparatus (for review see Cornelis 2002). Some of the Yops are involved in inhibiting phagocytosis and NF-κB activation, making the plasmid a well organized system of virulence. We have recently shown that YopJ is able to interact with NOD2 function (Meinzer *et al.* in press). Indeed, YopJ acetylates Rick, a NOD2 partner, and reduces its affinity for NOD2. As a consequence, NOD2 is free to interact with caspase-1, resulting in IL1β secretion. Finally, we were able to show that IL1β induces increased intestinal permeability, allowing the bacteria to colonize the gut. In cases of NOD2 deficiency, this phenomenon is deficient and the knock-out mice are more resistant to infection.

Conclusion

In summary, we propose the hypothesis that the recent development of refrigeration has increased exposure to low doses of *Yersinia* species present in refrigerated foods, especially meat and fish. Genetically predisposed people are characterized by increased reactivity toward *Yersinia*. As a result, inflammatory lesions occur at sites of host-bacterium interaction, namely the gut-associated lymphoid tissue including Peyer's patches (Table 1).

The cold chain is only one among many well-known hypotheses recently proposed to explain CD outbreaks in developed countries, including the hygiene hypothesis, food microparticles, the modern Western diet, *Mycobacterium avium paratuberculosis* (MAP), measles, enteroinvasive *E. coli*, loss of helminths, dysbiosis, Paneth cell deficiency, etc. (for review see Korzenik 2005). Some of these hypotheses are recent, e.g. Paneth cell deficiency, while others may be as old as the disease itself. For example, as early as 1913, Dalziel (1913) proposed that MAP is involved in CD, an idea that is still highly debated. Some infectious agents such as measles have been discarded while others are considered as very promising, such as enteroinvasive *E. coli* or *Faecalibacterium prausnitzii*, which have been shown to be associated with early relapse after ileocoecal resection in operated patients (Pineton de Chambrun *et al.* 2008; Sokol *et al.* 2008). Some proposals are relatively imprecise, e.g. the hygiene hypothesis (Koloski *et al.* 2008) and dysbiosis, while others such as MAP infection are relatively well formulated.

It is notable that the major weakness of most of proposals is that they explain special features of the disease but often fail to provide a global explanation of our knowledge about CD. For example, the helminth hypothesis is mainly supported by epidemiological data, but recent genetic discoveries do not provide additional support for it. The MAP hypothesis is well documented in terms of microbiology and even genetic factors, but epidemiological data and clinical observations (e.g. response to treatments) are difficult to reconcile with it. The Paneth cell hypothesis is rather well supported by molecular biology data but it does not explain the epidemiological observations (Gersemann *et al.* 2008).

In contrast, the cold chain hypothesis potentially reconciles the many aspects of CD in a single comprehensive account. It unifies independent epidemiological, clinical, pathological, microbiological and molecular findings. In this respect, the most important word in the phrase "cold chain hypothesis" may be "chain". Indeed, we do not propose a cause of CD but a chain of causality.

The second advantage of the cold chain hypothesis is that it is precise enough to lead to experimentally testable predictions. It is more than a conjecture. Furthermore, because the hypothesis is a chain of causality, it can be tested at several levels, from the molecule to human populations. This last point is important because, whatever the true CD environmental risk factors, no single study on its own will be able to demonstrate causality. Indeed, the complex question of causality will require a bundle of data before it can be resolved.

References

Autenrieth, I. B. and Firsching, R. (1996) Penetration of M cells and destruction of Peyer's patches by *Yersinia* enterolitica: an ultrastructural and histological study. *Journal of Medical Microbiology*, 44, pp. 285-294.

Barreau, F. *et al.* (2007) CARD15/NOD2 is required for Peyer's patches homeostasis in mice. *PLoS One*, 2, doi: 10.1371/journal.pone.0000523.

Barreau, F. *et al.* (2010) Nod2 regulates the host response towards microflora by modulating T cell function and epithelial permeability in mouse Peyer's patches. *Gut*, 59, pp. 207-217.

Binder, V. (2004) Epidemiology of IBD during the twentieth century: an integrated view. *Best Practice and Research Clinical Gastroenterology*, 18, pp. 463-479.

Bottone, E. J. (1999) *Yersinia* enterolitica: overview and epidemiologic correlates. *Microbes and Infection*, 1, pp. 323-333.

Carbonnel, F. *et al.* (2009) Environmental risk factors in Crohn's disease and ulcerative colitis: an update. *Gastroentérologie Clinique et Biologique*, 33[Suppl 3], pp. 145-157.

Cartun, R. W. *et al.* (1993)An immunocytochemical search for infectious agents in Crohn's disease. *Modern Pathology*, 6, pp. 212-219.

Champagne, C. P. *et al.* (1994) Psychrotrophs in dairy products: their effects and their control. *Critical Reviews in Food Science and Nutrition*, 34, pp. 1-30.

Chen, W. *et al.* (2000) Detection of Listeria monocytogenes by polymerase chain reaction in intestinal mucosal biopsies from patients with inflammatory bowel disease and controls. *Journal of Gastroenterology and Hepatology*, 15, pp. 1145-1150.

Chiba, M. *et al.* (1998) Listeria monocytogenes in Crohn's disease. *Scandinavian Journal of Gastroenterology*, 33, pp. 430-434.

Chiba, M. *et al.* (2010) Lifestyle-related disease in Crohn's disease: relapse prevention by a semi-vegetarian diet. *World Journal of Gastroenterology*, 16, pp. 2484-2495.

Cornelis, G. R. (2002) The *Yersinia* Ysc-Yop type III weaponry. *Nature reviews - Molecular Cell Biology*, 3, pp. 742-754.

Cosnes, J. *et al.* (2011) Epidemiology and natural history of inflammatory bowel diseases. *Gastroenterology*, 140, pp. 1785-1794.

Dalziel, T. K. (1913) Chronic intersticial enteritis. *British Medical Journal*, 2, pp. 1068-1070.

D'Souza, S. *et al.* (2008) Dietary patterns and risk for Crohn's disease in children. *Inflammatory Bowel Diseases*, 14, pp. 367-373.

Forbes, A. and Kalantzis, T. (2006) Crohn's disease: the cold chain hypothesis. *International Journal of Colorectal Disease*, 21, pp. 399-401.

Franchi, L. *et al.* (2009) Function of Nod-like receptors in microbial recognition and host defense. *Immunological Reviews*, 227, pp. 106-128.

Fujimura, Y. *et al.* (1996) Pathogenesis of aphtoid ulcers in Crohn's disease: correlative findings by magnifying colonoscopy, electron microscopy, and immunochemistry. *Gut*, 38, pp. 724-732.

Gent, A. E. *et al.* (1994) Inflammatory bowel disease and domestic hygiene in infancy. *The Lancet*, 343, pp. 766-767.

Gersemann, M. *et al.* (2008) Crohn's disease-defect in innate defence. World Journal of *Gastroenterology*, 14, pp. 5499-5503.

Gullberg, E. and Söderholm, J. D. (2006) Peyer's patches and M cells as potential sites of the inflammatory onset in Crohn's disease. *Annals of the New York Academy of Sciences*, 1072, pp. 218-232.

Hugot, J. P. *et al.* (2001) Association of Nod-2 leucine-rich repeat variants with susceptibility to Crohn's disease. *Nature*, 411, pp. 599-603.

Hugot, J. P. *et al.* (2003a) Clustering of Crohn's disease within affected sibships. *European Journal of Human Genetics*, 11, pp. 179-184.

Hugot, J. P. *et al.* (2003b) Crohn's disease: the cold chain hypothesis. *The Lancet*, 362, pp. 2012-2015.

Ibbotson, J. P. *et al.* (1992) Mucosal cell-mediated immunity to mycobacterial, enterobacterial and other microbial antigens in inflammatory bowel disease. *Clinical and Experimental Immunology*, 87, pp. 224-230.

Isberg, R. R. and Barnes, P. (2001) Subversion of integrins by enteropathogenic *Yersinia*. *Journal of Cell Science*, 114, pp. 21-28.

Janowitz, H. D. *et al.* (1998) The role of fecal stream in Crohn's disease : an historical and analytic review. *Inflammatory Bowel Diseases*, 4, pp. 29-39.

Jantchou, P. *et al.* (2010) Animal protein intake and risk of inflammatory bowel disease: The E3N prospective study. *American Journal of Gastroenterology*, 105, pp. 2195-2201.

Kalinowski, F. *et al.* (1998) Prevalence of enteropathogenic bacteria in surgically treated chronic inflammatory bowel disease. *Hepato-Gastroenterology*, 45, pp. 1552-1558.

Karlinger, K. *et al.* (2000) The epidemiology and the pathogenesis of inflammatory bowel disease. *Journal of Radiology*, 35, pp. 154-167.

Khor, B. *et al.* (2011) Genetics and pathogenesis of inflammatory bowel disease. *Nature*, 474, pp. 307-317.

Knösel, T. *et al.* (2009) Prevalence of infectious pathogens in Crohn's disease. *Pathology, Research and Practice*, 205, pp. 223-230.

Koloski, N. A. *et al.* (2008) Hygiene hypothesis in inflammatory bowel disease: a critical review of the literature. *World Journal of Gastroenterology*, 14, pp. 165-173.

Korzenik, J. R. (2005) Past and current theories of etiology of IBD: toothpaste, worms, and refrigerators. *Journal of Clinical Gastroenterology*, 39[Suppl 2], pp. 59-65.

Lamps, L. W. *et al.* (2003) Pathogenic *Yersinia* DNA is detected in bowel and mesenteric lymph nodes from patients with Crohn's disease. *The American Journal of Surgical Pathology*, 27, pp. 220-227.

Langman, J. M. and Rowland, R. (1986) The number and distribution of lymphoid follicles in the human large intestine. *Journal of Anatomy*, 149, pp. 189-194.

Langman, J. M. and Rowland, R. (1992) Density of lymphoid follicles in the rectum and at the anorectal junction. *Journal of Clinical Gastroenterology*, 14, pp. 81-84.

Lesage, S. *et al.* (2002) CARD15/NOD2 mutational analysis and genotype-phenotype correlation in 612 patients with inflammatory bowel disease. *American Journal of Human Genetics*, 70, pp. 845-857.

Liu, Y. *et al.* (1995) Immunocytochemical evidence of Listeria, Escherichia Coli and Streptococcus antigens in Crohn's Disease. *Gastroenterology*, 108, pp. 1396-1404.

Maconi, G. *et al.* (2010) Pre-illness changes in dietary habits and diet as a risk factor for inflammatory bowel disease: a case-control study. *World Journal of Gastroenterology*, 16, pp. 4297-4304.

Mahid, S.S. *et al.* (2006) Smoking and inflammatory bowel disease: a meta-analysis. *Mayo Clinic Proceedings*, 81, pp. 1462-1471.

Malekzadeh, F. *et al.* (2009) Crohn's disease and early exposure to domestic refrigeration. *PLoS One*, 4, doi: 10.1371/journal.pone.0004288.

Mayberry, J. F. and Rhodes, J. (1984) Epidemiological aspects of Crohn's Disease: a review of the literature. *Gut*, 25, pp. 886-899.

Mccormick, P. and Manning, D. (2001) Chronic inflammatory bowel disease and the "over clean" environment: rarity in the Irish traveller community. *Irish Medical Journal*, 94, pp. 203-204.

Meinzer, U. *et al.* (2005) Ileal involvement is age dependent in pediatric Crohn's disease. *Inflammatory Bowel Diseases*, 11, pp. 639-644.

Meinzer, U. *et al.* (2008) Nod2 mediates susceptibility to *Yersinia* pseudotuberculosis in mice. *PLoS One*, 3, doi: 10.1371/journal.pone.0002769.

Meinzer, U. *et al.* (in press) *Yersinia* pseudotuberculosis effector YopJ subverts the Nod2/Rick/Tak1/ pathway and elicits intestinal barrier dysfunction via caspase-1 activation. *Cell Host and Microbe*.

Odes, S. *et al.* (2006) Cost analysis and cost determinants in a European inflammatory bowel disease inception cohort with 10 years of follow-up evaluation. *Gastroenterology*, 131, pp. 719-728.

Ogura, Y. *et al.* (2001) A frameshift mutation in NOD2 associated with susceptibility to Crohn's disease. *Nature*, 411, pp. 603-606.

Parente, F. *et al.* (2000) Focal gastric inflammatory infiltrates in inflammatory bowel diseases: prevalence, immunohistochemical characteristics and diagnotic role. *The American Journal of Gastroenterology*, 95, pp. 705-711.

Penack, O. *et al.* (2010) Graft-versus-host disease: regulation by microbe-associated molecules and innate immune receptors. *Blood*, 115, pp. 1865-1872.

Pineton De Chambrun, G. *et al.* (2008) Pathogenic agents in inflammatory bowel diseases. *Current Opinion in Gastroenterology*, 24, pp. 440-447.

Podolsky, D. K. (2002) Inflammatory bowel disease. *The New England Journal of Medicine*, 347, pp. 417-429.

Polito, J. M. *et al.* (1996) Crohn's disease: influence of age at diagnosis on site and clinical type of disease. *Gastroenterology*, 111, pp. 580-586.

Probert, C. S. *et al.* (1992) Epidemiological study of ulcerative proctocolitis in Indian migrants and the indigenous population of Leicestershire. *Gut*, 33, pp. 687-693.

Qin, J. *et al.* (2010) A human gut microbial gene catalogue established by metagenomic sequencing. Nature, 464, pp. 59-65.

Rappaport, S. M. (2011) Implications of the exposome for exposure science. *Journal of Exposure Science and Environmental Epidemiology*, 21, pp. 5-9.

Saebo, A. *et al.* (2005) Inflammatory bowel disease associated with *Yersinia* enterocolitica O:3 infection. *European Journal of Internal Medicine*, 16, pp. 176-182.

Sakamoto, N. *et al.* (2005) Dietary risk factors for inflammatory bowel disease: a multicenter case-control study in Japan. *Inflammatory Bowel Diseases*, 11, pp. 154-163.

Smith, P. A. (2008) Nutritional therapy for active Crohn's disease. *World Journal of Gastroenterology*, 14, pp. 4420-4423.

Sokol, H. *et al.* (2008) Faecalibacterium prausnitzii is an anti-inflammatory commensal bacterium identified by gut microbiota analysis of Crohn disease patients. *Proceedings of the National Academy of Sciences of the United States of America*, 105, pp. 16731-16736.

Spehlmann, M. E. *et al.* (2012) Risk factors in German twins with inflammatory bowel disease: Results of a questionnaire-based survey. *Journal of Crohn's and Colitis*, 6, pp. 29-42.

Sukegawa, Y. *et al.* (2000) Induction of auto-immune colitis by *Yersinia* enterolitica 60-kilodalton Heat-Shock Protein. *Scandinavian Journal of Gastroenterology*, 35, pp. 1188-1193.

Swidsinski, A. *et al.* (2002) Mucosal flora in inflammatory bowel disease. *Gastroenterology*, 122, pp. 44-54.

Thévenot, R. (1978) *Essai pour une Histoire du Froid Artificiel dans le Monde*. Paris: Institut International du Froid.

van Kruiningen, H. J. *et al*. (1997) The role of Peyer's patches in the age-related incidence of Crohn's disease. *Journal of Clinical Gastroenterology*, 24, pp. 470-475.

Walmsley, R. S. *et al*. (1998) Absence of Escherichia coli, Listeria monocytogenes and Klebsiella pneumoniae antigens within inflammatory bowel disease tissues. *Journal of Clinical Pathology*, 51, pp. 657-661.

Wei, B. *et al*. (2002) Pseudomonas fluorescens encodes the Crohn's disease-associated I2 sequence and T-cell superantigen. *Infection and Immunity*, 70, pp. 6567-6575.

In: Hypotheses in Clinical Medicine
Editors: M.M. Shoja, P.S. Agutter et al.

ISBN: 978-1-62257-276-2

Chapter 6

Reflections on Pellagra: Lessons and Hypotheses for Diseases Ancient and Modern

Adrian C. Williams[1,*], Lisa J. Hill[2] and David B. Ramsden[2]
[1]Institute for Cognitive and Evolutionary Anthropology,
University of Oxford,Oxford, UK
[2]Neurotrauma and Neurodegeneration, School of Clinical
and Experimental Medicine, University of Birmingham,
Edgbaston, Birmingham, UK

Abstract

Optimal energy provision, the supply of nicotinamide adenine dinucleotide (NAD) and methyl groups, avoidance of hypo- and hyper-vitaminosis B3 (nicotinamide) and increasing the availability of choline, were important in our evolution and remain important for our healthy development and healthy aging avoiding Dementia and Parkinson's disease . Healthy energy, NAD and methyl budgets with feed-back and feed-forward systems that balance the external supply and the demand act like broad-spectrum "vaccines" against disease. Short-term internal homeostatic reactions accept risky trade-offs that can lead to uncontrolled chronic infections, such as tuberculosis, or uncontrolled autophagy/apoptosis, or excessive storage of energy in adipose tissue, or reversion to fermentation as happens in inflamed and cancerous tissues; NAD(P)(H) is redistributed in all these situations, but at a high long-term allostatic cost.

"Felix qui potuit cognoscere causas".
Virgil

"The past is a foreign country, where we come from".
Lowenthal

* E-mail: Adrian.Williams@uhb.nhs.uk.

Introduction

Very little is understood about the etiological mechanisms involved in degenerative and inflammatory diseases or in chronic infections and cancer, or aging phenomena in general. As the pastoralist Virgil said: "it is well to understand causes" and "fortunate also to comprehend the gods of the countryside". This requires us to appreciate the logic and energetics of our past survival strategies and invites an ecological, co-evolutionary and developmental approach to finding ultimate causes that may be simpler to correct than proximate mechanisms (currently hampered by slow progress in preventive therapy) (Bray 2009; Nurse 2008; Bocquet-Appel and Bar 2008; Stiner *et al.* 2009; Northcutt 2011). Human brain evolution has been closely linked with a change in diet from herbivory to omnivory and from hunting and gathering to farming and cooking, thus creating our own energetic, informatic and technological niche (Gaulin 1979; Palin and Quintana-Merci 2008; Cochran and Harpending 2009; Fish and Lockwood 2003; Navarrete *et al.* 2011; Sol 2009; Carmody and Wrangham 2009). This cultural niche greatly increased the somatic and exosomatic energy supply. Such micronutrients as nicotinamide and choline were captured through nutrigenomic and cultural innovations (concurrently, lactose tolerance in adults and more efficient salivary amylase contributed). This allowed cholinergic, dopaminergic and other systems to prosper, yet such systems remain at risk if the high quality energy or micronutrient supply either fails or becomes excessive (Csete and Doyle 2004; Williams and Ramsden 2005; Ungar and Sponheimer 2011; Raghanti *et al.* 2010; Raghanti *et al.* 2011). The supply of these evolutionary and developmentally key raw materials remains heterogeneous globally and in continual states of nutritional transition (mostly because meat, milk and eggs are expensive). Alongside other aspects of diet and social stress that could explain the striking geographic and temporal patterns of many common diseases with only a moderate effect from medical interventions, with the exception of preventive vaccination programs (McKeown 1976; Fogal 2004).

Redox energetic defects and aberrant mitochondrial dynamics, with consequent oxidative stress and loss of calcium, glutamate, proteosome and inflammasome homeostasis, are important proximate mechanisms of acute and chronic diseases and the physiological declines that are linked to aging (Adams and Klaidman 2011; Kapoginnus and Mattson 2011; Schrack *et al.* 2010; Fadini *et al.* 2010; Cunnane *et al.* 2011; Lazarov *et al.* 2010; van Leeuwen 2010; Kelly 2011; Kowald and Kirkwood 2011; Leloup *et al.* 2011; Perluigi *et al.* 2010). Some of these disease circuits may have particularly high energy requirements; for instance, diseases that affect higher intellectual and complex physical tasks and use cholinergic or dopaminergic neurons, which have a high metabolic energy cost in terms of adenosine triphosphate (ATP) and complex redox needs involving co-factors, metals and melanin (Surmeier *et al.* 2011; Adams *et al.* 2001). This fundamental and compartmentalized failure of the energy supply, often with impaired autophagy, was confirmed by studies of acute brain injury from hypoxia or hypoglycemia or direct trauma, mitochondrial mutations linked with chronic diseases of aging such as Alzheimer's (AD), Parkinson's (PD) and Huntington's disease and with complex I toxins (such as 1-methyl-4-phenyl-1,2,3,6-tetrahydropyridine (MPTP)) or rotenone, as well as physical tests of endurance such as polar and high altitude expeditions (Batlevi and Spada 2010; Luce *et al.* 2010; Wallace 2010; Szulc and Danoff 2011; Green *et al.* 2011; Bland and Birnbaum 2011; Speakman and Krol 2011; Noakes 2011).

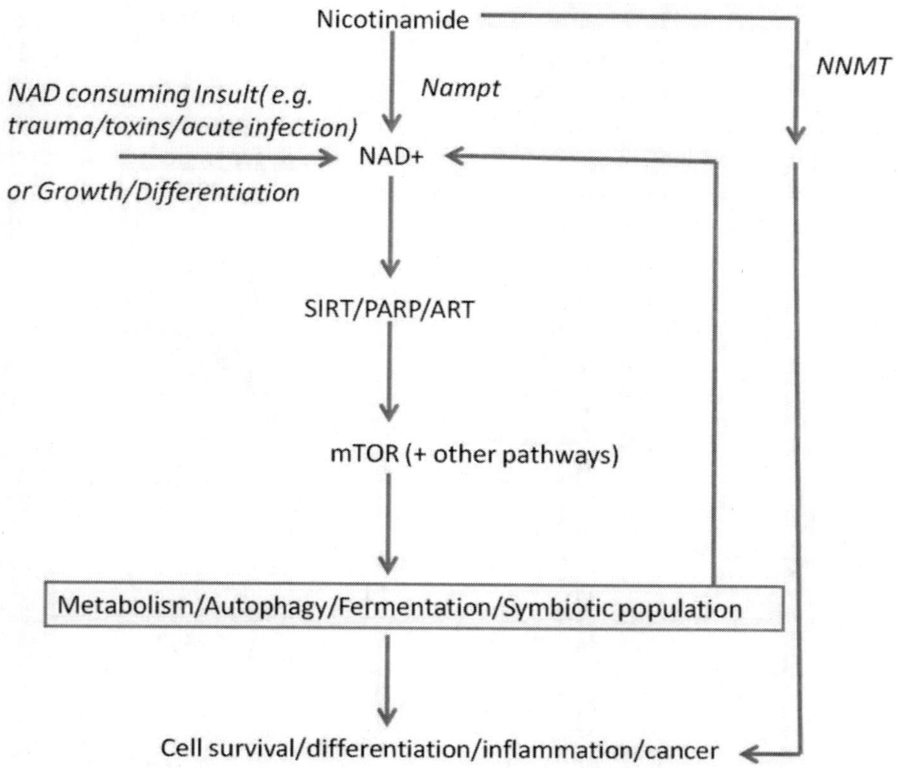

Figure 6.1. The central role of NAD(H) in cell survival and differentiation. Problems may arise when this buffered system is pushed too far and emergency homeostatic measures to maintain NAD and NADH levels fail. The allostatic cost then becomes too high in the medium to longer term, with autophagy and inflammation converting to uncontrolled degeneration or cancer or metabolic syndromes. Poor diet would lead to a deficiency of methyl donors as would excessive meat eating and nicotinamide through the over-induction of nicotinamide N-methyltransferase (NNMT). ART, ecto-ADP-ribosyltransferase; mTOR, mammalian target of rapamycin pathway; Nampt, nicotinamide phosphoribosyltransferase; PARP, poly-(ADP ribose) polymerases; SIRT, sirtuin.

Aging Diseases, Evolution and NAD (H)

Current theories on aging, lifetime behavior patterns, reproductive cycles, and inter-generational transfer of resource and stress responses invoke energy sources, sensors, regulators and trade-offs, as do wider theories on the astonishingly rapid metabolic evolution of big brains aided and driven by the social and cultural strategies used by man (Dunbar 1998; Domenico *et al.* 2010; Paul 2011; Drenos and Kirkwood 2005; Flatt and Schmidt 2009; Fontana *et al.* 2010; Krebs 2009). Thermodynamically open and phylogenomic models support the idea that nicotinamide adenine dinucleotide (reduced) (NADH) and nicotinamide adenine dinucleotide phosphate (reduced) (NADPH) have had a central role in cell differentiation and survival (Figure 6.1) as well as in evolution. Recent reviews of nicotinamide and nicotinamide adenine dinucleotide (NAD) metabolism, evolution and function concentrate on its pivotal role in gene silencing, development and aging. This role operates through recently-appreciated NAD consumers such as the sirtuins (SIRTs) (Vinciguerra *et al.*

2010; Wang *et al.* 2011; Finkel *et al.* 2009; Milner 2009; Brooks and Gu 2009; Feige and Auwerx 2008; Canto and Auwerx 2009; Bass and Takahashi 2010; Vassilopoulos *et al.* 2011), which evolved to work in large part as nutrient-sensing regulators, and poly-(ADP ribose) polymerases (PARPs) (Kauppinen and Swanson 2007; lmageed *et al.* 2012). Several reviews also emphasize the role of NAD(H) in Wallerian degeneration and neuronal death after a wide variety of insults (Avery *et al.* 2009; Li and Kazgan 2011; Verdin *et al.* 2010; Yahata *et al.* 2009; Zhang *et al.* 2011) (Figure 6.2).

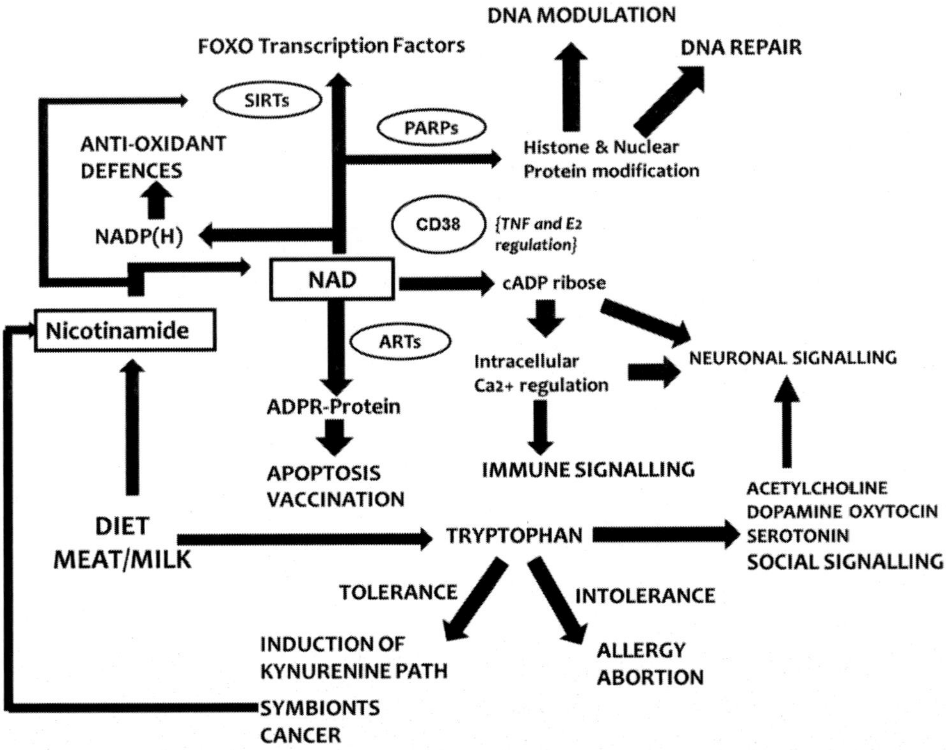

Figure 6.2. Nicotinamide and NAD(H) interactions with various cellular processes. NAD-consuming pathways influence a prodigious number of pathways involved in internal metabolism and connections with the external world(including several not shown here) such as social hormones, neurotransmitters and drugs. Internal NAD-mediated interactions place it at the hub of the survival of superorganisms such as humans. ADRP-protein, adenosine diphosphate ribosylated protein; ART2, T-cell ecto-ADP-ribosyltransferase; cADP, cyclic adenosine diphosphate; CD38, cluster differentiation 38 ectoenzyme; E2, prostaglandin E2; FOXO, forkhead transcription factors; PARP, poly-(ADP ribose) polymerases; Sirt2, sirtuin-2; TNF, tumor necrosis factor.

External Energy Environments: Internal Compensatory Mechanisms

Flow of energy largely determines the structure of ecosystems via food webs, and taste sensors with appetite and quality controls – and many ATP sensors - that enable individuals to balance energy budgets and avoid toxins (Watts and Donovan 2010; Chen *et al.* 2011;

Kaushik *et al.* 2011). Diet changed with concurrent domestication of crops and animals, and modified microbes (e.g., gut symbionts that break down proteins or indigestible starches or manufacture vitamins including nicotinamide and choline) co-evolved, helping to supply and translocate energy and information via circadian pulses of NAD (H) (Douglas 2010). Relinquishing the endogenous production of vitamins and some catabolic enzymes and relying instead on diet or symbionts appears to help capture hydrogen-based energy (Pester and Brune 2007).

Failure of the supply of NAD (H) as a consequence of malnutrition or starvation triggers attempts to compensate by autophagy, avoiding apoptosis or necrotic cell death, a tactic that is vital at least for neurons and other cells that are rarely renewed after birth (Rabinowitz and White 2010; Cheung 2011). Similarly, inflammasome and immune modulation is required in order to tolerate microorganisms that are potentially deleterious but are also capable of supplying NAD (H) or its precursors. Reversion to fermentation occurs in inflamed or cancerous tissue, favoring net export of NAD (P) H (and reducing equivalents such as lactate) even in oxygenated parts of the tumor, let alone the engineered hypoxic areas (the Warburg phenomenon). Many somatic oncogene mutations and other mechanisms, such as growth factor and endocrine signaling, are recruited to create this metabolic milieu, which often includes autophagosomes working in concert, sometimes active sometimes suppressed (Levine and Puzio-Kuter 2010; Richardson and Scott 2011; Cairns *et al.* 2011; Koppenol *et al.* 2011; Marie and Shinjo 2011). All the above, and several current therapies that induce cell death in and around the tumor lead to the secretion of energy substrates including ATP itself. These control the immune response to the tumor, but may really be short-term homeostatic attempts to correct a host environment that has been rendered locally energy and redox-poor by genetic, environmental or quite possibly stochastic factors.

Pellagra

A NAD (H) deficiency state, which illustrates the complexity of the co-evolved energy networks, was observed during epidemics of pellagra caused by economically determined suboptimal foraging of nicotinamide and tryptophan (tryptophan is converted metabolically to NAD and serotonin); these epidemics are now largely forgotten, or are overlooked, as is currently the case in Africa (Etheridge 1972; Rajakumar 2000; Passamonti *et al.* 2012; Seal *et al.* 2007). Such a dietary deficiency might still be important in sections of modern populations. Intracellular and microenvironmental deficiency states can also occur as a result of high NAD expenditure; NAD (H) ratios are also affected by any disorder that causes hypoxia or hypoglycemia.

Clinical Features of Pellagra

Scientific detectives investigating aging diseases and human evolution should revisit forks in the intellectual road at which we may have taken a predominantly genetic rather than an ecological turning. Clinically, this episode occurred exactly a century ago and was resolved scientifically a few decades later. Importantly, this was a real-life epidemic supporting many laboratory-based clues around the NADH/NAD-consumer axis: laboratory experiments in this area are however often controversial because they rely on genetic models that depend heavily on ecological context, as - in retrospect - should have been predicted (Couzin-Frankel 2011).

The last major human epidemic of pellagra (pellagra also occurs in several other carnivorous species such as dogs) occurred between 1910 and 1930 in the southeastern states of the United States, with a systems failure of NAD(H) and therefore of thermodynamic, NAD-Hub and methylome homeostasis at several discrete but interconnected hierarchical levels. The epidemic was started and ended socio-culturally. Hypovitaminosis B3 caused a premature aging condition with loss of robustness to chemical, physical and emotional stress, leading to Parkinsonism, dementia, metabolic disease and cancer. It was conquered by dietary supplementation. Classically, pellagra caused dementia, a characteristic photosensitive dermatitis (Casal's necklace), diarrhea and death. The cause was real world economics creating NAD (H) gradients across poor populations, and between sexes (it was twice as common in women as in men), in the cotton- and corn- dependent states of the southeastern USA. It reached epidemic proportions. Too much corn and molasses and too little meat led to a diet deficient in nicotinamide and probably other vitamins such as riboflavin and choline, though it was often adequate or even high in calories. Currently, a similar situation exists in parts of Africa. In the United States, familial aggregations were common, suggesting genetic predisposing factors and widespread epigenetic re-programming (Sassone-Corsi 2011). A diet with too much corn and too little meat caused deficiencies of nicotinamide and the essential amino acid tryptophan, though deficiencies in other vitamins such as choline and other methyl donors contributed to the malaise. Mental symptoms included more than dementia; depression, fatigue, psychomotor retardation, mania, obsessions and a whole range of psychoses with auditory and visual hallucinations were well described along with personality change and sociopathic and drug and alcohol addictive behaviors. Panic disorders were seen, as was a general inability to deal with physical or mental stress. Consequences of impaired brain development such as hydrocephalus or cerebral palsy were also common. Acute delirium or even coma occurred, with some patients having myoclonus and other extrapyramidal signs reminiscent of the spongiform encephalopathies. The dementias of pellagra included features akin to Lewy body, Alzheimer's, frontotemporal, vascular and prion diseases. Parkinsonism (PD) was also common and a festinant gait was in fact first described in pellagrins. Tremors of various descriptions, including asymmetric rest tremors, were noted and some patients had typical paralysis agitans. Pellagrins had a characteristically expressionless facies, so some signs of PD were present in most cases. Many features of pellagra closely resemble the non-motor aspects of PD.

There were further neurological manifestations; other degenerative conditions such as an amyotrophic lateral sclerosis-like picture were described, with fasciculation of the tongue and upper and lower motor neuron signs. Cerebellar syndromes occurred and vertigo was frequent. Headaches, sensory and pain syndromes, epilepsy and involuntary movements were noted as well as sleep disturbances. Cord lesions were also seen, as was optic atrophy, and there were multiple sclerosis (MS)-like variants.

Non-neurological effects included the diagnostic photosensitive and aging dermatitis along with diarrhea from multiple gut infections including helminths. Other infections including yeasts and tuberculosis (TB) were common, suggesting a general effect on the immune system. There were also profound metabolic effects on the endocrine and thermoregulatory systems. For instance, endocrine dysfunctions in the thyroid, cortisol and reproductive pathways were all clearly described. Cancer rates were increased but masked by a high premature death rate. Anergy was the rule.

Pellagra without dermatitis was commonplace and a frequently overlooked diagnosis. Young men from affected states had inordinate difficulty with intellectual tests that involved reading, writing and numeracy skills and the physical fitness tests required by the military, suggesting that subclinical disease was rife. Indeed, poor diet and health have been implicated in the Southern states having a tradition of violence (particularly toward the stealing of nicotinamide-rich livestock) and losing the American Civil War (Nisbett 1993).

The classic pathological sign was chromatolysis of the high energy-requiring pyramidal cells in the cortical gray matter, but Purkinje cells also degenerated and there was widespread cell loss in the basal and sympathetic ganglia. Demyelination was commonly seen in the spinal cord, particularly in the posterior and lateral columns. Much was made of pigmentary change, glial overgrowth, vascular change, amyloid deposition, cytoskeletal and mitochondrial abnormalities and signs of inflammation and atrophy in all organs. A systems failure with the degenerative pathology of premature senility was proposed by several pathologists in the late 19th century and clinicians commented on patients as "wrecks of humanity".

Pellagra is a wide-ranging systems failure, in that ecological dietary stress not only triggers developmental and degenerative effects on behavior but also impairs the transfer of resources and information between generations as well as cooperative work yields and survival. It triggered a vicious cycle that exacerbated the original economic stress. In addition, healthy members of society were phobic about pellagrins and showed them little if any sympathy (unlike most other disabilities) preferring explanations such as a poor gene pool or an infectious state to understanding the consequences of poverty. This picture, we suggest, may represent some aspects of human evolution in a down phase, given that not only individuals but also their recently-evolved social and symbiotic relationships were all "wrecked".

Is Subclinical Pellagra Relevant to Contemporary Chronic Degenerative and Infectious Diseases?

Many poor individuals and groups, even in rich communities, have low amounts of vitamins in their diet. This statement assumes that the recommended daily allowance (RDA) for vitamins should be taken to ensure good health and maintenance under all circumstances, as opposed to simply avoiding the classic deficiency states. Consequently, sub-pellagrous nicotinamide deficiency may have lifetime roles in a range of behavioral traits, neuropsychiatric diseases and dementias. Dietary choline deficiency exacerbates nicotinamide deficiency because the two agents are linked metabolically; N-methylnicotinamide blocks choline export and has other beneficial effects at most doses (Lamoureux *et al.* 2008; Meck *et al.* 2007). Currently, a trial of nicotinamide at high dosage is underway for AD, stroke and several other conditions, motivated by the following inferences from studies mostly undertaken during the past decade (Rafalski and Brunet 2011; Morris *et al.* 2004; Green *et al.* 2008; Chan *et al.* 2009; Chen *et al.* 2005; Adamczyk *et al.* 2005; Longpre *et al.* 2006; Julien *et al.* 2009; Kim *et al.* 2007; Fischer *et al.* 2007; Gao *et al.* 2010; Winder and Borrill 1998; Anstey *et al.* 2011; Filley and Anderson 2011; Garcia-Lara *et al.* 2010; Veeraraghavulu *et al.* 2010; Lee *et al.* 2010; Abeti *et al.* 2011; Fuso and Scarpa 2011; Koh 2011; Wen *et al.* 2011; Haar *et al.* 2011; Middleton *et al.* 2011; Colman *et al.* 2009; Hathorn *et al.* 2010; Kirkland 2009; Klawitter *et al.* 2006; Lui *et al.* 2009; Kaneko *et al.* 2006; Maiese 2008; Du *et al.* 2010; Drenos and Kirkwood 2010; Mastroeni *et al.* 2011; Milosavljevic 2011; Ali *et al.* 2011).

1. The brain uses a lot of energy in proportion to its weight. NADH modulates a highly evolved working memory, language and spatial domains amongst many other functions that are both constrained by the energy supply and lost if not used regularly.
2. In prospective studies, diets of AD patients were found to be deficient in nicotinamide premorbidly.
3. Nicotinamide reduces the accumulation of amyloid by an effect on secretases and ameliorates the toxic effects of amyloid on astrocytes by inhibiting poly(ADP-ribose) polymerase (PARP). The NAD synthase, nicotinamide mononucleotide adenylyl transferase (NMNAT), also has protein-protein chaperone activity that protects against tau-induced neurodegeneration by promoting clearance of hyperphosphorylated tau oligomers.
4. In transgenic mice, nicotinamide restores cognitive deficits by its effects on both dendrites and axons, reducing the levels of a phospho-species of tau linked to microtubule depolymerization (an effect also seen following the inhibition of Sirtuin 1 (SIRT1)), and increasing acetylated alpha-tubulin, which is linked to microtubule and tau stability.
5. In models of AD, over-expression of SIRT1 or PARP reduces memory loss and neurodegeneration.
6. Loss of SIRT1 is associated with the accumulation of amyloid-beta and hyperphosphorylated tau in the cortices of AD brains.
7. Recovery of learning and memory has been associated with chromatin remodeling induced by agents that affect SIRT.
8. Energy paths involving cyclic adenosine monophosphate (cAMP) and insulin-like growth factors are involved in memory consolidation and enhancement.
9. Dementia is linked with being both under- and over-weight and also with stress and exercise levels and the metabolic syndrome.
10. Nicotinamide administration and manipulation of NMNAT reduces ischemic and traumatic brain injury, a common factor in many forms of dementia.
11. Redox-active methylene blue affects dementia pathology and its clinical manifestations.
12. SIRT1 regulates Notch signaling, which is involved with mechanisms of action of mutations in the PSEN1 gene as well as the proliferation of neural progenitors in the subventricular zone. These progenitors are important in the evolution and development of large cortical mantles and are also essential for cell specification and tissue patterning.
13. Nicotinamide and SIRTs are involved in promoting DNA repair particularly under conditions of oxidative stress.

The degenerative neurology of human immunodeficiency virus/ acquired immune deficiency syndrome (HIV/AIDS), which includes premature aging, dementia and PD, has clinical, pathological and biochemical similarities with pellagra: many at-risk groups are nicotinamide deficient since monophagic corn-based diets are now common in Africa. Both AIDS sufferers and pellagrins suffer many parasitic infections, which may be dangerous homeostatic responses that boost NAD(H) in the host when dietary sources of energy are poor. The tuberculosis (TB) bacterium, for instance, excretes nicotinamide (used as a diagnostic test) and is inhibited by nicotinamide and related compounds such as isoniazid (manufactured originally as a nicotinamide analogue, as were several other anti-TB agents). Treatment of TB can precipitate pellagra; and other gut infections ("parasites") may break down otherwise indigestible celluloses, ultimately producing NAD(H). The HIV disease marker CD38 is a NADase that regulates intracellular NAD(H), implying disturbed nicotinamide-NAD(H)-tryptophan metabolism (Rozwarski *et al.* 1998; Murray 2003). SIRTs regulate the HIV transactivator Tat, promoting viral transcription and, through the NF-kappaB complex, induce T cell activation particularly in dendritic cells. There are other links between NAD and the immune system. In view of these effects, nicotinamide ought to be protective against AIDS and TB as a missing host factor, or, could be seen as a NAD-based vaccine affecting virulence by modulating immune responses via tryptophan-NAD and mTOR (mammalian target of rapamycin) pathways in dendritic cells and other T-cell pathways involved in the immune response and energy metabolism (Aksoy *et al.* 2006; Moell *et al.* 2009; Grahnert *et al.* 2010; Orabona and Grohmann 2011; Tracey 2011).

Hypervitaminosis B3 and Choline?

Macronutrients and micronutrients, which include nicotinamide, choline and other methyl sources, may all obey Bertrand's rule: an inverted "U" shaped dose-response curve with toxicity at either extreme, as was suggested by Waaler regarding increased mortality at both ends of weight/height ratio curves (Raubenheimer *et al.* 2005). At optimal nutrient levels, length of life may increase as has been noted in all economically successful populations, but a superabundant supply may generate several diseases of affluence. Affluent populations are exposed to diets with a historically high calorific content from refined sugars and fats relative to energy expenditure. In these populations, energy expenditure is relatively low because of limited exercise and the fact that body heat is maintained through clothing and living in artificial environments.

Injury is often assumed to occur from the effects of an obesogenic environment rather than the more direct effects of disturbed NAD^+:NADH ratios on a variety of dependent insulin, cortisol and other pathways (which are also affected by habits such as smoking, alcohol and stress); obesity can be seen as an attempt to sequester energy and actively metabolize nicotinamide, even if it comes at a price. The relationship between the dose of hydrogen source (caloric intake) and the dose of suppliers of the carrier (NAD) must be important for high-quality, biologically useful, energy- but it has never been investigated in detail. Recently, the possibility has been raised that vascular disease may be related to too little or too much choline in the diet, modified by gut flora and genetic factors (Zeisel 2011; West and Caudill 2011; Wang *et al.* 2011).

Extra choline and other methyl-group sources in the diet from vegetables, meat, milk and eggs, along with other key molecules such as nicotinamide, would have enabled us during evolution to develop cholinergic, glutaminergic and monoaminergic systems. These have actively evolved in primates; and through, for instance, the NADH-dependent recycling of an essential co-factor, tetrahydrobiopterin, they still depend on a good NADH supply (Yamamoto and Vernier 2011; Edwards and Self 2006; Bromberg-Martin and Hikosaka 2009; Fliessback *et al.* 2007; Previc 1999).

An evolutionary perspective is warranted, because aging of the cerebral cortex and basal ganglia is more prominent in humans than other primates, who do not suffer AD or PD naturally (though toxins such as MPTP produce a PD-like phenotype in the laboratory); living to old age arrived late in our evolution. The very existence of dementia and premature aging in cases of pellagra supports a role for nicotinamide; these patients also got PD, and there is extensive evidence that nicotinamide intake and manipulation of NADH levels is important in protecting against MPTP toxicity and other experimental Parkinsonian analogues, which whether they are toxic or genetic all affect mitochondrial function. Nevertheless, we propose that the nicotinamide dose may be a double-edged sword (Liu *et al.* 2008; Anderson *et al.* 2008; Yang *et al.* 2004; Outeiro *et al.* 2007a; Outeiro *et al.* 2007b; Barber-Singh *et al.* 2009; Choi *et al.* 2011; Park *et al.* 2011).

Affluence

Life spans have doubled in many economies over the last 200 years, partly because the incidence of previously common infectious diseases has been reduced. Better diet has increased resistance to acute infections that compete for NAD resources both directly and through many of their toxins, which transfer the ADP-ribose portion of NAD to specific host proteins, as do many synthetic vaccines (Deng and Barbieri 2008). In the so-called “infectious chronic unconquerables”, such as malaria and TB, there appears to be an immunological stand-off in which a degree of tolerance may have been traded for an increased supply of an essential nutrient. Many apparently healthy carriers present in the dietary deficient population, let alone the clinically affected, disappeared when dietary standards and the supply of meat improved in Europe and the USA ahead of Japan. The proposal that these are tropical diseases or related to poor hygiene might not be the only explanation (even malaria was formerly common in the UK and other temperate climates). Sanatoria for chronic infections such as TB were converted into sanatoria for allergic diseases within a single generation or two in several parts of the globe between the “hungry” 1850s and 1900. With an increasing quality of diet, some symbionts ceased to be necessary for providing supplements, and the immune system had to adapt (not so seamlessly) from trying to control the population size of a pathogen to controlling a valuable mutualist to rejecting a now unnecessary microbe. Recent information on the role of NAD in modulating innate immunity suggests complex energy-centered interactions between neuronal and immunological systems. Contextually useful organisms (as seen in cases of pellagra) that depend on ecological factors such as dietmay on a good diet no longer be advantageous. With the improved western diet, immunological reactions to formerly “useful” microbial antigens, or fall-back foods such as nuts, may be “confused” and may extend through molecular mimicry and nutrition-related and NADPH signals to antigens on gluten, nuts or pollen, initiating abnormal inflammatory and autoimmune allergic reactions. Some may mimic host-driven microbial pathology such as the granulomas of sarcoidosis and TB, or eosinophilic and immunoglobulin E pathology and helminths. (This explanation differs from the hygiene hypothesis, which proposes that lack of exposure, rather than a shunning of now-unwelcome "old friends" from lack of metabolic need, causes immunological hyper-reactivity).

Here, we suggest that since both nicotinamide and N-methylnicotinamide have an optimal range, a hypervitaminosis B3 state, resulting from a western diet over-rich in meat and vitamin supplements accompanied by calorific excesses, may be implicated in other modern disease phenomena. Meat eating is preferred where it is available, though during pregnancy it is a common dietary aversion, suggesting that it can be toxic in early development. This is consistent with the presence of the detoxification enzyme nicotinamide N-methyltransferase (NNMT) since some metabolites are (neuro) toxic in the context of kidney and liver failure, and with evidence of acute toxicity caused by nicotinamide overdose (Palacios *et al.* 2009; Fessler 2002; Daul and Beuhler 2011) - and with concerns about the relationship between red meat intake and various cancers such as colon cancer. Nicotinamide exposure can be high, well in excess of five times the RDA (15 mg/day), where the diet includes cereals, "high energy" drinks and other foodstuffs supplemented with the vitamin, and where there is an abundance of cheap meat and milk. This chronic overload can be envisioned as both unbalancing NAD (H)-dependent systems including SIRTs, PARPs and dehydrogenase pathways (for instance in cortisol metabolism) and exerting the direct effects of nicotinamide or N-methylated metabolites. NAD^+ is the substrate for SIRTs and nicotinamide is an inhibitor. Dietary levels of NAD (H) precursors could therefore act as both positive and negative influences on such systems. In the case of nicotinamide, dietary inputs are modulated in part by genetic determination of NNMT expression, which is high in 24% of the population. Non-genetic factors also modulate expression of this enzyme. These include nicotinamide itself, stress, and the demands imposed on NAD (H) availability by growth, tissue repair and exercise. Interestingly, NNMT and other components of NAD (H) pathways are markedly induced in a variety of currently common cancers as well as in the metabolic syndrome, obesity, PD and autism (Tang *et al.* 2011; Emanuelli *et al.* 2010; Yap *et al.* 2010; Riederer *et al.* 2009; van Driel *et al.* 2008; Zhang *et al.* 2007; Parsons *et al.* 2002; Pozzi *et al.* 2011).

An animal model of toxicity from excess dietary nicotinamide has been reported. In this model, dopaminergic neurons were injured and locomotor activity was reduced. This model also responded to L-DOPA (Lee *et al.* 2009). In other models, nicotinamide and novel derivatives such as N-nicotinoyl dopamine reduce melanin, as happens in PD (Bisaglia *et al.* 2010; Kim *et al.* 2011).

One consequence of NNMT induction and other methyltransferase reactions is a depletion of methyl stores and S-adenosylmethionine (SAM) that is ultimately dependent on an adequate dietary supply from expensive vegetables and meat rather than cheaper cereals such as maize (banned in 19th century France as unfit for human consumption, thus eliminating pellagra at a stroke) (Chan *et al.* 2008). Depletion of available methyl groups, whether from a poor diet or one with excessive nicotinamide, may be a common cause of epigenetic phenomena given the marked influence of methylation on gene expression in pluripotent and differentiated cells that maintain cellular identity (Kim *et al.* 2011). The methylome is an important mediator of information and modifies gene transcription and translation by various mechanisms, including riboswitches that affect RNA metabolism. It is also important in toxicology pathways in concert with NAD and the ATP-binding cassette, and all these effects appear to be involved in a number of diseases seen within the pellagra phenotype, such as motor neuron disease and many cancers and metabolic diseases (Bosco *et al.* 2011; Carroll *et al.* 2011; Batey 2011; Szyf 2011; Waring *et al.* 1989; Buratti 2011; Rottiers *et al.* 2011).

Longevity and Nutritional Balance

The NAD(H) energy path and NAD consuming hubs are involved in many key cellular processes and in the regulation of food intake and the phenomena of caloric restriction and hormesis, which are implicated in many diseases of aging (Belensky *et al.* 2007; Mentel and Martin 2008; Anderson *et al.* 2003; Lu *et al.* 2009; Kasting 1998; Shinmura *et al.* 2011; Bitterman *et al.* 2002; Estep *et al.* 2009; Calabrese *et al.* 2010; De Petrocellis and Di Marzo 2011; Rodgers *et al.* 2005; Chen *et al.* 2005b; Mineur *et al.* 2011; Balan *et al.* 2008; Suchankova *et al.* 2009; Salminen and Kaarniranta 2009; Kang and Hwang 2009; Sasaki and Kitamura 2010; Satoh *et al.* 2010; Malavasi *et al.* 2010; Noriega *et al.* 2011; Libert *et al.* 2011). These NAD hubs are easily amenable to therapeutic intervention and could have unwittingly contributed through a better overall diet to the recent unexplained increases in longevity in affluent countries. Age-related changes in NAD/NADH ratios have been noted and a world in which NAD is central has been proposed (Braidy *et al.* 2011; Imai 2011). Placebo effects that are so prominent in man have even been linked to energy pathways and are particularly effective when the energy future is perceived as healthy, allowing energy to be invested in healing rather than fire-fighting (Sauro and Greenburg 2005). Caloric restriction hints at the need for a nutritional stoichiometry to balance energy demand and supply throughout life. It is associated with telomeric stability and increased SIRT1 activity stabilizing PGC-1, and results in increased mitochondrial biogenesis, metabolic function, and the deacetylation and inactivation of p53. This balance may be more about NAD^+:NADH ratios than calories *per se*, which may explain the perplexing and contradictory effects of NAD-consumer agonists (such as resveratrol) and antagonists in disease models. SIRT1 knockouts show widespread p53 activation and shortened life expectancy (Cheng *et al.* 2003). Increased longevity as a result of caloric restriction and related genetic models fits with abundant evidence that nicotinamide is involved in neuroprotection.

Links between nicotinamide, acetyl and methyl metabolism and epigenetic phenomena are strong (Kaidi *et al.* 2010; Stover 2009). Other recently studied famines, such as the Dutch hunger winter of 1944-45 and the Chinese famine of 1958-61, not only had marked long-term and transgenerational effects on health such as risk of the metabolic syndrome but also induced psychiatric and antisocial behaviors via epigenetic mechanisms: those affected would have been NAD-deficient with an element of pellagra (Van Os *et al.* 2010; Roseboom *et al.* 2011). Optimizing choline and other aspects of methyl metabolism in embryonic life improves brain development and strikingly reduces age-related decline, perhaps through reducing epigenetic instability (Meck *et al.* 2007). Epigenomes, which may be marked by dietary, emotional and intellectual experiences working through neuroendocrine stress pathways that are themselves redox- and energy-regulated, are implicated in many "modern" diseases. These can be assimilated into the germline through several mechanisms and are unstable, creating somatic epimutations. Surviving epigenetic imprints may be the missing transgenerational elements, along with non-shared environments (thus merging nature and nurture) causing both familial clustering and sporadic cases of diseases such as AD and PD. Twin studies show low concordance in AD and PD, thereby demonstrating the importance of environmental dynamics and chance epigenetic drift over lifetimes (Poulsen *et al.* 2007).

Development to Decline: Managing Metabolic Expectations

Within the context of lifetime availability of NAD(H), where in adult life the net free energy or the availability of methyl groups is greater or less than that in early life or expected *a priori* on the basis of the individual's genome, an imbalance can occur between (epi) genetically-primed protein inductions such as NNMT (or equivalent enzymes involved in choline metabolism) and the nicotinamide/choline dose. This imbalance may not be attributable simply to the mismatch between modern diets and "thrifty gene" hangovers from the Pleistocene (Konner and Eaton 2010). Lack of moderation in meat intake across the globe, avoiding extreme lows and highs, may be the important mismatch with our past. Nutrigenomic and informatic adaptations and changes in trade-offs, resulting from knowing that the energy future is more likely than not to be benign, have occurred over the last 100,000 years and during individuals' lifetimes. Low levels of nicotinamide and choline in early life adversely affect neonatal brain development and later degeneration (Chen *et al.* 2010). Low NAD(H) levels in the fetal/neonatal period could result in a phenotype that might be re-enforced by low levels throughout life, giving rise to poor brain development and function. High early levels could lead to good brain development ("luxury" phenotype) but a fall in the supply later in life even to average levels, after NNMT has been induced, could trigger intracellular pellagra. If the NAD(H) and nicotinamide supply is superabundant throughout life, toxicity might result from excessive N-methyl-nicotinamide, a MPTP analogue (Figure 6.3).

This is plausible because nicotinamide and redox status have marked morphogenic effects that instruct internally-secreted morphogens, and protect against chemical teratogens and NADH anti-metabolites (and similar toxins later in life) which regulate all phases of neuronal development and - in effect - brain evolution (Libert *et al.* 2008; Noble *et al.* 2005; Prozorovski *et al.* 2008; Ullah *et al.* 2011; Ieraci and Herrera 2006; Kleinstreuer *et al.* 2011). The effects can become pathological when unexpected circumstances pertaining to energy and nicotinamide are encountered, as perhaps seen in the metabolic syndrome and, we propose, in neurological and cancerous diseases (Barker 1991).

Metabolic Fields

Accumulating evidence points to the probability that aging diseases such as AD, PD, cancers and metabolic diseases originate in mitochondrial depolarizations and uncouplings with disturbed electron-proton flows; such "protonopathies" have effects on ATP provision

(Soto and Sonnenschein 2011; Ganesan *et al.* 2009; Kenny *et al.* 2007; Czarnecka and Bartnik 2011). A unifying explanation imagines abnormally-spreading metabolic fields resulting from failure to meet the challenges of balancing NADH-dependent energy supply and demand with the need for optimal methyl group availability that arise during growth, reproduction, exercise and tissue repair. Most cancers, in return, have changed their energy metabolism and their methyl profiles even in pre-cancerous stages (Hansen *et al.* 2011).

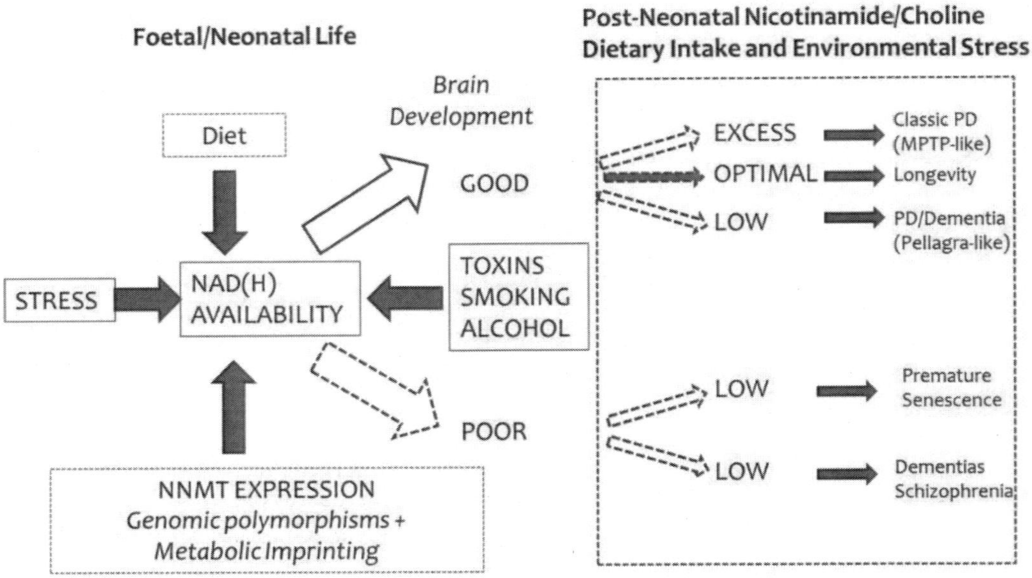

Figure 6.3. Nicotinamide homeostasis throughout life and its postulated role in aging and neurodegenerative diseases in man. NAD(H) availability is key to perfect brain evolution and development. The potential imbalance between nicotinamide and choline intakes and activity of nicotinamide N-methyltransferase (NNMT) in early and later life may increase the risk of such neurodegenerative conditions as AD and PD . The overinduction of NNMT by nicotinamide could paradoxically cause intracellular pellagra, perhaps explaining why nicotinamide can appear to help in short-term, even though it may be a long-term toxic trigger.

These challenges could happen at the same stage of life in diverse species, explaining why incidences of cancer and degeneration are similar despite large variations in numbers of cells, body size and longevity; this paradox is hard to explain on a random somatic mutational or purely immunological basis, which may be enabling and containing phenomena (Fassati and Mitchison 2010). The immune system is now seen by some authors as both suppressing and promoting cancers using the same tryptophan-NAD tolerogenic symbiosis-supporting mechanisms . There are overlaps with chronic infection, as cancer can be caused by infection or contained by introducing an infection such as live bacillus Calmette-Guerin (after William Coley 1891) and both can be prevented by vaccines that use NAD-based machinery (Deng and Barbieri 2008; Mellman *et al.* 2011; Sylvester 2011; Mellor and Munn 2004; Faccaibene *et al.* 2011; Schuler 2010; Schreiber *et al.* 2011).

Metabolism can be stabilized by excretion of NAD(P)H (essentially a waste product not a source of energy in cells using anaerobic metabolism) or other reducing equivalents (e.g. lactate). Reactions of this kind, such as autocarnivory and the Warburg effect and the additional fermentation happening in anoxic parts of tumors, could spread like a wave. NAD-metabolizing ecto-enzymes and salvage pathways appear to be important in shaping tumor-host interactions (Gatenby *et al.* 2010; Merlo *et al.* 2006; Peto *et al.* 1975; Vaisitti *et al.* 2011; D'Andrea *et al.* 2011; Albracht *et al.* 2011; Chandra *et al.* 2011; Bass and Takahashi 2011; Tang *et al.* 2011). When NNMT activity is decreased, cancer cell proliferation is affected; high activity affects radiation sensitivity and alters free radical production. These pathways have opened therapeutic possibilities for several tumors including glioblastoma. Many germline and somatic (epi) mutations in cancer cells continue to evolve as the cancer spreads, for example in p53 and relevant receptors such as those for multiple steroid receptor and growth factor signals, with many interacting with SIRTs (Moore *et al.* 2011). Thus, glucose and tryptophan uptake and mitochondrial and isocitrate dehydrogenase activity are affected, allowing oxidative metabolism to be switched to net NAD(P)H production in all parts of the tumor through all possible genetic means (van der Haiden 2011; Yan *et al.* 2009; Prendergast 2011; Dang *et al.* 2011; Griguer and Oliva 2011; Hamanaka and Chandel 2011; Metallo *et al.* 2011; Metallo and Van der Heiden 2010). From the cancer's point of view, it is hard to see the value of this, given the need for high energy efficiency for growth and proliferation (even if fermentation reactions are really quicker at producing ATP) - rather, cancers' sweet tooth may be seen as a dangerously short-sighted pseudo-symbiotic arrangement redistributing NAD(P)(H). Cancers cannot always be eliminated and often recur (though occasionally they spontaneously remit) or a second cancer develops, suggesting that the basic problem is not eliminated by simply killing cancer cells and their normal neighbors. Chemotherapy-induced DNA damage and autophagy, however, alter the local energy environment by releasing NADH and ATP, which in turn is a chemotactic ligand to purinergic receptors expressed by immune cells stimulating an antitumor vaccine-like immune response via dendritic cells and T-lymphocytes (Michaud *et al.* 2011).

Fetal implants develop PD pathology, illustrating in a different context the point that the niche microenvironment is key (Brundin *et al.* 2008; Segovia *et al.* 2009; Okuda *et al.* 2009; Stadtfeld and Hochedlinger 2010; Poss 2010; Lamour *et al.* 2010; Winner *et al.* 2011). Stem cell implants in PD and other conditions survive and connect but form strange connections, suggesting that lack of stem cells is not the real deficit. Rather, stem cell-based therapies, from hematological transplants to those for other organs, involve the efflux of NAD and ATP into the extracellular space or autocrine induction of NAD release. This activates purinergic and calcium pathways affecting growth-supporting and anti-apoptotic activities (Fruscione *et al.* 2011). Parabiotic fusions of young environments rejuvenate cells, even those expressing pro-cancerous somatic mutations or destined for apoptosis (Conboy *et al.* 2005) and changing the aging milieu alters neurogenesis and improves cognitive function. Stem cell fates toward both normal and abnormal differentiation or de-differentiation depend on their microenvironment and stochastic factors, and even cells that are already cancerous can be induced to behave normally (Ding *et al.* 2010; Capp 2011; Masip *et al.* 2010; Hochedlinger *et al.* 2004). Protein folding and the function of amyloid/ synuclein/ prion proteins and ionic and neurotransmitter gradients are exquisitely sensitive to energy landscapes, as are NAD-consumer-linked DNA repairs. Consequently, all these phenomena, when abnormal, may be secondary and late effects of abnormal NAD(H) ratios and methylation status whether in genetic or multifactorial diseases (Sorolla *et al.* 2011).

Conclusion

Classical pellagra is an archetypal energy and NAD supply-side premature-aging disease with excessive use of symbionts and degenerative or proliferative pathologies. It has been cured, but we have never checked whether sub-pellagrous NAD deficiency had been eliminated. An urgent need has arisen to improve our abilities to track suitable NAD(P)(H) and related methyl habitats from the social exterior of our redox "Russian Doll" to every internal compartment, cell type and organelle. Measurements in yeast suggest that NAD(P)(H) oscillations in mitochondria, which ultimately originate in the environment, provide an ultradian clock that coordinates the vast majority of events and processes in an organism's "reactome" (Sasidharan *et al.* 2012).

Sub-pellagrous NAD deficiency may be a socioeconomic "place" disease and rear its head episodically during lifetimes, triggering age-related degeneration and cancers. However, this type of socioeconomic illness does not seem to evoke sympathy, reducing the chances of resolving the situation (Harris and Fiske 2007). Interactions with other vitamins may be important, either with deficits or excesses, as we have implied for choline and other methyl donors. For example, the combination of low vitamin D intake and NAD supply along with at-risk genotypes and a changed relationship with micro-organisms may be important in the pathogenesis of multiple sclerosis (Penberthy and Tsunoda 2009). Intracellular pellagra may also be caused by other mechanisms such as high NAD expenditure after physical, emotional or toxic stress or acute infections (that compete for NAD) or inadvertent removal of key symbionts such as after antibiotic use; or, rarely, by mutations that affect autophagosome or other compensatory functions. Stress from loss of relative status is a powerful driver of ill health and provokes primates including man into reverting to a high glucose and low nicotinamide diet, or to addictive behaviors that, like stress, induce NNMT further lowering nicotinamide levels (Finger *et al.* 2011; Gesquiere *et al.* 2011).

On the other hand, populations should not be exposed to "too much of a good thing" with excessive supplies of nicotinamide or choline or calories, thereby perturbing NAD:NADH ratios to create a mirror image of pellagra, perhaps with an equally broad phenotype. Lowering nicotinamide intake would be much easier than most dietary interventions because in some affluent countries (with the least need for supplementation) it is inserted artificially into the diet, often partly by statute.

Poor worldwide distribution of NAD(H) supplies makes little sense if oversupply is dangerous. This is particularly so if undersupply is not only dangerous to those affected but also leads to acquiring novel or drug resistant symbionts, in metabolic desperation, that could infect the more affluent with the potential for pandemic harm (Sachs *et al.* 2011). Our current maladaptive group behavior needs the insight that, historically, we enhanced our cultural hunter-gatherer roots with a long teaching and learning childhood period for developing specialized (hunting) skills with divisions of labor and invention of new technology. However, we lost our egalitarian norm of sharing nicotinamide-rich meat with generalized strong reciprocity, involving not only kin (which does not calculate balances too carefully as a cognitive cushion against the risks of hunting - incapacitating injury and failure to kill) (Read 2011; Collings *et al.* 1998; Kaplan *et al.* 2000; Torrence 1989). "Stinginess" may date from a time when the natural meat supply declined and meat and the wherewithal to produce it came to be treated as property, making it an expensive rather than a risky item. Wars began as fighting and migration were preferred over starving: farming and trading promoted specialization, competition and inequality including of access to meat (Wiessner 2002). Resource allocation both of quality foods and of medicines is culturally driven, with choices as to whether those who earn the most or those with the greatest need are given preference. The former may now be a group-selected "Homo economicus" trap requiring conscious correction by political institutions that build human capacity and overcome ethno-religious and parochial concerns with appropriate sanctions (Hamann *et al.* 2011; Hrdy 2009; Murphy-Berman *et al.* 1984; Alexander and Christia 2011).

Fairer access to high quality energy or medicines allows all the options of Hippocratic style diets and exercise regimens, or parallel drug developments, which help build and maintain healthy interactive and innovative bodies and brains. Also, such regimens have hormetic and pre-conditioning effects that test the energy axis and clear cell debris through protein targeting and endoplasmic reticulum stress responses with controlled autophagythat simultaneously recycle energy sources in a win-win scenario (Haung *et al.* 2011). New treatments that quickly supply energy or save energy by inducing artificial hibernation, if employed after an unexpected insult such as trauma so that natural healing can take place, may also be beneficial (Turgut *et al.* 2011).

Now is the time to learn lessons from our evolutionary past as our minds engage with Virgil's "gods of the countryside" and we look for ultimate and preventable causes of disease at a population level (Marmot *et al.* 2008). We may find an energy/informatic-economy that matches supply and demand throughout life with fewer energy trade-offs or faulty methylation signals and in effect vaccinates through the NAD-axis against many ecological and genetic genetic eventualities. The stakes are high, if these hypotheses are correct, as the target is heightened robustness against insults, longer lives, and avoidance of losing intellectual or physical fitness traits whether from degenerative diseases, chronic infections, cancers or allergic diseases.

Acknowledgments

ACW thanks his evolution and anthropology tutors Robin Dunbar and Oliver Curry for their encouragement.

References

Abeti, R. *et al.* (2011) Beta-amyloid activates PARP causing astrocytic metabolic failure and neuronal death. *Brain*, 134, pp. 1658-1672.

Adamczyk, A. *et al.* (2005) Alzheimer's disease related peptides affected cholinergic receptor mediated poly (ADP-ribose) polymerase activity in the hippocampus. *Folia Neuropathologica*, 43, pp. 139-142.

Adams, J. D. *et al.* (2011) Parkinson's disease - Redox mechanisms. *Current Medicinal Chemistry*, 8, pp. 809-814.

Aksoy, P. *et al.* (2006) Regulation of intracellular levels of NAD: A novel role for CD38. *Biochemical Biophysical Research Communications*, 345, pp. 1386-1392.

Albracht, S. P. *et al.* (2011) Mammalian NADH: ubiquinone oxidoreductase (Complex I) and nicotinamide nucleotide transhydrogenase (Nnt) together regulate the mitochondrial production of $H_2)O_2$-Implications for their role in disease, especially cancer. *Journal of Bioenergetics Biomembranes*, 43, pp. 541-564.

Ali, Y. O. *et al.* (2011) NMNAT suppresses Tau-induced neurodegeneration by promoting clearance of hyperphosphorylated Tau oligomers in a Drosophila model of tauopathy. *Human Molecular Genetics*, DOI: 10.1093/hmg/ddr449.

Anastasiou, D. *et al.* (2011) Inhibition of pyruvate kinases M2 by reactive oxygen species contributes to cellular antioxidant responses. *Science*, 334, pp. 1278-1283.

Anderson, D. W. *et al* (2008). Broad neuroprotective profile of nicotinamide in different mouse models of MPTP-induced parkinsonism. *European Journal of Neuroscience*, 28, pp. 610-617.

Anderson, R. M. *et al.* (2003) Nicotinamide and PNC1 govern lifespan extension by calorie restriction in Saccharomyces cerevisiae. *Nature*, 423, pp. 181-185.

Anstey, K. J. *et al.* (2011) Body mass index in midlife and late-life as a risk factor for dementia: a meta-analysis of prospective studies. *Obesity Reviews*, 12, pp. 426-437.

Avery, M. A. *et al.* (2009) Wld (S) requires Nmnatl enzymatic activity and N16-VCP interactions to suppress Wallerian degeneration. *Journal of Cell Biology*, 184, pp. 501-513.

Balan, V. *et al.* (2008) Life span extension and neuronal cell protection by Drosophila nicotinamidase. *Journal of Biological Chemistry*, 283, pp. 27810-27819.

Barber-Singh, J. *et al.* (2009) Neuroprotective effect of long-term NDI1 gene expression in a chronic mouse model of Parkinson disorder. *Rejuvenation Research*, 12, pp. 259-267.

Barker, D. J. (1991) The foetal and infant origins of inequalities in health in Britain. *Journal of Public Health Medicine*, 13, pp. 64-68.

Bass, J. and Takahashi, J. S. (2010) Circadian Integration of Metabolism and Energetics. *Science*, 330, pp. 1349-1354.

Bass, J. and Takahashi, J. S. (2011) Redox redux. *Nature*, 469, pp. 476-478.

Batey, R. T. (2011) Recognition of S-adenosylmethionine by riboswitches. *Wiley Interdisciplinary Reviews – RNA*, 2, pp. 299-311.

Batlevi, Y. and La Spada, A. R. (2010) Mitochondrial autophagy in neural function, neurodegenerative disease, neuron cell death, and aging. *Neurobiology of Disease*, 43, pp. 46-51.

Belenky, P. *et al.* (2007) Nicotinamide riboside promotes Sir2 silencing and extends lifespan via Nrk and Urh1/Pnp1/Meu1 pathways to NAD(+). *Cell*, 129, pp. 473-484.

Berer, K. *et al.* (2011) Commensal microbiota and myelin autoantigen cooperate to trigger autoimmune demyelination. *Nature*, 479, pp. 538-541.

Bisaglia, M. *et al.* (2010) Molecular characterization of dopamine-derived quinines reactivity toward NADH and glutathione: implications for mitochondrial dysfunction in Parkinson's disease. *Biochimica et Biophysica Acta*, 1802, pp. 699-706.

Bitterman, K. J. *et al.* (2002) Inhibition of silencing and accelerated aging by nicotinamide, a putative negative regulator of yeast sir2 and human SIRT1. *Journal of Biological Chemistry*, 277, pp. 45099-45107.

Bland, M. L. and Birnbaum, M. J. (2011) Adapting to Energetic Stress. *Science*, 332, pp. 1387-1388.

Bocquet-Appel, J. R. and Bar-Yosef, O. (eds) (2008) T*he Neolithic Demographic Transition and its Consequences*. New York: Springer.

Bosco, D. A. *et al.* (2011) Proteostasis and movement disorders: Parkinson's disease amyotrophic lateral sclerosis. *Cold Spring Harbor Perspectives in Biology*, 3, doi: 0.1101/cshperspect.a007500.

Braidy, N. *et al.* (2011) Age related changes in NAD+ metabolism oxidative stress and sirt1 activity in wistar rats. *PLoS ONE*, 6, doi: 10.1371/journal.pone.0019194.

Bray, D. (2009) Wetware: *A Computer in Every Living Cell*. London: Yale University Press.

Bromberg-Martin, E. S. and Hikosaka, O. (2009) Midbrain dopamine neurons signal preference for advance information about upcoming rewards. *Neuron*, 63, pp. 119-126.

Brooks, C. L. and Gu, W. (2009) How does SIRT1 affect metabolism, senescence and cancer? *Nature Reviews Cancer*, 9, pp. 123-128.

Brundin, P. *et al.* (2008) Research in motion: the enigma of Parkinson's disease pathology spread. *Nature Reviews Neuroscience*, 9, pp. 741-745.

Buratti, E. (2011) TDP-43 and FUS in ALS/FTLD: Will common pathways fit all? *Neurology*, 77, 1588-1589.

Cairns, R. A. *et al.* (2011) Regulation of cancer metabolism. *Nature Reviews Cancer*, 11, pp. 85-95.

Calabrese, E. J. *et al.* (2010) Dose response biology: the case of resveratrol. *Human and Experimental Toxicology*, 29, pp. 1034-1037.

Canto, C. and Auwerx, J. (2009) PGC-1 alpha, SIRT1 and AMPK, an energy sensing network that controls energy expenditure. *Current Opinion in Lipidology*, 20, pp. 98-105.

Capp, J. P. (2011) Stochastic gene expression is the driving force of cancer. *Bioessays*, 33, pp. 781-782.

Carmody, R. N. and Wrangham, R. W. (2009) The energetic significance of cooking. *Journal of Human Evolution*, 57, pp. 379-391.

Carroll, J. S. *et al.* (2011) The DExD/H box ATPase Dhh1 functions in translational repsression, mRNA decay, and processing body dynamics. *Journal of Cell Biology*, 194, pp. 527-537.

Chan, A. *et al.* (2008) Dietary and genetic compromise in folate availability reduces acetylcholine, cognitive performance and increases aggression Critical role of S-adenosyl methionine. *Journal of Nutrition Health and Aging*, 12, pp. 252-261.

Chan, A. *et al.* (2009) Dietary deficiency increases presenilin expression, gamma-secretase activity, and Abeta levels: potentiation by ApoE genotype and alleviation by S-adenosyl methionine. *Journal of Neurochemistry*, 110, pp. 831-836.

Chandra, N. *et al.* (2011) Virtual screening, identification and experimental testing of novel inhibitors of PBEF1/Visfatin/NMPRTase for glioma therapy. *Journal of Clinical Bioinformatics*, 1, doi: 10.1186/2043-9113-1-5.

Chen, J. *et al.* (2005a) SIRT1 protects against microglia-dependent amyloid-beta toxicity through inhibiting NF-kappa B signaling. *Journal of Biological Chemistry*, 280, pp. 40364-40374.

Chen, J. H. *et al.* (2010) Early Growth and Aging. *Nestlé Nutrition Workshop Series - Paediatric Programme*, 65, pp. 41-54.

Chen, W. Y. *et al.* (2005b) Tumor suppressor HIC1 directly regulates SIRT1 to modulate p-53 dependent DNA-damage responses. *Cell*, 123, pp. 437-448.

Chen, X. *et al.* (2011) A Gustopic Map of Taste Qualities in the Mammalian Brain. *Science*, 333, pp. 1262-1266.

Cheng, H. L. *et al.* (2003) Developmental defects and p53 hyperacetylation in Sir2 homolog (SIRT1)-deficient mice. *Proceedings of the National Academy of Sciences of the United States of America*, 100, pp. 10794-10799.

Cheung, Z. H. and Ip, N.Y. (2011) Autophagy deregulation in neurodegenerative diseases – recent advances and future perspectives. *Journal of Neurochemistry*, 118, pp. 317-325.

Choi, W. S. *et al.* (2011) Loss of mitochondrial complex I activity potentiates dopamine neuron death induced by microtubule dysfunction in a Parkinson's disease model. *Journal of Cell Biology*, 192, pp. 873-882.

Cochran, G. and Harpending, H. (2009) *The 10,000 Year Explosion: How Civilization Accelerated Human Evolution*. New York: Basic Books.

Collings, P. *et al.* (1998) Modern food sharing networks and community integration in the Central Canadian Arctic. *Arctic*, 51, pp. 301-314.

Colman, R. J. *et al.* (2009) Caloric restriction delays disease onset and mortality in rhesus monkeys. *Science*, 325, pp. 201-204.

Conboy, I. M. *et al.* (2005) Rejuvenation of aged progenitor cells by exposure to a young systemic environment. *Nature*, 422, pp. 760-764.

Couzin-Frankel, J. (2011) Aging genes: the sirtuin story unravels. *Science*, 334, pp.1194-1198.

Csete, M. and Doyle, J. (2004) Bow ties, metabolism and disease. *Trends in Biotechnology*, 22, pp. 446-450.

Cunnane, S. *et al.* (2011) Brain Fuel Metabolism, Aging, and Alzheimer's Disease. *Nutrition*, 27, pp. 3-20.

Czarnecka, A. M. and Bartnik, E. (2011) The role of the mitochondrial genome in aging and carcinogenesis. *Journal of Aging Research*, 2011, doi: 10.4061/2011/136435.

dD'Andrea, F. P. *et al.* (2011) Cancer stem cell overexpression of nicotinamide N-methuyltransferase enhances cellular radiation resistance. *Radiotherapy and Oncology*, 99, pp. 373-378.

Dang, L. *et al.* (2011) Cancer-associated IDH1 mutations produce 2-hydroxyglutarate. *Nature*, 465, p. 966.

Daul, A. M. and Beuhler, M. C. (2011) Niacin Toxicity resulting from urine drug testing evasion. *The Journal of Emergency Medicine*, 41, pp. 65-68.

de Petrocellis, L. and Di Marzo, V. (2011) Cell Signalling: Why fasting worms age slowly. *Nature*, 473, pp. 161-163.

Deng, Q, and Barbieri, J. T. (2008) Molecular mechanisms of the cytotoxicity of ADP-ribosylating toxins. *Annuual Reviews Microbiology*, 62, pp. 271-288.

di Domenico, F. *et al.* (2010) Oxidative Damage in Rat Brain During Aging: Interplay Between Energy and Metabolic Key Target Proteins. *Neurochemistry Research*, 35, pp. 2184-2192.

Ding, L. *et al.* (2010) Genome remodelling in a basal-like breast cancer metastasis and xenograft. *Nature*, 464, pp. 999-1005.

Douglas, A. E. (2010) *The Symbiotic Habit*. New York: Princeton University Press.

Drenos, F. and Kirkwood, T. B. (2005) Modelling the disposable soma theory of aging. *Mechanisms of Aging and Development*, 126, pp. 99-103.

Drenos, F. and Kirkwood, T. B. (2010) Selection on alleles affecting human longevity and late-life disease: the example of apolipoprotein E. *PLoS One*, 5, doi: 10.1371/journal.pone.0010022.

Du, H. *et al.* (2010) Early deficits in synaptic mitochondria in an Alzheimer's disease mouse model. *Proceedings of the National Academy of Sciences of the United States of America*, 107, pp. 18670-18675.

Dunbar, R. I. (1998) The social brain hypothesis. *Evolutionary Anthropology*, 6, pp. 178-190.

Edwards, S. and Self, D.W. (2006) Monogamy: dopamine ties the knot. *Nature Neuroscience*, 9, pp. 7-8.

Elmageed, Z. Y. *et al.* (2012) The Poly (ADP-ribose) polymerases (PARPs): New roles in intracellular transport. *Cell Signalling*, 24, pp. 1-8.

Emanuelli, M. *et al.* (2010) Nicotinamide N Methyltransferase upregulation correlates with tumor differentiation in oral squamous cell carcinoma. *Histology and Histopathology*, 25, pp. 15-20.

Estep, P. W. *et al.* (2009) Short-term calorie restriction in male mice feminizes gene expression and alters key regulators of conserved aging regulatory pathways. *PLoS One*, 4, doi: 10.1371/journal.pone.0005242.

Etheridge, E. W. (1972) *The Butterfly Castle: A Social History of Pellegra in the South*. Connecticut: Greenwood.

Fadini, G. P. *et al.* (2010) At the crossroads of longevity and metabolism: the metabolic syndrome and lifespan determinant pathways. *Aging Cell*, 10, pp. 10-17.

Facciabene, A. *et al.* (2011) Tumor hypoxia promotes tolerance and angiogenesis via CCL28 and Treg cells. *Nature*, 475, pp. 226-230.

Fassati, A. and Mitchison, N. A. (2010) Testing the theory of immune selection in cancers that break the rules of transplantation. *Caner Immunology Immunotherapy*, 59, pp. 643-651.

Feige, J. N. And Auwerx, J. (2008) Transcriptional targets of sirtuins in the coordination of mammalian physiology. *Current Opinion in Cell Biology*, 20, pp. 303-309.

Fessler, D. M. (2002) Reproductive immunosupression and diet: An evolutionary perpective on pregnancy sickness and meat consumption. *Current Anthropology*, 42, pp. 19-61.

Filley, C. M. and Anderson, C. A. (2011) Dementia: five new things. *Neurology*, 76, pp. S26-30.

Finger, B. C. *et al.* (2011) High-fat diet selectively protects against the effects of chronic social stress in the mouse. *Neuroscience*, 192, pp. 351-360.

Finkel, T. *et al.* (2009) Recent progress in the biology and physiology of sirtuins. *Nature*, 460, pp. 587-591.

Fischer, A. *et al.* (2007) Recovery of learning and memory is associated with chromatin remodelling. *Nature*, 447, pp. 178-82.

Fish, J. L. and Lockwood, C. A. (2003) Dietary constraints on encephalization in primates. *Americal Journal of Physical Anthropology*, 120, pp. 171-181.

Flatt, T. and Schmidt, P. S. (2009) Integrating evolutionary and molecular genetics of aging. *Biochimica et Biophysica Acta*, 10, pp. 951-962.

Fliessback, K. *et al.* (2007) Social comparison affects reward-related brain activity in the human ventral striatum. *Science*, 318, pp. 1305-1308.

Fogal, R. W. (2004) *The Escape from Hunger and Premature Death, 1700-2100 Europe, America and the Third World.* Cambridge: Cambridge University Press.

Fontana, L. *et al.* (2010) Extending healthy life span -from yeast to humans. *Science*, 328, pp. 321-326.

Fruscione, F., *et al.* (2011) Regulation of Human Mesenchymal Stem Cell Functions by an Autocrine Loop Involving NAD+ Release and P2y11-Mediated Signaling. Ste*m Cells and Development*, 20, pp. 1183-1198.

Fuso, A. and Scarpa, S. (2011) One-carbon metabolism and Alzheimer's disease: is it all a methylation matter? *Neurobioogy of Aging*, 32, pp. 1192-1195.

Ganesan, A. *et al.* (2009) Epigenetic therapy: histone acetylation, DNA methylation and anti-cancer drug discovery. *Current Cancer Drug Targets*, 9, pp. 963-981.

Gao, J. *et al.* (2010) A novel pathway regulates memory and plasticity via SIRT1 and miR-134. *Nature*, 466, pp. 1105-1109.

Garcia-Lara, J. M. *et al.* (2010) The metabolic syndrome. Diabetes, and Alzheimer's disease. Revista de Investigacion *Clinica*, 62, pp. 343-349.

Gatenby, R. A. *et al.* (2010) The evolutionary dynamics of cancer prevention. *Nature Reviews Cancer*, 10, pp. 526-527.

Gaulin, S. J. (1979) A Jarman-Bell model of primate feeding niches. *Human Ecology*, 7, pp. 1-20.

Gesquiere, L. R. *et al.* (2011) Life at the top: rank and stress in wild male Baboons. *Science*, 333, pp. 357-360.

Grahnert, A. *et al.* (2010) NAD+: a modulator of immune functions. *Innate Immunity*, 17, pp. 212-213.

Green, D. R. (2011) Mitochondira and the autophagy-inflammation-cell death axis in organismal aging. *Science*, 333, pp. 1109-1112.

Green, K. N. *et al.* (2008) Nicotinamide restores cognition in alzheimer's disease transgenic mice via a mechanism involving sirtuin inhibition and selective reduction of thr231-phosphotau. *Journal of Neuroscience*, 28, pp. 11500-11510.

Griguer, C. E. and Oliva, C. R. (2011) Bioenergetics pathways and therapeutic resistance in gliomas: emerging role of mitochondria. *Current Pharmaceutical Design*, 17, pp. 2421-2427.

Haar, C. V. *et al.* (2011) Continuous nicotinamide administration improves behavioural recovery and reduces lesion size following bilateral frontal controlled cortical impact injury. *Behavioural Brain Research*, 224, pp. 311-317.

Hamanaka, R, B. and Chandel, N. S. (2011) Warburg effect and redox balance. *Science* 334, pp. 1219-1220.

Hamann, K. *et al* (2011) Collaboration encourages equal sharing in children but not chimpanzees. *Nature*, 476, pp. 328-330.

Hansen, K. D. *et al.* (2011) Increased methylation variation in epigenetic domains across cancer types. *Nature Genetics*, 43, pp. 768-775.

Harris, L. T. and Fiske, S. T. (2007) Social Groups that elicit disgust are differentially processed in mPFC. *Social Cognitive and Affective Neuroscience*, 2, pp. 45-51.

Hathorn, T. *et al* (2010) Nicotinamide improves motor deficits and upregulates PGC-1α and BDNF gene expression in a mouse model of Huntington's disease. *Neurobiology of Disease*, 41, pp. 43-50.

Haung, C. *et al.* (2011) Preconditioning involves selective mitophagy mediated by Parkin and p62/SQSTM1. *PLoS One*, 6, doi: 10.1371/journal.pone.0020975.

Hochedlinger, K. *et al.* (2004) Reprogramming of a melanoma genome by nuclear transplantation. *Genes Development*, 18, pp. 1875-1885.

Hrdy, S. B. (2009) *Mothers and others: the evolutionary origins of mutual understanding*. Massachusetts: Harvard University Press.

Ieraci, A. and Herrera, D. G. (2006) Nicotinamide protects against ethanol-induced apoptotic neurodegernation in the developing mouse brain. *PLoS Medicine*, 3, doi: 0.1371/journal.pmed.0030101.

Imai, S. I. (2011) Dissecting systemic control of metabolism and aging in the NAD world: the importance of SIRT1 and NAMPT mediated NAD biosynthesis. *FEBS Letters*, 585, pp. 1657-1662.

Julien, C. *et al.* (2009) Sirtuin 1 reduction parallels the accumulation of tau in Alzheimer disease. *Journal of Neuropathology and Experimental Neurology*, 68, pp. 48-58.

Kaidi, A. *et al.* (2010) Human SIRT6 promotes DNA end resection through CtIP deacetylation. *Science*, 329, pp. 1348-1353.

Kaneko, S. *et al.* (2006) Protecting axonal degeneration by increasing nicotinamide adenine dinucleotide levels in experimental autoimmune encephalomyelitis models. *Journal of Neuroscience*, 26, pp. 9794-9804.

Kang, H. T. and Hwang, E. S. (2009) Nicotinamide enhances mitochondria quality through autophagy activation in human cells. *Aging Cell*, 8, pp. 426-438.

Kaplan, H. *et al.* (2000) A theory of human life history evolution: diet, intelligence, and longevity. *Evolutionary Anthropology*, 9, pp. 156-185.

Kapoginnus, D. and Mattson, M. P. (2011) Disrupted energy metabolism and neuronal circuit dysfunction in cognitive impairment and Alzheimer's disease. *The Lancet Neurology*, 10, pp. 187-198.

Kasting, J. F. (1988) Runaway and moist greenhouse atmospheres and the evolution of Earth and Venus. *Icarus*, 74, pp. 472-494.

Kauppinen, T. M. and Swanson, R. A. (2007) The role of poly (ADP-ribose) polymerase-1 in CNS disease. *Neuroscience*, 145, pp. 1267-1272.

Kaushik, S. *et al.* (2011) Autophagy in hypothalamic AgRP neurons regulates food intake and energy balance. *Cell Metabolism*, 14, pp. 173-183.

Kelly, D. P. (2011) Aging theories unified. *Nature*, 470, 342-343.

Kenny, P. A. *et al* (2007) Targeting the tumor microenvironment. *Frontiers in Bioscience*, 12, pp. 3468-3474.

Kim, B. *et al.* (2011) N-Nicotinoyl dopamine, a novel niacinamide derivative, retains high antioxidant activity and inhibits skin pigmentation. *Experimental Dematology*, 20, pp. 950-952.

Kim, D. *et al.* (2007) SIRT1 deacetylase protects against neurodegeneration in models for Alzheimer's disease and amyotrophic lateral sclerosis. *EMBO Journal*, 26, pp. 3169-3179.

Kirkland, J. B. (2009) Niacin status impacts chromatin structure. *Journal of Nutrition*, 139, pp. 2397-2401.

Klawitter, V. *et al.* (2006) Plasticity of the central nervous system (CNS) following perinatal asphyxia: Does nicotinamide provide neuroprotection?. *Amino Acids*, 31, pp. 377-384.

Kleinstreuer, N. C. *et al.* (2011) Identifying developmental toxicity pathways for subset of ToxCast chemicals using human embryonic stem cells and metabolomics. *Toxicology and Applied Pharmacology*, 257, pp. 111-121.

Koh, P. O. (2011) Nicotinamide attenuates the ischemic brain injury-induced decrease of Akt activation and Bad phosphorylation. *Neuroscience Letters*, 498, pp. 105-109.

Konner, M. and Eaton, S. B. (2010) Paleolithic nutrition: twenty-five years later. *Nutrition in Clinical Practice*, 25, pp. 594-602.

Koppenol, W. H. *et al* (2011) Otto Warburg's contributions to current concepts of cancer metabolism. *Nature Reviews Cancer*, 11, pp. 325-337.

Kowald, A. and Kirkwood, T. B. (2011) 'Evolution of the mitochondrial fusion-fission cycle and its role in aging. *Proceedings of the National Academy of Sciences of the United States of America*, 108, pp. 10237-10242.

Krebs, J. R. (2009) The gourmet ape: evolution and human food preferences. American *Journal of Clinical Nutrition*, 90, pp. 707-711.

Lamour, G. *et al.* (2010) Neuronal adhesion and differentiation driven by nanoscale surface free-energy gradients. *Biomaterials*, 31, pp. 3762-3771.

Lamoureux, J. A. *et al.* (2008) Prenatal choline availability alters the context sensitivity of Pavlovian conditioning in adult rats. *Learning and Memory*, 15, pp. 866-875.

Lazarov, O. *et al.* (2010) When neurogenesis encounters aging and disease. *Trends in Neuroscience*, 33, pp. 569-579.

Lee, J. H. *et al.* (2010) Lysosomal proteolysis and autophagy require presenilin 1 and are disrupted by Alzheimer-relates PS1 mutations. *Cell*, 141, pp. 1146-1158.

Lee, J. Y. *et al.* (2009) Nicotinamide reduces dopamine in postnatal hypothalamus and causes dopamine-deficient phenotype. *Neurosience Letters*, 461, pp. 163-166.

Leloup, C. *et al.* (2011) Balancing mitochondrial redox signalling: a key point in metabolic regulation. *Antioxidants and Redox Signaling*, 14, pp. 519-530.

Levine, A. J. and Puzio-Kuter, A. M. (2010) The control of the metabolic switch in cancers by oncogenes and tumor suppressor genes. *Science*, 330, pp. 1340-1344.

Li, X. and Kazgan, N. (2011) Mammalian sirtuins and energy metabolism. International *Journal of Biollogical Science*, 7, pp. 575-587.

Libert, S. *et al.* (2008) Neurogenesis directed by Sirt1. *Nature Cell Biology*, 10, pp. 373-374.

Libert, S. *et al.* (2011) SIRT1 Activates MAO-A in the brain to mediate anxiety and exploratory drive. *Cell*, 147, doi: 10.1016/j.cell.2011.10.054.

Lin, S. J. and Guarente, L. (2003) Nicotinamide adenine dinucleotide, a metabolic regulator of transcription, longevity and disease. *Current Opinion in Cell Biology*, 15, pp. 241-246.

Liu, D. *et al.* (2009) Nicotinamide Prevents NAD(+) Depletion and protects neurons against excitotoxicity and cerebral ischemia: NAD(+) consumption by SIRT1 may endanger energetically compromised neurons. *Neuromolecular Medicine*, 11, pp. 28-42.

Liu, D. *et al.* (2008) Preventing NAD(+) depletion protects neurons against excitotoxicity: bioenergetic effects of mild mitochondrial uncoupling and caloric restriction. *Annals of the New York Academy of Sciences*, 1147, pp. 275-282.

Longpre, F. *et al.* (2006) Protection by EGb 761 against beta-amyloid-induced neurotoxicity: involvement of NF-kappaB, SIRT1, and MAPKs pathways and inhibition of amyloid fibril formation. *Free Radical Biology and Medicine*, 41, pp. 1781-1794.

Lu, S.P. *et al.* (2009) Assimilation of endogenous nicotinamide riboside is essential for calorie restriction-mediated life span extension in Saccharomyces cerevisiae. *Journal of Biological Chemistry*, 284, pp. 17110-17119.

Luce, K. *et al.* (2010) Mitochondrial protein quality control systems in aging and disease. *Advances in Experimental Medicine and Biology*, 694, pp. 108-125.

Maiese, K. (2008) Triple play: promoting neurovascular longevity with nicotinamide, WNT, and erythropoietin in diabetes mellitus. *Biomedicine and Pharmacotherapy*, 62, pp. 218-232.

Malavasi, F. *et al.* (2010) The hidden life of NAD+-consuming ectoenzymes in the endocrine system. *Journal of Molecular Endocrinology*, 45, pp. 183-191.

Marie, S. K. and Shinjo, S. M. (2011) Metabolism and brain cancer. *Clinics (Sao Paula)*, 66 [Suppl 1], pp. 33-43.

Marmot, M. *et al.* (2008) Closing the gap in a generation: health equity through action on the social determinants of health. *The Lancet*, 372, pp. 1661-1669.

Masip, M. *et al.* (2010) Reprogramming with defined factors: from induced pluripotency to induced transdifferentiation. *Molecular Human Reproduction*, 16, pp. 856-868.

Mastroeni, D. *et al.* (2011) Epigenetic mechanisms in Alzheimer's disease. *Neurobiology of Aging*, 32, pp. 1161-1180.

McKeown, T. (1976) *The role of medicine: dream, mirage or nemesis*. London, England: Nuffield Provincial Hosptials Trust.

Meck, W. H. *et al.* (2007) Developmental periods of choline sensitivity provide an ontogenetic mechanism for regulating memory capacity and age-related dementia. *Frontiers in Integrative Neuroscience*, 1, pp. 7-12.

Mellman, I. *et al.* (2011) Cancer immunotherapy comes of age. *Nature*, 480, pp. 480-488.

Mellor, A. L. and Munn, D.H. (2004) IDO expression by dendritic cells: tolerance and tryptophan catabolism. *Nature Reviews Immunology*, 4, pp. 762-744.

Mentel, M. and Martin, W. (2008) Energy metabolism among eukaryotic anaerobes in the light of Proterozoic ocean chemistry. *Philosophical Transactions of the Royal Society B-Biological Sciences*, 363, pp. 2717-2729.

Merlo, L. M. *et al.* (2006) Cancer as an evolutionary and ecological process. *Nature Reviews Cancer*, 6, pp. 924-935.

Metallo, C.. and Van der Heiden, M. G. (2010) Metabolism strikes back: metabolic flux regulates cell signaling. *Genes Development*, 24, pp. 2717-2722.

Metallo, C. M. *et al.* (2011) Reductive metabolism by IDH1 mediates lipogenesis under hypoxia. *Nature*, 481, pp. 380-384.

Middleton, L.. *et al.* (2011) Activity energy expenditure and incident cognitive impairment in older adults. *Archives of Internal Medicine*, 171, pp. 1251-1257.

Michaud, M. *et al.* (2011) Autophagy-dependent anticancer immune responses induced by chemotherapeutic agents in mice. *Science*, 334, pp. 1573-1577.

Milner, J. (2009) Cellular Regulation of SIRT1. *Current Pharmaceutical Design*, 15, pp. 39-44.

Milosavljevic, A. (2011) Emerging patterns of epigenomic variation. *Trends in Genetics*, 27, pp. 242-250.

Mineur, Y. S. *et al.* (2011) Nicotine decreases food intake through activation of POMC neurons. *Science*, 332, pp. 1330-1332.

Moëll, A. *et al.* (2009) Antiviral effect of nicotinamide on enterovirus-infected human islets *in vitro*: effect on virus replication and chemokine secretion. *Journal of Medical Virology*, 81, pp. 1082-1087.

Moore, R. *et al.* (2011) Sirtuin (SIRT) 1 and steroid hormone receptor activity in cancer. *Journal of Endocrinology*, doi: 10.1530/JOE-11-0217.

Morris, M. C. *et al.* (2004) Dietary niacin and the risk of incident Alzheimer's disease and of cognitive decline. Journal of Neurology, *Neurosurgery and Psychiatry*, 75, pp. 1093-1099.

Murphy-Berman, V. *et al.* (1984) Factors affecting allocation to needy and meritorious recipients: a cross cultural comparison. *Journal of Personality and Social Psychology*, 46, pp. 1267-1272.

Murray, M.. (2003) Tryptophan depletion and HIV infection: a metabolic link to pathogenesis. *Lancet Infectious Diseases*, 3, pp. 644-652.

Navarrete, A. (2011) Energertics and the evolution of human brain size. *Nature*, 480, pp. 91-93.

Nisbett, R. E. (1993) Violence and the U. S. regional culture. *American Psychologist*, 4, pp. 441-449.

Noakes, T. D. (2011) Time to move beyond a brainless exercise physiology: the evidence for complex regulation of human exercise performance. *Applied Physiology, Nutrition, and Metabolism*, 36, pp. 23-35.

Noble, M. *et al.* (2005) Redox regulation of precursor cell function: Insights and paradoxes. *Antioxidants and Redox Signaling*, 7, pp. 1456-1467.

Noriega, L. G. *et al.* (2011) CREB and ChREBP oppositely regulate SIRT1 expression in response to energy availability. *EMBO Reports*, 12, pp. 1069-1076.

Northcutt, R. G. (2011) Evolving large and complex brains. Science; 332, pp. 926-927.

Nurse, P. (2008) Life, logic and information. *Nature*, 454, pp. 424-426.

Okuda, H. *et al.* (2009) Environmental enrichment stimulates progenitor cell proliferation in the amygdala. *Journal of Neuroscience Research*, 87, pp. 3546-3553.

Orabona, C. and Grohmann, U. (2011) Indoleamine 2,3-dioxygenase and regulatory function: tryptophan starvation and beyond. *Methods Molecular Biology*, 677, pp. 269-280.

Outeiro, T. F. *et al.* (2007a) Pharmacological inhibition of PARP-1 reduces alpha-synucleinand MPP+-induced cytotoxicity in Parkinson's disease *in vitro* models. *Biochemical and Biophysical Research Communications*, 357, pp. 596-602.

Outeiro, T. F. *et al.* (2007b) Sirtuin 2 inhibitors rescue alpha-synuclein-mediated toxicity in models of Parkinson's disease. *Science*, 317, pp. 516-519.

Palacios, O. M. *et al.* (2009) Diet and exercise signals regulate SIRT3 and activate AMPK and PGC-1alpha in skeletal muscle. *Aging*, 1, pp. 771-783.

Park, G. *et al.* (2011) SIRT1 deficiency attenuates MPP+-induced apoptosis in dopaminergic cells. *FEBS Letters*, 585, 219-224.

Parsons, R. B. *et al.* (2002) Expression of nicotinamide N-methyltransferase (E.C. 2.1.1.1) in the Parkinsonian brain. *Journal of Neuropathology Experimental Neurology*, 61, pp. 111-124.

Passamonti, L. *et al.* (2012) Effects of acute tryptophan depletion on prefrontal-amygdala connectivity while viewing facial signals of aggression. *Biological Psychiatry*, 71, pp. 36-43.

Patin, E. and Quintana-Murci, L. (2008) Demeter's legacy: rapid changes to our genome imposed by diet. *Trends in Ecology and Evolution*, 23, pp. 56-59.

Paul, L. (2011) Diet, nutrition and telomere length. *Journal of Nutritional Biochemistry*, 22, pp. 895-901.

Penberthy, W. T. and Tsunoda, I. (2009) The importance of NAD in multiple sclerosis. *Current Pharmaceutical Design*, 15, pp. 64-99.

Perluigi, M. *et al.* (2010) Redox proteomics in aging rat brain: involvement of mitochondrial reduced glutathione status and mitochondrial protein oxidation in the aging process. *Journal of Neuroscience Research*, 88, pp. 3498-3507.

Pester, M. and Brune, A. (2007) Hydrogen is the central free intermediate during lignocellulose degradation by termite gut symbionts. *ISME Journal*, 1, pp. 551-565.

Peto, R. *et al.* (1975) Cancer and aging in mice and men. *British Journal of Cancer*, 32, pp. 411-426.

Poss, K. D. (2010) Advances in understanding tissue regenerative capacity and mechanism in animals. *Nature Reviews Genetics*, 11, pp. 710-722.

Poulsen, P. *et al.* (2007) The epigenetic basis of twin discordance in age-related diseases. *Pediatric Research*, 61, pp. 38-42.

Pozzi, V. *et al.* (2011) Inhibiting proliferation in KB cancer cells by RNA interference-medicated knockdown of nicotinamide n-methyitransferase expression. *International Journal of Immunopathology and Pharmacology*, 24, pp. 69-77.

Prendergast, G. (2011) Why tumours eat tryptophan. *Nature*, 478, pp. 192-194.

Previc, F. H. (1999) Dopamine and origins of human intelligence. *Brain Cognition*, 41, pp. 299-350.

Prozorovski, T. *et al.* (2008) Sirt1 contributes critically to the redox-dependent fate of neural progenitors. *Nature Cell Biology*, 10, pp. 385-395.

Rabinowitz, J. D. and White, E. (2010) Autophagy and metabolism. *Science*, 330, pp. 1344-1348.

Rafalski, V. A. and Brunet, A. (2011) Energy metabolism in adult neural stem cell fate. *Progress in Neurobiology*, 93, pp. 182-203.

Raghanti, M. A. *et al.* (2011) Comparative analysis of the nucleus basalis of meynert among primates. *Neuroscience*, 184, pp. 1-15.

Raghanti, M. A. *et al.* (2010) Cortical dopaminergic innervation among humans, chimpanzee, and macaque monkeys: a comparative study. *Neuroscience*, 506, pp. 203-220.

Rajakumar, K. (2000) Pellagra in the United States: a historical perspective. *Southern Medical Journal*, 93, pp. 272-277.

Raubenheimer, D. *et al.* (2005) Does Bertrand's rule apply to macronutrients?. *Proceedings of the Royal Society B-Biological Sciences*, 272, pp. 2429-2434.

Read, D. W. (2011) *How Culture Makes Us Human*. Canada: Left Coast Press Inc.

Richardson, A. D. and Scott, D. A. (2011) Reversing the Warburg effect through stromal autophagy. *Cell Cycle*, 10, pp. 2830-2831.

Riederer, M. *et al.* (2009) Adipose tissue as a source of nicotinamide N-methyltransferase and homocysteine. *Atherosclerosis*, 204, pp. 12-17.

Rodgers, J. T. *et al.* (2005) Nutrient control of glucose homeostasis through a complex of PGC-1α and SIRT1. *Nature* 434, pp. 113-118.

Roseboom, T. J. *et al.* (2011) Hungry in the womb: What are the consequences Lessons from the Dutch famine. *Maturitas*, 70, pp. 141-145.

Roth, J. *et al.* (2011) Energy, evolution, and human diseases: an overview. *American Journal of Clinical Nutrition*, 93, pp. S875-883.

Rottiers, V. *et al.* (2011) MicroRNAs in metabolism and metabolic diseases. *Cold Spring Harbor Symposia on Quantitative Biology*, doi: 10. 1101/sqb. 2011.76.011049.

Rozwarski, D. A. *et al.* (1998) Modification of the NADH of the Isoniazid Target (InhA) from Mycobacterium tuberculosis. *Science*, 279, pp. 98-101.

Sachs, J. L. *et al.* (2011) New paradigms for the evolution of beneficial infections. *Trends in Ecology and Evolution*, 26, pp. 153-210.

Salminen, A. and Kaarniranta, K. (2009) SIRT1: Regulation of longevity via autophagy. *Cellular Signalling*, 21, pp. 1356-1360.

Sasaki, T. and Kitamura, T. (2010) Roles of FoxO1 and Sirt 1 in the central regulation of food intake. *Endocrinology Journal*, 57, pp. 939-946.

Sasidharan, K. *et al.* (2012) 'Time-structure of the yeast metabolism *in vivo*. *Advances in Experimental Medicine and Biology*, 736, pp. 359-379.

Sassone-Corsi, P. (2012) NAD^+, a Circadian metabolite with an epigenetic twist. *Endocrinology*, 153, pp. 1-5.

Satoh, A. *et al.* (2010) SIRT1 promotes the central adaptive response to diet restriction through activation of the dorsomedial and lateral nuclei of the hypothalamus. *Journal of Neuroscience*, 30, pp. 10220-10232.

Sauro, M. D. and Greenburg, R. P. (2005) Endogenous opiates and the placebo effect: a meta-analytic review. *Journal of Psychosomatic Research*, 58, pp. 115-120.

Schrack, J. A. *et al.* (2010) The energetic pathway to mobility loss: an emerging new framework for longitudinal studies on aging. *Journal of the American Geriatrics Society*, 58, pp. 329-336.

Schreiber, R. D. *et al.* (2011) Cancer immunoediting: integrating immunity's roles in cancer suppression and promotion. *Science*, 331, pp. 1565-1570.

Schuler, G. (2010) Dendritic cells in cancer immunotherapy. *European Journal of Immunology*, 40, pp. 2123-2130.

Seal, A. J. *et al.* (2007) Low and deficient niacin status and pellagra are endemic in post-war Angola. *American Journal of Clinical Nutrition*, 85, 218-224.

Segovia, G. *et al.* (2009) Environmental enrichment, prefrontal cortex, stress, and aging of the brain. *Journal of Neural Transmission*, 116, pp. 1007-1016.

Shinmura, K. *et al.* (2011) Caloric restriction primes mitochondria for ischemic stress by deactelyating specific mitochondrial proteins of the electron transport chain. *Circulation Research*, 109, pp. 396-406.

Sol, D. (2009) Revisiting the cognitive buffer hypothesis for the evolution of large brains. *Biology Letters*, 5, pp. 130-133.

Sorolla, M. A. *et al.* (2011) Sir2 induced by oxidative stress in a yeast model of Huntington disease and its activation reduces protein aggregation. *Archives of Biochemistry and Biophysics*, 510, pp. 27-34.

Soto, A. M. and Sonnenschein, C. (2011) The tissue organization field theory of cancer: a testable replacement for the somatic mutation theory. *Bioessays*, 33, pp. 332-340.

Speakman, J. R. and Krol, E. (2011) Limits to sustained energy intake. XIII. Recent progress and future perspectives. *Journal of Experimental Biology*, 214, pp. 230-241.

Stadtfeld, M. and Hochedlinger, K. (2010) Induced pluripotency: history, mechanisms, and applications. *Genes Development*, 24, pp. 2239-2263.

Stiner, M. C. *et al.* (2009) Cooperative hunting and meat sharing 400-200kya at Qesem Cave, *Israel. Proceedings of the National Academy of Sciences of the United States of America*, 106, pp. 13207-13212.

Stover, P. J. (2009) One-carbon metabolism-genome interactions in folate-associated pathologies. *Journal of Nutrition*, 139, pp. 2402-2405.

Suchankova, G. *et al.* (2009) Concurrent regulation of AMP-activated protein kinase and SIRT1 in mammalian cells. *Biochemical and Biophysical Research Communications*, 378, pp. 836-841.

Surmeier, D. J. *et al.* (2011) The role of calcium and mitochondrial oxidant stress in the loss of substantia nigra pars compacta dopaminergic neurons in Parkinson's disease. *Neuroscience*, 198, pp. 221-231.

Syvester, R. J. (2011) Bacillus calmette-Guerin treatment of non-muscle invasive bladder cancer. *International Journal of Urology*, 18, pp. 13-120.

Szyf, M. (2011) The implications of DNA methylation for toxicology: toward toxicomethylomics, the toxicology of DNA methylation. *Toxicological Science*, 120, pp. 235-255.

Tang, S. W. *et al.* (2011) Nicotinamide N-methyltransferase induces cellular invasion through activating matrix metalloproteinase-2 expression in clear cell renal cell carcinoma cells. *Carcinogenesis*, 32, pp. 138-145.

Tracey, K. J. (2011) Cell biology. Ancient neurons regulate immunity. *Science*, 332, 673-674.

Torrence, R. (1989) Re-tooling: Towards a behavioural theory of stone tools. In: Torrence, R. (ed) *Time, Energy and Stone Tools*. Cambridge: Cambridge University Press, pp. 57-66.

Turgut, O. *et al.* (2011) Preconditioning, postconditioning, stunning and hibernation: towards an integrated insight into the mechanisms of hypoperfusion/reperfusion. *International Journal of Cardiology*, 146, pp. 442-443.

Ullah, N. *et al.* (2011) Nicotinamide inhibits alkylating agent-induced apoptotic neurodegeneration in the developing rat brain. *PLoS One*, 6, doi: 10.1371/journal.pone.0027093.

Ungar, P. S. and Sponheimer, M. (2011) The Diets of Early Hominins. *Science*, 334, pp. 190-193.

Vaisitti T., *et al.* (2011) NAD(+)-metabolizing ecto-enzymes shape tumor-host interactions: The chronic lymphocytic leukemia model. *FEBS Letters*, 585, pp. 1514-1520.

van Driel, L. M. *et al.* (2008) Eight-fold increased risk for congenital heart defects in children carrying the nicotinamide N-methyltransferase polymorphism and exposed to medicines and low nicotinamide. *European Heart Journal*, 29, pp. 1424-1431.

van Leeuwen, I. M. *et al.* (2010) Dynamic energy budget approaches for modelling organismal aging. *Philosophical Transactions of the Royal Society of London*, 12, pp. 3443-3454.

van Os, J. *et al.* (2010) The environment and schizophrenia. *Nature*, 468, 203-212.

van der Haiden, M. G. (2011) Targeting cancer metabolism: a therapeutic window opens. *Nature Reviews Drug Discovery*, 10, pp. 671-684.

Vassilopoulos, A. *et al.* (2011) The human sirtuin family: Evolutionary divergences and functions. *Human Genomics*, 5, pp. 485-496.

Veeraraghavulu, K. *et al.* (2010) Presenilin 1 mutants impair the self-renewal and differentiation of adult murine subventricular zone-neuronal progenitors via cell-autonomous mechanisms involving notch signaling. *Journal of Neuroscience*, 30, pp. 6903-6915.

Verdin, E. *et al.* (2010). Sirtuin regulation of mitochondria: energy production, apoptosis, and signalling. *Trends in Biochemical Science*, 35, pp. 669-675.

Vinciguerra, M. *et al.* N (2010) SirT1 in muscle physiology and disease: lessons from mouse models. *Disease Models and Mechanisms*, 3, pp. 298-303.

Wallace, D. C. (2010) Bioenergetics and the epigenome: interface between the environment and genes in common diseases. *Developmental Disabilities Research Reviews*, 16, pp. 114-119.

Wallace, T. C. *et al.* (2011) Human gut microbiota and its relationship to health and disease. *Nutritional Reviews*, 69, pp. 392-403.

Wan, P. *et al.* (2011) Pellagra: a review with emphasis on photosensitivity. *British Journal of Dematology*, 164, pp. 1188-1200.

Wang, Y. *et al.* (2011) SIRT1 and AMPK in regulating mammalian senescene: A critical review and a working model. *FEBS Letters*, 585, pp. 986-994.

Wang, Z. *et al.* (2011) Gut flora metabolism of phosphatidylcholine promotes cardiovascular disease. *Nature*, 472, pp. 57-63.

Waring, R. H. *et al.* (1989) S-methylation in motorneuron disease and Parkinson's disease. *Lancet*, 2, pp. 356-357.

Watts, A. G. and Donovan, C. M. (2010) Sweet talk in the brain: glucosensing, neural networks, and hypoglycemic counterregulation. *Frontiers in Neuroendocrinology*, 31, 32-43.

Wen, Y. *et al.* (2011) Nmnat exerts neuroprotective effects in dendrites and axons. *Molecular Cell Neuroscience*, 48, pp. 1-8.

West, A. A. and Caudill, M. A. (2011) Genetic Variation: Impact on Folate (and Choline) Bioefficacy. *International Journal of Vitamin Nutritional Research*, 80, pp. 319-329.

Wiessner, P. (2002) 'Hunting, Healing and hxaro exchange: a long term perspective on Kung (Hu/'hoansi) large-game hunting. *Evolution and Human Behavior*, 23, pp. 407-436.

Williams, A. C. and Ramsden, D. B. (2005) Nicotinamide homeostasis: a xenobiotic pathway that is key to development and degenerative diseases. *Medical Hypotheses*, 65, pp. 353-362.

Winder, R. and Borrill, J. (1998) Fuels for memory: the role of oxygen and glucose in memory enhancement. *Psychopharmacology*, 136, pp. 349-356.

Winner, B. *et al.* (2011) Neurodegenerative disease and adult neurogenesis. *European Journal of Neuroscience*, 33, pp. 1139-1151.

Yahata, N. *et al.* (2009) Nicotinamide Mononucleotide Adenylyltransferase Expression in Mitochondrial Matrix Delays Wallerian Degeneration. *Journal of Neuroscience*, 29, pp. 6276-6284.

Yamamoto, K. and Vernier, P. (2011) The evolution of dopamine systems in chordates. *Frontiers in Neuroanatomy*, 5, doi: 10.3389/fnana.2011.00021.

Yan, H. *et al.* (2009) Mutant metabolic enzymes are at the origin of gliomas. *Cancer Research*, 69, pp. 9157-9159.

Yang, J. *et al.* (2004) Early administration of nicotinamide prevents learning and memory impairment in mice induced by 1-methyl-4-phenyl-1,2,3,6-tetrahydropyridine. *Pharmacology, Biochemistry, and Behavior,* 78, pp. 179-183.

Yap, I. K. *et al.* (2010) Urinary metabolic phenotyping differentiates children with autism from their unaffected siblings and age-matched controls. *Journal of Proteome Research*, 9, pp. 2996-3004.

Zeisel, S. H. (2011) Nutritional genomics: defining the dietary requirements and effects of choline. *Journal of Nutrition*, 141, pp. 531-534.

Zhang, L. *et al.* (2007) The relation between nicotinamide N-methyltransferase gene polymorphism and plasma homocysteine concentration in healthy Japanese men. *Thrombosis Research*, 121, pp. 55-58.

Zhang, L. Q. *et al.* (2011) Nicotinamide phosphoribosyltransferase in human diseases. *Journal of Bioanalysis and Biomedicine*, 3, pp. 13-25.

In: Hypotheses in Clinical Medicine
Editors: M.M. Shoja, P.S. Agutter et al.

ISBN: 978-1-62257-276-2

Chapter 7

Population Genetics, Cancer Cell Growth and Cancer Evolution

Christopher Naugler*
Department of Pathology and Laboratory Medicine,
University of Calgary and Calgary Laboratory Services, Canada

Abstract

Darwinian evolution provides a powerful paradigm for the generation of new hypotheses in clinical medicine. Cancer cell growth and evolution is one area particularly amenable to this approach. This is largely because cancer cell clones behave like asexual sympatric species, evolving to higher levels of fitness while competing with other cancer cell clones and host tissues. The application of theoretical population genetics to the evolution of cancer cell clones leads to a number of novel, testable hypotheses. The first of these is that favorable mutations are expected to become established more rapidly in smaller populations. This suggests that cancer cell clonal evolution may be faster in smaller tumors or in tumors with greater clonal heterogeneity. Cancer cell clonal evolution could also occur as a result of genetic drift or of different intrinsic rates of increase among different cancer cell clones. The latter mechanism could be explored using mixed cell cultures. The relative importance of these differing drivers of clonal evolution could be explored by looking for genetic evidence of selection pressure as evidenced by varying rates of synonymous and non-synonymous base substitutions. Similarly, a number of techniques exist to reconstruct the clonal relationships of cancer cells and thereby reconstruct the evolutionary history of individual tumors. Finally, if we consider a stem cell model of clonal evolution, it is predicted that clonal evolution may be faster in such a model because there are relatively few stem cells compared to the bulk of non-stem (somatic) cells within the tumor.

* E-mail: christopher.naugler@cls.ab.ca.

Introduction

Darwinian evolution has provided a unifying concept in biology for a century and a half. As the geneticist Theodosius Dobzhansky (1973) wrote almost 40 years ago: "Seen in the light of evolution, biology is, perhaps, intellectually the most satisfying and inspiring science. Without that light it becomes a pile of sundry facts some of them interesting or curious but making no meaningful picture as a whole." Likewise, Darwinian evolution has the (largely unfulfilled) potential to be a unifying concept in medicine (Charlton 1997).

Aside from the potential as a theoretical foundation for medicine, there are two examples in clinical medicine where evolution by natural selection is not only relevant to treatment and prevention, but also occurs on a time scale rapid enough to be easily observable by clinicians. The first example involves the evolution of antibiotic resistance and pathogen virulence. This topic has been reviewed by a number of authors (Ewald 1994; Normark and Normark 2002; Wilkins 1996) and will not be expanded on here. Rather, the present offering will concentrate on a second clinically relevant example of Darwinian evolution in disease: the evolution of cancer cell clones. It may be useful at this point to clarify the distinction between cancer cells and cancer cell clones. Cancer cells are the individual neoplastic cells making up a tumor. They may be divided into one or more cell clones, which are populations of cancer cells derived from a common ancestor within the tumor, sharing similar genetic and phenotypic traits. It is the cancer cell clones that are presumed to be the units of selection within the cancer.

It is widely accepted that cancer cell clones evolve over the life span of a tumor and are under a number of selective pressures, which may include immune system attacks, treatment (surgery, radiation, chemotherapy), competition from other cells in the tumor, and competition from surrounding non-neoplastic cells (Merlo et al. 2006; Greaves 2006; Crespi and Summers 2005). The result is that cancer cells evolve to higher levels of "fitness", meaning greater ability to survive and reproduce, with the sequelae of increasing disruption of the host body. In fact, mutations "favorable" to a cancer cell may of course be detrimental to the ultimate survival of the host (because these mutations will commonly aid in overcoming anti-cancer defense mechanisms). As Merlo et al. (2006) argued, "It might be that most genes in the human genome are devoted to building and maintaining a multicellular body, and are therefore irrelevant to a neoplastic cell under selection for increased survival and proliferation".

Cancer is then, by definition, a problem of multicellularity. Elaborate constraints have evolved to control cell replication and maturation within the multicellular body. Once stripped of the fetters that control cell division, cancer cells embark on a wild Darwinian ride. Within a cancer, life is quite literally unleashed. In the remainder of this chapter, hypotheses are explored that follow from this line of thought and suggestions are given for ways in which some of these hypotheses could be tested.

Are Cancer Cells Separate Species?

Cancer cell clones can be thought of as analogous to sympatric asexual species (Crespi and Summers 2005). Some authors have taken this argument even further to assert that cancer cells do not merely behave like asexual species; they are in fact a different species. A review and theoretical background of this concept was recently presented by Vincent (2010) who wrote: "If the conventional wisdom is that cancers evolve, it is remarkable how rarely this is taken to its logical conclusion: that carcinogenesis is in fact a form of speciation and the clonal varieties of cancer cell which subsequently evolve (spontaneously or under treatment) are also novel species." Vincent (2010) goes on to argue that cancer cells may even constitute a separate major taxonomic group tentatively termed the dyskaryota (Vincent 2010).

There are, in fact, numerous examples where cancer cells have acted essentially like parasitic species, having been transmitted from one human to another. In one case, a malignant fibrous histiocytoma was accidentally transplanted into a surgeon's hand during an operation to remove the tumor from a patient (Gartner et al. 1996); in another, a colonic adenocarcinoma was transmitted via a needle-stick injury (Gugel and Sanders 1986). A number of cases of accidental transmission of cancer also exist in association with solid organ transplants (Moranth et al. 2005) and hematopoietic stem cell transplants (McMilan 2002). In these cases, approximately one third of accidentally transplanted cancers continue to grow in the new host (Welsh 2011). Tragically, fatal melanoma has been transplanted intentionally from a terminally ill woman to her mother with the intention of studying cancer immunity (Scanlon et al. 1965).

In addition to these cases of the accidental transplantation of cancer, two circumstances of transmissible cancer in nature are also relevant to this discussion. The first is canine transmissible venereal tumor (CTVT) (Murgin et al. 2006), a cancer cell line that is sexually transmitted among dogs. It has been suggested that the genetic distinctiveness of this cell line would qualify as a new canine species (Frank 2007).

A second example of a cancer directly transmitted from animal to animal is devil facial tumor disease (DFTD), a cancer cell line directly transmitted among the Tasmanian marsupial carnivores known as Tasmanian devils (Murchison et al. 2010). The disfiguring tumors of DFTD are concentrated around the animal's mouth and interfere with its ability to feed, resulting in death within a few months. This cancer appears to be transplanted directly from the face of one animal to the face of another by bites inflicted during feeding.

It may be an academic argument whether cancer cells behave like asexual sympatric species or actually are asexual sympatric species. However, if we accept that cancer cells at least behave like asexual sympatric species, it follows that hypotheses about the growth dynamics and evolution of cancer could be derived from population genetics as it pertains to asexual evolution. Models of so-called "island biogeography" provide an interesting analogy here. In evolutionary biology, models of island biogeography propose that islands acquire species through both immigration and speciation (Rosendell and Phillimore 2011). Cancer cell evolution primarily involves events analogous to speciation rather than immigration. However, the multiple examples of transmissible cancer reviewed above suggest that immigration may be a barrier primarily because of opportunity. In essence, the islands (human bodies) are too far apart to facilitate cancer cell immigration under most circumstances. But as described above, given the proper opportunity, the direct transmission of cancer cells is possible.

Evolution of Cancer Cells

In humans, as in other sexually reproducing organisms, meiosis randomly assorts mutations among offspring and natural selection then removes deleterious mutations through differential survival of those offspring. As Muller (1932) pointed out nearly 80 years ago, asexually reproducing organisms lack a mechanism to remove deleterious mutations from their ranks. The resulting tendency of asexual organisms to accumulate deleterious mutations is known as Muller's Ratchet. However, as pointed out previously, ostensibly "deleterious" mutations may not be deleterious to a cancer cell if they result in the shedding of an unnecessary metabolic process.

Population genetics theory predicts that following an initial favorable mutation in an asexual population, the establishment of a second favorable mutation is predicted by the equation $G = \log (N/s)$ (Smith 1978), where G = the number of generations, N = population size, and s = the selective advantage of the new mutation. From this equation, the hypothesis follows that the establishment of favorable mutations may be faster in smaller populations. In the context of cancer cell evolution, the logical corollary is that favorable mutations may become established more quickly in smaller tumors (Naugler 2010). Furthermore, the faster clonal evolution in smaller tumors could also mean that in the fragmented (i.e. smaller) subpopulations associated with genetic heterogeneity, new mutations may become established at a faster rate, thus adding to the malignant potential of genetically heterogeneic tumors. Indeed, several previous studies have reported an association between tumor heterogeneity and malignant potential (Maley et al. 2006; Park et al. 2010).

Mutations that are selectively neutral or deleterious to the cancer cell could still increase in the population due to genetic drift. For mutations that are deleterious, genetic drift will tend to fix a mutation if $U/s > 1$ (Smith 1978) where U = the total number of mutations per genome and s = the selection pressure against individual mutations. From this, we can derive the hypothesis that, even in the absence of positive selection pressure, tumors may be expected to accumulate unfavorable mutations (for instance mutations that decrease the aggressiveness of the tumor) over time by genetic drift alone.

Another mechanism by which one asexually reproducing species may come to replace another (or in this case one tumor cell clone replace another) is a difference in the relative rates of growth. In population genetics parlance the rate of population growth is known as the intrinsic rate of increase and is described by the equation $dx/dt = rx$ (Smith 1989) where dx is the change in the number of individuals over time, dt is the time interval, r is the intrinsic rate of increase and x is the starting population size. For two cancer cell clones (A and a) with overlapping generations, the rate of change expressed as the change in proportion of A to a is given by the equation $G = [\ln (P_t/(1-P_t) - \ln (P_0/(1- P_0)] / (r_A - r_a)$ (Felsenstein 2009), where G = the number of cell generations, P_0 = the starting proportion of the two clones, P_t = the final proportion of the two clones, r_A = the intrinsic rate of increase of clone A and r_a = the intrinsic rate of increase of clone a. Therefore, if we know the relative rates of growth of two different cancer cell clones, we should be able to predict how quickly one will come to replace the other within a cancer (Naugler 2010). An interesting *in vitro* test of this idea would be to measure the relative rates of increase of different cancer cell cultures and then grow the cell cultures under mixed population conditions.

It is widely believed that the clonal progression of cells within a cancer is driven by sequential bottlenecks at which selection for the best adapted cancer cell clones could occur (Merlo et al. 2006; Crespi and Summers 2005). Although the strength of natural selection among tumor cell clones has not been experimentally measured, hypothetical population changes in cancer cell clones can be modeled on the basis of varying levels of selection pressure. Selection is here defined as the relative advantage of one clone over another. Thus, if a given clone is said to have a selective advantage of 0.01, this means that, on average, members of that clone will pass on 1% more offspring to the next generation compared to a second clone. The change in clonal frequency (expressed as the change in proportion of clone A to clone a) is described by the equation $G = [\ln(P_A^{(t)}/P_a^{(t)}) - \ln(P_A^{(0)}/P_a^{(0)})] / \ln(1+s)$ (Felsenstein 2009), where G = the number of generations, $P_A^{(0)}$ = the initial proportion of clone A, $P_a^{(0)}$ = the initial proportion of clone a, $P_A^{(t)}$ = the final proportion of clone A, $P_a^{(t)}$ = the final proportion of clone a, and s = the selective advantage of clone A over clone a. Again, *in vitro* cell culture experiments utilizing cell clones with specific mutations could provide a very instructive test of this hypothesis.

Finally, mention should be made of the notion of quasispecies. Quasispecies can be defined as "stationary (equilibrium) mutant distributions of infinite size, centered around one or more master sequences" (Domingo 2002). Quasispecies theory developed to explain the evolutionary behavior of error-prone RNA virus replication. There may be analogies to cancer cell clones because of the frequent mutations present within cancer cell clones, which may therefore exhibit a consensus sequence in a similar sense to virus species. This concept has not been explored in the context of cancer clonal evolution but may warrant a closer look.

Inferring the Evolutionary History of Cancer Cells

Several studies have shown that cancers are often polyclonal (Khalique et al. 2009; Thirwell et al. 2010); at least some cancers begin as monoclonal collections of cells and become polyclonal over time (Khalique et al. 2009). There remains great scope for studies that attempt to reconstruct the clonal evolutionary histories of cancers surgically removed from patients. A number of methodologies have been employed to infer the evolutionary relationships of groups of cancer cells including immunohistochemistry/combined immunofluorescence staining and fluorescence in-situ hybridization (iFISH) (Park et al. 2010), DNA methylation pattern (Hong et al. 2010), microsatellite mutation (Shibata 2002; Tsao et al. 2000, Matsumoto et al. 2004), arbitrarily primed PCR (Tarafa et al. 2003; Arribas et al. 1997), comparative genomic hybridization (Tarafa et al. 2003; Desper et al. 2000; Jaing et al. 2000), and flow cytometry (Tarafa et al. 2003). In some studies, a combination of these techniques has been employed.

Some researchers have taken the innovative step of utilizing population biology measures of diversity such as the Shannon index and Simpson index to quantify intra-tumor clonal diversity (Park et al. 2010). In Park's study (2010), a number of associations were found between measures of diversity and histopathological variables such as nuclear polymorphism and tissue necrosis.

How Can Selection Be Measured in a Cancer?

Whether cancer clones replace each other because of different intrinsic rates of increase or because of differences in the level of selection may be of interest. A possible method to distinguish between these mechanisms is suggested by the prediction that a high level of selection among cancer cell clones would be expected to leave evidence of selection at the genetic level in the form of different rates of synonymous and non-synonymous base substitutions among different clones in the same tumor. The existence of such a difference in substitution rates would provide evidence of selection pressure on a given clone versus a difference in intrinsic rates of increase. This technique may offer a novel and powerful method for detecting positive selection in cancer cell clones. The caveat of course is that one could only comment on the strength of selection acting on the nucleotide sequence in question. Comparison of the strength of selection in early and late cancers could also provide a way of mapping the relative selection pressures of cancer cell clones as they evolve. Although we might expect that selection pressure acting on cancer cells would be in the form of purifying selection (to preserve gene function in the face of the anticipated large number of mutations within a cancer), the comparison of the relative rates of synonymous and non-synonymous base substitutions would also allow diversifying selection or neutral drift to be detected, each of which would provide valuable information regarding the selection processes acting on cancer cells.

Stem Cells

Cancer stem cell models posit that cancers, like normal tissues, are composed of a subset of relatively undifferentiated stem cells. Asymmetric division of these cells both maintains the stem cell pool and provides cells that differentiate further into the majority of cells in the tumor (Reya et al. 2001; Dick 2008). This process has been contrasted with the clonal evolution model where all cells may contribute to clonal progression of the tumor (Shackleton et al. 2009). Perhaps the nomenclature is somewhat misleading in this discussion as clonal evolution may be expected to occur in both models; however, in the stem cell model, it is only the stem cells rather than all cells in the cancer that participate in this evolution (Shackleton et al. 2009; Naugler 2010; Greaves 2010). If we consider a cancer stem cell model where clonal evolution is occurring only in a subset of the cancer cells (the stem cells), we can hypothesize that because of the much smaller number of stem cells, clonal evolution is predicted to be faster in stem cells than non-stem cells (Naugler 2010). Moreover, as cancer cells evolve into a more aggressive phenotype with greater inherent genomic instability, non-stem cells may acquire stem cell phenotypes and thereby blur the line between stem cells and non-stem cells (Shipitsin and Polyak 2008).

Conclusion

Darwinian evolution provides a rich theoretical background that can be applied to the generation of hypotheses in clinical medicine. The evolution of cancer cell clones is an area where this approach may prove especially fruitful. Here, hypotheses have been described that follow from the application of theoretical population genetics to the evolution of cancer cell clones, and some experimental ways to test these hypotheses have been suggested.

References

Arribas, R. et al. (1997) Assessment of genomic damage in colorectal cancer by DNA fingerprinting: prognostic applications. *Journal of Clinical Oncology*, 15, pp. 3230-3240.

Charlton, B. G. (1997) A syllabus for evolutionary medicine. *Journal of the Royal Society of Medicine*, 90, pp. 397-399.

Crespi, B. and Summers, K. (2005) Evolutionary biology of cancer. *Trends on Ecology and Evolution*, 20, pp. 545-552.

Desper, R. et al. (2000) Distance-based reconstruction of tree models for oncogenesis. *Journal of Computational Biology*, 7, pp. 789-803.

Dick, J. E. (2008) Stem cell concepts renew cancer research. *Blood*, 112, pp. 4793-4807.

Dobzhansky, T. (1973) Nothing in biology makes sense except in the light of evolution. *American Biology Teacher*, 35, pp. 125-129.

Domingo, E. (2002) Quasispecies theory in virology. *Journal of Virology*, 76, pp. 463-465.

Ewald, P. W. (1994) *Evolution of Infectious Disease*. Oxford: Oxford University Press.

Felsenstein, J. (2009) *Theoretical Evolutionary Genetics*. [www] University of Washington. Available from: http://rogov.zwz.ru/Macroevolution/felsenstein2.pdf[Accessed8/ 26/ 2011].

Frank, U. (2007) The evolution of a malignant dog. *Evolution & Development*, 9, pp. 521-522.

Gartner H. V. et al. (1996) Genetic analysis of a sarcoma accidentally transplanted from a patient to a surgeon. *The New England Journal of Medicine,* 335, pp. 1494-1496.

Greaves, M. (2006) *Cancer. The Evolutionary Legacy*. Cambridge and London: Oxford University Press.

Greaves, M. (2010) Cancer stem cells *Seminars in Cancer Biology, 20, pp. 65-70.*

Gugel, E. A. and Sanders, M. E. (1986) Needle-stick transmission of human colonic adenocarcinoma. *The New England Journal of Medicine*, 315, p. 1487.

Hong, Y. T. et al. (2010) Using DNA methylation patterns to infer tumor ancestry. *Public Library of Science One*, 5, doi: 10.1371/journal.pone. 0012002.

Jiang, F. et al. (2000) Construction of evolutionary tree models for renal cell carcinoma from comparative hybridization data. *Cancer Research*, 60, pp. 6503-6509.

Khalique, L. et al. (2009) The clonal evolution of metastases from primary serous epithelial ovarian cancers. *International Journal of Cancer*, 124, pp. 1579-1586.

Maley, C. C. et al. (2006) Genetic clonal diversity predicts progression to esophageal adenocarcinoma. *Nature Genetics*, 38, pp. 468-473.

Matsumoto, T. et al. (2004) Loss of heterozygosity analysis shows monoclonal evolution with frequent genetic progression and divergence in esophageal carcinocarcinoma. *Human Pathology*, 35, pp. 322-327.

Mcmilan, K. (2002) Allogeneic hematopoietic stem cell transplantation and the risk for transmission of heritable malignancy. *Transfusion,* 42, pp. 495-504.

Merlo, L. M. F. et al. (2006) Cancer as an evolutionary and ecological process. *Nature Reviews - Cancer*, 6, pp. 924-935.

Moranth, C. et al. (2005) Transmission of malignancy with solid organ transplants. *Transplantation*, 80 [Suppl1], pp. 164-166.

Murchison, E. P. et al. (2010) The Tasmanian devil transcriptome reveals Schwann cell origins of a clonally transmissible cancer. *Science,* 327, pp. 84-87.

Muller, H. J. (1932) Further studies on the nature and causes of gene mutations. In: Jones, D. F. (ed.) *Proceedings of the Sixth International Congress of Genetics.* Menagha, Wisconsin: Brooklyn Botanic Gardens, pp. 213-255.

Murgin, C. et al. (2006) Clonal origin and evolution of a transmissible cancer. *Cell,* 126, pp. 477-487.

Naugler, C. (2010) Population genetics of cancer cell clones: possible implications of cancer stem cells. *Theoretical Biology and Medical Modeling*, 7, doi: 10.1186/1742-4682-7-42.

Normark, B. H. and Normark, S. (2002) Evolution and spread of antibiotic resistance. *Journal of Internal Medicine*, 252, pp. 91-106.

Park, S. Y. et al. (2010) Cellular and genetic diversity in the progression of *in situ* human breast carcinomas to an invasive phenotype. *Journal of Clinical Investigation*, 120, pp. 636-644.

Reya, T. et al. (2001) Stem cells, cancer and cancer stem cells. *Nature*, 414, pp. 105-111.

Rosindell, J. and Phillimore, A. B. (2011) A unified model of island biogeography sheds light on zones of radiation. *Ecology Letters*, 14, pp. 552-560.

Scanlon, E. F. et al. (1965) Fatal homotransplanted melanoma: a case report. *Cancer*, 18, pp. 782-789.

Shackleton, M. et al. (2009) Heterogeneity in cancer: cancer stem cells versus clonal evolution. *Cell*, 138, pp. 822-829.

Shibata, D. (2002) Molecular tumor clocks and colorectal cancer: seeing the unseen. *Pathology*, 34, pp. 534-540.

Shipitsin, M. and Polyak, K. (2008) The cancer stem cell hypothesis: in search of definitions, markers, and relevance. *Laboratory Investigation*, 88, pp. 459-463.

Smith, J. M. (1978) The evolution of Sex. New York: Cambridge University Press.

Smith, J. M. (1989) *Evolutionary Genetics*. New York: Oxford University Press.

Tarafa, G. et al. (2003) Common genetic evolutionary pathways in familial adenomatous polyposis tumors. *Cancer Research*, 63, pp. 5731-5737.

Thirlwell, C. et al. (2010) Clonal assessment and clonal ordering of individual neoplastic crypts shows polyclonality of colorectal adenomas. *Gastroenterology*, 138, pp. 1441-1454.

Tsao, J. L. et al. (2000) Genetic reconstruction of individual colorectal tumor histories. *Proceedings of the National Academy of Science of the United States of America*, 97, pp. 1236-1241.

Vincent, M. D. (2010) The animal within: carcinogenesis *Evolution*, 64, pp. 1173-1183.

Welsh, J. S. (2011) Contagious cancer. *Oncologist*, 16, pp. 1-4.

Wilkins, A. S. (1996) Antibiotic resistance: origins, evolution and spread. Ciba Foundation Symposium, 16-18 July 1996, London. *BioEssays*, 18, pp. 847-848.

In: Hypotheses in Clinical Medicine
Editors: M.M. Shoja, P.S. Agutter et al.

ISBN: 978-1-62257-276-2

Chapter 8

Organism Mutation Stability and Cancer

Edward A. Rietman*[*], *J. Tyson McDonald and Lynn Hlatky
The Center of Cancer Systems Biology, St. Elizabeth's Medical Center,
Tufts University School of Medicine, Boston, Massachusetts, US

Abstract

We start with observational evidence to hypothesize that plants are more stable with respect to an energy threshold required for mutation than animals are. These observations include ploidy stability in plants, resulting in the fact that plants infrequently get cancer, and mutation hotspots, the existence of which imply some reproducible mechanism for mutation. We propose an experiment involving *Saccharomyces cerevisiae* as a model animal and *Chlamdomonas reinhardtii* as a model plant to evaluate our hypothesis. We further speculate that if we measure the genomic stability of a huge number of species of plants and animals, we would find a bimodal distribution not unlike those observed for nonthermal equilibrium states of bipartite systems.

"Nothing makes sense in biology except in the light of *thermodynamics*."
Apologies to *Theodosius Dobzhansky* (1964)

Introduction

Liquid-state Machine

The molecular network comprising a cell consists of the protein-protein interactome, DNA, RNA, small RNAs, small molecules, molecular signaling molecules, ATP, ADP,

[*] E-mail: erietman@gmail.com.

lipids, sugars, and many others. This is a complex interconnected molecular network. In addition, the internal environment of the cell consists of large molecular clusters or nanomachines, such as the proteasome, ATP synthase, and ribosomes. As shown in Figure 8.1, each of the molecular species, whether small or large, has its own potential energy surface representing the configuration energy (Atkins and de Paula 2006). This is important for not only the small molecules, as shown in Figure 8.1, but also for the larger molecular species that act as components in the nanomachines (Drexler 1992; Geggier and Vologodskii 2010). If a molecule (large or small) is not in an energetically favorable configuration, for instance due to protein misfolding, it may not participate in the appropriate chemical reaction(s), nor function properly as a molecular component in a machine.

In addition to potential energy surfaces playing a role in the energetics of a molecular network, perturbations in the number of molecules of a particular molecular species, *i,* affect the network energetics by changing the chemical potential, μ_i. The change in chemical potential can be expressed in terms of energy by using Gibbs relations. The chemical perturbation has the effect of being able to drive the reaction toward products or reactants; this is known as Le Chatleier's principle. We can also perturb the energy landscape of a cell by adding external sources of energy in the form of photons (e.g. ultraviolet, UV or ionizing radiation [IR]). These perturbations can be likened to a liquid-state machine (Maass *et al.* 2002), analogous to a pond. When we drop a pebble into the pond, it causes ripples throughout. These ripples or waves interfere with other objects floating on the surface, and cause further constructive and destructive interference in the waves. A biological cell behaves in the same way; when we perturb it with an energy pulse (or chemical potential pulse), the magnitude of that pulse ripples throughout the network, or may be deflected or absorbed. It will thus, one way or the other, affect the molecular network of the cell. When this occurs, as shown in the schematic of Figure 8.2, there will be a change in the energy landscape.

Observation 1. Genome Duplication and Ploidy

As an example of extreme perturbation of the molecular energy landscape, consider a genome duplication event such as polyploidy. In this situation, there is apparently an error during cell division, either during metaphase or mitosis, that results in one or more complete extra copies of the genome. In aneuploidy, there is duplication in only some of the chromosomes, not the complete chromosome set (Li 1997; Chen and Ni 2006). Ohno (1970) proposed that the key mechanism for evolution of the genome was by gene duplication. More recently, Wendel (2000) and Doyle and Gaut (2000) reviewed genome evolution in polyploids; and Zhang (2003) reviewed the mechanisms of gene divergence of paralogous genes after a duplication event occurs.

Keeping in mind the liquid-state machine analogy, when these duplications events occur, either with the whole genome or partial genome, they must produce significant changes in the overall molecular network, and thus the energy landscape. In the case of plants, the polyploidy events are not usually deleterious (Li 1997; Leitch and Leitch 2008). In non-deleterious cases, following the ploidy event there is typically an asynchronous differentiation of the duplicated genes. This is one of the key mechanisms by which genome complexity evolves (Langkjaer *et al.* 2003; Leitch and Leitch 2008). Zhang (2003) reviews this evolution and describes several mechanisms. One such mechanism is pseudogenization in which, through random mutations, the extra gene gradually becomes either unexpressed or non-functional. There are, for example, 2168 pseudogenes in *C. elegans*. In some organisms, e.g. chickens, a pseudogene serves the function of immunoglobulin diversity. Another possible outcome of a duplicated gene is that it is simply beneficial because of a high demand for the RNA or protein for which it codes. This so-called gene conservation increase in a molecular component boosts some molecular reactions by Le Chatleier's principle. A third mechanism, known as subfunctionalization, results in the duplicated gene, after some mutation drift, leading to better performance of the reactions for which it is a component. Finally, a fourth mechanism results in an entirely new, and beneficial, function, and is called neofunctionalization. All of these methods, pseudogene, gene conservation, subfunctionalization and neofunctionalization, are said to improve the fitness of the organism (Conant and Wolfe 2008). The concept of fitness must be describable by thermodynamics. A more "fit" chemical reaction is able to utilize free energy more effectively. In other words, the slope of some tangent on an energy manifold describing the molecular landscape is steeper for more fit organisms. Darwinian evolution can be expressed in terms of thermodynamics (Schneider and Sagan 2005; Martyushev and Seleznev 2006; Annila 2010).

The non-deleterious cases of gene duplication have been described above. More commonly, and in particular with aneuploidy, duplication is almost always lethal. Ganem *et al.* (2007, 2009) describe how tetraploidy often leads to aneuploidy through mitotic slippage. This imbalance leads to overall molecular system instability. Interestingly, even numbers of polyploids are more likely to be stable than odd numbers. This is probably due to mitosis-related mechanisms associated with simple separation and packing of physical components during mitosis. When there is a complete even number of polyploids, there is a balance in the number of molecular components in the molecular network comprising the cell. In the case of aneuploidy, the numbers of molecular components is not commensurate with the overall molecular network. This will lead to molecular system instability via Le Chatleier's principle. Often these instabilities lead to cancer (Ganem *et al.* 2007; Storchova and Pellman 2004).

In both lethal and non-lethal duplication, the extra gene products drive a chemical reaction towards either products or reactants. Depending upon the organism, the ploidy event may be stable and result in an organism able to reproduce the new set of chromosomes. Pavelka *et al.* (2010) used random meiotic segregation to create 38 stable fully isogenic aneuploid yeast strains with three to five extra copies of some chromosomes, in which they measured quantitative proteome changes in the phenotype. In such aneuploid stable cases, the new molecular species may interfere with some established chemical reaction, or interfere with some molecular machine, and again drive reactions forward or backward. This interference, of course, can either increase or decrease the velocity of entropy production (free energy utilization), and thus perturb the overall molecular energy landscape. Given that plants are more stable to changes in ploidy than animals (Li 1997; Chen and Ni 2006), this is one pointer to the possibility that plants are able to "absorb" molecular perturbations more easily than animals. It implies that there is a different threshold of minimum energy perturbation required to disturb the molecular energy landscape of plants and of animals.

We should add that ploidy-like phenomena are key steps in some tissue differentiation (Lee *et al.* 2009). The process known as endoreplication is when a cell enters the conventional G1-S-G2-M cycle without cell division. The genome is replicated, however. Endoreplication is crucial for normal development. For example, seeds and eggs are packed with an abundance of extra nucleic acids, proteins and mRNA, which are later "digested" during the embryogenesis and germination phase. Perturbation of the endoreplication phase may result in malfunction and pathogenesis including cancer. On the other hand, ploidy is believed to buffer against stresses such as radiation and drought. Beyond these early development needs for endoreplication, other ploidy phenomena serve a purpose in the homeostasis of certain tissues, such as trichome, specialized hair cells on plants and in megakaryocytes (Lee *et al.* 2009), and hepatocytes in the liver (Duncan *et al.* 2010).

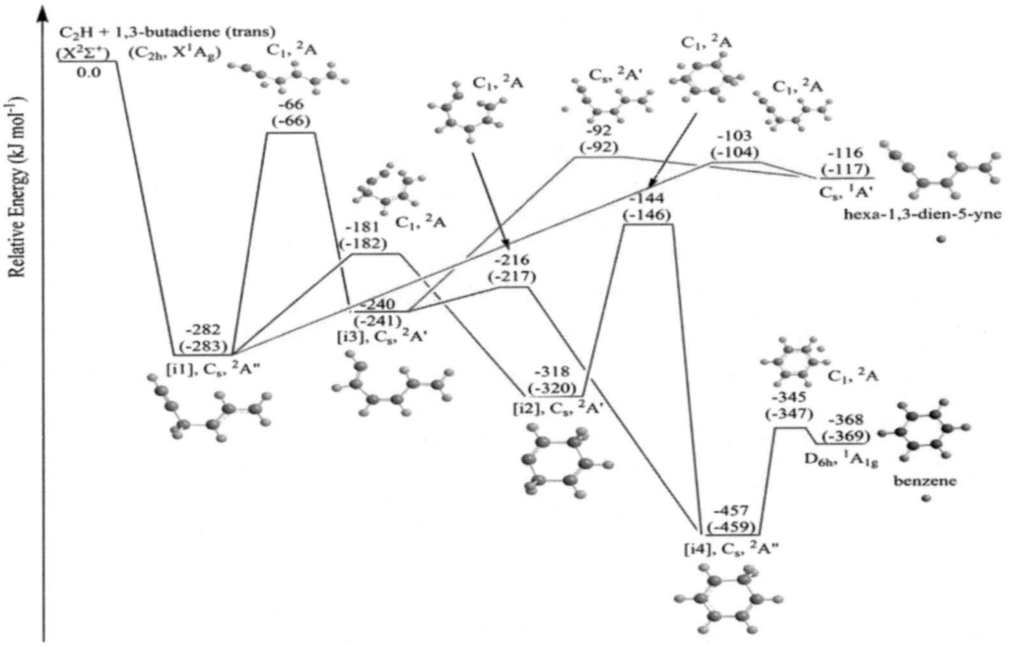

Figure 8.1. Schematic of potential energy surface and the configurations for a small molecule (from Jones et al. 2011 – reproduced with permission from Proceedings of the National Academy of Sciences of the United States of America).

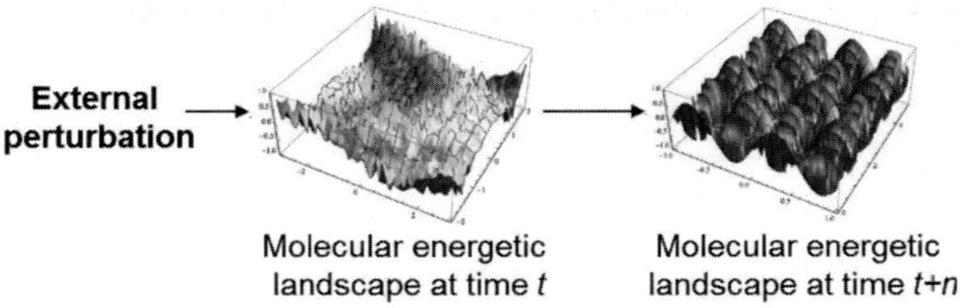

Figure 8.2. Schematic of perturbation of a molecular energy landscape.

Observation 2. Hotspots and Random Mutations

Mutations occur at hotspots during meiotic recombination, and these locations are beginning to be mapped in some model organisms. Mostly, these hotspots are related to recombination errors occurring at GC base pairs during DNA repair, and associated with meiotic recombination (Petes and Merker 2002; Segurado *et al.* 2002; Tsai *et al.* 2009). More recent work has shown that the hotspots occur in loci that express non-coding RNA, and are about 65 bp from the position where the double strand break (DSB) occurs for successful meiosis (Wahls *et al.* 2008). Gerton *et al.* (2000) found that the average spacing between hotspots is 54 kb. Chromosome pairing during meiosis can also result in mutations at different hotspots, in particular single point mutations. Aneuploidy has been described above as almost always being lethal, generally resulting in mitotic catastrophe. An analogy is heterozygotic indels. In this case, there is an indel in only one (or an odd number) of alleles. Tian *et al.* (2008) observed, from extensive bioinformatics analysis across multiple species, that in this heterozygotic indel allele, there will be a high probability of single nucleotide polymorphism (SNP) mutations. Seemingly, random point mutations also occur due to UV damage. However, sequence analysis of UV-induced mutations on *S. cerevisiae* indicates that there are certain hotspots. The majority (84%) occur at adjacent pyrimidine residues and transition mutations; with equal frequency at TC, CC, and TT sites. The substitution takes place opposite the 3' residue of the pyrimidine dinucleotide (Friedberg *et al.* 1995; Giroux *et al.* 1987). Though double strand breaks can occur during meiotic recombination, there is also an extreme example of multiple DSBs resulting in massive chromosome rearrangement, and almost always leading to cancer. Stephens *et al.* (2011) describe several cancer cell lines where a massive rearrangement of the chromosome has occurred. A mechanism for this is not given, but they speculate that ionizing radiation, which is known to produce hundreds of DSBs, could, when reassembled by the repair machinery, result in this massive rearrangement. Meyerson and Pellman (2011) suggest an alternative mechanism based on observations from Johnson and Rao (1970) and Sperling and Rao (1974). When a nucleus from a cell in S phase is transplanted into a cell in M phase, signals from the M nucleus will cause the S nucleus to shatter. Rearrangement could then result in massive numbers of assembly errors and, ultimately, cancer.

The Hypothesis

Plants are not mobile. They therefore need to adapt to stressful conditions (e.g. drought, salt) using innovative techniques such as ploidy, and the control of ploidy to adapt to stress. Doonan and Hunt (1996) argued, based on work of Doerner *et al.* (1996), that plants do not get cancer. Of course, plants can get tumors induced by, for example, gall-forming insects or the bacteria *Agrobacterium* and *Bacterium tumefaciens*. Counter arguments were made by Gaspar (1998) that plants can get oncogenic-like cancer, or the molecular equivalent of cancer. Smith (1917) demonstrated the chemical induction of crowngalls in plants. However, the literature concerning plant-cancer is very sparse. We will leave the debate open. The question we ask is: How does energy perturbation result in mutation? Uncovering the mechanism for this would be difficult, and no doubt, since it is a complex energy landscape, there are many mechanisms by which this may happen. We conjecture that understanding ploidy is a key to understanding the energetics of mutation. Combining the observations about ploidy and mutation, we hypothesize that plants are energetically more stable than animals. Figure 8.3 shows a conceptual energy diagram for this hypothesis. The graph shown on the left depicts a threshold required for phenotypic changes. Plants are at a lower energy or require larger perturbation to reach the phenotypic threshold. The plant cell shown in the diagram is *Chlamdomonas*. The same graph shows that animals require a smaller energy perturbation to reach the phenotypic threshold. The "animal" cell shown in the photo is *S. cerevisiae*. Since cancer cells are so aggressive in their growth, and since they are stable to ploidy and aneuploidy, cancer cells fall between the two extremes of plants and animals in genome stability. This stability of cancer suggests that cancer cells may be a separate species, a parasitic species that is cannibalizing the live organism it has invaded. Duesberg and Rasnick (2000) have suggested a similar concept, while Davies and Lineweaver (2011) have suggested that cancer cells are cells that have reverted to a more ancient phenotype, equivalent to metazoan 1.0. If we measured this threshold for a huge number of plant species and animal species, we conjecture we would find a bimodal distribution similar to the sketch on the right of Figure 8.3. In this case, cancer would likely be submerged in the background of the massive distribution.

Proposed Test of Hypothesis

Imagine we do an experiment where we measure the functional activity (or phenotypic outcome) of some molecule, and observe changes as a function of mutation(s) by DNA sequencing. We conjecture that, for a given energetic input and specific phase in the cell-cycle, we will most likely find the mutation(s) within the same region(s) of the genome. These regions(s) of the genome are more sensitive to alterations due to specific energy levels in the molecular network, including potential energy surface of the relevant molecular species. As the level of the energetic input increases (an increase in the chemical potential of that species, or the Gibbs free energy), the number of mutations in that region(s) of the genome will also increase. We are basically arguing that mutation is not random, but driven by chemical potential, stereochemistry, and Gibbs free energy.

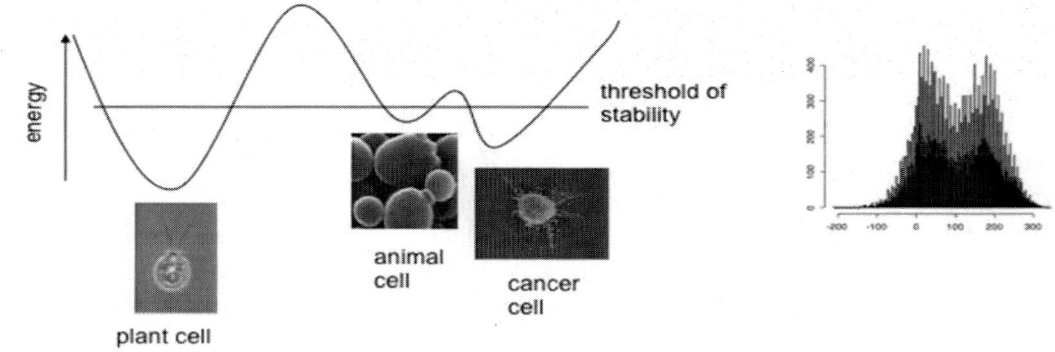

Figure 8.3. Schematic for hypothesis. Plants are energetically more stable to mutation than animals, and cancer cells are more energetically stable than animal cells. Threshold of stability would be a phenotypic difference. This, of course, is only a sketch of the hypothesis, and it remains to be tested empirically. Likely we would observe a bimodal distribution (shown on the right) representing plants and animals.

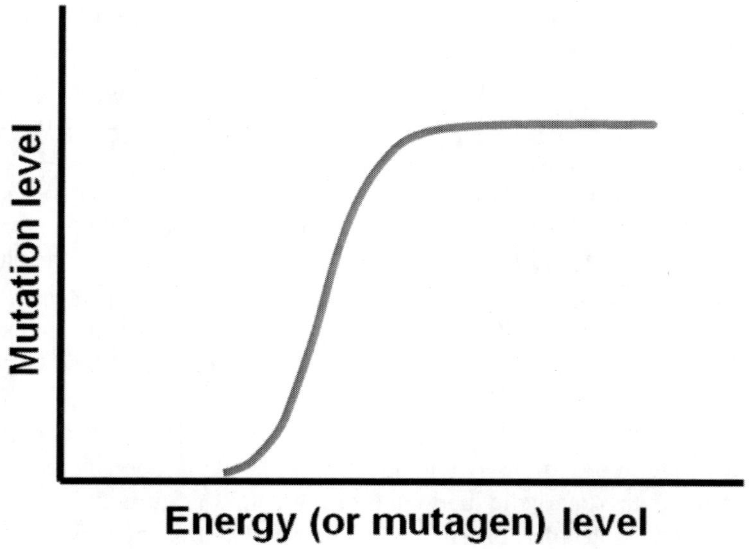

Figure 8.4. Typical graph showing dosage and yeast strain phenotypes. The graph is a schematic, and not real data, of the proposed measurements.

In this model, mutation hotspots on the functional activity of a protein would be a readout to probe the molecular disruption of exogenous energy on the biological system, starting from the genomic DNA blueprint to the functional protein. First, imagine all the possible mutations along a protein sequence, from the smallest SNP to larger more deleterious deletions. In the least damaging mutation, the SNP may simply result in a silent mutation that will not result in codon change, and thus not affect the functional outcome of protein synthesis. Alternatively, a SNP resulting in a missense mutation may result in a codon change that is physically similar to the original, and will also not affect functional activity. However, by mapping all the possible mutations of a protein that will result in a change in the codon sequence within a specific protein, a realistic prediction of all possible mutational events can be made. We assume deletion events will result in a nonfunctional protein. Second, to test the experimental relevance of these mutations in a controlled system, with nearly unlimited resources available, these mutations could be synthesized *in vitro* and tested for functional relevance. Finally, with this map, DNA sequencing within the biological system before and after energy perturbation can be made, and compared to predicted changes that result in the loss or attenuation of functional activity. Multiple events occurring simultaneously may also be categorized.

If we did this measurement with many different molecular species, ideally the entire genome, while sequencing,collecting expression data, and measuring functional activity at multiple timepoints, we would essentially be able to construct a map of energy level (Gibbs free energy or chemical potential) vs. gene ID, and this would give us a map of the *energome*. If an animal-system is more sensitive to energy perturbations than a plant-system, it will be reflected by the fact that receiving the same amount of external energy per mass will result in many more DNA mutations. In this way, if this is proven with *Chlamydomonas* versus *S. cerevisiae*, it explains why plant-systems are robust against cancer while the animal-systems are less robust, and suffer from cancer. The experiment should be done with, for example, UV or ionizing radiation and chemical perturbations.

Expanding beyond the irradiation at certain levels, we could also use different concentrations of chemical agents, and the concentration could be expressed in terms of chemical potential and thus to ergs, to put it on the same scale as electromagnetic radiation. We conjecture that at some low levels of damaging agent nothing happens; then, as we increase the concentration, we begin to see mutations (SNPs for example) at specific locations. As the concentration increases further, the mutation count increases until it reaches a lethal level (Moshinsky and Wogan 1997). Figure 8.4 shows a concept diagram for this.

If, in fact, we can view the cell as a complex chemical network with physio-chemical constraints such as potential energy surfaces and Le Chatelier's principle, then specific mutagens should cause only specific hot-spot mutations, and other mutagens should affect other regions. We should be able to map this out with some degree of resolution - albeit only with coarse resolution.

Our primary hypothesis is that plants mutate less easily than animals. Or, stated differently, plants are more robust to mutating agents. This conjecture is based on the supposition that the entire energetic landscape of the cell is perturbed, like a pebble thrown into a pond, when a molecular or energetic photon disturbs the network. As a further conjecture, if this disturbance re-occurs at the same time in the cell cycle, so that the cell is in the same state (as represented by the complete proteome and/or transcriptome), then this disturbance, if it is capable of causing a mutation, will be reproducible within the genome. Monitoring cellular toxicity as a function of increasing mutagen easily tests the main hypothesis proof-of-principle. The cellular viability of cultured samples can be measured by optical density in small cuvette-size chemostats, or at the single cell level by colony formation on an agar-based plate.

Imagine we carried out the experiment and collected data similar to the graph shown in Figure 8.4, where the y-axis is cell viability. What are the possible outcomes from this experiment, i.e. what are the possible overall shapes for the survival curves? From a DNA-target perspective taken from classical radiation biology measurements, as increasing energy is absorbed in the system, single cell survival is initially described by simple, single targeted exponential cell kill proportional to the input energy: y □ exp(□□E), where E is applied energy and α is constant. Increasing damage that results in irreparable damage from more than one event becomes exponential cell kill as a function of the square of the input energy: y □ exp(□□E^2). This experimental design is an indirect measure of the worst-case scenario of deleterious mutational events that result in the inability of the cell to survive. The radiation model, better known as the linear-quadratic, presumes that any energy will cause a slight decrease in cell survival. However, as postulated earlier, low levels may cause damage that is faithfully repaired. As energy levels increase, mutations become evident but are not lethal, until a tipping point can be reached, as described by the classic linear-quadratic model.

Conclusion and Future Directions

Finally, we raise several questions to expand this study beyond *Chlamydomonas* versus *S. cerevisiae*. As shown in Figure 8.3, we hypothesize that cancer cells are energetically more stable than healthy cells of the same tissue type. It may also be interesting to discover the energetic stability of a fungus, algae and their symbiont, lichen. Would more details of the energetic stability of symbionts provide any insight into the energetics of the virus-host interaction? Can knowledge of the energy levels for cells be exploited for reprogramming cells from a differentiated state to a pluripotent state? The ability to rapidly produce energomes on a genome-scale might open up new avenues of research and new insights into biology.

Acknowledgments

EAR has benefited from conversations with Javier De Las Rivas, Cancer Research Center (Centro de Investigacion del Cancer, University of Salamanca and Consejo Superior de Investigaciones Cientificas) Salamanca, Spain, and Kourosh Salehi-Ashtiani, New York University, Abu Dhabi, United Arab Emirates. This material is based on work supported by the U.S. Department of Energy Office of Science (BER) under award number DE-SC0001434 and by an award number U54CA149233 from the National Cancer Institute. The content is solely the responsibility of the authors and does not necessarily represent the official views of the U.S. Department of Energy, the National Cancer Institute, or the National Institutes of Health.

References

Annila, A. (2010) *Space, Time and Machines*. [www] Cornell University Library. Available from: http://arxiv.org/abs/0910.2629 [Accessed 1/25/12].

Atkins, P. and De Paula, J. (2006) *Physical Chemistry*. Oxford: Oxford University Press.

Bagley, T. J. *et al.* (2004) Hot spots for modulating toxicity identified by genomic phenotyping and localization mapping. *Molecular Cell*, 16, pp. 117-125.

Chen, Z. J. and Ni, Z. (2006) Mechanisms of genomic rearrangements and gene expression changes in plant ployloids. *Bioessays*, 28, pp. 240-252.

Conant, G. C. and Wolfe, K. H. (2008) Turning a hobby into a job: How duplicated genes find new functions. *Nature Reviews - Genetics*, 9, pp. 938-950.

Davies, P. C. W. and Lineweaver, C. H. (2011) Cancer tumors as Metazoa 1.0: tapping genes of ancient ancestors. *Physical Biology*, 8, doi: 10.1088/1478-3975/8/1/015001.

Dobzhansky, T. (1964) Biology, molecular and organismic. *American Zoologist*, 4, pp. 443-452.

Doerner, P. *et al.* (1996) Control of root growth and development by cyclin expression. *Nature*, 380, pp. 520-523.

Doonan, J. and Hunt, T. (1996) Cell cycle. Why don't plants get cancer?. *Nature*, 380, pp. 481-482.

Doyle, J. J. and Gaut, B. S. (2000) Evolution of genes and taxa: a primer. *Plant Molecular Biology*, 42, pp. 1-23.

Duesberg, P. and Rasnick, D. (2000) Aneuploidy, the somatic mutation that makes cancer a species of its own. *Cell Motility and the Cytoskeleton*, 47, pp. 88-107.

Duncan, A. W. *et al.* (2010) The ploidy conveyor of mature hepatocyes a source of genetic variation. *Nature*, 467, pp. 707-710.

Drexler, K. E. (1992) *Nanosystems: Molecular Machinery, Manufacturing, and Computation.* New York: Wiley.

Friedberg, E. C. *et al.* (1995) *DNA Repair and Mutagenesis*. Washington DC: ASM Press.

Ganem, N. J. *et al.* (2007) Tetraploidy, aneuploidy and cancer. *Current Opinion in Genetics and Development*, 17, pp. 157-162.

Ganem, N. J. *et al.* (2009) A mechanism linking extra centrosomes to chromosomal instability, *Nature*, 460, pp. 278-283.

Gaspar, T. (1998) Plants can get cancer. *Plant Physiology and Biochemistry*, 36, pp. 203-204.

Geggier, S. and Vologodskii, A. (2010) Sequence dependence of DNA bending rigidity. *Proceedings of the National Academy of Sciences of the United States of America*, 107, pp. 15421-15426.

Gerton, J. L. *et al.* (2010) Sequence dependence of DNA bending rigidity. *Proceedings of the National Academy of Sciences of the United States of America*, 107, pp. 15421-15426.

Giroux, C. N. *et al.* (1988) DNA Sequence Analysis of Spontaneous Mutations in the SUP4-o Gene of *Sacharomyces cerevisiae. Molecular and Cellular Biology*, 8, pp. 978-981.

Gerton, J. L. *et al.* (2000) Global mapping of meiotic recombination hotspots and coldspots in the yeast *Sacharomyces cerevisiae. Proceedings of the National Academy of Sciences of the United States of America*, 97, pp. 11383-11390.

Johnson, R. T. and Rao, P. N. (1970) Mammalian cell fusion: Induction of premature chromosome condensation in interphase nuclei. *Nature*, 226, pp. 717-722.

Jones, B. M. *et al.* (2011) Formation of benzene in the interstellar medium. *Proceedings of the National Academy of Sciences of the United States of America*, 108, pp. 452-457.

Langkjaer, R. B. *et al.* (2003) Yeast genome duplication was followed by asynchronous differentiation of duplicated genes. *Nature*, 421, pp. 848-852.

Lee, H. O. *et al.* (2009) Endoreplication: ploidy with a purpose. *Genes and Development*, 23, pp. 2461-2477.

Letch, A. R. and Letch, I. J. (2008) Genomic Plasticity and the diversity of ploypioid plants. *Science*, 320, pp. 481-483.

Li, W. H. (1997) *Molecular Evolution*. Sunderland, MA: Sinauer Associates.

Maass, W. *et al.* (2002) Real-time computing without stable states: A new framework for neural computation based on perturbations. *Neural Computation*, 14, pp. 2531-2560.

Martyushev, L. M. and Seleznev, V. D. (2006) Maximum entropy production principle in physics, chemistry and biology. *Physics Reports*, 426, pp. 1-45.

Meyerson, M. and Pellman, D. (2011) Cancer Genomes evolve by pulverizing single chromosomes. *Cell*, 144, pp. 9-10.

Moshinsky, D. J. and Wogan, G. N. (1997) UV-induced mutagenesis of human p53 in a vector replicated in *Sacharomyces cerevisiae. Proceedings of the National Academy of Sciences of the United States of America*, 94, pp. 2266-2271.

Ohno, S. (1970) *Evolution by Gene Duplication*. New York: Springer-Verlag.

Pavelka, N. *et al.* (2010) Aneuploidy confers quantitative proteome change and phenotypic variation in budding yeast. *Nature*, 468, pp. 321-325.

Petes, T. D. and Merker, J. D. (2002) Context dependence of meiotic recombination hotspots in yeast: the relationship between recombination activity and a reporter construct and base composition. *Genetics*, 162, pp. 2049-2052.

Schneider, E. D. and Sagan, D. (2005) *Into the Cool: Energy Flow, Thermodynamics and Life*. Chicago, IL: University of Chicago Press.

Segurado, M. *et al.* (2002) Increased recombination intermediates and homologous integration hot spots at dna replication origins. *Molecular Cell*, 10, pp. 907-916.

Smith, E. F. (1917) Chemically induced crowngalls. *Proceedings of the National Academy of Sciences of the United States of America*, 3, pp. 312-314.

Sperling, K. and Rao, P. N. (1974) Mammalian cell fusion. V. Replication behaviour of heterochromatin as observed by premature chromosome condensation. *Chromosoma*, 45, pp.121-131.

Stephens, P. J. *et al.* (2011) Massive genomic rearrangement acquired in a single catastrophic event during cancer development. *Cell*, 144, pp. 27-40.

Storchova, Z. and Pellman, D. (2004) From polyploidy to aneuploidy, genome instability and cancer. *Nature Reviews - Molecular Cell Biology*, 5, pp. 45-54.

Tian, D. *et al.* (2008) Single-nucletide mutation rate increases close to insertions/deletions in eukaryotes. *Nature*, 455, pp. 105-108.

Tsai, I. J. *et al.* (2009) Conservation of recombination hotspots in yeast. *Proceedings of the National Academy of Sciences of the United States of America*, 107, pp. 7847-7852.

Wahls, W. P. *et al.* (2008) Meiotic recombinatino hotspots of fusion yeast are directed to loci that express non-coding RNA. *PLoS One*, 3, doi: 10.1371/journal.pone.0002887.

Wendel, J. F. (2000) Genome evolution in polyploids. *Plant Molecular Biology*, 42, pp. 225-249.

Zhang, J. (2003) Evolution by gene duplication: and update. *Trends in Ecology and Evolution*, 18, pp. 292-298.

In: Hypotheses in Clinical Medicine
Editors: M.M. Shoja, P.S. Agutter et al.

ISBN: 978-1-62257-276-2

Chapter 9

The Growths of Most Cancers Are Driven by Tumor-stimulating Immune Reactions

Raúl A. Ruggiero[1], Paula Chiarella[1], Juan Bruzzo[1], Liisa M. Prehn[2] and Richmond T. Prehn[2,*]

[1]División Medicina Experimental, Instituto de Investigaciones Hematológicas, Academia Nacional de Medicina, Buenos Aires, Argentina
[2]Dept of Pathology, University of Washington, Seattle, Washington, US

Abstract

Recent data have shown that probably all malignant mouse cells, even those of spontaneous sporadic cancers, are endowed with tumor specific antigens. Stimulation, rather than inhibition, of cancers by the immune reaction is the prevalent effect in the autochthonous animal because small initial dosages of tumor antigen tend to produce persistently low stimulatory immune reactions rather than tumor inhibition. Thus, an immune response at a stimulatory level may be an essential growth-driving feature of cancer, and this may be why all cancers apparently have tumor-specific antigens.

Introduction

The following hypothesis is proposed: all cancers, even those overtly non-immunogenic, induce tumor-specific immune reactants, at least initially. A state of tolerance, caused by the tiny initial antigen load, probably induces an initial low stimulatory level of immunity in most non-transplanted (indigenous or autochthonous) cancers. The forces of immune selection probably maintain some low stimulatory level of immune reactivity to such autochthonous cancers (those growing in the animal of origin), no matter what their actual level of

* E-mail: prehn@u.washington.edu.

immunogenicity, as revealed by transplantation tests, might be. The extensive pertinent literature prior to 1971 has been discussed in detail and is still of considerable interest (Prehn and Lappé 1971; Prehn 1971). The facts of more current importance are presented in this chapter.

The Facts

The hypothesis is based largely upon the observation that the effects of immune reactants on tumor growth are not linear; small quantities of tumor-specific immune reactants are stimulatory to the growth of transplanted syngeneic tumors, while larger proportions of seemingly the same reactants are inhibitory. The mmune reaction curve (IRC) in Figure 9.1 was originally demonstrated, using 3-methylcholanthrene (MCA)-induced tumors, by Winn tests, in which different quantities of immunologically active anti-tumor spleen cells were mixed *in vitro* with tumor cells, and then inoculated into syngeneic mice that had been previously immunodepressed by radiation and thymectomy (Prehn 1972); the curve has been corroborated by a large number of subsequent studies (Prehn 2008). From the structure of the curve, it is deduced that the initial immune reactions to all tumor-specific transplantation antigens are stimulatory. Since all immune reactions presumably develop over time, these effects must be quantitatively small at first but they can become more pronounced later.

In line with these findings, it was recently shown that a dendritic cell-based vaccine against an established, overtly immunogenic tumor, or against the residual of that tumor after surgical debulking, produced inhibitory or stimulatory effects depending upon the putative ratio between the quantity of the immune response and the quantity of remaining target tumor cells (Chiarella *et al.* 2008). This observation is complicated by the fact that the apparent quantity of immune reactants depended, in part, on the size of the tumor before it was debulked. Another observation that supports our hypothesis is that the growths of even highly immunogenic methylcholanthrene-induced sarcomas, each growing in the very animal of origin, produce a specific immune tolerance and a probable stimulation of tumor growth rather than an inhibitory reaction (Basombrio and Prehn 1972; Stjernswärd 1968). Data support the hypothesis that this weak reaction to an autochthonous tumor is a consequence of the tolerance induced by the small size of the initial immunogenic dosage that occurs in the autochthonous animal, a tolerance that may be mediated by specific suppressor cells (McBride and Howie 1986). That the natural tumor tolerance of the autochthonous host can be, at least partially, broken by a superimmunization procedure was shown by the Karolinska group (Klein *et al.* 1960).

Furthermore, much evidence has been presented in recent years showing that an immune reaction favors the biological progression of syngeneic tumor implants (Prehn 2008; Hammond *et al.* 1995). Thus, it seems possible that the initial low immune reaction may remain low and stimulatory throughout most or all of the tumor's life, though this likelihood requires further substantiation.

Lastly, both Hewitt and Middle claimed that spontaneous, sporadic animal tumors, probably the best model for most human cancers, are non-immunogenic. In Hewitt's work, spontaneous mouse tumors (7 of 7) actually grew better, *i.e.*, showed a reduced LD_{50} (smallest dosage at which 50% of test tumors grew), when inoculated into putatively immunized syngeneic mice (Hewitt *et al.* 1976). In the work of Middle and Embleton, no inhibitory immunity could be detected among 28 transplanted, but originally spontaneous, rat tumors. However, the data permit evaluation of the LD_{50} in only four of these cases; in all four, the LD_{50} values suggest that the tumors were stimulated by immunity (Middle and Embleton 1981).

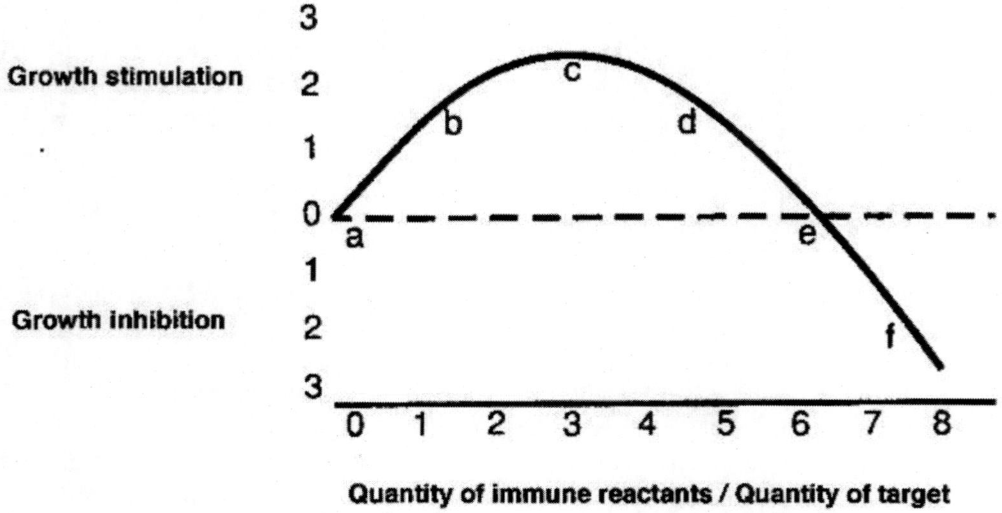

Figure 9.1. The immune reaction curve (IRC) - graph of idealized data of Prehn (1972) (reproduced from Prehn and Prehn (2010) with permission). The number and letters are arbitrary aids to discussion (see Discussion).

We predicted, based upon these varied observations, that sporadic, spontaneous tumors would, as a class, be weakly immunogenic rather than completely non-immunogenic, and that they would regularly engender a stimulatory immune reaction (Prehn and Prehn 2010). This prediction has now been substantiated, in that the majority (8 of 12) of a new collection of supposedly non-immunogenic tumors have also been shown to grow better (reduced LD_{50}) in specifically immunized mice (Bruzzo *et al.* 2011). There is no longer any class of tumor that can be considered to be totally without specific tumor antigens. The small percentage of supposedly nonimmunogenic tumors (four of a combined total of 23) that were neither stimulated nor inhibited by growth in putatively immune mice might, nonetheless, have tumor-specific antigens that were masked or neutralized by other factors, a possibility shown by the previously mentioned lack of inhibition induced by highly immunogenic tumors growing in the autochthonous tumor bearer.

The four apparently non-antigenic tumors discovered in the most recent study might have revealed some degree of antigenicity if different, or more stringent, immunization procedures had been carried out. This possibility has now been supported by the results that were obtained when one of the apparently nonantigenic tumors was examined in some detail (a T-lymphoma that arose spontaneously in a BALB/c mouse, called LB; for a more detailed description of this tumor see Ruggiero *et al.* 1985 and Zahalka *et al.* 1993). Upon *in vivo* treatments, using many putative immunization assays (such as pretreatment with irradiated tumor cells, pretreatment with dendritic cells (DCs) that were pulsed *in vitro* with LB tumor extracts, and many others), LB tumor implants were neither inhibited nor stimulated, suggesting that they had no tumor-specific antigens (Ruggiero *et al.* 1985; Franco *et al.* 1996; Franco *et al.* 2000; Bruzzo *et al.* 2011). On the other hand, when DCs were pulsed *in vitro* with an extract of a methylcholanthrene-induced, strongly immunogenic tumor (a fibrosarcoma called MC-C induced in a BALB/c mouse; for a more detailed description of this tumor see Franco *et al.* 1996), maturation of DCs (measured by enhanced expression of markers such as CD40, CD80 and CD86) was observed, along with strong *in vivo* protection against the growth of implants of the MC-C tumor (Reffo *et al.* 2008; Bruzzo *et al.* 2011). When, in five independent experiments *in vitro,* DCs were pulsed with both LB and MC-C extracts (proportion 50%-50%), some maturation of DCs still remained, and a weak but significant *in vivo* protection against LB tumor implants was achieved. Since no immune cross-reaction between the MC-C and LB tumors was ever observed, the most likely interpretation is that the LB tumor actually bears specific tumor antigens, but lacks other signals necessary to achieve DC maturation; these signals would have been provided by the MC-C extract, which enabled the DC to mature and to initiate an anti-LB immune response (Reffo *et al.* 2008).

Furthermore, in new experiments, DCs were pulsed *in vitro* with both LB and MC-C extracts, but in a proportion of 75%-25%, respectively. Although a lesser maturation of DCs was observed when these DCs were inoculated *in vivo*, a slight but significant stimulation of LB tumor growth was observed in both of the experiments that were performed (Bruzzo *et al.* 2011). The conclusion from these experiments would seem to be that a tumor antigen, present in an apparently non-antigenic spontaneous tumor (LB), can promote either inhibitory or stimulatory signals for tumor growth, depending upon the concentration of maturative signals for the DCs present in the environment of the tumor cells.

Discussion

Even highly immunogenic methylcholanthrene-induced sarcomas fail to show tumor inhibitory immunogenicity in the animal of origin unless the animal is hyper-immunized (Klein *et al.* 1960); instead, they are probably stimulated (Basombrio and Prehn 1972; Stjernswärd 1968). The additional findings that some, apparently non-immunogenic, tumors fail to immunize, despite the presence of tumor-specific antigens (Bruzzo *et al.* 2011), also show that the immunization/challenge test for tumor antigens is not always adequate; a tumor may be potentially highly antigenic, but the antigens may not be detected by the test. Thus, all tumors may carry specific tumor antigens, but appear, in rare cases, to be non-immunogenic. Overt immunogenicity is apparently dependent upon the effective size of the initial immunizing inoculum, as modulated by factors such as activated DCs or T-regulatory cells, in addition to the quantity and/or quality of tumor antigens *per se*.

The most likely place on the IRC where tumor immunization would produce accelerated growth and a lower LD_{50}, as was demonstrated in the majority of spontaneous, apparently non-immunogenic tumors of the mouse and the rat, is at the far left end of the curve, around "b" (Figure 1). In that tiny segment of the curve, any increase in the already weak immune response (a movement further to the right) would be expected to augment, rather than inhibit, tumor growth. Any tumor would probably be stimulated by an immune reaction if the initial exposure of the host to effective antigen is positive, but sufficiently small (McBride and Howie 1986).

Although some methylcholanthrene-induced sarcomas exhibit an increased incidence in immunodepressed mice (Smyth *et al.* 2001), most spontaneous murine tumors demonstrate no significant difference in tumor incidence as compared with immune competent controls (Stutman 1975; Prehn 2008). Similarly, in the human, immunodepression for allografting increases the incidence of a few common cancers (such as skin and lymphoreticular tumors), and decreases the incidence of some (such as mammary and rectal carcinomas), but most common human malignancies demonstrate no perceptible difference in their incidence as compared with immune competent individuals (Prehn 2008). These results have been interpreted as evidence that the immune system plays little, if any, role in the development of cancer. However, we think that it is because the initial reaction is effectively nearer "a" than "c" that so little effect on tumor incidence is seen in most studies of immune depression.

Although starting near "a", the very weak initial immune reaction may, with time, grow stronger, pushing the reaction toward "c" on the IRC; immune selection may then serve to keep the reaction from increasing beyond "c" to less stimulatory levels, unless the ratio of immunity to tumor size is somehow radically increased. However, it seems to us that, because of the tolerance to tumor antigens that is seen in the autologous host, almost all untransplanted tumors probably behave eventually as though near to point "c" on the IRC, regardless of how strong or weak their antigens may be when assayed in syngeneic transplantation tests. Furthermore, although at the early onset of most tumors the immune reaction is probably near "a", exceptions to this rule could also be explained according to the immunostimulatory theory. In effect, we can imagine that the initial reaction against mammary and rectal human tumors is placed near "b" (probably because of their intrinsically greater immunogenicity than most tumors), which might explain why the incidence of these particular tumors is perceptibly decreased by immune depression.

In the same way, the initial reaction to some murine methylcholanthrene-induced sarcomas, as well as human skin and lymphoreticular tumors, might be placed near "d" (probably because of their even stronger immunogenicity, as compared with the other tumors), which could explain why the incidence of these tumors is sometimes increased by immune depression. The location on the IRC of the immune reaction to human tumors could, perhaps, guide the type of immunological therapy (mitigation or enhancement of immunity) that might be useful in each particular case.

If some rare tumors are effectively non-immunogenic (Bruzzo *et al.* 2011) for whatever reason, the hypothesis that immune stimulation is an essential proximal cause of all cancers might still be retained (Prehn 2010). It might still be that effective stimulatory immunity could be essential for tumor initiation, but that this immunity, in rare instances, is lost during subsequent growth and transplantation. The hypothesis that stimulatory immunity is a major growth-driving force in most tumors remains viable, and is, indeed, reinforced by the work reported herein. The basic idea that much tumor growth is dependent upon immune stimulation appears to be similar to ideas developed and reviewed by Shevchenko *et al.* (2004).

Conclusion

It seems probable to us that the growth of perhaps all autochthonous cancers are driven by a weak stimulatory immune reaction, no matter how strong the immunogenicity of the tumor may be, as revealed by transplantation tests. During progression, we suggest that the initial weak immunity probably increases, but is constrained to the area around "c" on the IRC by the power of selection. Mitigation of the immunity from near "c" toward "a", if somehow possible, might be therapeutic.

On the other hand, the use of very stringent immunization therapies might be able, in certain cases, to transform the weak and stimulatory immune reaction into a stronger and tumor-inhibitory immunological force to break the tolerance (Klein *et al.* 1960). However, taking into account that the immune response against most autochthonous tumors could be placed towards the left end of the curve, probably between "a" and "b" in the IRC, anti-tumor vaccines may entail a real risk of doing harm if the immunity evoked by the vaccine were too weak to move the reaction into the tumor-inhibitory zone of the IRC.

Finally, inasmuch as autochthonous tumors behave immunologically so differently from most isogeneic transplants, more experimental work in autochthonous systems, or at least in systems initiated with minimal tumor dosages, is necessary.

References

Andrews, E .J. (1971) Evidence of nonimmune regression of chemically induced tumors in mouse skin. *Journal of the National Cancer Institute*, 47, pp. 653-665.

Basombrio, M. A. and Prehn, R. T. (1972) Immune status of autochthonous and adoptively protected mice toward spontaneous and chemically induced tumors. *Cancer Research*, 32, pp. 2545-2550.

Bruzzo, J. et al. (2011) On the immunostimulatory hypothesis of cancer. *Medicina (Buenos Aires),* 71, pp. 509-513.

Chiarella, P. et al. (2008) Therapeutic anti-tumor vaccines: from tumor inhibition to enhancement. *Clinical Medical Oncology*, 2, pp. 237-245.

Franco, M. et al. (1996) A serum-mediated mechanism for concomitant resistance shared by immunogenic and non-immunogenic murine tumours. *British Journal of Cancer*, 74, pp. 178-186.

Franco, M. et al. (2000) Two different types of concomitant resistance induced by murine tumors: morphological aspects and intrinsic mechanisms. *Oncology Reports*, 7, pp. 1053-1063.

Hammond, W. G. et al. (1995) Tumor progression by lung cancers growing in hosts of different immunocompetence. *Cancer Journal*, 8, pp. 130-138.

Hewitt, H. B. et al. (1976) A critique of the evidence for active host defenses against cancer, based on personal studies of 27 murine tumors of spontaneous origin. *British Journal of Cancer*, 33, pp. 241-259.

Klein, G. et al. (1960) Demonstration of resistance against methylcholanthrene-induced sarcomas in the primary autochthonous host. *Cancer Research*, 20, pp. 1561-1572.

Mcbride, W. H. and Howie, S. E. (1986) Induction of tolerance to a murine fibrosarcoma in two zones of dosage - the involvement of suppressor cells. *British Journal of Cancer*, 53, pp. 707-711.

Middle, J. G. and Embleton, M. J. (1981) Naturally arising tumors of the inbred WAB/Not rat strain. II. Immunogenicity of transplanted tumors. *Journal of the National Cancer Institute*, 67, pp. 637-643.

Prehn, R. T. and Lappé, M. A. (1971) An immunostimulation theory of tumor development. *Transplant Reviews*, 7, pp. 26-54.

Prehn, R. T. and Prehn, L. M. (2010) Cancer immunotherapy by immunosuppression. *Theoretical Biology and Medical Modelling*, 7, pp. 45-53.

Prehn, R. T. (1971) Perspectives on Oncogenesis: Does immunity stimulate or Inhibit Neoplasia? *Journal of the Reticularendothelial Society*, 10, pp. 1-16.

Prehn, R. T. (1972) The immune reaction as a stimulator of tumor growth. *Science*, 176, pp. 170-171.

Prehn, R. T. (2008) The flip side of immune surveillance: immune dependency. *Immunology Reviews*, 222, pp. 341-356.

Prehn, R. T. (2010) The initial immune reaction to a new tumor antigen is always stimulatory and probably necessary for a tumor's growth. *Clinical and Developmental Immunology*, 2010, doi: 10.1155/2010/851728.

Reffo, V. L. et al. (2008) Unveiling antigens in a non-immunogenic spontaneous murine tumor using a dendritic vaccine. *Medicina (Buenos Aires)*, 68, pp. 301-304.

Ruggiero, R. A. et al. (1985) Concomitant immunity in murine tumors of non-detectable immunogenicity. *British Journal of Cancer*, 51, pp. 37-48.

Shevchenko, A. V. et al. (2004) Specific Immune response of organism as initiator and promoter of carcinogenesis (hypothesis): A fundamentally new vision of the role of organism's immune response in pathogenesis of malignant tumors. *Journal of Medical Science Academy of Ukraine*, 10, pp. 50-84.

Smyth, M. J. et al. (2001) NK cells and NKT cells collaborate in host protection from methylcholanthrene-induced fibrosarcoma. *International Immunology*, 13, pp. 459-463.

Stjernswärd, J. (1968) Immune status of the primary host toward its own methylcholanthrene-induced sarcomas. *Journal of the National Cancer Institute*, 40, pp. 13-22.

Stutman, O. (1975) Immunodepression and malignancy. *Advances in Cancer Research,* 22, pp. 261-422.

Zahalka, M. A. et al. (1993) Blocking lymphoma invasiveness with a monoclonal antibody directed against the beta-chain of the leukocyte adhesion molecule (CD18). *Journal of Immunology,* 150, pp. 4466-4477.

In: Hypotheses in Clinical Medicine
Editors: M.M. Shoja, P.S. Agutter et al.

ISBN: 978-1-62257-276-2

Chapter 10

Complexity: Is It the Real Language of Prostate Cancer?

Fabio Grizzi[1,*], Gianluigi Taverna[1], Pier Carlo Muzzio[2,3] and Pierpaolo Graziotti[1]

[1]Humanitas Clinical and Research Center, Italy
[2] IRCCS Istituto Oncologico Veneto, Padua, Italy
[3]Department of Medical-Diagnostic Sciences and Special Therapies, University of Padua, Italy

Abstract

Despite years of intensive investigation into prostate cancer, it remains a major cause of death in men worldwide. Prostate cancer emerges from multiple alterations that induce changes in expression patterns of genes and proteins that function in networks controlling critical cellular events. Here, we briefly summarize several prognostic factors that have been proposed since serum prostate-specific antigen measurement was introduced over 20 years ago for predicting the outcome of patients with prostate cancer. We hypothesize prostate cancer as a complex dynamical disease using the basic principles of non-linear systems and chaos theory. Irrespective of whether it is confirmed, our hypothesis may help to clarify old concepts, categorize actual knowledge, and suggest alternative approaches to discovering additional markers with potential clinical value.

Introduction

Prostate cancer is the fifth most frequent cancer in the world and the second most commonly diagnosed non-cutaneous cancer in men in the United States (Michaelson et al. 2008). Although many prognostic factors have been proposed, no reliable index for predicting the outcome of prostate cancer patients has yet been identified. Currently, the quantification

[*] E-mail: Fabio.Grizzi@humanitasresearch.it.

of serum levels of prostate-specific antigen (PSA), a glycoprotein with serine protease activity that is secreted by the epithelial cells of the prostate gland, remains the most important tumoral marker because it has significant applications in all aspects of the management of prostatic diseases. Serum PSA has been used extensively in screening for prostate cancer on the basis of early studies showing that PSA levels greater than 4 ng/mL have predictive value for detecting this condition. Although PSA testing has led to a considerable increase in prostate cancer detection, it has important drawbacks and considerable efforts are in progress to improve performance, with emphasis directed primarily at enhancing its specificity and sensitivity (Andriole et al. 2009; Barry 2009; Concato 2009; Rosser 2008; Schroder et al. 2009). PSA is often elevated in non-neoplastic conditions, including benign prostatic hyperplasia, prostatitis or a prostate infarction (Loeb and Catalona 2007; Loeb et al. 2009). This has considerable clinical consequences, since this assessment forms the basis for primary clinical decisions (Loeb et al. 2009). The Prostate Cancer Prevention Trial has shown that even in patients with PSA levels < 4 ng/mL, >15% had biopsy-detectable prostate cancer (Meeks et al. 2009). It has also been reported that PSA screening reduced the rate of death from prostate cancer by 20% but was associated with a high risk of over-diagnosis (Schroder et al. 2009).

Apart from the serum PSA level, the Free-to-Total PSA (also called the PSA quotient) has been introduced into clinical practice. This is defined as the ratio between the unbound isoform of PSA (Free PSA) and the serum PSA (Total PSA) bound to α1-antichymotrypsin, α1-proteinase inhibitor, or α1-macroglobulin. Clinical studies have reported that the PSA quotient in patients with prostate cancer is less than that in patients with benign prostatic diseases. Additional tools have been proposed to evaluate the kinetics of PSA. They include:

1. PSA Doubling Time (PSADT), which evaluates the time required for the PSA level to double. It is calculated as $PSADT = \log_2 / [\log(PSA2 - PSA1)/time]$. Although it has been shown to be useful in the setting of relapse after therapy and in predicting metastatic disease and cancer-specific mortality, it is highly dependent on the baseline PSA measurement (Benecchi et al. 2008).
2. PSA Velocity (PSAV), which evaluates the rate of change in PSA time. It is obtained using the formula: $PSAV = (lastPSA - firstPSA)/\Delta t$ and is expressed as ng/mL/year. The clinical usefulness of PSAV has been intensively debated. Recently, it has been reported that different methods for calculating the PSAV, either simple arithmetic or linear regression, do not change the outcome (Benecchi 2006).
3. PSA slope, which is calculated with the least square fit (PSA versus time) using the equation: $y = a + bx$, where y represents the serum PSA level and a the intercept. Parameter b is the slope and reflects the increase of PSA in one year. The acceleration of PSA (lnPSA slope) is the slope of lnPSA versus time, where ln is the natural logarithm (Benson et al. 1992).

In 1992, to improve the accuracy of serum PSA, Benson and colleagues introduced the so-called PSA density (PSAD), which corresponds to the PSA serum level divided by the prostate volume (Benson et al. 1992). The concept underlying PSAD is that a given elevation of serum PSA is more likely to be caused by prostate cancer in a patient with a small prostate gland than in a man with a large gland. The limitations of PSAD are that it requires an estimation of the prostate volume, which is still made subjectively by transrectal ultrasonography (TRUS), it is time consuming and more expensive than a simple blood test, and morphological differences in gland shape may result in inaccurate evaluations.

Transrectal ultrasound-guided prostate biopsy remains the gold standard for detecting prostate cancer (Presti 2007). It is characterized by low sensitivity and high specificity, despite significant technical improvements such as color and power Doppler imaging, microbubble contrast agents and new post-processing techniques, especially real-time elastography (Lenkinski et al. 2008, Puech et al. 2009). Considerable advances have been made in the identification of organ-confined prostate cancer with multi-parametric magnetic resonance imaging (MRI) (Pondman et al. 2008). Kurhanewicz and colleagues showed that multi-parametric MRI techniques based on the anatomical, metabolic and physiological properties of prostate cancer provided the best characterization of the disease (Kurhanewicz et al. 2008). However, the clinical utility of such an examination is challenged by the need for appropriate tools to analyze and display the large amount of data acquired and to combine the data optimally to give the most accurate assessment of prostate cancer in the individual patient. Prostate biopsy has evolved from a paradigm of a small number of random biopsies to one of systematic, numerical, and anatomical strategy. Over recent years, several studies have demonstrated the importance of purposeful biopsy strategies for detecting, accurately grading, and staging prostate cancer in varying patient populations (Patel and Jones 2009). However, the efficiency of this practice is still debated and is limited in practice by patient tolerance and morbidity. Currently, clinical and pathological classifications are determined according to the World Health Organization criteria, the Gleason grade, and the Tumor-Node-Metastasis (TNM) staging system (Egevad 2008; Rubin 2008). The Gleason biopsy grade is used in conjunction with other clinical variables, including serum PSA level and clinical stage, to help make treatment decisions for prostate cancer and they are all incorporated into various nomograms to determine pre-operatively the risk of progression after specific therapy. Although several candidate tools with potential clinical value have been proposed, there is still no reliable index for predicting the outcome of prostate cancer patients. It is indubitable that in the management of prostate cancer the major challenge remains to distinguish men who need definite treatment from men who have latent disease. The limitations of serum PSA measurement and PSA kinetics indicate that better diagnostic and prognostic biomarkers for prostate cancer are needed.

The Hypothesis

The multifarious approaches adopted to discover more reliable diagnostic serum and urine biomarkers include genomics (Witte, 2009), proteomics (Steuber et al., 2008) and metabolomics (Sreekumar et al., 2009). This would lead us to reflect on the biological complexity underlying prostate cancer development, progression and metastasis. Here, we hypothesize prostate cancer as a complex dynamical disease using the basic principles of non-linear dynamics and chaos theory.

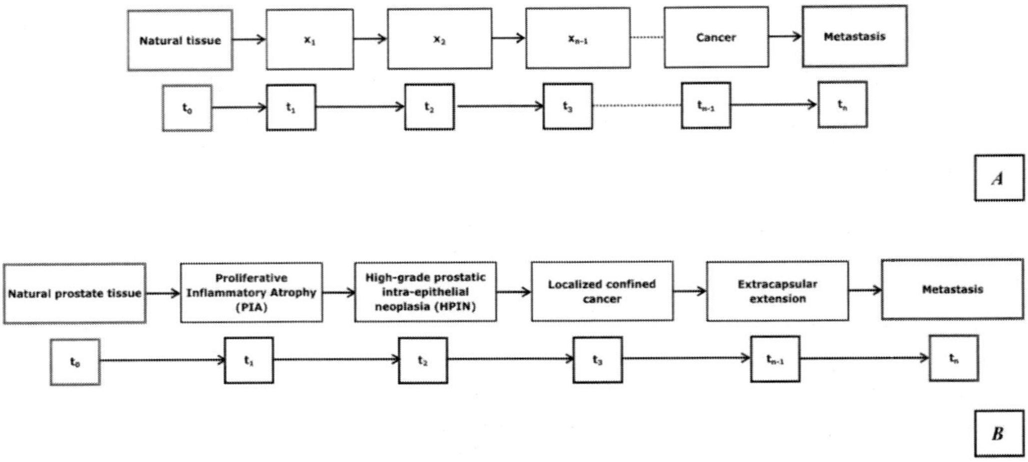

Figure 10.1. Multi-state prostate carcinogenesis: (a) progression of different qualitative states (x1, x2….xn-1, xn) identifiable in the development of cancer from normal tissue. The time parameter (t0, t1…….tn-1, tn) depends on a large number of variables interconnected in many ways in a non-linear manner. This makes it extremely difficult to predict the exact time interval between two successive states. Although carcinogenesis is a continuum, its differentiation into successive states is based on differences in histological and clinical data. (b) Simplified schema of dynamical view of prostate carcinogenesis. High-grade prostatic intra-epithelial neoplasia (HPIN) is currently regarded as the precursor lesion on the basis of pathological, epidemiological and cytogenetic evidence. HPIN is characterized by architecturally benign prostatic acini and ducts, lined by cytologically atypical cells. HPIN lesions can be subdivided into at least four different architectural patterns.

Prostate Cancer: A Complex Dynamical Disease

There is no doubt that cancer operates at different levels of the hierarchical organization making up a human, and evolves through an assortment of states (or possible pattern configurations) and a number of transitions between pairs of successive states (Figure 10.1) (Grizzi and Chiriva-Internati 2006; Grizzi et al. 2006).

The reductionist view of cancer expressed in myriads of molecular biology-based investigations claims that all of the information necessary for a cell to transform itself into a neoplastic cell can be attributed to changes at genomic level (Grizzi and Chiriva-Internati 2006; Grizzi et al. 2006). This "certainty" is based on the fact that the genome carries all of the information related to all cell processes, so any cellular modification is due to a specific genomic change.

Although this approach has offered what is still a fundamental means of generating knowledge, accumulated information has also raised a number of intriguing and still unsolved questions. How many distinct regulatory circuits within each type of target cell must be disrupted in order to make it become cancerous? Does the same set of regulatory circuits suffer disruption in the cells of all the disparate neoplasia arising in humans? And, if we had a complete description of all of the molecular reactions occurring within a living normal cell and its tumoral counterpart, would we understand that cell?

Cartesian reductionism seeks to explain the wide variety of natural phenomena on the basis of the behavior of a limited number of constituents subject to simple but rigorous laws

(Heng 2008). It has been a powerful driving force in science, as can clearly be seen from the impressive triumphs of molecular and cellular biology. However, the question remains as to how to transform this knowledge into an understanding of the complex phenomena existing in genes, subcellular entities, cells, tissues, organs, systems and the body as a complete hierarchical system (Grizzi and Chiriva-Internati 2006; Grizzi et al. 2006; Heng 2008; Nurse 1997; Rose 1998).

The need to tackle systemic complexity has become even more apparent since the completion of the various genome projects, which have stimulated a search for new ways of understanding the complex processes underlying cancer initiation, progression and metastasis (Grizzi and Chiriva-Internati 2006; Grizzi et al. 2006; Sogn et al. 2005).

Cancer is today recognized as a highly heterogeneous disease: more than 100 distinct types of human cancer have been described, and various tumor subtypes can be found within specific organs (Brafford and Herlyn 2005). This genetic and phenotypic variability is what primarily determines the self-progression of neoplastic disease and its response to therapy. Additionally, the asynchrony and self-progression of a cancer cell population suggests that the extent to which each neoplastic cell shares the properties of a normal cell may differ in time and in space. Individual cells from a clonal population respond differently to the same stimulus, some not responding at all (Bastiaens 2009). Variability in cell responses can have important implications. For instance, some tumor cells refuse to die in response to drugs that trigger programmed cell death (apoptosis), affecting the efficacy of chemotherapy (Bastiaens 2009; Spencer et al. 2009). Often, chemotherapy initially reduces tumor size but it also produces severe adverse effects leading to other complications (Heng 2008). It has also been shown that in a heterogeneous population, patients may display a multiplicity of genetic variations that respond differently to a given medical intervention. The same treatment could be of benefit to some patients yet harmful to others (Heng 2008; Mittra 2007).

It is now accepted that the complex environment in which a normal or cancer cell is embedded determines different cell-environment interchanges of matter, energy and information, thus inducing continuous qualitative or quantitative changes in their shared properties and/or behaviors (Anderson et al. 2006; Grizzi and Chiriva-Internati 2006; Grizzi et al. 2006; Mantovani 2009; Mantovani et al. 2008).

Prostate cancer is a highly heterogeneous disease encompassing a wide variety of pathological entities and a range of very different clinical behaviors. This is underpinned at the molecular level by a complex array of genetic alterations that affect cell processes, thus determining the dynamical progression of the neoplastic disease and its variable response to treatment (Liu et al. 2009). Clinical prostate cancer phenotypes range from indolent or clinically insignificant to locally aggressive or metastatic. Many gene expression profiling studies have been carried out in attempts to establish a molecular staging system, but no genetic markers that predict aggressive disease have yet been identified clinically (Golias et al. 2007; Konishi et al. 2005; Luo; Reynolds 2008; Sun). Molecular associations with prostate cancer phenotypes continue to be fragmentary and, in some cases, have been poorly substantiated by follow-up investigations. It can also be said that the optimal treatment for localized prostate cancer is still unknown (i.e. the current guidelines suggest that active surveillance or radical prostatectomy with lymphoadenectomy may be alternatives in the same patient), and published reports concerning the best treatment modality are conflicting.

In mathematical terms, prostate carcinogenesis may be depicted as a non-linear complex process, whose behavior follows no clearly predictable or repeatable pathway. In a linear system (Table 1), as the relationship with an environmental factor increases, the system behavior changes linearly in response. In contrast, the behavior of non-linear systems may be perceived as unpredictable. Periods of inactivity may be punctuated by sudden change, apparent patterns of behavior may disappear and new patterns unexpectedly emerge. Moreover, non-linear or chaotic systems do not react proportionally to the magnitude of their inputs, and depend on their initial conditions, i.e. small changes in the initial conditions may generate very different end-points. The behavior of chaotic systems, i.e. systems that exhibit variability, which is not necessarily random yet whose complex patterns are not discernible over a normal human time and spatial scale, may be perceived as unpredictable. This chaotic behavior does not indicate a lack of order. Rather, the order is difficult or impossible to describe in simple terms and requires complex description.

Table 1. Main characteristics of linear and non-linear systems

Linear Systems	Non-Linear Systems
React proportionally to their inputs.	Do not react proportionally to their inputs.
Do not depend on their initial conditions.	Depend on their initial conditions.
Their behavior is deterministic.	Their behavior is not deterministic.
Satisfy the superposition principle.[1]	Do not satisfy the superposition principle.
Satisfy a linear transformation that enlarges or diminishes objects (scaling).	Do not satisfy a linear transformation that enlarges or diminishes objects (scaling).
All the interrelationships among the quantities involved are expressed by linear equations that may be algebraic, differential, or integral.	Nonlinear equations are difficult to solve and give rise to interesting phenomena such as chaos.

[1] Superposition principle states that, for all linear systems, the net response at a given place and time caused by two or more stimuli is the sum of the responses that would have been caused by each stimulus individually.

Prostate carcinogenesis is a process involving anatomical structures, each consisting of a virtually infinite number of parts and being governed by a large number of biological sub-processes that differ in time and in space (i.e. multi-scale causality). In such a process: (a) the relationships between the parts are non-linear; (b) the variables influencing the behavior of the process are interconnected in a complex manner; (c) the individual component parts show systematic heterogeneity; (d) small alterations in variables can lead to completely different outcomes. The above features all are illustrated by the commonly-encountered differences in the progression or therapeutic response of prostate cancers, and the fact that cancer histopathology does not always reveal its underlying biological behavior.

The complexity of alterations in cancer presents a daunting problem with respect to treatment: how can we effectively treat cancers arising from such varied perturbations? A tumor consists of genetically distinct subpopulations of cancer cells, each with its own characteristic sensitivity profile to a given therapeutic agent. Each cancer therapy can be viewed as a filter that removes a subpopulation of cancer cells that are sensitive to this treatment while allowing other insensitive subpopulations to escape (Luo).

Conclusion

The above reflections make the following conclusions possible. Despite rapid advances in molecular and cellular biology, prostate cancer is still a complex dynamical disease in which normal organization breaks down and is replaced by abnormal and unpredictable dynamics. Prostate carcinogenesis is a non-linear process that depends on a large number of variables and is regulated at multiple spatial and temporal scales. Complex molecular events characterize prostate cancer development, progression and metastasis. To date, no single specific candidate gene or combinations of genes has been definitively assigned as responsible for prostate cancerogenesis (Golias et al. 2007; Konishi et al. 2005; Sun). Prostate cancer results from the accumulation of multiple genetic and epigenetic alterations that transform normal glandular epithelium to pre-neoplastic lesions and to invasive carcinoma (Reynolds 2008).

The natural history of prostate cancer is remarkably heterogeneous and still not completely understood. Many men who develop prostate cancer never have symptoms or undergo therapy and eventually die of other causes. Early detection of prostate cancer has proved difficult, and current detection tools are inadequate. The benefit of screening for prostate cancer with PSA testing, digital rectal examination (DRE) or any other screening test is still not clear. Lack of knowledge about the biology of prostate cancer has resulted in numerous controversies concerning the clinical management of early stages and the utility of population screening (Andriole et al. 2009; Barry 2009; Concato 2009; Rosser 2008; Schroder et al. 2009). A more specific method for detecting prostate cancer is required to enhance or replace screening with only serum PSA or its kinetics. The focus of recent research has been on creating cost-effective assays for circulating protein biomarkers in the blood, but because of the heterogeneity of prostate cancer, it has become clear that this will be a formidable challenge. Each marker will require proper validation to ensure clinical utility. The Biomarkers Definition Working Group (2001) defined with the term "biomarker" or biological marker as "a characteristic that is objectively measured and evaluated as an indicator of normal biological processes, pathogenic processes, or pharmacological responses to a therapeutic intervention". There are actually emerging markers at various stages of development that show some promise for prostate cancer diagnosis. These include kallikrein-related peptidase 2, early prostate cancer antigen, prostate cancer gene 3, hepsin, prostate stem cell antigen, and alpha-methylacyl-CoA racemase (Clarke et al. 2009; Fradet 2009; Lin 2009; Oh et al. 2009; Presti 2009; Sardana et al. 2008).

The Gleason biopsy score is widely used in conjunction with other clinical variables, including serum PSA level and clinical stage, to help make treatment decisions for prostate cancer and all these variables are incorporated into various nomograms to determine pre-operatively the risk of progression after specific therapy. However, prostate cancers are particularly intriguing with regard to their propensity to display multiple histological patterns within a single tumor (Ruijter et al. 1996). Although several studies have discussed grade heterogeneity, the nature and magnitude of this complex phenomenon have not been precisely documented (Ruijter et al. 1996).

The imaging of localized prostate cancer remains limited (Kelloff et al. 2009, Turkbey et al. 2009). TRUS is the most widely used imaging method, enabling the prostate size to be determined accurately and the zonal anatomy depicted, but its ability to delineate cancer foci is limited, with sensitivity and specificity around 40-50% (Turkbey et al. 2009). Future development of new imaging methods that interrogate the biological functions of tumors may aid risk assessment and therapy choice (Turkbey et al. 2009).

Prostate cancers are usually categorized as low-, intermediate- and high-risk disease on the basis of serum PSA level, Gleason grade, and clinical stage (Kelloff et al. 2009). These risk groups are used as a guide to treatment decisions. However, the percentage of incorrect categorization has led to unexpected results: approximately one-third of prostate cancer patients present with intermediate risk disease. While this risk group is clinically well defined, it demonstrates the most significant heterogeneity in PSA-based biochemical outcome. Additionally, the disparity between reported incidence and mortality rates strongly suggests that only a small proportion of diagnosed low-risk prostate cancers will progress to life-threatening disease during the lifetime of the patient (Komarova 2005).

In order to understand prostate cancer as a complex system that involves many interacting components, we need to determine the type of data that need to be collected at each level of organization, the boundary conditions to use when describing the disease (i.e. a perturbed system), and the technologies and approaches best suited to revealing its underlying biological behavior. Critical analysis of traditional clinical concepts is needed, as is reinterpretation of the clinical significance of failed therapies from the perspective of complexity. Two main concepts, multi-scale causality and heterogeneity, need to be considered when generating new medical interventions.

Modeling the development, progression and metastasis of prostate cancer using mathematics and biological data is a burgeoning area of cancer research. Mathematical models such as nomograms may offer more precise predictions of a prognosis or therapeutic response than staging alone. Models combining DRE, serum PSA level, and Gleason score have been shown to improve accuracy in predicting the risk of treatment failure compared with a single parameter alone. In addition, incorporating MRI or MRI-MR spectroscopy findings into nomograms has been shown to improve the prediction of insignificant cancer (Kelloff et al. 2009).

Mathematical methods and their derivatives have proved to be possible and practical in oncology (Anderson and Quaranta 2008; Baish and Jain 2000; Damber and Aus 2008; Grizzi and Chiriva-Internati 2005; Hessels and Schalken 2009; Joshua et al. 2008; Komarova 2005; Tanaka et al. 2010), but the current models are often simplifications that ignore vast amounts of knowledge; furthermore, most models struggle to resolve the 10-12 order-of-magnitude span of the timescales of systemic events, be they molecular (ion channel gating: 10^{-6} s), cellular (mitosis: 10^{2}-10^{3} s) or physiological (cancer progression: 10^{8} s) (Grizzi and Chiriva-Internati 2005).

Viewing prostate cancer as a system that is dynamically complex in time and space will probably reveal more about its underlying behavioral characteristics. It is encouraging that mathematicians, biologists and clinicians can contribute together towards a common quantitative understanding of prostate cancer complexity. This new way of thinking may help to clarify old concepts, categorize actual knowledge, and suggest an alternative approach to discovering biomarkers with potential clinical value.

References

Anderson, A. R. and Quaranta, V. (2008) Integrative mathematical oncology. *Nature Reviews: Cancer*, 8, pp. 227-234.

Anderson, A. R. *et al.* (2006) Tumor morphology and phenotypic evolution driven by selective pressure from the microenvironment. *Cell*, 127, pp. 905-915.

Andriole, G. L. *et al.* (2009). Mortality results from a randomized prostate-cancer screening trial. *The New England Journal of Medicine*, 360, pp. 1310-1319.

Baish, J. W. and Jain, R. K. (2000) Fractals and cancer. *Cancer Research*, 60, pp. 3683-3688.

Barry, M. J. (2009) Screening for prostate cancer - the controversy that refuses to die. *The New England Journal of Medicine*, 360, pp. 1351-1354.

Bastiaens, P. (2009) Systems biology: When it is time to die. *Nature*, 459, pp. 334-335.

Benecchi, L. (2006) PSA velocity and PSA slope. *Prostate Cancer and Prostatic Diseases*, 9, pp. 169-172.

Benecchi, L. *et al.* (2008) Optimal measure of PSA kinetics to identify prostate cancer. *Urology*, 71, pp. 390-394.

Benson, M. C. *et al.* (1992) Prostate specific antigen density: a means of distinguishing benign prostatic hypertrophy and prostate cancer. *The Journal of Urology*, 147, pp. 815-816.

Biomarkers Definitions Working Group. (2001) Biomarkers and surrogate endpoints: preferred definitions and conceptual framework. *Clinical Pharmacology and Therapeutics*, 69, pp. 89-95.

Brafford, P. and Herlyn, M. (2005) Gene expression profiling of melanoma cells - searching the haystack. *Journal of Translational Medicine*, 3, doi: 10.1186/1479-5876-3-2.

Clarke, R. A. *et al.* (2009). New genomic structure for prostate cancer specific gene PCA3 within BMCC1: implications for prostate cancer detection and progression. *PloS One*, 4, doi: 10.1371/journal.pone.0004995.

Concato, J. (2009) What will the emperor say? Screening for prostate cancer as of 2008. *Cancer Journal*, 15, pp. 7-12.

Damber, J. E. and Aus, G. (2008) Prostate cancer. *Lancet*, 371, pp. 1710-1721.

Egevad, L. (2008) Recent trends in Gleason grading of prostate cancer: I. Pattern interpretation. *Analytical and quantitative cytology and histology / the International Academy of Cytology [and] American Society of Cytology*, 30, pp. 190-198.

Fradet, Y. (2009) Biomarkers in prostate cancer diagnosis and prognosis: beyond prostate-specific antigen. *Current Opinion in Urology*, 19, pp. 243-246.

Golias, C. *et al.* (2007) Molecular profiling and genomic microarrays in prostate cancer. *Experimental Oncology*, 29, pp. 82-84.

Grizzi, F. and Chiriva-Internati, M. (2005) The complexity of anatomical systems. *Theoretical Biology and Medical Modelling*, 2, doi: 10.1186/1742-4682-2-26.

Grizzi, F. and Chiriva-Internati, M. (2006) Cancer: looking for simplicity and finding complexity. *Cancer Cell International*, 6, doi: 10.1186/1475-2867-6-4.

Grizzi, F. *et al.* (2006) Cancer initiation and progression: an unsimplifiable complexity. *Theoretical Biology and Medical Modelling*, 3, doi: 10.1186/1742-4682-3-37.

Heng, H. H. (2008) The conflict between complex systems and reductionism. *JAMA: the journal of the American Medical Association*, 300, pp. 1580-1581.

Hessels, D. and Schalken, J. A. (2009) The use of PCA3 in the diagnosis of prostate cancer. *Nature Reviews - Urology*, 6, pp. 255-261.

Joshua, A. M. *et al.* (2008) Prostatic preneoplasia and beyond. *Biochimica et Biophysica Acta*, 1785, pp. 156-181.

Kelloff, G. J. *et al.* (2009) Challenges in clinical prostate cancer: role of imaging. *American Journal of Roentgenology*, 192, pp. 1455-1470.

Komarova, N. L. (2005) Mathematical modeling of tumorigenesis: mission possible. *Current Opinion in Oncology*, 17, pp. 39-43.

Konishi, N. *et al.* (2005) Molecular pathology of prostate cancer. *Pathology International*, 55, pp. 531-539.

Kurhanewicz, J. *et al.* (2008) Multiparametric magnetic resonance imaging in prostate cancer: present and future. *Current Opinion in Urology*, 18, pp. 71-77.

Lenkinski, R. E. *et al.* (2008) An illustration of the potential for mapping MRI/MRS parameters with genetic over-expression profiles in human prostate cancer. *Magma*, 21, pp. 411-421.

Lin, D. W. (2009) Beyond PSA: utility of novel tumor markers in the setting of elevated PSA. *Urologic Oncology*, 27, pp. 315-321.

Liu, W. *et al.* (2009) Copy number analysis indicates monoclonal origin of lethal metastatic prostate cancer. *Nature Medicine*, 15, pp. 559-565.

Loeb, S. And Catalona, W. J. (2007) Prostate-specific antigen in clinical practice. *Cancer Letters*, 249, pp. 30-39.

Loeb, S. *et al.* (2009) Exclusion of inflammation in the differential diagnosis of an elevated prostate-specific antigen (PSA). *Urologic Oncology*, 27, pp. 64-66.

Luo, J. *et al.* (2009) Principles of cancer therapy: oncogene and non-oncogene addiction. *Cell*, 136, pp. 823-837.

Mantovani, A. (2009) Cancer: Inflaming metastasis. *Nature*, 457, pp. 36-37.

Mantovani, A. *et al.* (2008) Cancer-related inflammation. *Nature*, 454, p. 436-444.

Meeks, J. J. *et al.* (2009) Characteristics of prostate cancers detected at prostate specific antigen levels less than 2.5 ng/ml. *The Journal of Urology*, 181, pp. 2515-2518.

Michaelson, M. D. *et al.* (2008) Management of complications of prostate cancer treatment. *CA: A Cancer Journal for Clinician*s, 58, pp. 196-213.

Mittra, I. (2007) The disconnection between tumor response and survival. *Nature Clinical Practice - Oncology*, 4, p. 203.

Nurse, P. (1997) Reductionism. The ends of understanding. *Nature*, 387, p. 657.

Oh, J. H. *et al.* (2009) Prostate cancer biomarker discovery using high performance mass spectral serum profiling. *Computer Methods and Programs in Biomedicine*, 96, pp. 33-41.

Patel, A. R. and Jones, J. S. (2009) Optimal biopsy strategies for the diagnosis and staging of prostate cancer. *Current Opinion in Urology*, 19, pp. 232-237.

Pondman, K. M. *et al.* (2008) MR-guided biopsy of the prostate: an overview of techniques and a systematic review. *European Urology*, 54, pp. 517-527.

Presti, J. C. Jr. (2007) Prostate biopsy strategies. Nature clinical practice. *Urology*, 4, pp. 505-511.

Presti, J. C. Jr. (2009) Repeat prostate biopsy--when, where, and how. *Urologic Oncology*, 27, pp. 312-314.

Puech, P. *et al.* (2009). Imaging of organ-confined prostate cancer: functional ultrasound, MRI and PET/computed tomography. *Current Opinion in Urology*, 19, pp. 168-176.

Reynolds, M. A. (2008) Molecular alterations in prostate cancer. *Cancer Letters*, 271, pp. 13-24.

Rose, S. (1998) What is wrong with reductionist explanations of behaviour? N*ovartis Foundation Symposium*, 213, pp. 176-186.

Rosser, C. J. (2008) Prostate cancer - to screen, or not to screen, is that the question? *BMC urology*, 8, doi: 10.1186/1471-2490-8-20.

Rubin, M. A. (2008) Targeted therapy of cancer: new roles for pathologists--prostate cancer. *Modern Pathology*, 21[Suppl 2], pp. 44-55.

Ruijter, E. T. *et al.* (1996). Histological grade heterogeneity in multifocal prostate cancer. Biological and clinical implications. *The Journal of Pathology*, 180, pp. 295-299.

Sardana, G. *et al.* (2008). Emerging biomarkers for the diagnosis and prognosis of prostate cancer. *Clinical Chemistry*, 54, pp. 1951-1960.

Schroder, F. H. *et al.* (2009) Screening and prostate-cancer mortality in a randomized European study. *The New England Journal of Medicine*, 360, pp. 1320-1328.

Sogn, J. A. *et al.* (2005). Meeting report: NCI think tanks in cancer biology. *Cancer Research*, 65, pp. 9117-9120.

Spencer, S. L. *et al.* (2009) Non-genetic origins of cell-to-cell variability in TRAIL-induced apoptosis. *Nature*, 459, pp. 428-432.

Sreekumar, A. *et al.* (2009) Metabolomic profiles delineate potential role for sarcosine in prostate cancer progression. *Nature*, 457, pp. 910-914.

Steuber, T. *et al.* (2008) Serum markers for prostate cancer: a rational approach to the literature. *European Urology*, 54, pp. 31-40.

Sun, J. *et al.* (2007) Genetic variability in inflammation pathways and prostate cancer risk. *Urologic Oncology*, 25, pp. 250-259.

Tanaka, G. *et al.* (2010) Mathematical modelling of prostate cancer growth and its application to hormone therapy. *Philosophical Transactions: Series A, Mathematical, Physical, and Engineering Sciences*, 368, pp. 5029-5044.

Turkbey, B. *et al.* (2009) Imaging localized prostate cancer: current approaches and new developments. *American Journal of Roentgenology*, 192, 1471-1480.

Witte, J. S. (2009) Prostate cancer genomics: towards a new understanding. *Nature Reviews: Genetics*, 10, pp. 77-82.

In: Hypotheses in Clinical Medicine
Editors: M.M. Shoja, P.S. Agutter et al.

ISBN: 978-1-62257-276-2

Chapter 11

New Hypotheses Concerning Cancer Carriage with Special Reference to Intracranial Lymphatic Connection

Wilson I. B. Onuigbo *
Medical Foundation and Clinic, Enugu, Nigeria

Abstract

The history of the discovery of the blood circulation to the brain is a success story. Will such success be reaped from research concerning lymphatic connections with the brain? Hitherto, strong voices have been denying lymph-borne cancer carriage to the brain on the basis that it lacks lymphatic connections with the rest of the body. However, history does throw considerable light on this elusive issue with anatomical experiments and pathological observations. The solution lies in employing the recent immuno-histochemical staining technique, which ensures differential staining of lymph vascular and blood vascular epithelia. It is predicted that perspicacious processing and strict staining of human autopsy materials that encompass (a) the skull base, (b) the suprajacent meninges and brain, and (c) the uppermost invaded neck portion will ensure the visual identification without any iota of doubt of nature's lymph-borne footsteps in the brain axis.

Introduction

The field of medicine contains several examples of diverse phenomena that were denied at one time but later recognized as part of the body of established knowledge. For example, there is the intriguing story of the ups and downs of the cerebral circulation and the measurement of cerebral blood flow (Bell 1984).

* E-mail: wilson.onuigbo@gmail.com.

Consider this quotation from Le Gros Clark (1957):

> "It was not till Harvey many years later applied experimental methods to the study of the circulation, and more particularly made calculations of the output of the blood from the heart with each heart beat, that the fact of a true circulation of the blood was established. And even then this remained in some measure a hypothesis until the existence of the capillary vessels linking arteries and veins was eventually demonstrated histologically by Malpighi and Leeuwenhoek and the movement of blood through the capillaries actually seen."

Seen with dim light even nowadays is another circulatory system. I refer to the curious conclusions concerning cancer carriage with respect to the lymphatics and cranial cavity. As Wilson (1940) concluded regarding this cavity, "modes of propagation have been much in dispute". Therefore, this disputed frontier of knowledge should be reviewed. The existence of any lymphatic connections between the cranial contents and the rest of the body was denied by Le Gross Clark (1965):

> "In the central nervous system they are entirely absent – indeed they have never been observed inside the skull or the vertebral canal. It should be noted, in this connection that perivascular channels and other spaces in connective tissue have sometimes been referred to as 'lymph spaces.' This designation is quite erroneous, for they form no part of the lymphatic vascular system and do not contain lymph."

With lymph being excluded from this supposedly alien axis, there are those who deny the possibility of cancer spreading by way of its own vessels to the brain. In other words, they accept the spread occurs through the blood vessels only. In fact, the permutations and combinations of their assertions necessitate listing as follows:

- Rich (1930) – *"the brain was not connected with the general lymphatic system of the body, precluding spread by that channel."*
- Christensen (1949) – *"we may reckon exclusively with metastasis by way of the blood stream, as there are no lymphatics in the central nervous system."*
- Anderson (1951) – *"cerebral metastatic lesions are blood-borne since no lymphatics are present in the brain."*
- West *et al.* (1972) – *"the central nervous system (CNS) does not contain lymphoid tissue, and CNS invasion by leukemic blast cells is presumed to occur from the blood."*
- Potter *et al.* (1983) – *"The CNS lacks lymphatics, and neoplasms cannot spread by this pathway so long as they are confined to brain tissue."*

International RadioSurgery Association (2008) – "Since the brain has no lymphatic systems, all tumors metastasizing to the brain do so by spreading through the bloodstream."

The bloodstream rather than the lymph stream is accepted as the route of transmission of ordinary infections to the brain. "It is anatomically impossible," asserted Atkinson (1934), "for an infection to reach the intracranial contents by a lymphatic route"; and Mackenzie (1948) wrote: "The brain has no lymphatic system, so spread of infection by this means is an anatomical impossibility". Impossibility is a word that should not to be used in science.

Perhaps many are unaware of the historical data concerning intracranial lymphatic connections. This makes it necessary to present various developments in this field, with reference to anatomical experiments and pathological observations.

Anatomical Experiments

The great John Hunter (1861) reported as follows:

> "I observed in a dog, whose carotid artery I tied, that the lymphatics were likewise tied, and that by next morning the lymphatics were very turgid with clear lymph. It is most likely that every cavity of the body has absorbents."

Absorbents, i.e. lymphatics, had been the subject of research by many anatomists. Commenting on the results obtained by some of the old masters, Horner (1846) had this to say:

> "The deep-seated absorbents of the head have been followed to the membranes of the brain, but not farther. Ruysch observed them between the tunica arachnoidea and the pia mater. Lanciscus, Pacchioni, and others, assert their having found them in the pia mater. Doubts are cast upon these several observations, owing to such vessels not having been injected with quicksilver, and from the want of a valvular appearance in them; also from the want of lymphatic glands in the cavity of the brain."

Brain elements were included among the experimental results discussed at length by Morton (1849):

> "Notwithstanding the profusion with which lymphatics are distributed to some and indeed to most of the organs, they are not demonstrable in all. In some tissues, for example, their presence can only be inferred from reason and analogy. Thus they have not been seen in the interior of the brain and spinal cord, in the cartilages, tendons and ligaments, nor in the membranes of the ovum. Yet that they exist in these parts there can be no question; for it is only of recent time that Fohmann detected them on the surface of the brain and in its membranes, in the plexus choroids, placenta and umbilical cord. They were long denied to the eye, but Arnold has found them there also; and they have moreover been traced into the interior of the bones. In these several tissues no lymphatics could be detected even by the critical eye of Mascagni, and we may therefore suppose that they will yet be discovered in the few remaining exceptions."

Exceptions were looked into by Professor His (1867). He was interested in the connection between the perivascular canals in the central nervous system and the peripheral lymphatic system:

> "If an injection of the (perivascular) network… be placed side by side with injected networks which are undoubtedly lymphatic, it is seen fully to accord with these last in respect of the width of the canals, the manner in which they are connected and the lack of an independent fibrous membrane separable from the surrounding tissue… It will only be fully settled as to the lymphatic nature of our network of tubes when we are able to demonstrate its connection with undoubted lymphatic vessels."

Amongst the anatomists who in the first ten years of the 20th century employed themselves in the injection of lymphatics, none succeeded in filling lymph-spaces within the brain or spinal cord. On the other hand, Fohmann and Arnold have observed undoubted lymphatic vessels in the pia mater (and arachnoid?), which are not difficult to display in man. But are the perivascular canals of the brain in communication with the lymphatics of the pia mater?

Pia mater was positively identified by Professor His (1867): "I think," he said, "that I am able to maintain for the brain, then, that the perivascular spaces are lymph spaces…" MacAlister (1889) accepted this. Scientists were well aware of the pitfalls of injection experiments. Rolleston (1873) confidently accepted the existence of intracranial lymphatic connections after personally comparing various investigative methods. Incidentally, Rouvière (1938) drew attention to the doubts cast on the work of Professor His, such doubts having been made "in spite of the proofs brought forward by Bevan Lewis, Obersteiner, Binswanger and Berger". Then he added:

> "Beside these lymph sheaths, the idea of a possible existence of true lymph vessels in the brain substance itself must be entertained."

Therefore, Kronthal observed canaliculi in the brain cortex, which were too small to permit the passage of blood cells, and may have been lymph capillaries. Before Kronthal, Riedel had observed similar canaliculi that connected the intra-adventitial sheaths of neighboring blood vessels. Animal experiments such as those reported by Orr and Rows (1914) are of interest in this context. In their own view, the investigation "leaves no room for doubt that the lymph-stream in nerves is an ascending one, and that toxins and organisms can be carried to the (spinal) cord by that path". Indeed, they were convinced of similar ascent to the brain. Similarly, in the words of Bruce (1928-9), "The key to many of the problems of inflammatory lesions in the central nervous system that appear so obscure will be found by a study of infection up the lymphatic channels of the peripheral nerves".

Nerves were in the research field of Brierley and Field (1948). They injected Indian ink into the cranial subarachnoid space of the rabbit and observed the presence of that ink in the cervical lymph node within four hours. They put their result in historical perspective as follows:

> "The first clear evidence of a connection between the cranial subarachnoid space and the cervical lymphatic system was provided by Schwalbe in 1869, and the existence of such a connection is now generally accepted, although detailed knowledge of the precise pathway is still incomplete. In general, it is believed that the route is from the subarachnoid space, along the perineural spaces of the olfactory nerves to the tissue spaces of the nasal mucosa and thence, via fine lymph vessels, to the deep cervical lymph nodes."

Nodes interested Orosz and his co-workers (1957). They used radioactive dyes and reported that "a lymphatic communication exists between the mucosa of the nasal septum and the cranial cavity, inasmuch as the lymph flowed from the middle and posterior thirds of the septal mucosa toward the cranial cavity… (and) the dye reached not only the subarachnoid space, but also the hypothalamus…" That such connections do exist was described as being "highly significant anatomically, physiologically and pathologically" by Rusznyak and co-authors (1960). That decade saw Foldi and his group (1966) surveying new contributions to the anatomical connections of the brain and the lymphatic system. In an elegant experiment using Congo red solution in dogs, they applied back pressure to the cervical lymphatics to obtain retrograde flow toward and within the skull. The tissues were removed *en bloc,* fixed in formalin, decalcified, embedded in paraffin, and cut serially, starting from the brain and proceeding caudally. In this way, they demonstrated the existence of lymphatics connecting intracranial tissues with cervical structures.

Pathological Observations

Structures in diseased states have been observed through the centuries. Little wonder that many have been struck by the manifestations of intracranial lymphatic connections as revealed by pathological processes. Long ago, Cruikshank (1790), a protégé of John Hunter, was "perfectly certain" that the brain has lymphatics:

> "The glands of the neck swell in some diseases of the brain: I have seen this particularly in scrophulous abscess of the brain; I found the glands of the neck swelled with affection of the brain, in the living, and I found the abscess after death; nor should I believe any vessel to be an absorbent which, coming from the brain, did not terminate in the glands of the neck."

Neck nodes impressed Velpeau (1853) when he saw them to be swollen in scrofulous persons "in consequence of some previous disease of the head". Three decades later, Ziegler (1883) appreciated that inflammatory mischief may be wrought on the brain through the lymphatics. As he wrote: "The central nervous system is thus not only surrounded on all sides by lymph-spaces but also traversed in all directions by lymph channels, and its blood-vessels all lie in lymph-sheaths". William MacEwen (1893) also believed this, and his penetrating observation is worth recalling: "Intracranial irritation shows itself first in the swelling of the deep cervical glands, but, as they lie under the cervical fascia, their enlargement is apt to be concealed unless specially looked for…"

For Colomiatti (1877), it was "an axiom that one of the means by which cancer spreads is the lymphatic system of nerves quite independent of the other nervous elements". In the opinion of Wagstaffe (1871), with reference to intracranial meningeal lesions, this was a direct result of Nature's own experiments. "Now," as he averred, "the artificial injections have been made by Professor His, and an example of the natural one is shown in the accompanying cases of tubercular meningitis". Furthermore, his forecast is worthy of recall: "It would be interesting to examine more carefully into the condition of the vessels and perivascular canals in all cases of similar or allied tumors of the brain, but I am not aware of attention having been given to this point".

The point of view of Hassin (1919), another who believed in the existence of intracranial lymphatic connections, is material. His analogy in respect of cancerous invasion of the meninges was apt: "In this case the injection was, as it were, done with cancer cells, and not by hands, but by nature herself, and must, therefore, be considered a much superior experiment and of greater scientific value". Value was probably added to the ongoing discourses, with the striking example of the 10th case in the M.D. thesis of Stewart (1908). In it, breast cancer was reported to have spread intracranially. Moreover, "the extension to the brain was obviously along the perivascular lymphatics" that follow the carotid artery, the line of spread being "visible to the naked eye". In a contemporaneous M.D. thesis, Frew (1910) traced comparable perivascular lymphatic connection in the intracranial spread of neuroblastomatous tumor.

Tumor spread with regard to the role of the lymphatics in intracranial deposition was problematic. Therefore, it is significant that those who believed in its possibility varied widely in their points of view. For example, Taylor *et al.* (1984) combined all possibilities: "Tumor cells may spread to intracranial structures as blood-borne deposits, as retrograde metastases through lymphatic vessels, or as extensions from metastatic foci in adjacent skull or soft tissue". Pochedly (1976) pronounced: "It should be noted that lymphatic connections exist between many parts of the brain and the extracranial lymph nodes and that a considerable amount of CSF is reabsorbed into the lymphatic system".

The system of lymph transportation, which is related to the nerves, i.e. *perineural* lymphatics, was accepted by Cornwall (1927), Alpers and Smith (1938), Barnard and Robb-Smith (1945), Brain (1955), Carter *et al.* (1979) and Strauss and Cohen (1981). Carter *et al.* (1982) distinguished the practical point that taking at minimum of between four and six tissue blocks – and sometimes many more – increased the incidence of perineural spread in a series. However, variability is such that the pendulum swung from Delafield and Prudden (1928), who accepted the probability that "most" brain metastases are the result of retrograde invasion of the perineural lymphatics of the cranial nerves, to Earle (1955), who described as "uncommon" the spread through these channels. Again, there is the swing between Elkington (1936), who saw "much more rarely a diffuse carcinomatous invasion of the meninges... which is probably due to a lymphatic spread", and Grain and Karr (1955) whose "main thesis is the support of the theory of perineural lymphatic invasion in leptomeningeal carcinomatosis". Indeed, as Davison and Horwitz (1930) exemplified: "The involvement of the glands in the neck and the solitary metastatic nodule to the brain are in favor of a direct extension of the mass from the cervical lymph glands and the lymphatic spaces of the neck by a backward flow of the lymph".

A lymph-oriented pattern was established in respect of the brain when there was an intimate *perivascular* relationship (Biggart, 1940). Earlier, Muir (1924) had described this beautifully: "The cells of the growth have a great tendency to spread along the perivascular lymphatics, so that vessels, including even the capillaries, may be ensheathed by them". Perhaps these spaces should not be called perivascular "lymphatics" as Carmichael *et al.* (1939) argued. However, what are they? Fischer-Williams *et al.* (1955) and his associates related a case in which "the blood vessels in the subarachnoid space were surrounded by carcinoma cells, which continued on the penetrating vessels as a perivascular cuff for a short distance into the substance of the brain". Muir (1924) was strongly affirmative; knowing that there is "a great tendency to spread along the perivascular lymphatics, so that vessels, including even the capillaries, may be ensheathed by them". Courville (1953) accepted their invading "to varying degrees in the nervous structure". Scheinker (1948) and Biggart (1940, 1961) designated the phenomenon as "cuffing" in their pathology textbooks. Likewise, Hassin and Singer (1922), Hassin (1933), Swinburne (1948), Johnston and Whillis (1950), and Keele and Neil (1965) observed this. Olson *et al.* (1974) recognized that metastatic deposits originating in the perivascular spaces of the penetrating vessels could extend directly across the pial-glial membrane to form a nodular parenchymal mass. Therefore, this is a disputed issue whose enigmatic nature is best illustrated with the solution offered by Globus and Meltzer (1942):

> "Mention is often made of the probability that lymphatics may serve as channels for the transportation of tumor cells to the brain. In such discussion no clear distinction is made between the perivascular system of Virchow and Robin and true lymphatics. Certainly, these two systems are independent in the main and are not to be confused."

A confused area worthy of notice is the invasion of skull bones. Biggart (1961) observed that some carcinomas "grow into the skull cavity along the cranial nerves, and spread along the dura or into the brain itself". Mikhail *et al.* (1986) reminisced that bone acts as a natural barrier to the direct spread of basal cell carcinoma. As they put it: "Invasion through the full thickness of the calvarium results in involvement of the meninges and brain that is serious and life-threatening". Reynolds (1930) in his M.D. thesis was of the view that intracranial structures were linked with the system "consisting of blood vessels with their accompanying lymph vessels and loose connective tissue". Little wonder that Symonds and Cairns (1950) mentioned that occasionally the neoplastic process is limited to the pia arachnoid but that "tumors in the middle or posterior fossa sometimes arise by direct spread from a squamous carcinoma of the nasopharynx". In the words of Ewing (1942): "The dura and skull may be affected when the brain is free, suggesting an access by cranial lymphatics". In what he called "Lymphatic Manifesto," Casley-Smith (1984) considered that "in the brain and retina these communications lie outside the skull". Carter (1985) reflected on the incidence of "direct invasion" of the skull. In this vein, it is interesting to note that there is a definition problem regarding *direct* spread and *metastatic* spread. Lack of appreciation of their inter-relationship, in my view (Onuigbo 1973; Onuigbo 1975), constitutes a stumbling block in the theories of cancer carriage. Hence, as I see it (Onuigbo 1958), specific aspects of cancer carriage require concerted research including hypotheses.

Hypotheses and Conclusion

To reminisce, Willis (1973) was authoritative: "Some writers have supposed that discrete secondary tumors in the brain may arise by retrograde lymphatic embolism from affected cervical lymph glands… Since no lymphatics exist in central nervous tissue and since no tangible evidence for their hypothesis has ever been advanced by its supporters, the suggestion may be dismissed". Admittedly, it has been demonstrated that the history of the possible existence of intracranial lymphatic connections is a long standing enigma. Incidentally, although several modern authors are under the impression that these connections have never been observed, their existence cannot be altogether ruled out. Perhaps part of the problem is that original observations are not followed up. For instance, Frew (1911) reported a case in which a chain of invaded lymph nodes "passed upwards, along the carotid sheath, and could be traced passing through the base of the skull, along with the internal carotid artery, whilst in one case a small gland was found in the wall of the cavernous sinus". Has such an opening ever been pursued? Be that as it may, it was necessary in this chapter to begin by pointing out the elements of the befogged beliefs in the existence of lymphatic linkages. Certainly, they were recorded, not only by the old masters but by researchers today.

Continuing to pursue such leads requires fresh hypotheses. In particular, just as was the case with animal experiments, Foldi *et al.* (1966) called for *serial* cutting, "starting from the brain and proceeding caudally", that is imitated with human autopsy materials. Incidentally, this was carried out to a limited extent with reference to the debated issue of the spread of cancer along the lymph node-pancreas axis.

An axis of great importance evoked supreme surprise in a recent review in the *Journal of Pathology*, whose Editor-in-Chief, Peter Hall (2011), called it the pathology journal with the highest impact factor. Therein, Mohammed *et al.* (2011) assessed data concerning lymphatic and blood vascular invasion in lymph node-negative breast carcinomas. Based on a large case series, they wrote "results raise some important questions" concerning the three questions that they had posed, the second being: "How do tumor cells reach organs known to have very few or no lymphatics, such as the brain?"

The brain connection or lack of it has long occupied a precarious position in the way in which researchers assess lymph-borne metastasis. More than half a century ago, I tackled that dilemma in terms of history (Onuigbo 1961b) and topography (Onuigbo 1958). The latter article marshaled several points of interest concerning the spread of lung cancer to the brain:

i. The probability of an even distribution of metastases expected from the hematogenous theory does not occur. Instead, there is statistically significant ipsilateral preponderance, which is in keeping with the lymphogenous route.
ii. The nearer a tumor is to the brain, the more likely it is to spread there, i.e. centrifugal spread occurs.
iii. The cerebellum is seen to be a site of predilection when compared with the rest of the much larger brain.
iv. Solitary brain deposits are relatively common, thereby indicating that this phenomenon is not due to chance but to the localization role of the lymphogenous route.
v. Cases were featured to indicate surprising one-sided preponderance of deposits that is more in keeping with lymphogenous predisposition. Take the Record of Aberdeen Royal Infirmary, No 92/1952, which was abstracted thus: "*Right* lung origin. The *right* paratracheal lymph nodes are extensively invaded by tumor and form a large mass extending up into the neck above the clavicle; on the left, one of the paratracheal nodes is invaded. Two small tumor nodules are seen, on section, in the *right* frontal lobe; a similar nodule is found in the *right* occipital lobe. On section, numerous secondary deposits of varying size are found scattered throughout the liver, more especially in the *right* lobe. The *right* adrenal is extensively invaded and weighs 130 g. The left is free."

Free use of a new technique is quintessential. I refer to the development of immunohistochemical staining that differentiates lymph vasculature from its blood vascular counterpart (Mohammed *et al.* 2007). The availability of such markers has increased the probability of developing a decisive model. A model worthy of development hinges partly on the fact that Carter *et al.* (1983) worked with major surgical *resections* for squamous carcinomas of the head and neck and discovered that: "Infiltrating carcinomas frequently invade perineural spaces, which provide a route of further dissemination, notably to the intracranial cavity". In fact, Kyzas *et al.* (2005) found that lymph vessels naturally sprout outwards from squamous cell carcinomas of the head and neck. Therefore, whenever such growths exist in the upper neck and the suprajacent brain, their interconnections should be stained with perspicacity and precision. In short, the next step should be to employ the more copious materials that are obtainable at *autopsy*. Since lymph-borne metastasis tends to be unilateral or to preponderate on one side (Onuigbo 1961a), the redoubtable research blocks need to be handily unilateral. Accordingly, wide enough samples should encompass (i) the skull base, (ii) the invaded suprajacent meninges or brain, and (iii) the uppermost invaded neck tissues. It is hypothesized that exploiting such triple tissue blocks will expose the panoramic patterns of any underlying lymphogenous or hematogenous pathways.

Pathways have recently been categorically distinguished as either lymphatic or blood vascular by means of the new staining marker techniques. I am persuaded that these same markers will provide the breakthrough in the elusive field of lymphatic connections existing along the body-brain axis. Hopefully, Hospital Ethical Committees will welcome such a promising prospect of answering this long standing question in human oncology. Thus, as Cochran (2001) maintained, the practicing pathologist is in a prime position to advance knowledge by developing novel techniques, and such techniques should be welcomed as they emerge.

Finally, the role of tumor lymphangiogenesis in spread of metastasis is receiving growing attention (Stacker *et al.* 2002; Onuigbo 2010). Elsewhere, I fully documented twelve human models for research concerning cancer carriage (Onuigbo 2011). It is predicted that the present model will prove that when the old postmortem methods and the new immuno-histochemical staining techniques are effectively combined, the quoted questionings of the role of the lymphatics in the realm of cancer carriage to the brain will be finally answered.

References

Alpers, B. J. and Smith, O. N. (1938) Carcinomatosis of the meninges of the spinal cord and base of brain without involvement of the parenchyma, secondary to carcinoma of the lung. *American Journal of Cancer*, 32, pp. 361-366.

Anderson, R. (1951) Diodrast studies of the vertebral and cranial venous systems to show their probable role in cerebral metastases. *Journal of Neurosurgery*, 8, pp. 411-422.

Atkinson, E. M. (1934) *Abscess of the Brain: Its Pathology, Diagnosis and Treatment*. London: Medical Publications Ltd., p. 28.

Barnard, W. G. and Robb-Smith, A. H. T. (1945) *Kettle's Pathology of Tumours*. London: H.K. Lewis, p. 28.

Bell, B. A. (1984) A history of the study of the cerebral circulation and the measurement of cerebral blood flow. *Neurosurgery*, 14, pp. 238-246.

Biggart, J. H. (1940) *Pathology of the Nervous System, Edition* 2. Edinburgh: Livingstone, p. 323.

Biggart, J. H. (1961). *Pathology of the Nervous System, Edittion 3*. London: Livingstone, p. 334.

Brain, R. (1955) *Disease of the Nervous System*. London: Oxford University Press, p. 235.

Brierley, J. B And Field, E. J. (1948) The connections of the spinal sub-archnoid space with the lymphatic system. *Journal of Anatomy*, 72, pp. 153-166.

Bruce, A. N. (1928-9) Lymphogenous infection of the central nervous system, with a review of malarial therapy. *Transactions of the Medical-Chirurgical Society of Edinburgh*, 43, pp. 111-127.

Carmichael, F.A. *et al.* (1939) Histopathogenesis of cerebral abscess. *Archives of Neurology and Psychiatry*, 42, pp. 1001-1029.

Carter, R. L. (1985) Patterns and mechanisms of localized bone invasion by tumors: studies with squamous carcinomas of the head and neck. *Critical Reviews of Clinical Laboratory Science*, 22, pp. 275-315.

Carter, R. L. *et al.* (1979) Perineural spread in squamous cell carcinomas of the head and neck: a clinicopathological study. *Clinical Otolaryngology*, 4, pp. 271-281.

Carter, R. L. *et al.* (1982) Pain and dysphagia in patients with squamous carcinomas of the head and neck: the role of perineural spread. *Journal of the Royal Society of Medicine*, 75, pp. 598-605.

Carter, R. L. *et al.* (1983) Perineural spread by squamous carcinomas of the head and neck: a morphological study using antiaxonal and antimyelin monoclonal antibodies. *Journal of Clinical Pathology,* 36, pp. 269-275.

Casley-Smith, J. R. (1984) Lymphatic manifesto. *Lymphology*, 17, pp. 109-110.

Christensen, E. (1949) Intracranial carcinomatous metastases in a neurosurgical clinic. *Acta Psychiatrica et Neurologica Scandinavica*, 24, pp. 353-361.

Cochran, A. J. (2001) The role of practising pathologists in the generation of novel and original observations. *Journal of Pathology*, 193, pp. 1-2.

Colomiatti, V. (1877) The spread of cancer. *Edinburgh Medical Journal*, 22, p. 1041.

Cornwall, L. H. (1927) Metastatic meningo-encephalic carcinoma without tumefaction. *Archives of Neurology and Psychiatry*, 17, pp. 467-470.

Courville, C. B. (1953) *Essentials of Neuropathology*. Los Angeles: San Lucas Press, pp. 247-252.

Cruikshank, W. (1790) T*he Anatomy of the Absorbing Vessels of the Human Body, Edition 2*. London: Nicol, p. 204.

Davison, C. and Horwitz, W. H. (1930) Primary carcinoma of the lungs with metastases to the central nervous system. *Archives of Internal Medicine*, 46, pp. 680-704.

Delafield, F. and Prudden, T. M. (1928) *Textbook of Pathology, Revised by F. C. Wood*. Edinburgh: Livingstone, p. 732.

Earle, K. M. (1955) Metastatic brain tumours. *Diseases of the Nervous System*, 17, pp. 86-92.

Elkington, J. C. (1936) Metastatic brain tumours. *St. Thomas Hospital Report*, 1, pp. 97-108.

Ewing, J. *Neoplastic Diseases*. Philadelphia: Saunders, p 586.

Fischer-Williams, M. *et al.* (1955) Carcinomatosis of the meninges: A report of 3 cases. *Brain*, 78, pp. 42-58.

Foldi, M. *et al.* (1966) New contributions to the anatomical connections of the brain and the lymphatic system. *Acta Anatomica*, 44, p. 498.

Frew, R. S. (1910) *On Carcinoma Originating in the Suprarenal Medulla in Children*. M. D. thesis, Edinburgh University.

Frew, R. S. (1911) On carcinoma originating in the suprarenal medulla in children. *Quarterly Journal of Medicine*, 4, pp. 123-140.

Grain, G. O. and Karr, J. P. (1955) Diffuse leptomeningeal carcinomatosis. Clinical and pathologic characteristics. *Neurology*, 5, pp. 706-722.

Globus, J. H. and Meltzer, T. (1942) Metastatic tumors of the brain. *Archives of Neurology and Psychiatry*, 48, pp. 163-226.

Hall, P. A. (2011) Getting your paper published: an editor's perspective. *Annals of Saudi Medicine*, 31, pp. 72-76.

Hassin, G. B. (1919) Histopathology of the cerebral meninges. *Archives of Neurology and Psychiatry*, 1, pp. 705-716.

Hassin, G. B. (1933) *Histopathology of the Peripheral and Central Nervous Systems*. London: Bailliere, Tindoll and Cox, p. 409.

Hassin, G. B. and Singer, H. D. (1922) Histopathology of cerebral carcinoma. *Archives of Neurology and Psychiatry*, 8, pp. 155-171.

His, W. (1867) On a system of perivascular canals in the nerve centres, and on their relationship to the lymphatic system. *Journal of Anatomy and Physiology*, 7, pp. 347-352.

Horner, W. E. (1846) *Special Anatomy and Histology, Edition 7, Volume 2*. Philadelphia: Lea and Blanchard, p. 321.

Hunter, J. (1861) *Essays and Observations (Edited by. By R. Owen), Volume 1*. London: John vas Hoorst, p. 151.

International Radiosurgery Association (2008) Radiosurgery practice guideline report, no. 5-08.

Johnston, T. B. and Whillis, J. (1950) *Gray's Anatomy*. London: Longmans, Green & Co Ltd, p. 858.

Keele, C. E. and Neil, E. (1965) *Samson Wright's Applied Physiology*. London: Oxford University Press, p. 48.

Kyzas, P. A. *et al.* (2005) Evidence for lymphangiogenesis and its prognostic implications in head and neck squamous cell carcinoma. *Journal of Pathology*, 206, pp. 170-177.

Le Gros Clark, W. (1957) *Lectures in the Scientific Basis of Medicine*. London: Athlone Press.

Le Gros Clark, W. (1965) *The Tissues of the Body, Edition 5*. Oxford: Clarendon Press, p. 246.

Macalister, A. (1889) *A Text-book of Human Anatomy*. London: Charles Griffin, p. 88.

Mackenzie, K. G. (1948) Brain abscess. *British Surgical Practice*, 2, p. 325.

Macewen, W. (1893) *Pyogenic Infective Diseases of the Brain and Spinal Cord*. Glasgow: Maclehose, p. 39.

Mikhail, G. R. et al. (1986) Cranial invasion by basal cell carcinoma. *The Journal of Dermatologic Surgery and Oncology*, 12, pp. 459-464.

Mohammed, R. A. *et al.* (2007) Improved methods of detection of lymphovascular invasion demonstrate that it is the predominant method of vascular in breast cancer and has important clinical consequences. *American Journal of Surgical Pathology*, 31, pp. 1825-1833.

Mohammed, R. A. A. *et al.* (2011). Objective assessment of lymphatic and blood vascular invasion in lymph node-negative breast carcinoma: findings from a large case series with long-term follow-up. *Journal of Pathology*, 223, pp. 358-365.

Morton, S. G. (1849) *An Illustrated System of Human Anatomy, Special, General and Microscopic*. Philadelphia: Grigg, Eliot & Co, p. 471.

Muir, R. (1924) *Textbook of Pathology*. London: Arnold, p. 626.

Olson, M. E. *et al.* (1974) Infiltration of the leptomeninges by systemic cancer. A clinical and pathologic study. *Archives of Neurology*, 30, pp. 122-137.

Onuigbo, W. I. B. (1958) The spread of lung cancer to the brain. *British Journal of Tuberculosis and Diseases of the Chest*, 52, pp. 141-148.

Onuigbo, W. I. B. (1961a) Patterns of metastasis in lung cancer: a review. *Cancer Research*, 21, pp. 1077-1085.

Onuigbo, W. I. B. (1961b) Cerebral lymphatics. *British Medical Journal*, 1, pp. 505-506.

Onuigbo, W. I. B. (1973) Fundamental differences between direct and metastatic spread clarified with lung cancer. *British Journal of Diseases of the Chest*, 67, pp. 131-140.

Onuigbo, W. I. B. (1975) A definition problem in cancer metastasis. *Neoplasma*, 22, pp. 547-550.

Onuigbo, W. I. B. (2010) Lymphangiognesis may explain adrenal selectivity in lung cancer metastases. *Medical Hypotheses*, 75, pp. 185-186.

Onuigbo, W. I. B. (2011) *Human Models in Cancer Metastasis Research*. Saarbrucken: Lambert Academic Publishing, GmbH & Co.

Orosz, A. *et al.* (1957) Radioactive isotope studies of the connection between the lymph circulation of the nasal mucosa, the cranial cavity and cerebrospinal fluid. *Acta Physiologica Hungarica*, 11, pp. 75-81.

Orr, D and Rows, R. G. (1914) Lymphogenous infection of the central nervous system. *Brain*, 36, pp. 271-340.

Pochedly, C. (1976) Untitled reprint. *Postgraduate Medicine*, 59, pp. 101-105.

Potter, C. R. *et al.* (1983) Glioblastoma multiforme metastatic to the neck. *American Journal of Otolaryngology*, 4, pp. 74-76.

Reynolds, F. E. (1930) *A Pathological Study of the Pathways of Infection to the Intracranial Structures from Foci of Inflammation on the Face and in the Nasal and Nasal Accessory Cavities*. MD thesis, Edinburgh University, pp. 17-18.

Rich, G. J. (1930) The distribution of metastatic tumors in the cerebrum. *Archives of Neurology and Psychiatry*, 51, pp. 423-425.

Rolleston, G. (1873) *The Harveian Oration*. London: Macmillan, p. 21.

Rouvière, H. (1938) *Anatomy of the Human Lymphatic System (Translated by M. J. Tobias)*. Michigan: Edward Brothers, pp. 238-239.

Rusznyak, I. *et al.* (1960) *Lymphatics and Lymph Circulation*. Oxford: Pergamon, p. 156.

Scheinker, I. M. (1948) *Neurosurgical Pathology*. Springfield: Thomas, p. 270.

Stacker, S. A. *et al.* (2002) Lymphangiogenesis and cancer metastasis. *Nature Reviews - Cancer*, 2, pp. 573-583.

Stewart, H. G. (1908) *Notes and Observations on Forty Consecutive Cases of New Growth*. MD thesis, Birmingham University, p. 79.

Strauss, M. and Cohen, C. (1980) Perineural invasion of the facial nerve: a case report with extension from cutaneous squamous cell carcinoma. *Head and Neck Surgery*, 89, pp. 831-835.

Swinburne, G. (1948) The surgical pathology of brain abscess. *Medical Journal of Australia*, 2, pp. 157-183.

Symonds, C. and Cairns, H. (1950) Brain tumors. In: Horder, L. (ed.) *The British Encylopaedia of Medical Practice, Edition 2, Volume 3*. London: Butterworths, p. 96.

Taylor, H. G. *et al.* (1984) Intracranial metastases in prostate cancer. *Cancer*, 53, pp. 2728-2730.

Velpeau, A. (1853) Diseases of the lymphatics. *London Medical and Surgical Journal*, 7, p. 352.

Wagstaffe, W. W. (1871) Remarks on the healthy and morbid anatomy of the perivascular system of the brain. *St. Thomas Hospital Reports*, 2, pp. 149-164.

West, R. J. *et al.* (1972) Factors in pathogenesis of central nervous system leukaemia. *British Medical Journal*, 3, pp. 311-314.

Willis, R. A. (1973) *The Spread of Tumours in the Human Body*. London: Butterworths, p. 252.

Wilson, S. A. K. (1940) *Neurology, Volume 2*. London: Edward Arnold, pp. 1211-1213.

Ziegler, E. (1883) *A Text-Book of Pathological Anatomy and Pathogenesis, Volume 2 (translated by D. MacAlister)*. London: Macmillan, p. 221.

In: Hypotheses in Clinical Medicine
Editors: M.M. Shoja, P.S. Agutter et al.

ISBN: 978-1-62257-276-2

Chapter 12

A Proposal for a New Strategy in the Treatment of Head and Neck Cancer: Combination Chemotherapy Targeting the PI3kinase/Akt and EGFR Signaling Pathways

Yuh Baba[1,*], Masato Fujii[2], Yutaka Tokumaru[2] and Yasumasa Kato[3]

[1]Ohtawara Red Cross Hospital, Ohtawara City, Tochigi, Japan
[2]National Institute of Sensory Organs, National Tokyo Medical Center, Higashigaoka, Meguro, Tokyo, Japan
[3]Department of Oral Function and Molecular Biology, Ohu University, Tomita-machi, Koriyama City, Fukushima, Japan

Abstract

Epidermal growth factor receptor (EGFR) is expressed at high levels in head and neck squamous cell carcinoma (HNSCC), but EGFR inhibitor monotherapy has limited success. The PI3kinase/Akt pathway is responsible for cellular survival and inhibition of phosphatidylinositol (PI) synthesisprovides anti-proliferative, anti-invasive and anti-angiogenesis effects on HNSCC. There is molecular cross-talk between EGFR and insulin-like growth factor-1 receptor (IGF1R) signaling through the PI3kinase/Akt pathway in HNSCC. Therefore, combination therapy that targets PI3kinase/Akt and EGFR signaling pathways should provide clinical benefits to patients with HNSCC.

[*] E-mail: yuh_baba@hotmail.com.

Introduction

Head and neck squamous cell carcinoma (HNSCC) is the sixth most common neoplasm worldwide (Cripps *et al.* 2010). Approximately 600,000 new cases are reported each year (Cripps *et al.* 2010), and in the past 30 years, recurrent and/or metastatic HNSCC has had a poor prognosis (Khuri *et al.* 2000; Forastiere *et al.* 2001). More than 50% of newly diagnosed patients do not achieve complete remission, and in approximately 10% of HNSCC cases, relapse with metastasis to distant organs has been reported (van Houten *et al.* 2000). Therefore, research focused on gaining a better understanding of this disease and the development of novel treatment strategies is required.

Epidermal growth factor receptor (EGFR), a ubiquitously expressed transmembrane glycoprotein belonging to the ErbB/HER family of receptor tyrosine kinases (TK), is composed of an extracellular ligand-binding domain, a hydrophobic transmembrane segment and an intracellular TK domain. When ligands bind to EGFR, the receptor undergoes a conformational change that promotes homo- or hetero-dimerization with other members of the ErbB/HER family of receptors; subsequent autophosphorylation and activation of the TK domain ensues (Ciardiello and Tortora 2003). Activation of EGFR leads to the activation of intracellular signaling pathways that regulate cell proliferation, invasion, angiogenesis and metastasis.

EGFR is expressed at high levels in the majority of epithelial malignancies including HNSCC. Elevated expression of EGFR in HNSCC correlates with poor prognosis, and it has long been a target of anti-cancer treatments owing to its critical role in cell survival and proliferation. Numerous tyrosine kinase inhibitors with FDA approval have been developed to target EGFR including gefitinib, erlotinib and lapatinib (Carter *et al.* 2009). These molecules are reversible competitors, competing with adenosine triphosphate (ATP) for the tyrosine kinase binding domain of EGFR. By inhibiting receptor activation, downstream signaling pathways are inhibited, leading to a decrease in cell proliferation and survival. EGFR signaling activates a number of downstream effectors including the phosphatidylinositol-3-kinase (PI3kinase)/Akt pathway.

Rare EGFR Mutations in HNSCC

Somatic mutations in the TK domain of the EGFR gene (in-frame deletion in exon 19, L858, G719X and L861Q) are associated with increased sensitivity to EGFR tyrosine kinase inhibitors (TKIs) and are present in 10~30% of non-small cell lung carcinoma (NSCLC) cases depending on ethnic origin. These mutant EGFRs selectively activate signal transduction and activator of transcription (STAT) signaling pathways and Akt, which promote cell survival. However, they have no effect on extracellular signal-regulated kinase signaling, which induces proliferation. Furthermore, mutant EGFRs selectively transduce survival signals, and inhibition of those signals by TKIs could contribute to the efficacy of a drug used to treat NSCLC (Sordella *et al.* 2004). However, molecular analysis of HNSCC tumor samples has not revealed the same spectrum of mutations (Loeffler-Ragg *et al.* 2006; Taguchi *et al.* 2008; Ozawa *et al.* 2009).

A resistance mutation has emerged in EGFR and is known as T790M. It is a missense mutation in the kinase domain that could help to explain resistance to TKIs in NSCLCs exhibiting L858R (Wong 2008). However, we did not detect this mutation in 86 HNSCC tumor samples (unpublished data).

Inhibition of Phosphatidylinositol (PI) Synthesis in HNSCC

a) Anti-proliferation

An imbalance between G1 cyclin and CDK (cyclin-dependent kinase) inhibitors (CKIs) contributes to tumorigenesis and tumor progression. Cyclin D1/PRAD1 acts as a positive regulator of the cell cycle via phosphorylaton of pRB (Rb protein), and the formation of a cyclin D1-CDK4 complex. When pRB is hyperphosphorylated by CDKs, pRB releases E2F, and free E2F is available to transcriptionally active genes encoding proteins critical for S-phase functions.

CKIs are classified into two groups: members of the Ink4 family (p15, p16, p18, and p19) for cyclin D/CDK4 or cyclin D/CDK6, and the cip/kip family (p21, p27, and p57) for cyclin D/CDK4 and cyclin E/CDK2. Over-expression of cyclin D1 in HNSCC is an important prognostic marker, predicting sensitivity to chemotherapy and radiotherapy. Furthermore, imbalance between cyclin D1 and its inhibitors (p16 and p27) could be critical in the development of HNSCC. Strategies to block cyclin D1 function have been studied extensively; for example, Nakashima and Clayman (2000) reported that the introduction of an anti-sense cyclin D1 expression vector into cells reduced their growth rate *in vitro* and decreased tumorigenicity in athymic nude mice. We have previously reported that inhibition of PI synthesis caused G1 arrest of HNSCC accompanied by decreased levels of cyclin D1, cyclin E and phosphorylated pRB (Baba *et al.* 2001).

b) Inhibition of MMP (Matrix Metalloproteinase) Production/Activity

Tumor metastasis is a complex multistep process including growth at the primary site, entry into the circulation (intravasation), adhesion to the basement membranes (BM) of target organs, extravasation and growth at secondary sites. Among these steps, the intravasation and extravasation processes involve degradation of the BM by proteinases, normally MMPs. MMP-9/gelatinase B and MMP-2/gelatinase A have specificity for type IV collagen, which acts as the backbone of BM, and therefore probably plays a major role in degrading the BM. In HNSCC, MMP-2 and MMP-9 are associated with metastatic potential. Therefore, MMPs are attractive therapy targets and many drugs have been developed to prevent their extracellular matrix-degrading activities during metastasis and angiogenesis. We have previously demonstrated that the inhibition of PI synthesis affects production of MMP-2 and MMP-9 in HNSCC cell lines (Baba *et al.* 2000).

c) Anti-angiogenesis

Angiogenesis, the formation of new blood vessels from pre-existing capillaries or incorporating bone marrow-derived endothelial precursor cells into growing vessels, is associated with the malignant phenotype of cancer. In addition, it plays a role in diverse diseases such as diabetic retinopathy, age-related macular degeneration, rheumatoid arthritis, psoriasis, atherosclerosis and restenosis (Cherrington *et al.* 2000). Clinical association of tumor vascularity with tumor aggressiveness has been demonstrated in a wide variety of tumor types including HNSCC. Therefore, determining microvessel density in tumor tissues can be useful in the estimation of a patient's prognosis. Inhibition of angiogenesis can repress the growth rate of tumor cells and lead to cell death resulting from reduced nutrition and oxygen supply to the tumor. Vascular endothelial growth factor (VEGF), which plays a major role in many angiogenic processes, binds to its receptor Flk-1/KDR in order to stimulate EC (endothelial cell) proliferation through the phospholipase Cγ-protein kinase C-ERK (extracellular signal-regulated kinase) pathway, but not via Ras (Takahashi *et al.* 1999). In addition, VEGF stimulates EC migration through p38 MAPK (mitogen-activated kinase) independently of ERK (Rousseau *et al.* 1997). Therefore, these two major MAPK pathways are eligible targets for therapeutic reduction of angiogenesis in HNSCC.

Most clinical trials concerning anti-angiogenic agents have been conducted in patients with advanced disease that had become resistant to conventional therapies. Phase III trials of these agents have compared the efficacy of standard chemotherapy alone and in combination with an experimental angiogenesis inhibitor (Gotink and Verheul 2010). The results of some studies have been negative or controversial, but several recent clinical trials in which VEGF signaling was blocked demonstrated a significant clinical benefit (Ho and Kuo 2007). SU11248, a tyrosine kinase inhibitor of the Flk-1/KDR receptor (VEGF receptor) and bevacizumab, a monoclonal antibody to VEGF, have been approved by the FDA (Ho and Kuo 2007). Furthermore, we have demonstrated that the inhibition of PI abrogated stimulation by VEGF on the growth and migration of human umbilical vein ECs through the ERK-cyclin D1 and p38 pathways, respectively (Baba *et al.* 2004). Increased PI synthase expression is an early event in HNSCC (Kaur *et al.* 2010), so inhibition of PI synthesis could be a potent therapeutic strategy for HNSCC (Baba *et al.* 2010).

Resistance to EGFR TKIs

HNSCC is almost always associated with the expression of EGFR and the extremely rare mutation T790M, and EGFR signaling activates a number of downstream effectors including the PI3Kinase/Akt pathway. Inhibition of PI synthesis could be a potent therapeutic strategy for HNSCC, but treatment with anti-EGFR agents has had limited results in patients. In a phase II trial, gefitinib was administered to patients with recurrent or metastatic HNSCC and the overall response rate was 11% (Cohen *et al.* 2003). Furthermore, in a similar study carried out on patients with recurrent and /or metastatic HNSCC, the response rate to erlotinib was 4% (Soulieres *et al.* 2004).

a) Ras Mutations

Previous reports have indicated that activating K-*ras* mutations could induce activation of the Ras/mitogen activated protein kinase (MAPK) pathway independently of EGFR, which in turn induces resistance to TKIs (Eberhard *et al.* 2005). The data suggests that K-*ras* mutation causes insensitivity to TKIs. In HNSCC, H-*ras* mutations are more common than K-*ras* mutations and may play an important role in resistance to EGFR-targeted therapies (Anderson *et al.* 1994).

b) Epithelial-mesenchymal Transition (EMT)

EMT, a change in the morphology and motility of cells that is indicated by increased vimentin expression, decreased expression of E-cadherin and increased expression of claudins 4 and 7, has been associated with gefitinib resistance in HNSCC (Frederick *et al.* 2007).

c) Upregulation of Cyclin D1

Upregulation of cyclin D1 in HNSCC cell lines is specifically associated with resistance to gefitinib; retinoblastoma protein (pRb) is hyperphosphorylated by cyclin D1-cyclin dependent kinase 4 (CDK4) (Kalish *et al.* 2004).

d) Cortactin

Recently, increased expression of cortactin, a protein that increases the formation of actin networks critical for cell motility and receptor-mediated endocytosis, has been associated with gefitinib resistance and increased metastasis in HNSCC (Timpson *et al.* 2007).

Akt has been implicated in EMT by integrin-linked kinase (ILK). The PI3Kinase/Akt pathway not only regulates the transcriptional activity of cyclin D1, but also increases its accumulation by inactivating glycogen synthase kinase-3 (GSK3), which targets cyclin D1 for proteasomal degradation. The effect of cortactin on cancer cell proliferation is associated with increased activation of Akt (Timpson *et al.* 2007). Therefore, factors related to resistance to EGFR TKIs are associated with the PI3kinase/Akt pathway.

PI3kinase/Akt Pathway

a) Activation of the PI3kinase/Akt Pathway

Signaling through the PI3kinase/Akt pathway can be initiated by several mechanisms, all of which increase activation of the pathway in cancer cells. Once activated, the PI3kinase/Akt pathway can be propagated to various substrates including mTOR, a master regulator of protein translation. The pathway is initially activated at the cell membrane, where the signal for activation is propagated through class IA PI3kinase. Activation of PI3kinase can occur through tyrosine kinase growth factor receptors such as EGFR and insulin-like growth factor-1 receptor (IGF-1R), cell adhesion molecules such as integrins, G-protein-coupled receptors (GPCRS) and oncogenes such as Ras. PI3kinase catalyzes phosphorylation of the D3 position on phosphoinositides to generate the biologically active moieties phosphatidylinositol-3,4,5-triphosphate (PI(3,4,5)P3) and phosphatidylinositol-3,4-bisphosphate (PI(3,4)P2). PI(3,4,5)P3 binds to the pleckstrin homology (PH) domains of PDK-1 (3'-phosphoinositide-dependent kinase 1) and Akt, resulting in the proteins being translocated to the cell membrane where they are subsequently activated. The tumor suppressor PTEN (phosphatase and tensin homolog deleted on chromosome 10) antagonizes PI3kinase by dephosphorylating PI (3,4,5)P3 and (PI(3,4)P2), thereby preventing activation of Akt and PDK-1. Akt exists as three structurally similar isoforms, Akt1, Akt2 and Akt3, which are expressed in most tissues. Activation of Akt1 occurs through two crucial phosphorylation events. The first, carried out by PDK-1, occurs at T308 in the catalytic domain. Full activation requires a subsequent phosphorylation at S473 in the hydrophobic motif, which can be mediated by several kinases including PDK-1, ILK, Akt itself, DNA-dependent protein kinase and mTOR; phosphorylation of homologous residues in Akt2 and Akt3 occurs by the same mechanism. Phosphorylation of Akt at S473 is controlled by a recently described phosphatase, PHLPP (PH domain leucine-rich repeat protein phosphatase), which has two isoforms that preferentially decrease activation of specific Akt isoforms (Brognard *et al.* 2007). Amplification of Akt1 has been described in human gastric adenocarcinoma, and amplification of Akt2 has been described in ovarian, breast and pancreatic carcinoma (Bellasosa *et al.* 1995; Cheng *et al.* 1996). Akt mutations are rare, but Carpten *et al.* (2007) recently described somatic mutations occurring in the PH domain of Akt1 in a small percentage of human breast, ovarian and colorectal cancers.

b) Downstream Substrates of Activated Akt

Akt recognizes and phosphorylates the consensus sequence RXRXX (S/T) when it is surrounded by hydrophobic residues. This sequence is present in many proteins resulting in numerous Akt substrates being identified and validated. These substrates control key cellular processes such as apoptosis, cell cycle progression, transcription and translation. For example, Akt phosphorylates the FoxO subfamily of forkhead family transcription factors, inhibiting transcription of several pro-apoptotic genes including Fas-L, IGF Binding Protein1 (IGFBP1) and Bim. Additionally, Akt can directly regulate apoptosis by phosphorylating and inactivating pro-apoptotic proteins such as BAD, which controls the release of cytochrome c from mitochondria, and ASK1 (apoptosis signal-regulating kinase-1), a mitogen-activated protein kinase kinase involved in stress- and cytokine-induced cell death. In contrast, Akt can phosphorylate IKK, which indirectly increases the activity of nuclear factor kappa B (NF-κB) and stimulates the transcription of pro-survival genes. Cell cycle progression can also be affected by Akt; inhibitory phosphorylation of the cyclin-dependent kinase inhibitors p21 and p27, and inhibition of GSK3β by Akt, stimulates cell cycle progression by stabilizing cyclin D1 expression. A novel pro-survival Akt substrate, PRAS40 (proline-rich Akt substrate of 40kDa), has been described recently (Vander Haar *et al.* 2007). Phosphorylation of PRAS40 by Akt attenuates its ability to inhibit mTORC1 kinase activity. It has been suggested that PRAS40 could be a specific substrate of Akt3 (Madhunapantula *et al.* 2007). Therefore, Akt inhibition could have pleiotropic effects on cancer cells that contribute to an anti-tumor response. The most-studied downstream substrate of Akt is the serine/threonine kinase mTOR (mammalian target of rapamycin). Akt can directly phosphorylate and activate mTOR, and indirectly activate it by phosphorylating and inactivating TSC2 (tuberous sclerosis complex 2, also called tuberin), which normally inhibits mTOR through the GTP binding protein Rheb (Ras homolog enriched in the brain) (Inoki *et al.* 2003). When TSC2 is inactivated by phosphorylation, the GTPase Rheb is maintained in its GTP-bound state, allowing increased activation of mTOR (Inoki *et al.* 2005). mTOR exists in two complexes: the TORC1 complex, in which mTOR is bound to Raptor; and the TORC2 complex, in which mTOR is bound to Rictor. In the TORC1 complex, mTOR signals to its downstream effectors S6 kinase/ribosomal protein and 4EBP-1/eIF-4E to control protein translation (Inoki *et al.* 2005). mTOR is generally considered to be a downstream substrate of Akt, but it can phosphorylate Akt when bound to Rictor in TORC2 complexes (Sarbassov *et al.* 2005), and this could provide positive feedback in the pathway. In addition, the downstream mTOR effector S6 kinase-1 (S6K1) can regulate the pathway by catalyzing an inhibitory phosphorylation on insulin receptor substrate (IRS) proteins. This prevents IRS proteins from activating PI3kinase, thereby inhibiting activation of Akt (Harrington *et al.* 2004).

c) Rationale for Targeting the PI3kinase/Akt Pathway

In addition to preclinical studies, clinical observations support the targeting of the PI3kinae/Akt/mTOR pathway in human cancer (Vogt *et al.* 2009). Immunohistochemical studies using antibodies that recognize Akt phosphorylated at S473 have demonstrated that activated Akt is detectable in cancers including multiple myeloma, lung cancer, head and neck cancer, breast cancer, brain cancer, gastric cancer, acute myelogenous leukemia, endometrical cancer, melanoma, renal cell carcinoma, colon cancer, ovarian cancer and prostate cancer (Yuan *et al.* 2000; Hsu *et al.* 2001; Kanamori *et al.* 2001; Kurose *et al.* 2001; Nakayama *et al.* 2001; Sun *et al.* 2001; Alkan and Izban 2002; Ermoian *et al.* 2002; Gupta *et al.* 2002; Malik *et al.* 2002; Perez-Tenorio and Stal 2002; Roy *et al.* 2002; Choe *et al.* 2003; Horiguchi *et al.* 2003; Nam *et al.* 2003; Schlieman *et al.* 2003; Terakawa *et al.* 2003; Kreisberg *et al.* 2004; Min *et al.* 2004; Dai *et al.* 2005). Immunohistochemical analysis has demonstrated the prognostic significance of Akt activation. Phosphorylation of Akt at S473 has been associated with poor prognosis in cancers of the skin, pancreas, liver, prostate, breast, endometrium, stomach, brain and blood (Ermoian *et al.* 2002; Perez-Tenorio and Stal 2002; Nam *et al.* 2003; Schlieman *et al.* 2003; Terakawa *et al.* 2003; Kreisberg *et al.* 2004; Min *et al.* 2004; Dai *et al.* 2005; Nakanishi *et al.* 2005). Tsurutani *et al.* (2006) recently extended these studies using antibodies against S473 and T308, two sites of Akt phosphorylation. This study demonstrated that Akt activation is selective for NSCLC versus normal tissue, and that phosphorylation of Akt at both sites is a better predictor of poor prognosis in NSCLC than phosphorylation of S473 alone. In addition, amplification of Akt isoforms has been observed in some cancers, albeit at a lower frequency. Another frequent genetic event occurring in human cancer is loss of function of the tumor suppressor PTEN. PTEN normally suppresses activation of the PI3kinase/Akt/mTOR pathway by functioning as a lipid phosphatase. Loss of PTEN function in cancer can occur through mutation, deletion or epigenetic silencing. In tumor types where PTEN mutations are rare such as lung cancer, epigenetic silencing can occur (Forgacs *et al.* 1998). Several studies have demonstrated the prognostic significance of PTEN loss in multiple human cancers where mutation, deletion or epigenetic silencing of PTEN correlates with poor prognosis and reduced survival (Bertram *et al.* 2006). Collectively, these studies have established that the loss of PTEN is a common mechanism for activation of the PI3kinase/Akt/mTOR pathway and a poor prognostic factor in human cancer. Activation of PI3kinase has been described in human cancers. It can result from amplification, over-expression, or mutations in the p110 catalytic or p85 regulatory subunits. Amplification of the 3q26 chromosomal region, which contains the gene PI3KCA that encodes the p110α catalytic subunit of PI3K, occurs in 40% of ovarian and 50% of cervical carcinomas (Shayesteh *et al.* 1999; Ma *et al.* 2000). Somatic mutations of this gene have been detected in several cancer types and result in increased kinase activity of mutant PI3K relative to wild type PI3K (Samuels and Ericson 2006). Mutations in the regulatory p85 subunit have also been detected. Any of the aforementioned alterations in individual components would result in activation of the PI3 kinase/Akt pathway, and studies suggest that pathway activation is one of the most frequent molecular alterations that occur in cancer (Samuels and Ericson 2006).

Cross-talk between the IGF1R and EGFR Pathways

The phenomenon of growth factors switching from one pathway to another has an adaptive component, which could be induced by blocking the dominant growth factor receptor pathway. Blockade of EGFR signaling has been demonstrated to result in the enhancement of the growth-promoting effects of the peptide growth factor ligands basic fibroblast growth factor and IGF-1 in DU145 and PC-3 human prostate cancer cells, respectively (Jones *et al.* 1997). More recently, substantial growth inhibitory effects of the EGFR-selective tyrosine kinase inhibitor gefitinib have been demonstrated in EGFR-positive MCF-7-derived tamoxifen-resistant breast cancer cells. Furthermore, this effect can be subverted by additionally exposing cells to non-EGF ligands such as heregulin-β and IGF-II (Knowlden *et al.* 2005). The reversal of the anti-tumor effects of gefitinib by IGF-II, acting through the IGF-1R, is accompanied by a reactivation of the previously reduced activity of Akt and extracellular-regulated kinase (ERK); ERK signaling contributes to the re-establishment of tumor cell growth. Therefore, in the presence of a dominant growth pathway, cancer cells are capable of responding to other growth factors that are present, thereby compromising the anti-tumor activity of agents designed specifically to inhibit EGFR. Importantly, a previous study demonstrated that following blockade of EGFR signaling, switching to the IGF-1R pathway is a common mechanism used to promote resistance to anti-EGFR treatment (Choi *et al.* 2010). For example, gefitinib initially inhibited the growth of the EGFR-positive cell lines DU145 (prostate cancer cells) and MCF-7-derived tamoxifen- and fulvestrant-resistant breast cancer cell lines, but chronic challenge with the inhibitor resulted in the development of gefitinib-resistant variant sub-lines, all of which presented with upregulation of multiple IGF-1R signaling components when compared with the parental cell lines (Jones *et al.* 2004). This resulted in increased production and elevated expression of the IGF-1R ligand IGF-II, increased activity of IGF-1R and increased levels of Akt activity. In addition, the A549 lung cancer cell line, which displays a partial sensitivity to gefitinib, was chronically challenged with the inhibitor; the resistant variant that emerged presented with a marked adaptive increase in the activity of elements of the IGF-1R pathway (Jones *et al.* 2006a). The importance of IGF-1R signaling in these various cell types with acquired gefitinib resistance was further supported by the observation that they demonstrated an enhanced dependency on IGF-1R signaling; they were subsequently more sensitive to growth inhibition by IGF-1R-selective tyrosine kinase inhibitors (Jones *et al.* 2004). Therefore, the dominance of the EGFR pathway in parental cells is replaced by the elevated use of the IGF-1R in gefitinib-resistant cells. However, such growth factor pathway switching can not only result from changes occurring during the development of acquired resistance, but also, critically, can occur rapidly and modulate initial sensitivity to EGFR-blockade resulting in *de novo* or intrinsic resistance to anti-EGFR agents such as gefitinib. Indeed, although the EGFR and IGF-1R pathways are classically regarded as separate entities, promoting growth by utilizing overlapping downstream signal transduction molecules indicates that these receptors can affect each other's signaling abilities, although the precise mechanisms involved in this cross-talk have not been fully elucidated. For example, gefitinib only partially blocks EGFR activity in A549 lung cancer cells and this is accompanied by a dramatic increase in the activity but not the expression of IGF-1R (Jones *et al.* 2006a). Moreover, IGF-1R can transphosphorylate EGFR in these cells, maintaining EGFR activity in the presence of gefitinib (Jones *et al.* 2006a). Therefore, gefitinib limits its own efficacy by facilitating IGF-1R activity in these cells. Interestingly, it was observed that in *de novo* gefitinib-resistant LoVo colorectal cancer cells, which are defective in terms of ability to produce mature IGF-1R and predominantly express insulin receptor-isoform A (InsR-A), a close family member of the IGF-1R, insulin receptor activity is increased and downstream activated Akt levels are elevated in the presence of gefitinib (Jones *et al.* 2006b). Furthermore, InsR can modulate and maintain EGFR phosphorylation in these cells. Such rapid and dynamic interplay between EGFR and IGF-1R or InsR could play an important role in limiting the anti-tumor activity of gefitinib; partial and *de novo* resistance to the inhibitor have been demonstrated in A549 and LoVo cells, respectively.

Future Prospects

Signaling of multiple receptor tyrosine kinases (RTKs) is propagated through Akt. Therefore, simultaneous inhibition of EGFR using pathway components such as Akt or mTOR could circumvent the feedback activation observed with either approach alone. The most extensive data concerning proximal and distal signaling inhibition relates to combining PI3kinase/Akt/mTOR pathway inhibitors with EGFR antagonists. Several PI3kinase inhibitors can restore sensitivity to EGFR inhibitors. For example, the selective pI3kinase inhibitor PX-866 and p110α can abolish gefitinib resistance in NSCLC xenografts (Ihle *et al.* 2005). Synergistic effects of rapamycin and EGFR TKIs have been observed in several *in vitro* systems including glioblastoma multiforme, prostate cancer, pancreatic cancer, squamous cell carcinoma, renal cell carcinoma, leukemia, cervical carcinoma and NSCLC (Mohi *et al.* 2004; Birle and Hedley 2006; Buck *et al.* 2006; Costa *et al.* 2007; Hjelmeland *et al.* 2007; Jimeno *et al.* 2007). Several of these studies extended the efficacy of these combinations to xenograft experiments. Buck *et al.* (2006) noted re-sensitization and synergistic growth inhibition with the combination of rapamycin and erlotinib in cell lines that were previously resistant to erlotinib. Li *et al.* noted significant regression of lung tumors in transgenic mice possessing the secondary resistance mutation T790M when treated with a combination of rapamycin and the irreversible EGFR TKI, HKI-272 (Li *et al.* 2007). In human glioma cell lines with mutant PTEN, addition of the dual PI3kinase/mTOR inhibitor PI-103 to erlotinib was necessary to induce growth arrest (Fan *et al.* 2007), suggesting that the activation of the PI3kinase/Akt/mTOR pathway by EGFR-independent mechanisms confers resistance to EGFR inhibitors, which can nonetheless be overcome by the addition of pathway inhibitors. Collectively, this data suggests that the use of EGFR antagonists with pathway inhibitors could be beneficial to patients who have developed resistance to EGFR TKIs.

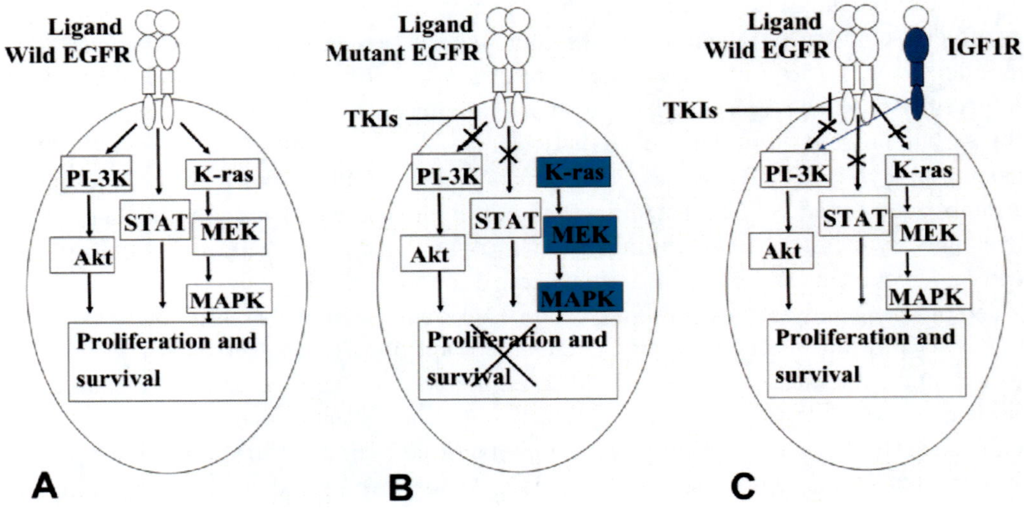

Figure 12.1. The hypothesis concerning combination therapy targeting PI3kinase/Akt and EGFR signaling pathways in HNSCC. (A) EGFR signaling in cancer cells. (B) Mutant EGFRs selectively activate Akt and signal transduction and activator of transcription (STAT) signaling pathways, which promote cell survival, but have no effect on extracellular signal-regulated kinase signaling, which induces proliferation. Mutant EGFRs selectively transduce survival signals, and inhibition of those signals by TKIs contributes to the efficacy of drugs (NSCLC). (C) HNSCC can exhibit extremely rare EGFR mutations, and HNSCC have resistance to TKIs by activating PI3Kinase/Akt signaling through IGF1R.

Conclusion

EGFR is expressed at a high level in HNSCC but EGFR inhibitor monotherapy has limited success. Previous studies have demonstrated that EGFR mutations are extremely rare in HNSCC; inhibition of PI synthesis provides anti-proliferative, anti-invasive and anti-angiogenesis effects on HNSCC. The PI3kinase/Akt pathway is responsible for cellular survival and there is molecular cross-talk between EGFR and IGF1R signaling through PI3kinase/Akt in HNSCC. Therefore, combination therapy targeting the PI3kinase/Akt and

EGFR signaling pathways should provide clinical benefit for patients suffering with HNSCC (Figure 12.1). Although various Akt-specific inhibitors have been developed, we recommend using a combination of an EGFR antagonist with numerous chemopreventive compounds that inhibit the activation of Akt, as natural compounds have little effect. Curcumin, selenium and the flavonoids quercetin, genistein, apigenin, and silibinin have been shown to have effects *in vitro*, but normally with doses far above those that are physiologically achievable. However, several *in vivo* studies have correlated chemopreventive actions with diminution of Akt signaling. Suppression of intestinal tumor formation by sulforaphane (Hu *et al.* 2006) and epigallocatechin gallate (Ju *et al.* 2005) in $Apc^{min/+}$ mice was associated with decreased activation of Akt. In the latter study, oral administration of epigallocatechin gallate markedly suppressed levels of pAkt in intestinal tumors without significantly altering total Akt levels. Another chemopreventive agent whose effects on Akt signaling have been studied in some detail is the rotenoid deguelin. Deguelin is a rotenoid from the African plant *Mundulea sericea* (Leguminosae), which was identified as a potent chemopreventive agent on the basis of its action against chemically-induced preneoplastic lesions in a mammary organ culture, and its inhibition of papillomas in a two-stage mouse skin carcinogenesis model (Nair *et al.* 2006).

Furthermore, deguelin suppresses the formation of carcinogen-induced aberrant crypt foci in mouse colon (Murillo *et al.* 2003). More recently, this rotenoid was shown to suppress cigarette smoke-induced lung carcinogenesis (Lee *et al.* 2005), and it enhances the sensitivity of leukemia cells to chemotherapeutic agents (Bortul *et al.* 2005). How deguelin mediates its chemopreventive and chemosensitizing effects is not yet fully understood, but various mechanisms have been proposed including the suppression of the PI3kinase/Akt pathway (Chen *et al.* 2009). In Akt-inducible transgenic mice, deguelin was competent at suppressing Akt activation in the lung. At doses achievable *in vivo*, it reduced pAkt levels, induced apoptosis and suppressed proliferation of premalignant and malignant human bronchial epithelial cells; minimal effects were observed in normal bronchial cells (Chun *et al.* 2003). Blockade of Akt activation is likely to contribute to the pro-apoptotic actions of deguelin in breast cancer cell lines and anti-angiogenic effects *in vitro*. Deguelin inhibited formation of murine lung tumors in conjunction with suppression of Akt activation *in vivo* (Hecht 2005). The cruciferous vegetable component indole-3-carbinol has chemopreventive activity that could be associated with downregulation of Akt signaling (Chinni and Sarkar 2002). SR13688, a drug designed to optimize the anti-cancer activities of indole-3-carbinol and minimize its undesirable metabolic, estrogenic and toxicological characteristics, demonstrates growth-inhibitory effects in breast, ovarian and prostate xenografts *in vivo* and cell lines *in vitro*, and this correlates with a decrease in pAkt expression (Chao *et al.* 2007).

SR13668 is orally available and has no adverse effects on the fasting glucose levels in mice at a 10-fold higher dose than that required for anti-tumor activity. Resveratrol, trans-3,5,4'-trihydroxystibene, was first isolated in 1940 as a constituent of the root of white hellebore (*Veratrum grandiflorum O. Loes*), but has since been found in various plants including grapes, berries and peanuts. In addition to cardioprotective effects, resveratrol exhibits anti-cancer properties as suggested by its ability to suppress proliferation of a wide variety of tumor cells. The growth-inhibitory effects of resveratrol are mediated through cell-cycle arrest: upregulation of p21, p53 and Bax, and downregulation of survivin, cyclin D1, cyclin E, Bcl-2, Bcl-xl and cIAPs, and activation of caspases. Resveratrol suppresses the activation of several protein kinases including Akt (Banerjee *et al.* 2010) and limited data from humans suggests that it is pharmacologically safe. Honokiol, used as a muscle relaxant, is derived from the stem and bark of the plant *Magnolia officinalis,* which is used in traditional Chinese and Japanese medicine. Extensive research has demonstrated that honokiol inhibits skin tumor promotion, nitric oxide synthesis and TNF expression and also inhibits invasion. Furthermore, it downregulates the anti-apoptotic protein bcl-xl, inhibits angiogenesis and tumor growth *in vivo*, induces caspase-dependent apoptosis in B-cell chronic lymphocytic leukemia cells through downregulation of the anti-apoptotic protein Mcl-1, and overcomes drug resistance in multiple myeloma. Honokiol inhibits EGFR signaling involving Akt and enhances the anti-tumor effects of EGFR inhibitors (Leeman-Neill *et al.* 2010).

Acknowledgments

We thank Dr. Masaya Imoto (Keio University, Japan) for the generous gift of inostamycin. This study was supported in part by a grant-in-aid from the Ministry of Education, Culture, Sports, Science and Technology of Japan (to Y.K.).

References

Alkan, S., Izban, K.F. (2002) Immunohistochemical localization of phosphorylated AKT in multiple myeloma. *Blood*, 99, pp. 2278-2279.

Anderson, J.A. *et al.* (1994) H-ras oncogene mutation and human papillomavirus infection in oral carcinomas. *Archives of Otolaryngology - Head and Neck Surgery*, 120, pp. 755-760.

Baba, Y. *et al.* (2000) Inostamycin, an inhibitor of cytidine5'-diphosphate1, 2-diacyl-sn-glycerol (CDP-DG): inositol transferase, suppresses invasion ability by reducing productions of matrix metalloproteinase-2 and -9 and cell motility in HSC-4 tongue carcinoma cell line. *Clinical and Experimental Metastasis*, 18, pp. 273-279.

Baba, Y. *et al.* (2001) Cytostatic effect of inostamycin, an inhibitor of cytidine5'-diphosphate1, 2-diacyl-sn-glycerol(CDP-DG): inositol transferase, on oral squamous cell carcinoma cell lines. *Cell Biology International*, 25, pp. 613-620.

Baba, Y. *et al.* (2004) Inostamycin suppresses vascular endothelial growth factor-stimulated growth and migration of human umbilical vein endothelial cells. *Cell Biology International*, 21, pp. 419-425.

Baba, Y. *et al.* (2010) Inostamycin prevents malignant phenotype of cancer: inhibition of phosphatidylinositol synthesis provides a therapeutic advantage for head and neck squamous cell carcinoma. *Cell Biology International*, 34, pp. 171-175.

Banerje-Mustafi, S. *et al.* (2010) Modulation of Akt and ERK1/2 pathways by resveratrol in chronic myelogenous leukemia (CML) cells results in the downregulation of Hsp70. *PLoS One*, 5, doi: 10.1371/journal.pone. 0008719.

Bellacosa, A. *et al.* (1995) Molecular alterations of the AKT2 oncogene in ovarian and breast carcinomas. *International Journal of Cancer*, 64, pp. 280-285.

Bertram, J. *et al.* (2006) Loss of PTEN is associated with progression to androgen independence. *Prostate*, 66, pp. 895-902.

Birle, D.C., Hedley, D.W. (2006) Signaling interactions of rapamycin combined with erlotinib in cervical carcinoma xenografts. *Molecular Cancer Therapeutics*, 5, pp. 2494-2502.

Bortul, R. *et al.* (2005) Deguelin, A PI3K/AKT inhibitor, enhances chemosensitivity of leukaemia cells with an active PI3K/AKT pathway. *British Journal of Haematology*, 129, pp. 677-686.

Brognard, J. *et al.* (2007) PHLPP and second isoform, PHLPP2, differentially attenuate the amplitude of Akt signaling by regulating distinct Akt isoforms. *Molecular Cell*, 25, pp. 917-931.

Buck, E. *et al.* (2006) Rapamycin synergizes with the epidermal growth factor receptor inhibitor erlotinib in non-small-cell lung, pancreatic, colon and breast tumors. *Molecular Cancer Therapeutics*, 5, pp. 2676-2684.

Carpten, J.D. *et al.* (2007) A transforming mutation in the pleckstrin homology domain of AKT1 in cancer. *Nature*, 448, pp. 439-444.

Carter, C.A. *et al.* (2009) Small-molecule inhibitors of the human epidermal receptor family. *Expert Opinion on Investigational Drugs*, 18, pp. 1829-1842.

Chao, W.R. *et al.* (2007) Computer-aided rational drug design: a novel agent (SR13688) designed to mimic the unique anti-cancer mechanisms of dietary indole-3-carbinol to block Akt signaling. *Journal of Medicinal Chemistry*, 50, pp. 3412-3415.

Chen, Y. *et al.* (2009) Deguelin blocks cells survival signal pathways and induces apoptosis of HL-60 cells *in vitro*. *International Journal of Hematology*, 89, pp. 618-623.

Cheng, J.Q. *et al.* (1996) Amplification of AKT2 in human pancreatic cells and inhibition of AKT2 expression and tumorigenicity by antisense RNA. *Proceedings of the National Academy of Sciences of the United States of Americ*a, 93, pp. 3636-3641.

Cherrington, J.M. *et al.* (2000) New paradigms for the treatment of cancer: the role of anti-angiogenesis agents. *Advances in Cancer Research*, 79, pp. 1-38.

Chinni, S.R.,Sarkar, F.H. (2002) Akt inactivation is a key event in indole-3-carbinol-induced apoptosis in PC-3 cells. *Clinical Cancer Research*, 8, pp. 1228-1236.

Choe, G. *et al.* (2003) Analysis of the phosphatidylinositol 3' -kinase signaling pathway in glioblastoma patients *in vivo*. *Cancer Research*, 63, pp. 2742-2746.

Choi, Y.J. *et al.* (2010) Combined inhibition of IGFR enhances the effects of gefitinib in H1650: a lung cancer cell line with EGFR mutation and primary resistance to EGFR-TK inhibitors. *Cancer Chemotherapy and Pharmacology*, 66, pp. 381-388.

Chun, K.H. *et al.* (2003) Effects of deguelin on the phosphatidylinositol3-kinase/Akt pathway and apoptosis in premalignant human bronchial epithelial cells. *Journal of the National Cancer Institut*e, 95, pp. 291-302.

Ciardiello, F., Tortora, G. (2003) Epidermal growth factor receptor (EGFR) as a target in cancer therapy: understanding the role of receptor expression and other molecular determinants that could influence the response to anti-EGFR drugs. *European Journal of Cancer*, 39, pp. 1348-1354.

Cohen, E.E. *et al.* (2003) Phase II trial of ZD1839 in recurrent or metastatic squamous cell carcinoma of the head and neck. *Journal of Clinical Oncology*, 21, pp. 1980-1987.

Costa, L.J. *et al.* (2007) Upstream signaling inhibition enhances rapamycin effect on growth of kidney cancer cells. *Urology*, 69, pp. 596-602.

Cripps, C. *et al.* (2010) Epidermal growth factor receptor targeted therapy in stages III and IV head and neck cancer. *Current Oncology*, 17, pp. 37-48.

Dai, D.L. *et al.* (2005) Prognostic significance of activated Akt expression in melanoma: a clinicopathologic study of 292 cases. *Journal of Clinical Oncology*, 23, pp. 1473-1482.

Eberhard, D.A. *et al.* (2005) Mutations in the epidermal growth factor receptor and in KRAS are predictive and prognostic indicators in patients with non-small-cell lung cancer treated with chemotherapy alone and in combination with erlotinib. *Journal of Clinical Oncology*, 23, pp. 5900-5909.

Ermoian, R.P. *et al.* (2002) Dysregulation of PTEN and protein kinase B is associated with glioma histology and patient survival. *Clinical Cancer Research*, 8, pp. 1100-1106.

Fan, Q.W. *et al.* (2007) A dual phosphoinositide-3-kinase alpha/mTOR inhibitor cooperates with blockade of epidermal growth factor receptor in PTEN-mutant glioma. *Cancer Research*, 67, pp. 7960-7965.

Forastiere, A. *et al.* (2001) Head and neck cancer. *The New England Journal of Medicine*, 345, pp. 1890-1900.

FORGACS, E. *et al.* (1998). Mutation analysis of the PTEN/MMAC1 gene in lung cancer. *Oncogene*, 17, pp. 1557-1565.

Frederick, B.A. *et al.* (2007) Epithelial to mesenchymal transition predicts gefitinib resistance in cell lines of head and neck squamous cell carcinoma and non-small cell lung carcinoma. *Molecular Cancer Therapeutics*, 6, pp. 1683-1691.

Gotink, K.J., Verheul, H.M. (2010) Anti-angiogenic tyrosine kinase inhibitors: what is their mechanism of action? *Angiogenesis*, 13, pp. 1-14.

Gupta, A.K. *et al.* (2002) Local recurrence in head and neck cancer: relationship to radiation resistance and signal transduction. *Clinical Cancer Research*, 8, pp. 885-892.

Harrington, L.S. *et al.* (2004) The TSC1-2 tumor suppressor controls insulin-PI3K signaling via regulation of IRS proteins. *The Journal of Cell Biology*, 166, pp. 213-223.

Hecht, S.S. (2005) Deguelin as a chemopreventive agent in mouse lung tumorigenesis induced by tobacco smoke carcinogens. *Journal of the National Cancer Institute*, 97, pp. 1634-1635.

Hjelmeland, A.B. *et al.* (2007) The combination of novel low molecular weight inhibitors of RAF (LBT613) and target of rapamycin (RAD001) decreases glioma proliferation and invasion. *Molecular Cancer Therapeutics*, 6, pp. 2449-2457.

Ho, Q.T., Kuo, C.J. (2007) Vascular endothelial growth factor: biology and therapeutic applications. *International Journal of Biochemistry and Cell biology*, 39, pp. 1349-1357.

Horiguchi, A. *et al.* (2003) Elevated Akt activation and its impact on clinicopathological features of renal cell carcinoma. *Journal of Urology*, 169, pp. 710-713.

Hsu, J. *et al.* (2001) The AKT kinase is activated in multiple myeloma tumor cells. *Blood*, 98, pp. 2853-2855.

Hu, R. *et al.* (2006) Cancer chemoprevention of intestinal polyposis in ApcMin/+mice by sulforaphane, a natural product derived from cruciferous vegetable. *Carcinogenesis*, 27, pp. 2038-2046.

Ihle, NT. *et al.* (2005) The phosphatudylinositol-3-kinase inhibitor PX-866 overcomes resistance to the epidermal growth factor receptor inhibitor gefitinib in A-549 human non-small cell lung cancer xenografts. *Molecular Cancer Therapeutics*, 4, pp. 1349-1357.

Inoki, K. *et al.* (2003) Rheb GTPase is a direct target of TSC2 GAP activity and regulates mTOR signaling. *Genes and Development*, 17, pp. 1829-1834.

Inoki, K. *et al.* (2005) Signaling by target of rapamycin proteins in cell growth control. *Microbiology and Molecular Biology Reviews*, 69, pp. 79-100.

Jimeno, A. *et al.* (2007) Dual EGFR and mTOR targeting in squamous cell carcinoma models, and development of early markers of efficacy. *British Journal of Cancer*, 96, pp. 952-959.

Jones, H.E. *et al.* (1997) New EGF-R selective tyrosine kinase inhibitor reveals variable growth responses in prostate carcinoma cell lines PC-3 and DU-145. *International Journal of Cancer*, 71, pp. 1010-1018.

Jones, H.E. *et al.* (2004) Insulin-like growth factor-I receptor signaling and acquired resistance to gefitinib (ZD1839; Iressa) in human breast and prostate cancer cells. *Endocrine-Related Cancer*, 11, pp. 793-814.

Jones, H.E. *et al.* (2006a) Growth factor receptor interplay and resistance in cancer. *Endocrine-Related Cancer*, 13, pp. 45-51.

Jones, H.E. *et al.* (2006b) Inhibition of insulin receptor isoform-A signaling restores sensitivity to gefitinib in previously de novo-resistant colon cancer cells. *British Journal of Cancer*, 95, pp. 172-180.

Ju, J. *et al.* (2005) Inhibition of intestinal tumorigenesis in Apcmin/+mice by (-)-epigallocatechin-3-gallate, the major catechin in green tea. *Cancer Research*, 65, pp. 10623-10631.

Kalish, L.H. *et al.* (2004) Deregulated cyclin D1 expression is associated with decreased efficacy of the selective epidermal growth factor receptor tyrosine kinase inhibitor gefitinib in head and neck squamous cell carcinoma cell lines. *Clinical Cancer Research*, 10, pp. 7764-7774.

Kanamori, Y. *et al.* (2001) Correlation between loss of PTEN expression and Akt phosphorylation in endometrial carcinoma. *Clinical Cancer Research*, 7, pp. 892-895.

Kaur, J. *et al.* (2010) Clinical significance of Phosphatidyl Inositol Snthase overexpression in oral cancer. *BMC Cancer*, 10, pp. 1-11.

Khuri, F.R. *et al.* (2000) Treatment of patients with recurrent or metastatic squamous cell carcinoma of the head and neck: current status and future directions. *Seminars in Oncology*, 27, pp. 25-33.

Knowlden, J.M. *et al.* (2005) Insulin-like growth factor-I receptor signaling in tamoxifen-resistant breast cancer: a supporting role to the epidermal growth factor receptor. *Endocrinology*, 146, pp. 4609-4618.

Kreisberg, J.I. *et al.* (2004) Phosphorylation of Akt (Ser473) is an excellent predictor of poor clinical outcome in prostate cancer. *Cancer Research*, 64, pp. 5232-5236.

Kurose, K. *et al.* (2001) Frequent loss of PTEN expression is linked to elevated phosphorylated Akt levels, but not associated with p27 and cyclinD1 expression, in primary epithelial ovarian carcinomas. *The American Journal of Pathology*, 158, pp. 2097-2106.

Lee, H.Y. *et al.* (2005) Chemopreventive effects of deguelin, a novel Akt inhibitor, on tobacco-induced lung tumorigenesis. *Journal of the National Cancer Institute*, 97, pp. 1695-1699.

Leeman-Neill, R.J. *et al.* (2010) Honokiol inhibits epidermal growth factor receptor signaling and enhances the antitumor effects of epidermal growth factor receptor inhibitors. *Clinical Cancer Research*, 16, pp. 2571-2579.

Li, D. *et al.* (2007) Bronchial and peripheral murine lung carcinomas induced by T790M-L858R mutant EGFR respond to HKI-272 and rapamycin combination therapy. *Cancer Cell*, 12, pp. 81-93.

Loefflerr-RAGG, J. *et al.* (2006) Low incidence of mutations in EGFR kinase domain in Caucasian patients with head and neck squamous cell carcinoma. *European Journal of Cancer*, 42, pp. 109-111.

Ma, Y.Y. *et al.* (2000) PI3CA as an oncogene in cervical cancer. *Oncogene*, 19, pp. 2739-2744.

Madhunapantula, S.V. *et al.* (2007) PRAS40 deregulates apoptosis in malignant melanoma. *Cancer Research*, 67, pp. 3626-3636.

Malik, S.N. *et al.* (2002) Immunohistochemical demonstration of phospho-Akt in high Gleason grade prostate cancer. *Clinical Cancer Research*, 8, pp. 1168-1171.

Min, Y.H. *et al.* (2004) Cytoplasmic mislocalization of p27Kip1 protein is associated with constitutive phosphorylation of Akt or protein kinase B and poor prognosis in acute myelogenous leukemia. *Cancer Research*, 64, pp. 5225-5231.

Mohi, M.G. *et al.* (2004) Combination of rapamycin and protein tyrosine kinase (PTK) inhibitors for the treatment of leukemias caused by oncogenic PTKs. *Proceedings of the National Academy of Sciences of the United States of America*, 101, pp. 3130-3135.

Murillo, G. *et al.* (2003) Deguelin suppresses the formation of carcinogen-induced aberrant crypt foci in the colon of CF-1 mice. *International Journal of Cancer*, 104, pp. 7-11.

Nair, A.S. *et al.* (2006) Deguelin, an Akt inhibitor, suppresses IkappaBalpha kinase activation leading to suppression of NF-kappaB-regulated gene expression, potentiation of apoptosis, and inhibition of cellular invasion. *Journal of Immunology*, 177, pp. 5612-5622.

Nakanishi, K. *et al.* (2005) Akt phosphorylation is a risk factor for early disease recurrence and poor prognosis in hepatocellular carcinoma. *Cancer*, 103, pp. 307-312.

Nakashima, T., Clayman, G. L. (2000) Anti-sense inhibition of cyclin D1 in human head and nek squamous cell carcinoma. *Archives of Otolaryngology - Head and Neck Surgery*, 126, pp. 957-961.

Nakayama, H. *et al.* (2001) High expression levels of nuclear factor kappaB, IkappaB kinase alpha and Akt kinase in squamous cell carcinoma of the oral cavity. *Cancer*, 92, pp. 3037-3044.

Nam, S.Y. *et al.* (2003) Akt/PKB activation in gastric carcinomas correlates with clinicopathologic variables and prognosis. *Acta Pathologica, Microbiologica, et Immunologica Scandinavica*, 111, pp. 1105-1113.

Ozawa, S. *et al.* (2009) Restoration of BRAK/CXCL14 gene expression by gefitinib is associated with antitumor efficacy of the drug in head and neck squamous cell carcinoma. *Cancer Science*, 100, pp. 2202-2209.

Perez-Tenorio, G., Stal, O. (2002) Activation of AKT/PKB in breast cancer predicts a worse outcome among endocrine treated patients. *British Journal of Cancer*, 86, pp. 540-545.

Rousseau, S. *et al.* (1997) P38MAP kinase activation by vascular endothelial growth factor mediates actin reorganization and cell migration in human endothelial cells. *Oncogene*, 15, pp. 2169-2177.

Roy, H.K. *et al.* (2002) AKT proto-oncogene overexpression is an early event during sporadic colon carcinogenesis. *Carcinogenesis*, 23, pp. 201-205.

Samuels, Y., Ericson, K. (2006) Oncogenic PI3K and its role in cancer. *Current Opinion in Oncology*, 18, pp. 77-82.

Sarbassov, D.D. *et al.* (2005) Phosphorylation and regulation of Akt/PKB by the rector-mTOR complex. *Science*, 307, pp. 1098-1101.

Schlieman, M. G. *et al.* (2003) Incidence, mechanism and prpgnostic value of activated AKT in pancreas cancer. *British Journal of Cancer*, 89, pp. 2110-2115.

Shayesteh, L. *et al.* (1999) PIK3CA is implicated as an oncogene in ovarian cancer. *Nature Genetics*, 21, pp. 99-102.

Sordella, R. *et al.* (2004) Gefitinib-sensitizing EGFR mutations in lung cancer activate anti-apoptotic pathways. *Science*, 305, pp. 1163-1167.

Soulieres, D. *et al.* (2004) Multicenter phase II study of erlotinib, an oral epidermal growth factor receptor tyrosine kinase inhibitor, in patients with recurrent or metastatic squamous cell cancer of the head an neck. *Journal of Clinical Oncology*, 22, pp. 77-85.

Sun, M. *et al.* (2001) AKT1/PKBalpha kinase is frequently elevated in human cancers and its constitutive activation is required for oncogenic transformation in NIH3T3 cells. *The American Journal of Pathology*, 159, pp. 431-437.

Taguchi, T. *et al.* (2008) Involvement of EGFR in the response of squamous cell carcinoma of the head and neck cell lines to gefitinib. *Oncology Reports*, 19, pp. 65-71.

Takahashi, T. *et al.* (1999) VEGF activates protein kinase C-dependent, but Ras-independent Raf-MEK-MAP kinase pathway for DNA synthesis in primary endothelial cells. *Oncogene*, 18, pp. 2221-2230.

Terakawa, N. *et al.* (2003) Loss of PTEN expression followed by Akt phosphorylation is a poor prognostic factor for patients with endometrial cancer. *Endocrine-Related Cancer*, 10, pp. 203-208.

Timpson, P. *et al.* (2007) Aberrant expression of cortactin in head and neck squamous cell carcinoma cells is associated with enhanced cell proliferation and resistance to the epidermal growth factor receptor inhibitor gefitinib. *Cancer Research*, 67, pp. 9304-9314.

Tsurutani, J. *et al.* (2006) Evaluation of two phosphorylation sites improves the prognostic significance of Akt activation in non-small-cell lung cancer tumors. *Journal of Clinical Oncology*, 24, pp. 306-314.

van Houten, V.M. *et al.* (2000) Molecular diagnosis of head and neck cancer. *Recent Results in Cancer Research*, 157, pp. 90-106.

van der Haar, E. *et al.* (2007) Insulin signaling to mTOR mediated by the Akt/PKB substrate PRAS40. *Nature Cell Biology*, 9, pp. 316-323.

Vogt, P.K. *et al.* (2009) PI3-kinase and cancer: changing accents. *Current Opinion in Genetics and Development*, 19, pp. 12-17.

Wong, K.K. (2008) Searching for a magic bullet in NSCLC: the role of epidermal growth factor receptor mutations and tyrosine kinase inhibitors. *Lung Cancer*, 60[Suppl2], pp. 10-18.

Yuan, Z.Q. *et al.* (2000) Frequent activation of AKT2 and induction of apoptosis by inhibition of phosphoinositide-3-OH kinase/Akt pathway in human ovarian cancer. *Oncogene*, 19, pp. 2324-2330.

In: Hypotheses in Clinical Medicine
Editors: M.M. Shoja, P.S. Agutter et al.
ISBN: 978-1-62257-276-2

Chapter 13

Individualized Cancer Chemotherapy

Da-Yong Lu[1,*], Ting-Ren Lu[2], Xue-Liang Chen[3] and Jian Ding[4]
[1]School of Life Sciences, Shanghai University, Shanghai, PR China
[2]College of Science, Shanghai University, Shanghai, PR China
[3]Devision of Oncology and Thermal therapy,
Central Hospital of Jing-An District, Shanghai, PR China
[4]Shanghai Institute of Materia Medica,
Chinese Academy of Sciences, Shanghai, PR China

Abstract

One of the major obstacles to controlling cancer growth and metastases is the inappropriate use of anticancer drugs. Treatment using individualized cancer chemotherapy (ICC) has been attracting increasing attention and will continue to show beneficial outcomes in the future. In this chapter, this issue is addressed by discussing specific strategies for ICC, including drug sensitivity testing, biomarker detection, biomarker-oriented therapy, pharmacogenetics, cancer metastasis-targeted therapy, combined chemotherapy and biotherapy, adjunctive therapy, mathematical techniques, and computational analysis. Many longstanding key debates and future trends are also discussed.

Introduction

One of the major obstacles to controlling cancer growth and metastases in patients is the inappropriate use of anticancer drugs. As increasing numbers and types of anticancer drugs are developed, clinicians become more and more likely to misuse them in their practice. The norm is to use a chemotherapeutic regimen that is "randomized" or "standard" in relation to the target organ or tumor origin. Since tumors originate from a wide variety of phenotypically or genetically abnormal tissues, they are sensitive to different anticancer drugs. Thus, most cancer patients are unsuited to the use of such "uniform" or "standardized" chemotherapy. As

* E-mail: ludayong@sh163.net.

no single drug or combination has so far been found to be optimal for cancers of all origins, developing a good and clinically practical drug selection system is no less important than the discovery of new drugs. Researchers are now beginning to focus on "individualized cancer chemotherapy" (ICC), which improves therapeutic quality by selecting and prescribing well-matched drugs and avoiding ineffective ones. Given a knowledge of the drug responses and pathogenic status of a specific tumor, physicians can prescribe the best-matched drugs in succeeding trials. The first experiments relating to this issue date back to the early 1950s (Black and Speer 1954; Wright *et al.* 1957). Those reports provided the experimental basis for evaluating drug sensitivity in tumor samples from humans. Systematic investigations of drug sensitivity tests in clinics began in the late 1970s (Hamburger and Salmon 1977; Salmon *et al.* 1978; Bodegen *et al.* 1978). Since then, drug sensitivity tests have been the mainstream of ICC strategy and continue to be one of the best ways of selecting chemotherapeutic agents in current clinical practice.

At the start of the 21st century, the genetic disorders related to cancer etiology and therapeutics have become easier to identify and detect accurately (Weir *et al.* 2004; Williams *et al.* 2003; Pusztai *et al.* 2003; Guo 2003), and there has been a new trend towards utilizing these bioinformatics data as selective criteria for ICC (Lu *et al.* 2006a; Dalton and Friend 2006). Benefiting from the Human Genome Project, these techniques are growing rapidly (Lander *et al.* 2001; Pritchard and Przeworski 2001; Venter *et al.* 2001; Sachidanandam *et al.* 2001; Gibbs *et al.* 2003; Collins *et al.* 2003; Carlson *et al.* 2004; Bentley 2004). Using bioinformatics data and modern experimental techniques, tumor cells can be genetically detected more easily than ever before. Pharmacogenetics also addresses which drug might work in an individual patient, and at what dosage (Watters and McLeod 2003; Efferth and Vom 2005; Huang and Ratain 2009). Further information will be outlined and discussed in the following sections.

In Vivo and *In Vitro* Drug Sensitivity Testing

ICC was pioneered in drug sensitivity tests half a century ago (Black and Speer 1954; Wright *et al.* 1957). It gained more notice and was promoted during the 1970s (Hamburger and Salmon 1977; Salmon *et al.* 1978; Bodegen *et al.* 1978). Drug sensitivity testing compares the anticancer activities of candidate drugs on surgically removed tumor samples, and those showing the best responses are selected for use in succeeding treatments. Drug sensitivity tests can be conducted *in vivo* (Bodegen *et al.* 1978; Lu *et al.* 2006a) and *in vitro* (Hamburger and Salmon 1977; Salmon *et al.* 1978; Morioka *et al.* 2001; Tanino *et al.* 2001; Takamura *et al.* 2002; Lu *et al.* 2006a; Ulukaya 2006).

The subrenal capsule (SRC) assay is the earliest and best known *in vivo* method. It involves transplanting surgically removed tumors into the renal capsules of mice and evaluating the candidate drugs within 4-11 days. *In vitro* drug sensitivity testing methods involve cytological tests and include the micro-culture tetrazolium (MTT) method (Morioka *et al.* 2001; Tanino *et al.* 2001), the ChemoFx method (Ness *et al.* 2002), the ATP luminescence assay (Kawamura *et al.* 1997; Kurbacher *et al.* 1998; Ulukaya 2006) and the collagen gel droplet-embedded culture method (Takamura *et al.* 2002). Usually, the effects of drugs on tumor enzymes and energy are assessed. For example, Kondo and colleagues described a test involving effects on succinate dehydrogenase activity in tumors (Kondo *et al.* 1966); this was the prototype of the MTT method. To reduce interference by normal cells collected along with the neoplastic tissue, serum-free culture is recommended to promote tumor growth selectively (Kawamura *et al.* 1997).

The major advantage of the SRC assay is that the drug sensitivity testing is conducted on a tumor within a living body. The environment of the renal capsule is proposed to be the most relevant to clinical situations among all drug sensitivity tests. This method was once widely practiced but its use has declined now. Its disadvantages are as follows: (i) It is labor intensive and technically demanding. A routine SRC assay needs three skilled personnel working for 2-4 h. The high cost of hiring skilled personnel makes it difficult to use widely. In addition, a sufficiently pathogen-free laboratory space for large-scale animal breeding and other operations is seldom available in conventional hospitals. Therefore, only small numbers of nude mice can be provided and very limited numbers of patients can be tested. (ii) Low drug sensitivity or response rates make it difficult to select well-matched drugs from the candidate panel (Venesmaa and Ylikorkala 1991). The maximum number of drugs tested in one screening for SRC assay is 4-6, and it is dubious whether the best-suited drugs are among those 4-6. So, the likelihood of selecting the best options is less than optimal. (iii) Use of the SRC assay compared to other methods does not always improve chemotherapy in clinical practice (Akao *et al.* 1996; Gazdar et al. 1990). The main contributor to the financial burden of the SRC assay is the utilization of immunodeficient nude mice (Bodegen *et al.* 1978). Several attempts to supersede the utilization of normal mice have been proposed (Aamdal *et al.* 1985; Bodegen *et al.* 1978; Cunningham *et al.* 1986; Levi *et al.* 1984; Lu *et al.* 2010c). There is a longstanding controversy whether athymic nude mice differ from immunocompetent normal mice in this regard. It was found that xenografts of primary surgical explants showed positive growth rates more frequently in 4-6 days in immunocompetent mice (82%) than in an 11-day SRC assay in nude mice (30%) (Aamdal *et al.* 1985; Bodegen *et al.* 1979; Cunningham *et al.* 1986; Levi *et al.* 1984). We have suggested that drug response rates are the same in normal and nude mice if the experiment is terminated in similar periods of time (~ 7 days) (Lu *et al.* 2010c). It is likely that the differences between SRC assay results are more closely related to the duration of the experiment than to the immunological status of the tumor recipient. However, the duration should be no longer than seven days in immunocompetent mice as immune rejection may then ensue (Lu *et al.* 2006a).

The advantage of many *in vitro* drug sensitivity tests is that they are easier to perform and implement in a routine hospital, so it is less difficult to use them in daily hospital routine and practice. For these reasons, they are now the preferred methods. The disadvantage of *in vitro* drug sensitivity tests is that they lack a matrix and other environmental resources to support solid tumor growth. However, most patients undergoing therapy in clinics carry solid tumors. Some types of anticancer drugs targeting aspects of the tumor matrix, such as the fibrinogen-related pathway, will elicit little or no response in *in vitro* drug sensitivity systems. More recently, some types of *in vitro* drug sensitivity tests have been supplemented with a tumor matrix in culture (Takamura *et al.* 2002). With further scientific and technological developments, these types of drug sensitivity tests will meet clinical requirements more perfectly and will be used to test drug responses in environments resembling the natural ones.

Technical Analysis

In vitro drug sensitivity tests are advantageous owing to labor-saving and technical feasibility and are currently more popular than *in vivo* ones. Comparing *in vivo* with *in vitro* methods, the former often require longer experimental duration, delaying the production of data, and are technically more difficult. Transplantation success rates for both *in vivo* and *in vitro* methods have increased from the initial 25-45% to more than 50%, especially for *in vitro* systems. *In vivo* methods commonly show no obvious advantage over *in vitro* methods in clinical practice. *In vitro* methods can be used to evaluate greater numbers of drugs in a single test; also, they require much less labor and are quicker to perform. Since *in vivo* methods routinely screen only 2-3 drugs in one test, the number of drug groups compared in such a sensitivity test is small, markedly diminishing the value of the test for drug selection. From a theoretical standpoint, the quality of treatment is likely to be higher when the range of drugs available for selection is greater. *In vitro* drug sensitivity testing seems advantageous over *in vivo* methods in this respect. Some *in vitro* techniques such as the ATP-tumor chemo-sensitivity assay can evaluate more than 10 anticancer drugs in a single test (Kawamura *et al.* 1997; Ulukaya 2006). To address the commonly-occurring problems of false-positive or false-negative data, it is advisable to examine more than two concentrations of each drug if dose-response relationships are available (Lu *et al.* 2006a). More importantly, *in vitro* methods can be used for blood samples from leukemic patients; in contrast, only solid tumor material surgically removed from patients is appropriate for *in vivo* tests. It should also be mentioned that a combination of *in vivo* and *in vitro* methods is presumed to be more useful because the two approaches may provide complementary data (Lu *et al.* 2006a).

Cytotoxic and Cytostatic Anti-cancer Drugs

Most anticancer drugs can be divided into two categories: cytotoxic and cytostatic (Millar and Lynch 2003). Cytotoxic anticancer drugs often appear strongly effective in drug sensitivity tests or in clinical situations when they are initially used. However, they readily induce multidrug resistance (MDR) and are often useless in terms of a patient's survival benefits. Cytostatic anticancer drugs, which mainly inhibit tumor growth by targeting tumorigenic molecules, show low sensitivity rates in drug sensitivity tests. However, they show better survival benefits than cytotoxic drugs if they are well-matched. Therefore, it is optimal to utilize both cytotoxic and cytostatic drugs on a single patient in order to reduce the tumor and prolong survival. It is therefore appropriate to involve both cytotoxic and cytostatic anticancer drugs in drug sensitivity tests and obtain drug response information about both categories.

The less than optimal performances of cytotoxic anticancer drugs in patients result mainly from the induction of MDR. Different cytotoxic anticancer drugs often show cross-resistance. For example, it has been reported that a neoplasm that induces resistance to doxorubicin may also induce resistance to other cytotoxic anticancer drugs (Efferth *et al.* 2008). This issue should be considered in drug sensitivity tests. When such tests are used, patients benefit by avoiding ineffective drugs in a trial, reducing hemotoxicity and drug expenditure (Bosanquet *et al.* 2002; Breidenbach *et al.* 2003). The ineffective drugs can also induce cross-resistance, treatment delays and unnecessary treatment-related morbidity (Tewari and Maretta 1999).

Bioinformatics and Pharmacogenetics for ICC

Various molecules have been widely reported to have diagnostic and/or prognostic value in cancer patients. Such molecules range from immunoregulatory and inflammatory factors (interleukins and cytokines) and signal transduction regulators (tyrosine kinase, cycloxygenase-2, MAPK, etc.) to factors related to tumor pathology (metastases, angiogenesis and apoptosis) such as vascular epithelial growth factor and its receptor (VEGF and VEGFR), epidermal growth factor receptor (EGFR) and fibrinogen. These pathogenic markers in tumors are specific targets for drug antagonism or disruption. It has been shown that in patients who have elevated plasma levels of tumorigenic molecules but lack grossly recognizable tumors, the tumorigenic factor levels return to normal following targeted chemotherapy (unpublished data). Small tumor nodules (diameter less than 0.3 mm) are more sensitive to drugs and therefore therapeutic outcomes are much better (unpublished data). Before initiating monotherapy (treatment with monoclonal antibodies, a type of cytostatic anticancer drug), it is ideal to know the levels of targeted antigen in tumors in order to provide a rational basis for the treatment. Tumor biomarker detection methods can be conducted without the prerequisite for obtaining fresh tumor samples. Routine blood tests can be useful (Eikelboom and Mehta 2000; Lu *et al.* 2000; Lu *et al.* 2007c). With the increasing production of highly selective drugs (cytostatic anticancer drugs), cancer patients can be treated with targeted agents chosen by reference only to pathobiological data without drug sensitivity tests. Successful examples are fluoropyrimidine-based chemotherapy for metastatic colon cancers over-expressing dihydropyrimidine dehydrogenase and thymidylate synthase (Ichikawa *et al.* 2003), and treatment of the deadliest lung cancers resulting from EGFR mutation with the monoclonal antibody Iressa (Marx 2004).

In tumor marker detection, bioinformatics methods are best suited to identifying tumorigenic initiators and promoters, and further deciding which cytostatic anticancer drugs are most likely to target the neoplasm. Since tumors are progressive conditions (Nowell 1976; Hanahan and Weinberg 2000; Futreal *et al.* 2001) with more than a hundred genetic changes accumulating in a single cell (Stoler *et al.* 1999; Jongeneel *et al.* 2003), high-throughput methods are needed to identify or pinpoint the underlying abnormalities.

Cancers have different etiological bases but share the same pathological characteristic of unlimited growth. They result from genetic malfunctions and molecular disturbances. More than a thousand types of genetic abnormality can cause about one hundred different tumor types and more than one hundred different anticancer drugs are available for treatment. Even with a certain tumor type, the responses to the same anticancer drugs may vary from patient to patient. Bioinformatics is a genomics-based approach and provides a variety of techniques for analyzing abnormalities in DNA, RNA, proteins and glycoligands in tumors. In the earliest era of bioinformatics development, clinical cancer practice was to predict patients' prognoses (Van de Vijver *et al.* 2002) or classify tumor origins (Gordon *et al.* 2002). Presently, the best use of bioinformatics for predicting anticancer drug responses is to decide on monotherapy (treatment of cancer patients with monoclonal antibodies). If a tumorigenic biomarker has been detected at an abnormally high level, it is reasonable to assume that the monoclonal antibodies specifically targeting that biomarker will be ideally effective. Numerous reports have addressed this issue and some successful results have been obtained (Diehl 2007; Geyer *et al.* 2006; Vermorken *et al.* 2008; Younes *et al.* 2010; The Lancet Oncology 2010). On the other hand, the monoclonal antibodies are very expensive and doses costing thousands of dollars can be used only in a single therapeutic cycle. Usually, only a few months of survival benefit is all that can be expected. Some authors have reported no survival benefit after monotherapy (Tol *et al.* 2009; Miller *et al.* 2007).

Bioinformatics methods are important for identifying the original and causative biomarkers in any individualized chemotherapy. To attain this goal, many more basic and clinical investigations are needed to establish good routines and paradigms for clinical practitioners to follow. These routines and paradigms need to be easy to handle, less costly, high-throughput, and as effective as possible. Currently, there are bioinformatics techniques to select amongst and no single technique seems advantageous over the rest. It is recommended that an international committee should be encouraged to work on this issue, and standard chips or techniques be designed and made uniform by manufacturers in order to safeguard the quality and cost of investigations.

Apart from monotherapy, some small-molecular cytostatic anticancer drugs can also be chosen by consulting biomarker information. Choice of this type of drug chemotherapy depends on implementing a sophisticated system to analyze high-throughput data. The exact tumorigenic pathways that a drug inhibits or blocks need to be understood (Knight and Shokat 2007). It must also be known how far a drug acts and what possible toxicities it has, so the balance between efficacy and risk can be evaluated (Lu *et al.* 2007b), and whether it is cost-effective in therapeutic application (Hasenclever *et al.* 2001; Brown *et al.* 2001; Bayoumi *et al.* 2000; Lyman 2000). This requires the retrieval and interpretation of pharmacogenetics data.

Pharmacogenetics

It is known that the plasma concentrations, drug responses and toxicities of anticancer drugs can vary more than ten-fold among patients who are given the same dosages because of genetic variations or polymorphisms in drug metabolism enzymes. The purpose of pharmacogenetics is to predict the metabolism and required dosage of a drug and the possible sensitivity of tumors to it (Evans and Relling 2004; Goldstein *et al.* 2003) by analyzing the genetic status of the drug metabolism enzymes in patients or the biomarker status of the cancer tissues. Large inter-individual variation is observed in both the response and toxicity associated with anticancer therapy. Pharmacogenetics and pharmacogenomics studies have successfully identified genetic variants that contribute to these variations in the susceptibility and toxic response to chemotherapeutics. For more information, the readers are referred to the systematic reviews available on this topic (see Watters and McLeod 2003; Efferth and Volm 2005; Huang and Ratain 2009).

Combining Small Molecular Drugs with Biotherapy

Presumably, the best strategy for anticancer therapy is the combinatory use of chemicals and biotherapies. If chemicals kill 70% to 90% of tumor cells, the highly specific biotherapies can kill the rest. It is expected that this strategy will be a paradigm of future cancer chemotherapy. It is well known that anticancer drugs rarely kill all tumor cells. If several cancer cells survive, they can in time re-grow to a large volume of cancer. Therefore, patients' immunosurveillance systems or specific biotherapies (Lechleider *et al.* 2008; Gillespie *et al.* 2007) will determine the long-term effectiveness of a given chemotherapy. So far, some attempts have been made to combine cytotoxic anticancer chemicals with monoclonal or polyclonal antibodies for treatment of the cancers (Diehl 2007; Geyer *et al.* 2006; Vermorken *et al.* 2008; Younes *et al.* 2010; The Lancet Oncology 2010). The patients are first given cytotoxic anticancer drugs to shrink the tumor mass and are then given biotherapy (e.g., monoclonal antibodies). These patients are likely to survive longer. It is suggested that future ICC strategies should be designed according to such a protocol.

Mathematical Modeling and Computational Networks

Mathematics is becoming increasingly pervasive in various fields of biology and medicine (Pennisi 2003). Mathematical modeling and computational networks are powerful tools for decision-making and for meeting the ultimate goals of ICC. These tools will help to select crucial targets from the wealth of tumorigenic factors, weigh the importance of each variable and finally coordinate matched drugs to rectify the problem. In general, since mathematical techniques can coordinate and integrate multi-variant data, a mathematical approach that helps to optimize therapeutic efficiency will become an indispensable part of ICC. Currently, mathematical studies for cancer chemotherapy only focus on the requisite plasma drug concentration and cost-effectiveness in terms of the controlling budget, but mathematical approaches can potentially do far more. As quantitative data are superior to qualitative descriptions for decision-making, mathematical methods will be used to perform more quantitative calculations and handle sophisticated bioinformatics data in the future. The current use of mathematics in ICC is to process and extract drug sensitivity testing data and/or biomarker-orientated therapy data with long term follow-up of the patient's survival and quality of life.

Cost-effectiveness Problems and Budget Control

Cost-effectiveness is a long-standing medical problem and is also an early concern of mathematics in ICC. Increasing efforts to develop ICC are generally paralleled by rising diagnostic costs. Systematic evaluation of the relationship between the running costs and benefits of ICC is crucial for updating the ICC system and making it available in the long term, since the cost of therapy is a critical matter to consider. The balance between cost and effectiveness is an unavoidable ICC research project (Hasenclever *et al.* 2001; Brown *et al.* 2001; Bayoumi *et al.* 2000; Lyman 2000; Smith and Hillner 2011) and cannot be overlooked. Optimizing the cost-and-effect of a therapy and providing the best medical service is an important task awaiting study.

Finding Tumorigenic Markers from the Genome

Finding tumorigenic markers from tumor tissue genomes is an important statistical and mathematical challenge in ICC. It is known that there are some 35,000 genes in normal human cells. Each individual has a distinctive genetic makeup, and expression of some of the 35,000 genes will be higher or lower than normal in a tumor cell. Only one or two of them are likely to be the original genetic abnormalities that caused tumorigenesis and led to further and more widespread abnormalities of gene expression. When the genetic status of a tumor is assessed, only an average or total picture of gene expression is obtained, which concerns the general genetic status of the tumor. Thus, the original genetic abnormalities have to be extracted from this wealth of data using mathematical procedures. Currently, only a few biomarkers are detected in routine assays. Hence, the origin of a tumor is unlikely to be identified by the routine approaches. More comprehensive approaches to mapping the genetic polymorphisms and cytological levels of biomarkers as well as application of increasingly sophisticated mathematical means will be required to pinpoint the real culprit from the wealth of bioinformatics data in order to optimize the efficacy of the anticancer drugs. The mathematical approach to genes and their interrelationships (cf. Friedman 2004; Hoh and Ott 2003; Hu *et al.* 2007) will be indispensable parts of future ICC.

Future Directions

Four types of clinical investigation will help to perfect the ICC strategy: (1) validating and pinpointing the intermediate processes and biomarkers that are neglected in current standard treatment, and establishing the relationship between individual biomarker changes and effectiveness of relevant anticancer drugs; (2) technical improvements in the analytical capacity for biomarker detection, decreasing the cost of such detection, and finally validation and identification of key biomarkers from the whole genome by mathematical means; (3) evaluation and prediction of tumor responses to each anticancer drug in different pathological conditions with varying genetic abnormalities; and finally (4) design of a genetic rectification system compatible with the real-time situations of patients (Benenson *et al.* 2004).

Treatments of Tumor Metastases and MDR by ICC

Pathology of Tumor Metastases

Tumor metastases involve a cascade of pathophysiological processes (Poste and Fidler 1980; Fidler 1990, 2003; Dong *et al.* 2009) and are responsible for more than 60% of cancer deaths worldwide. Currently, tumor metastases can be only partially treated or controlled by anti-cancer drugs. Metastases and MDR are two major pathological aspects of tumors that are now regarded as mechanistically linked (Yang *et al.* 2003) and are responsible for poor prognoses for patients.

Metastatic Therapy in Clinics

Since neoplasm metastases are pathologically more complicated than primary tumors, therapy for them needs to be more selective and personalized. Morphological or biochemical information is needed to ascertain the pathological stage of a metastasis in an individual. Since heterogeneity of metastatic tumors is a common feature of experimental models (Fidler 1990, 2003), primary tumors and metastatic nodules in a single patient may differ in their drug responses (Von Hoff *et al.* 1986, 1990). Indeed, many reports indicate that large-volume primary tumors and small metastatic nodules must be treated differently; the cytostatic agents often target small tumor nodules, while cytotoxic or apoptotic drugs are more likely to target large-volume tumors (Folkman 1996; Taraboletti and Margosio 2001; Lu and Lu 2010b).

Antimetastatic drugs are important for prolonging the life-spans of cancer patients who have suffered metastases after the initiation of treatment. Individualized therapy for cancer metastases requires appropriate use of antimetastatic agents, so the characteristics of those agents must be clearly known. Current antimetastatic agents fall into two main categories: antivascular agents and matrix metalloproteinase (MMP) inhibitors (Tarabotti 2001; Sava *et al.* 1999; Lu *et al.* 2006b). In the future, antimetastatic agents targeting other types of metastatic molecules such as sialic acids (Lu and Lu 2010b; Lu *et al.* 2011) or inhibiting tumor cell movement (Lu *et al.* 2010d) might also be studied and developed. These endeavors will increase the range of drugs available for selection according to clinical situations.

Bisdioxopiperazine compounds (*Biz*) including ICRF-154, razoxane (ICRF-159, (±)1,2-di(3,5-dioxopiperazin-1-yl) propane or *Raz*), ICRF-186 and ICRF-187 (two stereoisomers of Raz) and ICRF-193, developed in the UK, were among the earliest agents found to be effective against a model of spontaneous metastasis: Lewis lung carcinoma (3LL) (Hellmann and Burrage 1969; Herman *et al.* 1982). *Biz* compounds are unique in their pharmacological action in inhibiting metastases, which is conserved among the different compounds. But the important area of key targeting is not well defined especially regarding their antimetastatic mechanisms. Other bisdioxopiperazine compounds probimane (*Pro*) and bimolane (*Bim*) have been synthesized at the Shanghai Institute of Materia Medica, Chinese Academy of Sciences.

It is hypothesized that many anticancer or antimetastatic drugs might act differently at different substages and well-chosen combinations could achieve better therapeutic outcome (Lu *et al.* 2010a). A study showed that *Pro* and *Bim* significantly inhibited the pulmonary metastasis of 3LL in mice if administered either from day 2 or day 8 post-inoculation of the tumor, but *Raz* required early administration from day 2 to reduce tumor metastasis significantly (Lu *et al.* 2010a). The pathogenesis of tumor metastasis has been categorized into three critical steps: (i) tumor detachment from its primary location; (ii) flow of tumor cells in the blood or lymphatic vessels; (iii) tumor cell attachment and penetration through blood vessels of distant organs (Poste and Fidler 1980). From the report of James and Salsbury (1974), the detachment of 3LL began on day 6-8; the inhibition of metastasis by *Raz* is due to the inhibition of neovascularization in the tumor tissues. These data indicate that *Raz* is effective only against early tumor detachment, and remains ineffective against the pulmonary metastatic foci of 3LL. This can also explain why *Raz* is reportedly more effective against spontaneous metastatic tumors than artificial ones. On the other hand, *Pro* and *Bim* might be equally effective in both cases. Our early data concerning the tracing and autoradiography of ^{14}C-probimane showed an obviously greater accumulation of *Pro* in tumor tissues, especially in metastatic foci. This helps to explain why *Pro* is a more effective inhibitor than *Raz* in the established metastatic foci through its stronger antiproliferative effect (Lu and Lu 2010b). The design of antimetastatic therapy should also take account of different stages of metastasis and mechanism of its initiation and growth to help in developing the most effective antimetastatic regimens.

Multidrug resistance (MDR) is an unavoidable detrimental circumstance affecting the quality of chemotherapy. Drug sensitivity tests and characterization of the genetic status of the members of the ABC (ATP-binding cassette) superfamily (Ulukaya 2006; Ross and Doyle 2004; Szakacs *et al.* 2004) can provide information about potential drug resistance as well as transmembrane drug transport systems, and the patients can be provided with alternative drugs to overcome MDR (Sargent *et al.* 2001; Steinbach *et al.* 2003). Again, the treatment of cancer metastases and MDR should ideally be personalized according to the clinical situations and circumstances of individual patients.

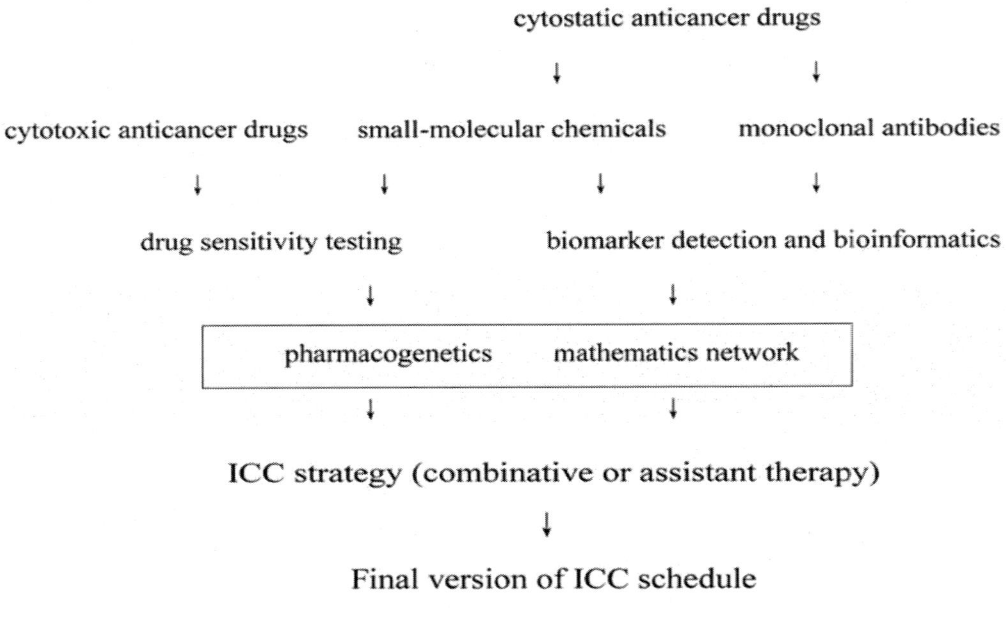

Figure 13.1. The proposed sketch for the development of an individualized cancer chemotherapy schedule.

Adjunctive Therapy

There are many causes of death in cancer patients. Apart from direct causes from tumor progression, other clinical complications or psychiatric factors will more or less aggravate the prognosis. Several adjunctive therapies are available for patients with clinical complications or psychiatric problems. For example, it has been suggested that cancer patients should benefit from anticoagulants such as warfarin and heparin and/or fibrinolytic agents (recommended for those at particular risk for thrombosis) (Costantini and Zacharski 1992; Lu *et al.* 2007a; Eikelboom and Mehta 2000) or the antifungal antibiotic oxalysine, which has immunomodulatory and anticancer activities (Lu *et al.* 1999, 2007a). It is known that the fear of death in cancer patients implies a poor prognosis and antidepressants can provide adjunctive therapy for psychiatrically disturbed patients (Lieb 2007; Lu and Lu 2008). With these types of adjunctive therapy, a longer survival in cancer can be expected.

Conclusion

In the past, cancer clinicians made therapeutic decisions on an empirical basis rather than by thorough individualized evaluation of the pathological features of the cancer and/or anticancer drug sensitivity patterns. When tumors acquire MDR and become refractory or recurrent after first line chemotherapy, a poor clinical prognosis seems inevitable. The ICC strategy seems to be beneficial for these cancer patients (Lu *et al.* 2006a; Ugurel *et al.* 2006). The utility of ICC can be portrayed by another example. It is said that there is a marginal benefit in terms of overall survival for colon cancer patients with normal prognoses, but there are marked survival benefits for colon cancer patients with poor prognoses, especially those with tumors over-expressing HER2 (Kim *et al.* 2003). In such a scenario, ICC is optimal in both situations, and is best suited for the latter.

Numerous studies show the favorable or beneficial effects of employing drug sensitivity tests in clinics. The drug response rates of patients are improved by approximately 10%, but survival benefits are reported to be relatively small (Cortazar and Johnson 1999; Ness *et al.* 2002; Ugurel *et al.* 2006; Gazdar *et al.* 1990). This is the main reason why the effectiveness of the ICC strategy is contentious. Although drug sensitivity tests have not been routinely used in clinics, the pro and con debates about them continue and reports on their benefits vary from patient to patient, we should remain optimistic about their future advancement and utility. More clinicians should be encouraged and trained to use the ICC strategy. With such an approach, the strategy will be transferred from bench to bedside. Several important considerations in developing ICC strategies need to be taken into account in future:

1. *The number of drugs available for choosing*: Increasing the number of drugs available for choice on the basis of a single drug sensitivity test will help to select in the drugs that are best suited for chemotherapy (Lu *et al.* 2006a).
2. *The simplification of drug sensitivity tests*: It is expected that the drug sensitivity tests in future would be simplified (Lu *et al.* 2006a). Ulukaya (2006) challenges this view by arguing that simplification of the drug sensitivity test protocol would lead to poor test performance. However, there may be no relationship between the therapeutic outcome and simplicity of protocol. We argue here again that with a deeper understanding of the nature of cancer cells following scientific investigations, we can utilize more appropriate and simpler conditions for tumor cells to grow and be tested. In ordinary hospitals, it is impractical to support very sophisticated protocols. The shortening and simplification of drug-sensitivity tests without compromising their

effects will become a future trend. The simpler the drug sensitivity test protocol, the more hospitals can implement an ICC strategy.

3. *The advancement of biomarker detection*: Whether there is a relationship between biomarker levels in individual tumor specimens and drug response outcomes among cancer patients is controversial. The central point in this issue is to identify the original or causative biomarkers in a specific tumor tissue.
4. *The utility of bioinformatics*: There are two important approaches to bioinformatics-based ICC. The first is to detect as many polymorphisms or cytological levels of biomarkers as possible at the least possible cost. The second is to pinpoint the original or causative biomarkers as clearly as possible by mathematical means. The more successfully we pinpoint these genes, the more appropriate will be our choice of anticancer drugs, especially for monotherapy or ribonucleic acid interference (RNAi) agents. These two approaches need to be systemized, e.g. standard chips and techniques and genetic analysis software are waiting to be developed and perfected. Finally, the following priorities for improving ICC strategy are emphasized: (i) to sketch routine ICC procedures in a diagram (Figure 13.1); (ii) to develop novel applicable equations and calculating systems; (iii) to design automatic protocols to save labor and to be universally usable in conventional hospitals (Lu *et al.* 2006a).

Finally, it should be considered for every cancer patient to have his/her own unique chemotherapy trial based on consultation of pathogenic profiles and drug sensitivity testing data. Research and application of ICC is encouraged by growing patient demand, scientific advances and medical ethics. The ICC system is not a luxury but an absolute necessity, and a powerful strategy that we cannot overlook.

References

Aamdal, S. *et al.* (1985) Characteristics of human tumour xenografts transplanted under the subrenal capsule of immunocompetent mice. *British Journal of Cancer*, 51, pp. 347-356.

Akao, S. *et al.* (1996) Evaluation of subrenal capsule assay (SRC) for clinical cancers. *Gan To Kagaku Ryoho (Japanese Journal of Cancer and Chemotherapy)*, 23, pp. 607-613.

BAYOUMI, A.M. *et al.* (2000) Cost-effectiveness of androgen suppression therapies in advanced prostate cancer. *Journal of the National Cancer Institute*, 92, pp. 1731-1739.

Bentley, D. R. (2004) Genomes for medicine. *Nature*, pp. 440-445.

Black, M. M. and Speer, F. D. (1954) Further observations on the effects of cancer chemotherapeutic agents on the *in vitro* dehydrogenase activity of cancer tissue. *Journal of the National Cancer Institute,* 14, pp. 1147-1158.

Bodegen, A. E. *et al.* (1978) A rapid screening method for testing chemotherapeutic agents against human tumor xenograft. In: Houcheus, D. P. and Ovejera, A. A. (eds) *Proceedings of the Symposium on the Use of Athymic (Nude) Mice in Cancer Research.* New York: Gustav Fischer Inc., pp. 231-250.

Bosanquet, A. G. *et al.* (2002) Parameters affecting the ex vivo cytotoxic drug sensitivity of human hematopoietic cells. *Journal of Experimental Therapeutics and Oncology*, 2, pp. 53-63.

Breidenbach, M. *et al.* (2003) Hematological side-effect profiles of individualized chemotherapy regimen for recurrent ovarian cancer. *Anticancer Drugs*, 14, pp. 341-346.

Brown, R. E. *et al.* (2001) Cost effectiveness of treatment options in advanced breast cancer in the UK. *Pharmacoeconomics*, 19, pp. 1091-1102.

Carlson, C. S. *et al.* (2004) Mapping complex disease loci in whole-genome association studies. *Nature*, 429, pp. 446-452.

Collins, F. S. *et al.* (2003) A vision for the future genomic research. *Nature*, 422, pp. 835-847.

Cortazar, P. and Johnson, B. E. (1999) Review of the efficacy of individualized chemotherapy selected by *in vitro* drug sensitivity testing for patient with cancer. *Journal of Clinical Oncology*, 17, pp. 1625-1631.

Costantini, V. and Zacharski, L. R. (1992) The role of fibrin in tumor metastasis. *Cancer Metastasis Review*, 11, pp, 283-290.Cunningham, D. *et al.* (1986) The 6 day subrenal capsule assay is of no value with primary surgical explants from gastric cancer. *British Journal of Cancer*, 54, pp. 519-523.

Dalton, W. S. and Friend, A. S. H. (2006) Cancer biomarkers-an invitation to the table. *Science*, 312, pp. 1165-1168.

Diehl, V. (2007) Hodgkin's disease from pathology specimen to cure. *The New England Journal of Medicine*, 357, pp. 1968-1971.

Dong, F. *et al.* (2009) Translating the metastasis paradigm from scientific theory to clinical oncology. *Clinical Cancer Research*, 15, pp, 2588-2593.

Efferth, T. and Volm, M. (2005) Pharmacogenetics for individualized cancer chemotherapy. *Pharmacology and Therapeutics*, 107, pp.155-176.

Efferth, T. *et al.* (2008) Prediction of broad spectrum resistance of tumors towards anticancer drugs. *Clinical Cancer Research*, 14, pp. 2405-2412.

Eikelboom, J. W. and Mehta, S. R. (2000) Venous thromboembolism and cancer. *The New England Journal of Medicine*, 343, pp. 1337-1338.

Evans, W. E. and Relling, M. V. (2004) Moving towards individualized medicine with pharmacogenomics. *Nature*, 429, pp. 464-468.

Fidler, I. J. (1990) Critical factors in the biology of human cancer metastasis: Twenty-eight GHA Clowes memorial award lecture. *Cancer Research*, 59, pp. 6130-6138.

Fidler, I. J. (2003) The pathogenesis of cancer metastasis: the "seed and soil" hypothesis revisited. *Nature Review of Cancer*, 3, pp, 453-458.

Folkman, J. (1996) New perspectives in clinical oncology from angiogenesis research. *Europe Journal of Cancer*, 32A, pp, 2534-2539.

Friedman, N. (2004) Inferring cellular networks using probabilistic graphical models. *Science*, 303, pp. 799-805.

Futreal, P. A. *et al.* (2001) Cancer and genomics. Nature, 409, pp. 850-852.

Gazdar, A. F. *et al.* (1990) Correlation of *in vitro* drug-sensitivity testing results with response to chemotherapy and survival in extensive-stage small cell lung cancer: a prospective clinical trial. *Journal of the National Cancer Institute*, 82, pp. 117-124.

Geyer, C. E. *et al.* (2006) Lapatinib plus capecitabine for HER2-positive advanced breast cancer. *The New England Journal of Medicine*, 355, pp. 2733-2743.

Gibbs, R. A. *et al.* (2003) The international HapMap project. *Nature*, 426, pp. 789-796.

Gillespie, D. L. *et al.* (2007) Silencing of hypoxia inducible factor-1α by RNA interference attenuates human glioma cell growth *in vivo*. *Clinical Cancer Research*, 13, pp. 2441-2448.

Goldstein, D. B. *et al.* (2003) Pharmacogenetics goes genomic. *Nature Reviews - Genetics*, 4, pp. 937-947.

Gordon, G. J. *et al.* (2002) Translation of microarray data into clinically relevant cancer diagnostic tests using gene expression ratios in lung cancer and mesothelioma. *Cancer Research*, 62, pp. 4963-496.

Guo, Q. B. M. (2003) DNA microarray and cancer. *Current Opinion in Oncology*, 15, pp. 36-43.

Hamburger, A. W. and Salmon, S. E. (1977) Primary bioassay of human tumor stem cells. *Science*, 197, pp. 461-463.

Hanahan, D. and Weinberg, R. A. (2000) The hallmarks of cancer. *Cell*, 100, pp. 57-70.

Hasenclever, D. *et al.* (2001) Modeling of chemotherapy: the effective dose approach. *Annals of Hematology*, 80[Suppl 3], pp. 89-94.

Herman, E. H. *et al.* (1982) Properties of ICRF-159 and related Bis(dioxopiperazine) compounds. *Advances in Pharmacology and Chemotherapy,* 19, pp. 249-290.

Hellmann, K. and Burrage, K. (1969) Control of malignant metastases by ICRF-159. *Nature*, 224, pp, 273-275.

Hoh, J. and Ott, J. (2003) Mathematical multi-locus approaches to localizing complex human trait genes. *Nature Reviews - Cancer*, 3, pp. 701-709.

Hu, P. Z. *et al.* (2007) Computational prediction of cancer-gene function. *Nature Reviews - Cancer*, 7, pp. 23-34.

Huang, R. S. and Ratain, M. J. (2009) Pharmacogenetics and pharmacogenomics of anticancer drugs. *CA: A Cancer Journal for Clinicians*, 59, pp. 42-55.

Ichikawa, W. *et al.* (2003) Combination of dihydropyrimidine dehydrogenase and thymidylate synthase gene expressions in primary tumors as predictive parameters for the efficacy of fluoropyrimidine-based chemotherapy for metastatic colorectal cancer. *Clinical Cancer Research*, 9, pp. 786-791.

James, S. E. And Salsbury, A. J. (1974). Effect of (plus or minus)-1,2-bis(3,5-dioxopiperazin-1-yl)propane on tumor blood vessels and its relationship to the antimetastatic effect in the Lewis lung carcinoma. *Cancer Research*, 34, pp. 839-842.

Jongeneel, C. V. *et al.* (2003) Comprehensive sampling of gene expression in human cell lines with massively parallel signature sequencing. *Proceedings of the National Academy of Sciences of the United States of America*, 100, pp. 4702-4705.

Kawamura, H. *et al.* (1997) The usefulness of the ATP assay with serum-free culture for chemosensitivity testing of gastrointestinal cancer. *European Journal of Cancer*, 33, pp. 960-966.

Kim, R. *et al.* (2003) Chemosensitivity testing for gastrointestinal cancer: survival benefit potential and limitations. *Anti-Cancer Drugs*, 14, pp. 715-723.

Knight, Z. A. and Shokat, K. M. (2007) Chemical genetics: where genetics and pharmacology meet. *Cell*, 128, pp. 425-430.

Kondo, T. *et al.* (1966) *In vitro* test for sensitivity of tumor to carcinostatic agents. *Gann*, 57, pp. 113-121.

Kurbacher, C. M. *et al.* (1998) Use of an ex vivo ATP luminescence assay to direct chemotherapy for recurrent ovarian cancer. *Anticancer Drugs*, 9, pp. 51-57.

The Lancet Oncology (2010) New hope for advanced gastric cancer. The Lancet Oncology, 11, p. 211.

Lander, E. S. *et al.* (2001) Initial sequencing and analysis of the human genome. *Nature*, 409, pp. 860-921.

Lechleider, R. J. *et al.* (2008) Ixabepilone in combination with capecitabine and as monotherapy for treatment of advanced breast cancer refractory to previous chemotherapies. *Clinical Cancer Research*, 14, pp. 4378-4384.

Levi, F. A. *et al.* (1984) A four-day subrenal capsule assay for testing the effectiveness of anticancer drugs against human tumors. *Cancer Research*, 44, pp. 2660-2667.

Lieb, J. (2007) Antidepressants, prostaglandins and the prevention and treatment of cancer. *Medical Hypotheses*, 69, pp. 684-689.

Lu, D.Y. *et al.* (1999) Comparison of some antineoplastic drugs on inhibiting thrombin catalyzing fibrinogen clotting *in vitro*. *Chinese Medical Journal*, 112, pp. 1052-1053.

Lu, D. Y. *et al.* (2000) Effects of cancer chemotherapy on the blood fibrinogen concentrations of cancer patients. *The Journal of International Medical Research,* 28, pp. 313-317.

Lu, D. Y. *et al.* (2006a) Individualized cancer chemotherapy integrating drug sensitivity tests, pathological profile analysis and computational coordination-an effective strategy to improve clinical treatment. *Medical Hypotheses*, 66, pp. 45-51.

Lu, D. Y. *et al.* (2006b) Recent advances in anti-metastatic drug development. *Acta Pharmacologica Sinica*, 27[Suppl], pp. 66-67.

Lu, D. Y. *et al.* (2007a) Treatment of solid tumors and metastases by fibrinogen-targeted anticancer drug therapy. *Medical Hypotheses*, 68, pp. 188-193.

Lu, D. Y. *et al.* (2007b) Employing new mathematical models and equations to evaluate risk-benefit criteria of clinical therapeutics. *OnLine Journal of Biological Sciences*, 7, pp. 1-2.

Lu, D. Y. *et al.* 2007c, Relationship between blood fibrinogen concentration and pathological features of cancer patients: a 139-case clinical study. *OnLine Journal of Biological Sciences,* 7, pp. 8-11.

Lu, D. Y. and Lu, T. R. (2008) Antidepressants can be only used as assistant therapy in cancer treatment. *Medical Hypotheses*, 70, pp. 204-205.

Lu, D. Y. *et al.* (2010a) Different spontaneous pulmonary metastasis inhibitions against Lewis lung carcinoma in mice by Bisdioxopiperazine compounds of different treatment schedules. *Scientia Pharmaceutica*, 78, pp. 13-20.

Lu, D. Y. and Lu, T. R. (2010b) Antimetastatic activities and mechanisms of Bisdioxopiperazine compounds. *Anti-Cancer Agents in Medicinal Chemistry*, 10, pp. 564-570.

Lu, D. Y. *et al.* (2010c) Similarity of drug sensitivity test results on human pulmonary adenocarcinoma xenografts transplanted under the subrenal capsules between normal immunocompetent and immunodeficient athymic mice. *International Journal of Pharmacy and Therapeutics*, 1, pp. 106-109.

Lu, D. Y. *et al.* (2010d) Cell biological manifestations of Bisdioxopiperazines: treatment of human tumor cell lines in culture. *Anti-Cancer Agents in Medicinal Chemistry*, 10, pp. 657-660.

Lu, D. Y. *et al.* (2011). Antimetastatic therapy targeting aberrant sialylation profiles in cancer cells. *Drugs and Therapy Studies*, 1, doi: 10.4081/dts.2011.e12.

Lyman, G. H. (2000) A novel approach to maintain planned dose chemotherapy on time: a decision-making tool to improve patient care. *European Journal of Cancer*, 36[Suppl 1], pp. 15-21.

Marx, J. (2004) Why a new cancer drug works well in some patients. *Science*, 304, pp. 657-658.

Millar, A. W. and Lynch, K. P. (2003) Rethinking clinical trials for cytostatic drugs. *Nature Reviews - Cancer*, 3, pp. 540-545.

Miller, K. *et al.* (2007) Paclitaxel plus bevacizumab versus paclitaxel alone for metastatic breast cancer. *The New England Journal of Medicine*, 357, pp. 2666-2676.

Morioka, H. *et al.* (2001) *In vitro* chemosensitivity of human soft tissue sarcoma. *Anticancer Research*, 21, pp. 4147-4152.

Ness, R. B. *et al.* (2002) Cell viability assay for drug testing in ovarian cancer: *In vitro* kill versus clinical response. *Anticancer Research*, 22, pp. 1145-1150.

Nowell, P. C. (1976) The clonal evolution of tumor cell populations. *Science*, 194, pp. 23-28.

Pennisi, E. (2003) Tracing life's circuitry. *Science*, 302, pp. 1646-1649.

Poste, G. and Fidler, I. J. (1980) The pathogenesis of cancer metastasis. *Nature*, 283, pp, 139-146.

Pritchard, J. K. and Przeworski, M. (2001) Linkage disequilibrium in humans: Models and data. *American Journal of Human Genetics*, 69, pp. 1-14.

Pusztai, L. *et al.* (2003) Clinical application of cDNA microarrays in oncology. *Oncologist*, 8, pp. 252-258.

Ross, D. D. and Doyle, L. A. (2004) Mining our ABCs: pharmacogenomics approach for evaluating transporter function in cancer drug resistance. *Cancer Cell*, 6, pp. 105-107

Sachidanandam, R. *et al.* (2001) A map of human genome sequence variation containing 1.42 million single nucleotide polymorphisms. *Nature*, 409, pp. 928-933.

Salmon, S. E. *et al.* (1978) Quantitation of differential sensitivity of human-tumor stem cells to anticancer drugs. *The New England Journal of Medicine*, 298, pp. 1321-1327.

Sargent, J. M. *et al.* (2001) Dexrazoxane significantly impairs the induction of doxorubicin resistance the human leukemia, K562. *British Journal of Cancer*, 84, pp. 959-964.

Smith, T. J. and Hillner, B. E. (2011) Bending the cost curve in cancer care. *The New England Journal of Medicine*, 364, pp. 2060-2065.

Steinbach, D. *et al.* (2003) Response to chemotherapy and expression of the genes encoding the multidrug resistance-associated protein MRP2, MRP3, MRP4, MRP5, and SMRP in childhood acute myeloid leukemia. *Clinical Cancer Research*, 9, pp. 1083-1086.

Stoler, D. L. *et al.* (1999) The onset and extent of genomic instability in sporadic colorectal tumor progression. *Proceedings of the National Academy of Sciences of the United States of America*, 96, pp. 15121-15126.

Szakacs, G. *et al.* (2004) Predicting drug sensitivity and resistance: Profile ABC transporter genes in cancer cells. *Cancer Cell*, 6, pp. 129-137.

Takamura, Y. *et al.* (2002) Prediction of chemotherapeutic response by collagen gel droplet embedded culture-drug sensitivity test in human breast cancers. *International Journal of Cancer*, 98, pp. 450-455.

Tanino, H. *et al.* (2001) Acquisition of multidrug resistance in recurrent breast cancer demonstrated by the histoculture drug response assay. *Anticancer Research*, 21, pp. 4083-4086.

Taraboletti, G. and Margosio, B. (2001) Antiangiogenic and antivascular therapy for cancer. *Current Opinion in Pharmacology*, 1, pp. 378-384.

Tol, J. *et al.* (2009) Chemotherapy, bevacizumab, and cetuximab in metastatic colorectal cancer. *The New England Journal of Medicine*, 360, pp. 564-572.

Ugurel, S. *et al.* (2006) *In vitro* drug sensitivity predicts response and survival after individualized sensitivity-directed chemotherapy in metastatic melanoma: a multicenter phase II trial of dermatologic cooperative oncology. *Clinical Cancer Research*, 12, pp. 5454-5463.

Ulukaya, E. (2006) Drug response assay: an increasing trend in designation of tailored-chemotherapy for more rational management of cancer patients. *Advances in Molecular Medicine*, 2, pp. 53-58.

Van De Vijver, M. J. *et al.* (2002) A gene-expression signature as a predictor of survival in breast cancer. *The New England Journal of Medicine*, 347, pp. 1999-2009.

Venesmaa, P. and Ylikokala, O. (1991) Subrenal capsule assay in selection of chemotherapy after operation for recurrent ovarian cancer. *British Journal of Cancer*, 63, pp. 84-86.

Venter, J. C. *et al.* (2001) The sequence of the human genome. *Science*, 291, pp. 1304-1351.

Vermorken, J. B. *et al.* (2008) Platinum-based chemothgerapy plus cetuximab in head and neck cancer. *The New England Journal of Medicine*, 359, pp. 1116-1127.

von Hoff, D. D. *et al.* (1986) Simultaneous *in vitro* drug sensitivity testing on tumors from different sites in the same patient. *Cancer*, 58, pp. 1007-1013.

von Hoff, D. D. *et al.* (1990) Selection of cancer chemotherapy for a patient by an *in vitro* assay versus a clinician. *Journal of the National Cancer Institute*, 82, pp. 110-116.

Watters, J. W. and Mcleod, H. L. (2003) Cancer pharmacogenomics: current and future applications. *Biochimica et Biophysica Acta*, 1603, pp. 99-111.

Weir, B. *et al.* (2004) Somatic alterations in the human cancer genome. *Cancer Cell*, 6, pp. 433-438.

Williams, N. S. *et al.* (2003) Identification and validation of genes involved in the pathogenesis of colorectal cancer using cDNA microarrays and RNA interference. Clinical *Cancer Research*, 9, pp. 931-946.

Wright, J. L. *et al.* (1957) Investigation of the relation between clinical and tissue-culture response to chemotherapeutic agents on human cancer. *The New England Journal of Medicine*, 257, pp. 1207-1211.

Yang, J. M. *et al.* (2003) Overexpression of extracellular matrix metalloproteinase in nultidrug resistant cancer cells. *Molecular Cancer Research*, 1, pp. 420-427.

Younes, A. *et al.* (2010) Brentuximab vedotin (SGM-35) for relapsed CD30-positive lymphomas. *The New England Journal of Medicine*, 363, pp. 1812-1821.

In: Hypotheses in Clinical Medicine
Editors: M.M. Shoja, P.S. Agutter et al.

ISBN: 978-1-62257-276-2

Chapter 14

The Potential Evolutionary Significance of the Pineal Gland

***Paul S. Agutter*[1], *R. Shane Tubbs*[2], *Marios Loukas*[3], *Mehdi Farhoudi*[4], *Alireza Ghaffari*[5], *Martin M. Mortazavi*[6], *Kamyar Ghabili*[7] and *Mohammadali M. Shoja*[6,8,9,*]**

[1]Theoretical Medicine and Biology Group, Glossop, Derbyshire, UK
[2]Pediatric Neurosurgery, Children's Hospital, Birmingham, Alabama, US
[3]Department of Anatomical Sciences,
St. George's University,Grenada, West Indies
[4]Neurosciences Research Center (NSRC),
Tabriz University of Medical Sciences, Tabriz, Iran
[5]Tuberculosis and Lung Disease Research Center,
Tabriz University of Medical Sciences, Tabriz, Iran
[6]Division of Neurological Surgery, Department of Surgery,
University of Alabama at Birmingham, Birmingham, Alabama, US
[7]Medical Philosophy and History Research Center,
Tabriz University of Medical Sciences, Tabriz, Iran
[8]Pediatric Neurosurgery, Children's Hospital, Birmingham, Alabama, US
[9]Tuberculosis and Lung Disease Research Center,
Tabriz University of Medical Sciences, Tabriz, Iran

Abstract

Although during the early 20th century the pineal gland was considered to have little functional significance, the activity of its secretory product, melatonin, has been increasingly appreciated during recent decades. Melatonin has a role in the sleep-wake cycle and recent studies have shown that it acutely enhances mating behaviour and libido. Since reproductive activity is obviously of primary importance for the survival of species,

[*] E-mail: shoja.m@gmail.com.

this could plausibly suggest a circadian control of mating behaviour. In this chapter, we argue that the coupling of mating behaviour to light-dark shifts by melatonin might have influenced the survival of species, and this could throw fresh light on the evolutionary significance of the pineal gland.

Introduction

The evolutionary significance of the pineal gland has not been fully elucidated. Melatonin, the hormone secreted by the pineal gland cells (pinealocytes), has been shown to play a key regulatory role in physiological circadian rhythms. It is very widely distributed among taxa (Tan *et al.* 2010), and in mammals and other groups it is secreted in response to light-dark shifts, secretion being up-regulated by darkness (McIntyre *et al.* 1989). In some species, melatonin is also produced in the retina (Cahill *et al.* 1991) and, at least in goldfish, it is produced locally in the gut and the liver, where synthesis seems to follow a circadian rhythm not entrained by light-dark stimuli (Velarde *et al.* 2010).

A review by Falcón *et al.* (2009) highlighted the differences in circadian clocks between lower and higher vertebrates. In fish and amphibia, the pineal gland, retina and perhaps other parts of the brain form a network of complete circadian systems, which is probably synchronized by melatonin, so photoperiodic control of the clock is direct: the clock and the phototransduction processes are housed in the melatonin-producing pinealocytes. In birds and mammals, the eyes contain the photoreceptive units and the suprachiasmatic nuclei (SCN) in the hypothalamus house the clocks; the pineal, which is the main or sole source of melatonin in these taxa, is separate from both. Photoperiodic control is therefore indirect. The SCN controls the pineal via a multisynaptic pathway (Teclemariam Mesbah *et al.* 1999).

In humans, the circadian rhythm of melatonin secretion starts at the end of the neonatal period (one month after birth) with the highest secretion between 12 p.m. and 8 a.m. (Ardura *et al.* 2003). Bellavía *et al.* (1993) showed that neonatal rats kept in 24-hour darkness retained the circadian rhythm of alpha-amylase secretion from the parotid gland, even when their mothers had been kept in constant darkness during pregnancy. However, no such rhythm was found in the pups if the mothers had undergone bilateral ablation of the cervical superior ganglia (which provide the nerve supply to the pineal), unless they were given melatonin supplements. It therefore appears that the pineal gland, and its secretion of melatonin, is essential for the transfer of circadian rhythm information from the mother to the fetus or the neonate.

This chapter is organized as follows: We first consider the evolution of the pineal gland as a producer of melatonin, and then discuss the organization of clock genes in the hypothalamus and the molecular basis of rhythmic melatonin production. This is followed by a brief comment on the role of melatonin in seasonal mating and libido. We then discuss the evolutionary change from nocturnal to diurnal lifestyles in some mammalian species, and draw attention to the link between the circadian clock and seasonal reproductive activity. In the concluding section we draw together these lines of evidence and propose that the pineal gland, and its secretory product, played a crucial role in the evolutionary change to a diurnal lifestyle.

Pinealocytes, Photoreceptors and Melatonin: Evolutionary Aspects

Retinal photoreceptors and pinealocytes have much in common. The mammalian retina produces melatonin and this production follows a circadian rhythm (Cahill *et al.* 1991). Pinealocytes in lower vertebrates are photosensitive (Dodt 1963). Pinealocytes and retinal photoreceptors are histologically similar, being highly polarized and equipped with cilia (Eakin 1973). Although pinealocytes do not have these features in adult mammals, they are apparent during embryonic development and even in neonates (Zimmerman and Tso 1975; Araki *et al.* 1988); also, the pineal gland and the retina develop from adjacent regions of the neural plate (reviewed by Ekström and Meissl 2003). Many genes expressed in photoreceptors are also highly expressed in the pineal gland (reviewed by Klein 2006). Tumors of the pineal region are histologically very similar to retinoblastomas (Jakobiec *et al.* 1977).

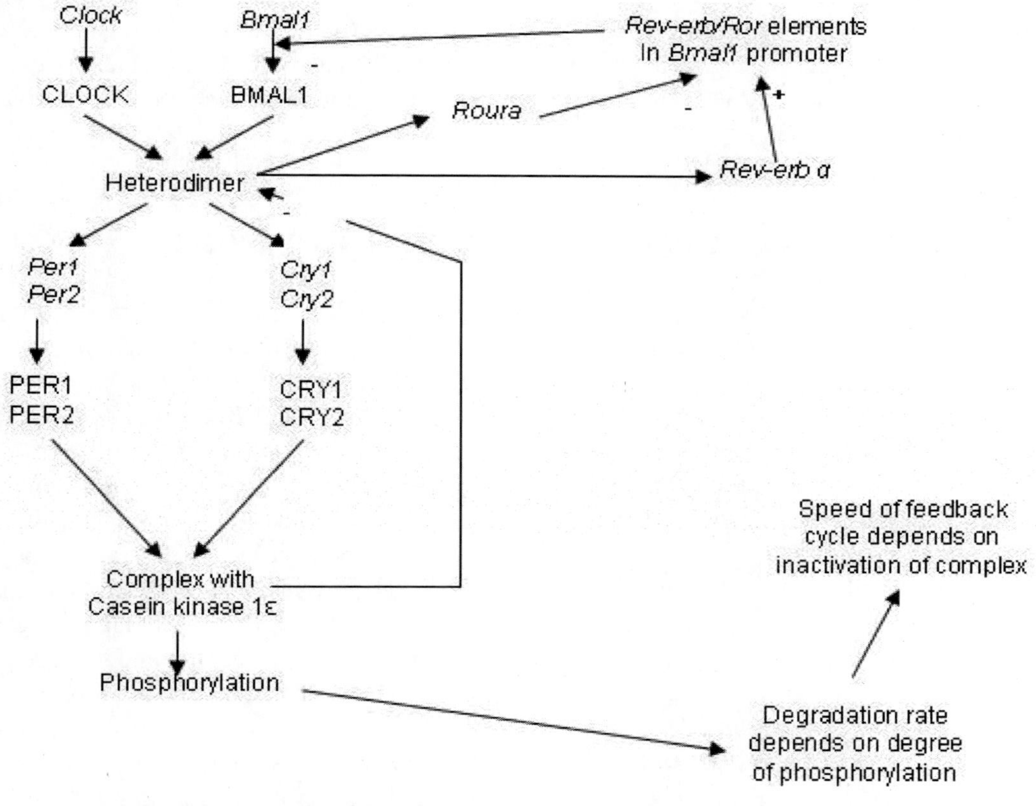

Figure 14.1. Interrelationships among the clock genes in the superchiasmatic nucleus. The protein products of Clock (circadian locomotor output cycle kaput) and Bmal1 (brain and muscle ARNT-like protein 1) form a heterodimer, which promotes the transcription of the Per and Cry genes. The products of those genes bind to casein kinase 1ε and are phosphorylated. The complex blocks the binding of the heterodimer to the Per and Cry promoters. The heterodimer also stimulates the expression of Rev-erb α and Roura , which have opposing effects on the transcription of Bmal1. The rate of degradation of PER and CRY depends on the degree of phosphorylation by casein kinase 1ε, and this alters the speed of the feedback cycle.

Collectively, these observations suggest that retinal photoreceptors and the pineal gland have a common ancestry. Eakin (1973) found that the structure of the photoreceptor cell of the urochordate *Ciona* is very similar to both mammalian structures, and since *Ciona* and vertebrates have a common ancestor, the ancestral cell was probably of this type. However, *Ciona* does not have genes encoding the melatonin biosynthetic enzymes or melatonin receptors. Klein (1976) suggested that the acquisition of these enzymes in the chordate line was the preliminary step in the evolution of the vertebrate pineal gland, and further proposed that the key enzyme in melatonin biosynthesis, arylalkylamine-N-acetyltransferase (AANAT), was initially acquired (perhaps by lateral gene transfer from bacteria) as a mechanism for detoxifying amines that could remove retinaldehyde by Schiff base formation, impairing the visual system. The other enzyme in the biosynthetic pathway, hydroxyindole-O-methyltransferase (HIOMT), could also have served a protective function originally, since O-methylation renders hydroxyl-containing xenobiotics less reactive.

Melatonin itself probably served a protective function originally. It is an antioxidant and its primary function in prokaryotes, protists and fungi seems to be as a free radical scavenger, affording protection against environmental insults; indeed, it has anti-inflammatory and immunomodulatory effects in vertebrates (Tan *et al.* 2010). During the evolution of vertebrates, however, it has been recruited to other biological functions, including sexual signaling in some fish species and birds, and the seasonal regulation of reproductive activity in many mammals (see below).

Generation of Circadian Rhythms

Studies in various laboratories beginning in the late 1990s have established the feedback relationships among the clock genes in the SCN, which are responsible for the central control of circadian rhythms. These studies, and the significance of the clock gene system for reproductive behaviour in mammals, were reviewed by Boden and Kennaway (2006) and Mahoney (2010). The feedback relationships described in those reviews are summarized in Figure 14.1. The clock genes and their interconnections have also been identified in a number of peripheral tissues, including female reproductive tract structures such as the ovary (Fahrenkrug et al. 2006), and are functional in cultures of gonadotrophin releasing hormone (GnRH)-containing neurons derived from the SCN (Chappell *et al.* 2003). They are also present in the pineal gland itself, at least in fish (Huang *et al.* 2010). Although there is substantial redundancy in the clock gene system, so that loss of some of the component genes has no major pathological consequences, gene knockout studies indicate some perturbation of the reproductive system, and *Bmal1* in particular is crucial for successful mating and its physiological concomitants (Klein 2006; Boden and Kennaway 2006). Expression of some of the clock genes, notably *Per1* and *Cry2*, is sensitive to estrogen (Nakamura *et al.* 2001, 2005).

Various subtypes of melatonin receptors are widely distributed among mammalian organs, including the pars temporalis of the pituitary (Confente *et al.* 2010). Melatonin affects the expression of clock genes in peripheral tissues of mice with arthritis induced by anti-type II collagen antibody (Bang *et al.* 2012) and in prostate cancer cells (Jung-Hynes *et al.* 2010). More pertinently to the present argument, it has a marked effect on clock gene expression in the pars tuberalis of the pituitary (Unfried *et al.* 2010) and in many central neurons (Imbesi *et al.* 2009). The resetting of the circadian clock by different light-dark regimes (Cermakian and Boivin 2009) could therefore be effected via melatonin receptors in the relevant parts of the brain, though orally administered melatonin could not be shown to alter clock gene expression in the SCN of hypertensive rats (Zeman *et al.* 2009). It is well established that melatonin synchronizes the sleep-wake cycle in most mammalian species (Escames and Acuña-Castroviejo 2009).

Rhythmic Melatonin Biosynthesis

In pinealocytes, melatonin is formed from serotonin in two enzyme-catalyzed steps. First, serotonin is N-acetylated by the action of AANAT; second, the N-acetylserotonin is methylated on the ring hydroxyl group by HIOMT. There are circadian changes in the activity of the key enzyme AANAT (Falcón *et al.* 2009). In the dark, sympathetic neurons from the SCN stimulate cyclic-AMP production in pinealocytes via α_1 and β_1 receptors (Klein 2006). AANAT undergoes protein kinase A-dependent phosphorylation of residues close to the N and C termini, flanking the catalytic region, and the phosphorylated groups bind 14-3-3 proteins (Ganguly *et al.* 2005). This stabilizes and activates the AANAT so the rate of melatonin production rises. When a mammal is exposed to light, the 14-3-3 proteins dissociate and the enzyme undergoes proteolysis, decreasing melatonin production.

The level of melatonin output from the mammalian pineal, which decreases as day length increases, establishes long-term changes in the immune system, the autonomic nervous system, the hypothalamo-hypophyseal axis, brain-gut interactions and other physiological variables (Walton *et al.* 2010). Its importance for species survival is therefore clear. In mammals and other organisms, melatonin production declines with increasing age, and this may be related to the age-related malfunctioning of the circadian clock (Tan *et al.* 2010).

Melatonin and Libido/Mating

It is well established that seasonal changes in melatonin output affect the synchronization of libido, reproductive activity and behavior, and fecundity. Experimental studies have shown that an acute low dose (10-100 μg/kg) or chronic administration of melatonin enhances sexual activity and libido in male rats (Drago and Busá 2000; Brotto and Gorzalka 2000). Melatonin-treated ewes mated more readily with rams than control ewes, had higher circulating progesterone levels, and lambed earlier, though there was no significant effect on fertility or litter size (Abecia *et al.* 2006). Similarly, melatonin enhanced conception in Saanen goats (du Preez *et al.* 2001) and was shown to be involved in the seasonal reproductive activity of the flying fox, *Pteropus poliocephalus* (McGuckin and Blackshaw 1992). However, melatonin is not the sole determinant of seasonal mating, as demonstrated in the carnivorous marsupial *Antechinus stuartii* (McAllan *et al.* 2008).

When the cervical superior ganglia of mink were ablated bilaterally, denervating the pineal gland, the animals ceased to respond to changes in an artificial light-dark cycle. Long light periods no longer increased the secretion of progesterone and prolactin or stimulated the molting that is characteristic of wild mink during spring, and long dark periods did not promote the autumn-like molting or the increase in body mass that is normal at the end of summer (Martinet and Allain 1985). Melatonin treatment restored these responses to light-dark cycle changes. The pineal gland therefore seems to be necessary for transducing perception of light-dark changes into physiological responses via the secretion of melatonin, though it does not modulate these responses once they are initiated. In many female mammals, disruption of the normal light-dark cycle – e.g. by shift work or jet lag in humans – has adverse effects on many aspects of physiology including reproductive functions. Successful mating and conception seem to be dependent on entrainment to the light-dark cycle (Endo and Watanabe 1989).

Changes in the Timing of Mating during Mammalian Evolution

The neuroendocrine and behavioral mechanisms involved in mating must have undergone changes when day-activity first evolved in mammals; it is generally agreed that ancestral mammals were largely or wholly nocturnal. Until the last decade, only nocturnal animals were used in research on circadian rhythms, so this evolutionary issue had not been addressed. Recently, however, more diurnal mammals such as squirrels and grass rats have been studied, so some insights have been gained into the evolution of circadian patterns of mating (Smale *et al.* 2003).

Species differ in the way in which the reproductive process is organized in time. Successful mating depends on synchronization between the female's reproductive physiology and behavior and the provision of sperm by the male. This synchronization depends primarily on endogenous circadian rhythms, which in mammals are entrained by stimulation of the SCN by signals originating from the retina (Moore-Ede *et al.* 1983; Klein *et al.* 1991). In some species, the circadian rhythm only indirectly influences the timing of estrus-related behavior during the day, but in others the SCN directly affects the neuroendocrine and behavioral concomitants of successful mating (Schwartz 2000). In these latter species, direct projections from the SCN to hypothalamic cells containing estrogen receptors may be involved in the precise timing of mating behavior and its neuroendocrine correlates (De la Iglesia *et al.* 1995; Watson *et al.* 1995). Some of these projections contain vasoactive intestinal polypeptide (VIP) and vasopressin (VP) and connect with hypothalamic neurons containing gonadotrophin releasing hormone (GnRH) (Palm *et al.* 1999; van der Beek *et al.* 1999); the appositions appear to be functional synapses (Lee 2004).

Many nocturnal mammals mate more or less exclusively during twilight, after sunset. In nocturnal rats, this timing correlates with female steroid hormone levels (Sodersten *et al.* 1981), and it persists in animals kept in constant darkness; however, it is destroyed if the SCN are ablated (Alleva *et al.* 1971; Sodersten *et al.* 1981). About four hours before the onset of darkness on the day of proestrus, when ovarian hormone levels are high, there is a lutenizing hormone (LH) surge (Schwartz 2000) gated by the circadian clock. However, in a diurnal murid rodent, the unstriped Nile grass rat (*Arvicanthis niloticus*) of sub-Saharan Africa, this LH surge is 12 hours out of phase with the nocturnal species: it occurs approximately four hours before the onset of light, and mating takes place predominantly at dawn

(McElhinny *et al.* 1997, 1999). This is a striking example of the evolutionary shift in diurnal patterns of mating among mammals that cease to be nocturnal.

The divergence is general among mammals: the LH surge predominantly occurs just before the onset of light in diurnal species and just before the onset of darkness in nocturnal species (Sodersten 1989; McElhinney *et al.* 1999).

The Circadian Clock Is Linked to Seasonal Changes in Reproductive and Other Aspects of Physiology and Behavior in Mammals

Dardente *et al.* (2010) have found evidence for a molecular connection between seasonal changes in melatonin output by the pineal and the circadian clock in homeothermic vertebrates. Expression of the gene encoding the β subunit of thyrotrophin (TSHβ) in the pituitary is controlled through a D element in the promoter for this gene, which is controlled by thyrotroph embryonic factor. Melatonin adjusts the expression of eyes absent 3 in the pituitary, which serves as a coactivator with thyrotroph embryonic factor, so that expression is maximal 12 hours after the onset of darkness. Therefore, during long periods of light, there is high expression of eyes absent 3 early in the morning, and therefore increased expression of TSHβ. Although the D element in the TSHβ promoter is highly conserved, there are species differences in its responsiveness to eyes absent 3, so species differ in the ways they respond to photoperiod changes. Thus, there is evidence for a molecular-level connection between the circadian secretion of melatonin by the pineal gland and the seasonal pattern of reproductive behavior in some mammals.

Conclusion

The molecular basis of the clock mechanism in the SCN is now well understood. The SCN is connected to the pineal by a multisynaptic pathway, and it is also crucial for the cyclic nature of reproductive activity and function, notably in controlling the timing of the LH surge. However, melatonin has been shown to affect clock gene function in many cell types, including neurons and pituitary cells, that have the requisite receptors; and its pattern of secretion from the pineal gland is known to reset the clock mechanism in response to exogenous signals (zeitgeber), notably light-dark regimes. On this basis, we propose that the pineal gland played a pivotal evolutionary role during the change from nocturnal to diurnal lifestyles in some mammalian species, by resetting the clock mechanism that regulates the timing of the LH surge and *ipso facto* of mating and fertilization.

References

Abecia, J. A. *et al.* (2006) The effect of melatonin treatment on the ovarian response of ewes to the ram effect. *Domestic Animal Endocrinology*, 31, pp. 52-62.

Alleva, J. J. *et al.* (1971) A biological clock controlling the estrous cycle of the hamster. *Endocrinology*, 88, pp. 1368-1379.

Araki, M. *et al.* (1988) Phenotypic expression of photoreceptor and endocrine cell properties by cultured pineal cells of the newborn rat. *Cell Differentiation and Development*, 25, pp. 155-163.

Ardura, J. *et al.* (2003) Emergence and evolution of the circadian rhythm of melatonin in children. *Hormone Research*, 59, pp. 66-72.

Bang, J. *et al.* (2012) Melatonin attenuates clock gene Cryptochrome1, which may aggravate mouse anti-type II collagen antibody-induced arthritis. *Rheumatology International*, 32, pp. 379-385.

Bellavía, S. L. *et al.* (1993) Effect of sympathetic denervation of the pineal gland on maternal co-ordination of the circadian rhythm of alpha-amylase in parotid gland from young rats. *Archives of Oral Biology*, 38, pp. 1121-1125.

Boden, M. J. and Kennaway, D. J. (2006) Circadian rhythms and reproduction. *Reproduction*, 132, pp. 379-392.

Brotto, L. A. and Gorzalka, B. B. (2000) Melatonin enhances sexual behavior in the male rat. *Physiology and Behavior*, 68, pp. 483-486.

Cahill, G. M. *et al.* (1991) Rhythmic regulation of retinal melatonin: metabolic pathways, neurochemical mechanisms, and the ocular circadian clock. *Cellular and Molecular Neurobiology*, 11, pp. 529-560.

Cermakian, N. and Boivin, D. B. (2009) The regulation of central and peripheral circadian clocks in humans. *Obesity Reviews*, 10[Suppl 2], pp. 25-36.

Chappell, P. E. *et al.* (2003) Circadian gene expression regulates pulsatile gonadotropin-releasing hormone (GnRH) secretory patterns in the hypothalamic GnRH-secreting GT1-7 cell line. *Journal of Neuroscience*, 23, pp. 11202-11213.

Confente, F. *et al.* (2010) Melatonin receptors in a pleuronectiform species, *Solea senegalensis*: Cloning, tissue expression, day-night and seasonal variations. *General and Comparative Endocrinology*, 167, pp. 202-214.

Dardente, H. *et al.* (2010) A molecular switch for photoperiod responsiveness in mammals. *Current Biology: CB*, 20, pp. 2193-2198.

de la Iglesia, H. *et al.* (1995) The suprachiasmatic area in the female hamster projects to neurons containing estrogen receptors and GnRH. *Neuroreport*, 6, pp. 1715-1722.

Dodt, E. (1963) Photosensitivity of the pineal organ in the teleost, *Salmo irideus* (Gibbons). *Experientia*, 19, pp. 642-643.

Du Preez, E. R. *et al.* (2001) Out-of-season breeding of milk goats - the effect of light treatment, melatonin and breed. *Journal of the South African Veterinary Association*, 72, pp. 228-231.

Drago, F. and Busá, L. (2000) Acute low doses of melatonin restore full sexual activity in impotent male rats. *Brain Research*, 878, pp. 98-104.

Eakin, R. M. (1973) *The Third Eye*. Berkeley: University of California Press.

Endo, A. and Watanabe, T. (1989) Effects of non-24-hour days on reproductive efficacy and embryonic development in mice. *Gamete Research,* 22, pp. 435-441.

Escames, G. and Acuña-Castroviejo, D. (2009) Melatonin, synthetic analogs, and the sleep/wake rhythm. *Revista de Neurologia*, 48, pp. 245-254.

Falcón, J. *et al.* (2009) Structural and functional evolution of the pineal melatonin system in vertebrates. *Annals of the New York Academy of Sciences*, 1163, pp.101-111.

Fahrenkrug, J. *et al.* (2006) Diurnal rhythmicity of the clock genes Per1 and Per2 in the rat ovary. *Endocrinology*, 147, pp. 3769-3776.

Ganguly, S. *et al.* (2005) Melatonin synthesis: 14-3-3-dependent activation and inhibition of arylalkylamine N-acetyltransferase mediated by phosphoserine-205. *Proceedings of the National Academy of Sciences of the United States of America*, 102, pp. 1222-1227.

Huang, T. S. *et al.* (2010) Diurnal expression of clock genes in pineal gland and brain and plasma levels of melatonin and cortisol in Atlantic salmon parr and smolts. *Chronobiology International*, 27, pp. 1697-1714.

Imbesi, M. *et al.* (2009) The melatonin receptor MT1 is required for the differential regulatory actions of melatonin on neuronal 'clock' gene expression in striatal neurons *in vitro*. *Journal of Pineal Research*, 46, pp. 87-94.

Jakobiec, F. A. *et al.* (1977) Retinoblastoma and intracranial malignancy. *Cancer*, 39, pp. 2048-2058.

Klein, D. C. (2006) Evolution of the vertebrate pineal gland: the AANAT hypothesis. *Chronobiology International*, 23, pp. 5-20.

Klein, D. *et al.* (1991) *Suprachiasmatic Nucleus: the Mind's Clock*. New York: Oxford University Press.

Lee, T. M. (2004) *Octodon degus:* A Diurnal, Social, and Long-lived Rodent. *ILAR Journal/National Research Council, Institute of Laboratory Animal Resources*, 45, pp. 14-24.

Mahoney, M. M. (2010) Shift work, jet lag and female reproduction. *International Journal of Endocrinology*, doi: 10.1155/2010/813764.

Martinet, L. And Allain, D. (1985) Role of the pineal gland in the photoperiodic control of reproductive and non-reproductive functions in mink (*Mustela vison*). *Ciba Foundation Symposium*, 117, pp. 170-187.

McAllan, B. M. *et al.* (2008) Sex, season and melatonin administration affects daily activity rhythms in a marsupial, the brown antechinus, Antechinus stuartii. *Physiology and Behavior*, 93, pp. 130-138.

McElhinny, T. M. *et al.* (1997) Patterns of body temperature, activity, and reproductive behaviour in a tropical murid rodent, *Arvicanthis niloticus*. *Physiology and Behavior*, 62, pp. 91-96.

McElhinny, T. L. *et al.* (1999) A morning surge in plasma luteinizing hormone coincides with elevated fos expression in gonadotropin-releasing hormone-immuno-reactive neurons in the diurnal rodent, *Arvicanthis niloticus*. *Biology of Reproductiom*, 61, pp. 1115-1122.

McGuckin, M. A. and Blackshaw, A. W. (1992) Effects of photoperiod on the reproductive physiology of male flying foxes, *Pteropus poliocephalus*. *Reproduction, Fertility and Development*, 4, pp. 43-53.

McIntyre, I. M. *et al.* (1989) Human melatonin suppression by light is intensity dependent. *Journal of Pineal Research*, 6, pp. 149-156.

Moore-Ede, M. *et al.* (1983) T*he Clocks that Time Us: Physiology of the Circadian Timing System*. Cambridge, MA: Harvard University Press.

Nakamura, T. J. *et al.* (2001) Effect of estrogen on the expression of Cry1 and Cry2 mRNAs in the suprachiasmatic nucleus of female rats. *Neuroscience Research*, 41, pp. 251-255.

Nakamura, T. J. *et al.* (2005) Estrogen differentially regulates expression of Per1 and Per2 genes between central and peripheral clocks and between reproductive and nonreproductive tissues in female rats. *Journal of Neuroscience Research,* 82, pp. 622-630.

Palm, I. *et al.* (1999) Vasopressin induces a luteinizing hormone surge in ovariectomized, estradiol-treated rats with lesions of the suprachiasmatic nucleus. *Neuroscience*, 93, pp. 659-666.

Schwartz, N. B. (2000) Neuroendocrine regulation of reproductive cyclicity. In: Conn, P. M. and Freeman, M. E. (eds) *Neuroendocrinology in Physiology and Medicine*. New Jersey: Humana Press, pp. 135-145.

Smale, L. *et al.* (2003) Mammalian diurnality: some facts and gaps. *Journal of Biological Rhythms*,18, pp. 356-366.

Sodersten, P. (1989) Hormonal and behavioural rhythms related to reproduction. In: Balthazart, J. (ed) *Advances in Comparative and Environmental Physiology,* Volume 3. New York, NY: Springer, pp. 1-29. (Molecular and Cellular Basis of Social Behaviour in Vertebrates).

Sodersten, P. *et al.* (1981) Neuroendocrine control of daily rhythms in rat reproductive behaviour. In: Sodersten, P. *et al.* (ed) *Steroid Hormonal Regulation of Brain*. New York: Pergamon, pp. 301-315.

Tan, D. X. *et al.* (2010) The changing biological roles of melatonin during evolution: from an antioxidant to signals of darkness, sexual selection and fitness. *Biological Reviews of The Cambridge Philosophical Society*, 85, pp. 607-623.

Teclemariam Mesbah, R. *et al.* (1999) Anatomical demonstration of the suprachiasmatic nucleus–pineal pathway. *The Journal of Comparative Neurology*, 406, pp. 171-182.

Unfried, C. *et al.* (2010) Melatonin receptor 1-dependent gene expression in the mouse pars tuberalis as revealed by cDNA microarray analysis and *in situ* hybridization. *Journal of Pineal Research*, 48, pp. 148-156.

van der Beek, E. M. *et al.* (1999) Central administration of antiserum to vasoactive intestinal peptide delays and reduces luteinizing hormone and prolactin surges in ovariectomized, estrogen-treated rats. *Neuroendocrinology*, 69, pp. 227-237.

Velarde, E. *et al.* (2010) Melatonin-synthesizing enzymes in pineal, retina, liver, and gut of the goldfish (*Carassius*): mRNA expression pattern and regulation of daily rhythms by lighting conditions. *Chronobiology International*, 27, pp. 1178-1201.

Walton, J. C. *et al.* (2010) Influence of photoperiod on hormones, behavior, and immune function. *Frontiers in Neuroendocrinology*, 32, pp. 303-319.

Watson, R. *et al.* (1995) Estrogen-receptive neurons in the anteroventral periventricular nucleus are synaptic targets of the suprachiasmatic nucleus and peri-suprachiasmatic region. *Brain Research*, 689, pp. 254-264.

Zeman, M. *et al.* (2009) Effect of rhythmic melatonin administration on clock gene expression in the suprachiasmatic nucleus and the heart of hypertensive TGR (mRen2) 27 rats. *Journal of Hypertension Supplement*, 27, pp. 21-26.

Zimmerman, B. L. and Tso, M. O. (1975) Morphologic evidence of photoreceptor differentiation of pinealocytes in the neonatal rat. *The Journal of Cell Biology*, 66, pp. 60-75.

In: Hypotheses in Clinical Medicine
Editors: M.M. Shoja, P.S. Agutter et al.

ISBN: 978-1-62257-276-2

Chapter 15

Cytoskeletal Proteins as Drug Development Targets for Various Diseases

***Nancy J. Woolf*[1]*, Avner Priel*[2] *and Jack A. Tuszynski*[2,3*]**
[1]Behavioral Neuroscience, Department of Psychology,
University of California, Los Angeles, California, US
[2] Department of Physics, University of Alberta, Edmonton, Alberta, Canada
[3] 3–336 Cross Cancer Institute, Department of Oncology,
University of Alberta, Edmonton, Alberta, Canada

Abstract

In this chapter, we stress the importance of the cytoskeleton for various functions of all eukaryotic cells. We outline how the impairment of key proteins of the cytoskeleton can be implicated in the development of various diseases. Consequently, these aberrant proteins should become targets for drug development. Particular attention is paid to neurological disorders and cancer. In the latter case, various drugs have been used in cancer chemotherapy, and many more are currently in development stages. A few examples are given to illustrate these concepts.

Introduction

The cytoskeleton is a major biomechanical operator enabling key functions in all eukaryotic cells (Tuszynski 2008; Woolf *et al.* 2009). Typical roles played by the cytoskeleton include organizing chromosomes during cell division, orchestrating cell motility, transporting materials to specific sites in the cell, and giving a cell its characteristic shape, structure and mechanical stability. The key molecular components of the cytoskeleton are

[*] E-mail: jackt@ualberta.ca.

actin filaments, microtubules, intermediate filaments and a host of proteins collectively referred to as motor proteins.

Microtubules (MTs) are long hollow cylindrical filaments made from heterodimers consisting of bound α-tubulin and β-tubulin monomers. Assembled microtubules have outer diameters of 25 - 26 nm and inner diameters of 15 nm and typically contain 13 protofilaments when assembled in living cells (Dustin 1984). MTs represent dynamic protein polymer assemblies and are often cross-linked in cells, especially neurons, via microtubule-associated-proteins (MAPs). Such MT-MT connections form tracks along which organelles and other structures are transported around the cell via motor proteins (mostly from the kinesin and dynein families), such as in the transport of neuronal vesicles from the cell body to the synapse in nerve cells.

The building block of MTs, tubulin protein, is a heterodimer composed of α-tubulin and β-tubulin monomers, which are highly homologous with an average molecular weight of 50-55 kilodaltons. Based on 3.5-3.7 Å resolution X-ray crystallographic images (Nogales *et al.* 1998; Lowe *et al.* 2001), the αβ-tubulin dimer has been computationally reconstructed as having a β-sheet core surrounded by α-helices. Each monomer is composed of approximately 450 amino acids, or about 7000 atoms. On average each αβ-heterodimer has dimensions of 46 x 80 x 65 Å, and is a polar molecule with its positive end near the β tubulin monomer. The monomer structures, composed of a double β-sheet core encircled by several α-helices, can be separated into three functional domains: the amino-terminal domain containing a nucleotide-binding region, the intermediate domain containing the taxol and colchicine drug binding sites, and the carboxy-terminal domain containing the suggested motor protein binding region. Both monomers can bind a molecule of GTP, but only the β-tubulin will hydrolyze it to GDP in a process that is believed to build up excess energy in the MT lattice that eventually causes MT depolymerization through so-called catastrophe events. Two different conformational states of the heterodimer are known to depend on this GTP hydrolysis such that hydrolysis causes a small angle distortion between the original centre-to-centre line joining the monomers, releasing 0.42 eV of energy per molecule in free tubulin and a few times less that amount when embedded in a MT. Henceforth, unless it is otherwise stated, 'tubulin' will be used to refer to the αβ-heterodimer.

Tubulin dimers assemble in a GTP-dependent process, whereby GTP-tubulin dimers add to the growing ends of microtubules (Walker 1991). Under certain experimental conditions individual protofilaments can form first and then co-assemble into mature MTs. Microtubules depolymerize by losing GDP-tubulin dimers after protofilaments separate and curve away from one another forming structures resembling "ram's horns". Like actin filaments, microtubules have plus- and minus-ends. Polymerization or elongation typically occurs at plus-ends and depolymerization or shortening occurs at minus-ends. Under very specific conditions of tubulin concentration, pH and temperature, the net result may be no appreciable change in MT length - a process called treadmilling, which also occurs in actin filaments (Margolis and Wilson 1981).

The major microtubule-associated proteins (MAPs) found in human brain include various isoforms of the stabilizing proteins MAP1, MAP2, and tau, which have been shown to be correlated with various disorders. Other MAPs include motor proteins. MAPs are developmentally regulated and compartmentalized in accordance with their specialized cellular roles. These binding proteins determine, to a large degree, the arrangement of MTs in a given part of the neuron and the function played by the MTs in that neuronal compartment.

Microtubule binding proteins determine the architecture of MTs and are also dysfunctional in many neurodegenerative and neurodevelopmental disorders. MTs in adult dendrites bind MAP2 preferentially, whereas MTs in axons prefer tau. The process by which this adult pattern is achieved is gradual and follows a distal-to-proximal gradient. Growing axons contain both MAP2 and tau, but the amount of MAP2 begins to diminish from the distal tip of the axon to the proximal part, finally disappearing altogether.

The functions of MTs in neurons differ markedly from those in other cells in the human body. Key to their function is how MTs link many neuronal compartments together. For example, only MTs carry synaptic vesicles manufactured in the Golgi apparatus of the cell body all the way down the axon to the actin filaments in the axon terminal or developing growth cone. Similarly, only MTs provide a direct conduit from the cell body carrying protein and mRNA granules to dendritic spines and other non-spinous postsynaptic sites along the dendritic membrane. It is quite possible that MT transport lies at the core of higher cognitive function. Transport is one of the main functions of MT tracks.

Pharmacological agents of various types (small molecule inhibitors, aptamers, antibodies, biologics, etc.) that can either stabilize or destabilize the cytoskeleton (Jordan and Wilson 2004) offer great potential for treating a wide spectrum of diseases. These include neurodegenerative diseases, neurodevelopmental disorders, neuropsychiatric illnesses, heart disease, a wide spectrum of cancers, bone disease, and sensory impairments. Specific examples in each category are listed in the sections that follow.

Cytoskeleton and Neurodegenerative Diseases

A common finding across this category of disorders is a deteriorating cytoskeleton. Bioengineered cytoskeletal protein products have enhanced capacities to stabilize, or alternatively destabilize, the existing cytoskeletal matrix, and thereby stand to prevent neuronal degeneration resulting from multiple causes. Products include modified tubulins and actins deriving from known animal and plant sequences (as well as from completely novel sequences), gene vectors for modified tubulins and actins, biohybrid tubulins and actins (e.g., nanoparticle-bound protein units), coated microtubules and actin filaments (e.g., metalized-cytoskeletal polymers), and biologically-inspired cytoskeletal-like nanomaterials (e.g., modified nanotubes that effectively interface with microtubules or actin filaments). These products range from biomolecular and biohybrid complexes that can be introduced into a targeted part of the body, to nanopharmaceuticals that can be administered orally, intraperitoneally or intraveneously, to dietary supplements. Specific neurodegenerative diseases include but are not limited to:

- *Alzheimer's disease* – Being one of the most prevalent neurodegenerative disorders today, Alzheimer's disease illustrates both the neuronal and cognitive consequences of cytoskeletal protein disruption. Cortical neurons in Alzheimer's diseased brain accumulate hyperphosphorylated tau, a MAP, which in turn triggers the formation of neurofibrillary tangles (Pei *et al.* 2008). Neurons in Alzheimer's disease brain also demonstrate impaired axonal transport and compromised microtubule matrices, even in the absence of neurofibrillary tangles (Cash *et al.* 2003). Recent evidence suggests that preventing neurofibrillary tangle accumulation is more likely to protect against dementia or cognitive impairment than is targeting amyloid-β plaques (Sigurdsson 2009). Accordingly, measures to stabilize the microtubule cytoskeleton would be expected to prevent or diminish the neural degradation associated with Alzheimer's disease.

- *Parkinson's disease* – Mutations in genes for α-synuclein and parkin proteins lead to familial Parkinson's disease, and these proteins may also contribute to sporadic cases (Gasser *et al.* 2009). Altered α-synuclein and parkin proteins result in impaired axonal transport of dopamine-containing vesicles (Mizuno *et al.* 2001). As a result, dopamine is released and subsequently degraded into toxic by-products that selectively kill dopamine-containing neurons in the nigrostriatal pathway (Feng 2006). Stabilizing the cytoskeleton, which is pivotally responsible for axonal transport, would be expected to prevent this type.
- *Huntington's chorea* – This autosomal dominant disorder is caused by mutations in huntingtin protein characterized by polyglutamine repeat expansion (Sugars and Rubinsztein 2003). Polyglutamine repeats in huntingtin protein disrupt its binding to microtubules resulting in impaired axonal transport (Gauthier *et al.* 2004). Stabilized microtubules would be expected to remedy this condition.
- *Stroke and brain injury* – The neuronal cytoskeleton is disrupted here following ischemia due to blood hemorrhage, occlusion, or injury (Lingwood *et al.* 2008). Stabilizing the cytoskeletal fibers would be expected to counter these effects.
- *Epilepsy* – Microtubule-associated protein, MAP2, shows decreased phosphorylation in parts of the brain where epileptic seizure activity is prevalent (Sanchez *et al.* 2001). This is indicative of impaired cytoskeletal dynamics. Stabilizing the cytoskeleton would be expected to aid in the recovery of damaged brain regions.
- *Amyotropic lateral sclerosis* – Axonal transport is compromised in this movement disorder as a result of cytoskeletal disruption (Vickers *et al.* 2009). Stabilizing the cytoskeletal fibers would be expected to ameliorate such conditions.
- *Charcot-Marie-Tooth disease* – An underlying cause of the impaired axonal transport found in this disease may be stalled microtubules that assume a hyperstabilized state due to mutated dynamin2 protein (Tanabe and Takei 2009).
- *Multiple sclerosis* – This demyelinating disease appears to involve fundamental disruption to the underlying axon and its cytoskeleton (Vickers *et al.* 2009). Stabilizing the cytoskeletal fibers would be beneficial.

Cytoskeleton and Neurodevelopmental Disorders

These disorders, which are frequently associated with mental retardation, show disrupted actin dynamics and abnormal microtubule-associated protein processing. These cytoskeletal abnormalities interfere with proper neuronal growth and development, and contribute to cognitive disturbances. Enhanced dynamism engineered into actin and tubulin subunit proteins would be expected to ameliorate many of the structural and cognitive deficits, especially if introduced during early development. As enumerated above, examples include modified tubulins and actins, gene vectors for modified tubulins and actins, biohybrid designs for tubulin and actin, coated microtubules and actin filaments, and biologically-inspired cytoskeletal-like nanomaterials. Specific neurodevelopmental disorders include but are not limited to:

- *Fragile X syndrome* – Deletion of the fragile X mental retardation protein results in misregulation of MAP1B and impaired transport due to overly stabilized microtubules (Lu *et al.* 2004). Deletion of fragile X mental retardation protein also results in less dynamic actin filaments due to down-regulation of actin depolymerizing factor/cofilin (Castets *et al.* 2005).
- *Turner syndrome* – The failure of dendrite pruning in this disorder indicates a flaw in cytoskeletal protein dynamics (Cutter *et al.* 2006).
- *Williams' syndrome* – This disorder is associated with genetic deletion of two proteins that regulate the dynamics of the cytoskeleton, LIMK1 and CLIP115 (Hoogenraad *et al.* 2004).
- *Autism spectrum* – Some of these diverse patient populations show single nucleotide polymorphisms linking the disorder to the cytoskeleton (Maussion *et al.* 2008).
- *Rett syndrome* – The genetic deletion present in this syndrome causes downstream effects on MAP2 (Armstrong 2005).
- *Down syndrome* – Chromosomal non-disjunction, the cause of Down syndrome, may be due to maternal microtubule dysfunction (Dotan and Avivi 1986). Down's syndrome patients are also vulnerable to early cytoskeletal deterioration as occurs in Alzheimer's disease at a later age (Pollack *et al.* 2003).

Cytoskeleton and Neuropsychiatric Illnesses

Drugs that interact with neurotransmitters are effective in treating mental illnesses such as schizophrenia, bipolar disorder, depression, and anxiety; however, this need not implicate brain imbalances of neurotransmitters. A new perspective is that neuropharmaceutical agents impact on neuroplasticity. This fits with the routine observation that antipsychotics, antidepressants, and mood stabilizers usually take weeks to exert therapeutic effects – about the same time course that information is consolidated into long-term memory according to a process orchestrated by dynamic interactions between actin filaments and microtubules (Woolf *et al.* 2009). Accordingly, altering the dynamics assumed by actin and tubulin subunit proteins would be expected to ameliorate many of the structural and cognitive deficits associated with neuropsychiatric illnesses. As enumerated above, examples of such products include modified tubulins and actins, gene vectors for modified tubulins and actins, biohybrid designs for tubulin and actin, coated microtubules and actin filaments, and biologically-inspired cytoskeletal-like nanomaterials. The advantage of modifying the cytoskeleton is that many of the current neuropharmaceutical agents have unacceptable side effects in the long term (e.g., tardive dyskinesia). Recurrent or chronic courses of illness are also not adequately addressed by neuropharmaceutical interventions alone.

Specific neuropsychiatric illnesses include (but are not limited to):

- *Schizophrenia* – Recent evidence suggests that schizophrenia may be reduced in severity or even prevented by early invention that reverses the development of abnormal neuronal structure (Piontkiewitz *et al.* 2009). Neuronal structure is essentially determined by dynamic interactions between actin filaments and microtubules, both of which appear to be compromised in schizophrenia. The disrupted-in-schizophrenia 1 (DISC1) gene, for example, shows variation in certain cases of schizophrenia and other mental illnesses, and the protein regulates the expression of cytoskeleton proteins (Hennah and Porteous 2009). Genetic variations in dysbindin and neuregulin-1 are also implicated in schizophrenia, and like DISC1, lead to impaired axonal transport and impaired neurogenesis (Alaerts *et al.* 2009; Jaaro-Peled *et al.* 2009).
- *Bipolar disorder* – This affective disorder is associated with genetic variation for DISC1, dysbindin, and neuregulin-1, leading to impaired axonal transport and impaired neurogenesis, similar to the case for schizophrenia (Goes *et al.* 2008).
- *Depression and anxiety* – Neuroplasticity-based theories particularly stand to modify older neurotransmitter-based theories when it comes to future treatments of depression (Costa e Silva 2004). Neuroplasticity can be measured as altered receptor efficacy or as reorganized neuronal structure, both of which are mediated by microtubules and actin filaments. Antidepressant drugs, most of which increase serotonin and/or norepinephrine at the synapse, are the third most commonly prescribed type of drug in the U.S., with prescriptions rising (McDevitt 2009). While these drug actions are interpreted as having a strictly synaptic basis, effects on neuroplasticity are prevalent. For example, activation of the serotonin receptor (5-HT1A) inhibits N-methyl-D-aspartate (NMDA) receptor activity, whereupon signal transduction cascades result in the depolymerization of microtubules (Yuen *et al.* 2005). The breakdown of the microtubule matrix subsequently results in fewer NMDA receptors being transported to the neuronal membrane. Future antidepressants need not act at the synapse to be effective. A more direct approach is to affect the dynamic state of microtubules and actin filaments.
- *Alcohol and substance abuse* – Since alcohol and substance abuse are common co-morbidities found in patients diagnosed with affective disorders, any effective treatments for affective disorder could be appropriate for select populations having substance abuse issues.

Cytoskeleton and Heart Disease

Muscle contraction in heart tissue is mediated by dynamic interactions between actin filaments and microtubules, with intermediate filaments playing an auxiliary role (Hein et al. 2000). Heart disease results when muscle tissue is compromised by ischemia, hypertrophy, or congenital defects. Modifying dynamic interactions between actin and tubulin subunit proteins would be expected to address many of the physiological and structural defects arising with heart disease. As mentioned above, such products include modified tubulins and actins, gene vectors for modified tubulins and actins, biohybrid designs for tubulin and actin, coated microtubules and actin filaments, and biologically inspired cytoskeletal-like nanomaterials. Specific heart diseases include but are not limited to:

- *Congestive heart failure* – A key underlying factor in cardiac hypertrophy and consequent heart failure is an increased density of the microtubule matrix in cardiac myocytes (Tsutsui *et al.* 1993). In addition to structural remodeling of the heart, the electrical and mechanical properties of cardiac myocytes directly depend on cytoskeleton protein dynamics (Calaghan *et al.* 2004). Cardiac hypertrophy need not necessarily be maladaptive (Cooper 2006). Hence altering the dynamics among cytoskeletal proteins has the potential to alter remodeling to the benefit of cardiac function.
- *Cardiac arrest* – Heart attacks are triggered by ischemia caused by atherosclerosis, among other factors (O'Keefe *et al.* 2006; Kloner 2006). Stabilizing microtubules in cardiac myocytes with tubulin-binding taxanes increases resistance to ischemia (Devillard *et al.* 2008). Thus, stabilizing microtubules with enhanced tubulin products would similarly be expected to increase resistance to ischemic injury, without the toxic side effects of taxanes. This approach would be of benefit in reducing risk of future heart attack.
- *Heart transplant and heart valve replacement* – A concern in heart transplantation and bioprosthetic valve replacement is damage to heart tissue during cold storage or perfusion. Microtubules, in particular, are sensitive to the cold. Tubulin-binding taxanes protect cardiac myocytes from cold-induced cytoskeletal damage (Devillard *et al.* 2008). Stabilizing microtubules with enhanced tubulin products would similarly be expected to reduce cold-induced damage.
- *Congenital heart disease* – Structural abnormalities present at birth give rise to an increased incidence of cardiac arrest, some of which could be addresses with enhanced cytoskeletal protein products.

Cytoskeleton and Cancer

The dynamic properties of MTs are especially critical during mitosis, when a delicate equilibrium of distances and forces is necessary for proper chromosome alignment prior to segregation (Margolis and Wilson 1981; Melki *et al.* 1989; Walker *et al.* 1991; Zheng *et al.* 1995). During mitosis, microtubule dynamics is essential for constructing the mitotic spindle, which is responsible for the segregation of aligned chromosomes prior to cell division. MTs constitute much of the mitotic spindle apparatus and its proper assembly is essential, as it likely provides the substantial mechanical force for mitotic chromosome segregation. Assembly failure of the mitotic spindle generally results in mitotic arrest, apoptosis, and eventually cell death. As such, MTs have become the target for a large number of anti-mitotic agents including antitumor drugs such as the taxanes, epothilones, colchicine and *vinca* alkaloids, including vinblastine and vincristine (Jordan. The method of action of these drugs is to promote or inhibit microtubule polymerization by binding at specific sites on the interface of α/β tubulin heterodimers. For example, the vinca alkaloid vinblastine binds at the inter-tubulin dimer interface, ultimately resulting in microtubule de-polymerization. On the other hand, binding of the taxanes results in an overall increase in the spindle microtubule mass with a concurrent reduction in microtubule dynamics. The resulting cellular phenotype of these drugs is the induction of mitotic arrest leading to apoptosis, making them effective chemotherapeutic agents for targeting rapidly dividing cells. Nevertheless, even the most successful chemotherapy drugs have undesirable side effects that limit their utility. Their drawback is that when these drugs are given systemically, they bind tubulin indiscriminately, leading to the destruction of both cancerous and healthy cells.

Paclitaxel, which continues to be one of the most successful cancer therapeutic agents, has a unique mechanism of action as it binds to and results in the stabilization of MTs within all cells (Schiff and Horwitz 1980). Derivatives of paclitaxel, such as docetaxel, have been synthesized to address the limited solubility of paclitaxel and show increased binding to β-tubulin. Two additional families of similar tubulin-binding drugs are the epothilones and dolastatins, which share a similar mode of binding. Interest in the epothilones over existing MT stabilizing agents such as paclitaxel is primarily due to their ability to retain cytotoxicity in multidrug resistant (MDR) cells (Bollag *et al.* 1995). Compounds such as discodermolide and sarcodictyin have been shown to inhibit the proliferation of human cells through a mechanism similar to that of the taxanes. These compounds seem to selectively stabilize MTs during cell division, and outcompete paclitaxel for tubulin binding (Klein *et al.* 2005). In the absence of paclitaxel, it has been predicted that the energy stored in longitudinal contacts is greater than that stored in lateral contacts (VanBuren *et al.* 2002). Recent results using hydrogen/deuterium exchange coupled with mass liquid chromatography have demonstrated that increased rigidity in paclitaxel-stabilized MTs was distinct from stabilization as a result of GTP-induced polymerization (Xiao *et al.* 2006). The authors suggest that paclitaxel increases the overall energy associated with polymerization while maintaining the same differential between lateral and longitudinal contacts in the microtubule lattice. Through structural studies, both the taxanes and epothilones were shown to bind to a unique site within the β subunit of the α/β-tubulin heterodimer (Lowe *et al.* 2001; Nettles *et al.* 2004). Unfortunately, neither of the structures has been able to reveal the precise mechanism of MT stabilization by these drugs.

The *vinca* alkaloids include vincristine, vinblastine and vinorelbine and are used most commonly in combination chemotherapy regimes. Vinblastine was shown to bind at the inter-tubulin dimer interface, ultimately resulting in the net reduction of polymerized tubulin concentration (Gigant *et al.* 2005). At high concentrations, vinblastine binds to MTs and results in their depolymerization. However, at low concentrations, it is thought to bind to MT tips and suppresses their dynamic instability, leading to stabilization (Toso *et al.* 1993). We suggest that this may be a result of vinblastine's ability to maintain the tubulin dimer at the end of the growing MT in a slightly bent conformation (Wang and Nogales 2005). If the tip of a protofilament were maintained with a slightly bent conformation, due to the positioning of vinblastine between the dimers, then at low enough concentrations, a small amount of drug bound to the end of the MT would mimic the presence of a GTP cap, thereby resulting in MT stabilization.

The third observed drug site within β-tubulin was shown to bind colchicine, a water-soluble alkaloid that, like paclitaxel, binds to α/β tubulin dimers and blocks cell division by inhibiting mitosis (Ravelli *et al.* 2004). Unlike paclitaxel or vinblastine at low concentration, the binding of colchicine does not result in MT stabilization, but instead results in MT destabilization since colchicine binds only to free tubulin and not to tubulin polymerized into MTs.

Following exposure to all of the drugs discussed above, cells experience mitotic arrest, which eventually leads to apoptosis. This makes these drugs extremely effective chemotherapeutic agents for targeting all rapidly-dividing cancerous cells. Nevertheless, even the most successful chemotherapy drugs have undesirable side effects that limit their utility. The anti-tubulin chemotherapeutic agents' main flaw is that they bind tubulin indiscriminately, leading to the widespread destruction of both cancerous and healthy cells, resulting in unwanted side-effects such as neuropathy (Rowinsky *et al.* 1989). The ultimate goal of chemotherapy research is to develop a drug or treatment regimen that will target only cancer cells and will target them selectively. In the case of paclitaxel, this would require determining the differences between tubulin as observed in cancerous cells and non-cancerous cells. Fortunately there are slight differences within several β-tubulin isotypes expressed in a range of cell types that may afford a foundation for the development of anti-tubulin drug derivatives with increased specificity for particular cancer cells. Unfortunately, as the precise binding modes of these compounds within β-tubulin cannot yet fully explain how these drugs affect MT stabilization, our ability to create a precise molecular model of their effects is limited.

The two most problematic features found in many types of cancer are prolific growth and invasion of surrounding tissue, both of which are mediated by the cytoskeleton (Hall 2009; Yilmaz *et al.* 2009). Accordingly, microtubule-stabilizing drugs such as taxanes, epothilones and discodermolides are in current use or are being investigated in clinical trials (Zhao *et al.* 2009). As an alternative - products such as modified tubulins and actins, gene vectors for modified tubulins and actins, biohybrid designs for tubulin and actin, coated microtubules and actin filaments, and biologically inspired cytoskeletal-like nanomaterials - offer the advantage of modifying the cytoskeleton without having the unacceptable side effects of the current chemotherapeutic agents. Specific types of cancer (among others) implicate involvement of the cytoskeleton as follows:

- *Breast cancer* – Epothilones, tubulin stabilizers distinct from taxanes, show promise in treating breast cancer (Buzdar 2008). Also, a significant percentage of breast cancers are estrogen-dependent, and estrogen increases the expression particularly of the βIII-tubulin subunit (Saussede-Aim *et al.* 2009). The cytoskeletal products outlined here enable specific cytoskeletal protein subunits to be targeted.
- *Lung cancer* – As is the case for breast cancer, βIII-tubulin subunit over-expression accounts for acquired resistance to taxane chemotherapy for non-small cell lung cancer (Dumontet *et al.* 2009). A viable alternative approach is to specifically target cytoskeletal protein subunits using products described here.
- *Prostate cancer* – Resistance to taxane chemotherapy develops during the treatment of prostrate cancer (Mathew and Dipaola 2007). Increased tau expression is also correlated with chemotherapeutic drug resistance during prostate cancer treatment (Souter and Lee 2009). Target-specific products can circumvent these problems.
- *Brain cancer* – Glioblastoma multiforme, the most deadly form of brain cancer in adults, presents with abnormal patterns of γ-tubulin and βIII-tubulin expression (Katsetos *et al.* 2009a; Katesetos *et al.* 2009b). Such subunits can be specifically targeted with the products outlined here.

Other Diseases

- *Bone disease* – Bone growth and healing depend on cellular mechanotransduction, which is mediated by actin filaments and microtubules (Myers *et al.* 2007). Thus, enhanced cytoskeletal proteins are likely to be effective as primary or adjunctive treatments of bone injury, fractures, and osteoporosis.
- *Sensory impairments and human capabilities enhancement* – The actin cytoskeleton in particular is implicated in congenital and acquired forms of deafness and blindness (Li *et al.* 2004; Kremer *et al.* 2006; Mogensen *et al.* 2007; Lee *et al.* 2008). Actin cytoskeletal subunit products described here have the potential to correct certain visual and hearing defects at the cellular level. These products have additional potential applications in sensory processing enhancement - for example, reversing age-related hearing loss.

This is not an exhaustive list of diseases, disorders, illnesses, or conditions that could be aided by the cytoskeletal products described in this chapter.

Restoring Transport with Tubulin Gene Therapy

There are rational designs of cytoskeletal protein subunit sequences that insert into the cytoskeleton of adult neurons to repair and restore normal cell functions, particularly transport and structural stability. These products, when administered alone or in conjunction with neurotrophic factors, serve to repair or prevent neuronal dysfunction secondary to interrupted transport or dysfunctional neuroplasticity (i.e., lack of growth, overgrowth, failed maintenance, loss of function) (Woolf 2009; Woolf *et al.* 2009). Alzheimer's disease and Parkinson's disease (among other developmental and degenerative disorders) are excellent candidate illnesses for these products. One available mode for introducing such a product is through gene therapy, although advances in nanotechnology will undoubtedly soon give rise to drug delivery methods as means of introducing these bioengineered subunits without the necessity of invasive surgery. There is a clear need for these types of products and our market analysis indicates several large patient populations exist in addition to Alzheimer's disease and Parkinson's disease.

In one application, genes for bioengineered tubulins are administered along with genes expressing neurotrophins. Current clinical evidence indicates that gene therapy (e.g., introducing AAV2-neurturin) to Parkinson's patients is successful, but does not result in the neurotrophin traveling from the target site (striatum) to parent cell bodies (nigral area); this means injections of the gene vector are necessary at both the target site and the cell body of origin region (Bartus *et al.* 2011). Various custom-bioengineered tubulin subunit sequences could restore transport of neurotrophins from target (striatum) to the parent cells bodies, and could be easily added to the mix of neurotrophin genes in such a therapeutic approach. In this manner, a dual injection could be avoided. Perhaps even more importantly, restoring transport along the nigrostriatal pathway would presumably permit normal functional connectivity in that pathway.

Gene therapies delivering nerve growth factor (NGF) into the nucleus basalis of Meynert have been successful in experimental animals and show promise in Alzheimer's disease patients (Bishop *et al.* 2008; Mandel 2010). Nonetheless transport is a problem, which could be corrected by custom-bioengineered tubulins that would facilitate the transport of nerve growth factor from cortical targets back to cell bodies in the basal forebrain. Restored transport would enable surgeons to avoid the need to inject the genes into the nucleus basalis of Meynert, which is a highly vascularized brain area posing surgical risk. Restored transport along the basolocortical pathways would furthermore restore functional connectivity between the two brain regions.

Tubulin-targeting Drugs in Development

Paclitaxel and its mimetics represent a standard of care in the treatment of solid tumors of the breast, ovary and lung (de Bree *et al.* 2006; Paz-Ares *et al.* 2008). These drugs bind to microtubules in a manner that distorts the dynamic assembly properties of this protein polymer, leading to mitotic arrest and variable cell fates including apoptosis. The pivotal role of microtubules in cell division has rendered the assembly unit - the α/β-tubulin dimer - an enduring target for the development of chemotherapeutic drugs. Clinical inadequacies of the taxoids, including severe and persistent peripheral neuropathies, drug resistance and vehicle-related toxicities, continue to drive new ligand development (Argyriou 2005). Unfortunately, the diffuse nature of the taxoid binding site has presented roadblocks to pharmacophore modeling and rational ligand design (Nettles *et al.* 2004), prompting a search for alternative therapeutic entry points.

Table 1. Some compounds targeting tubulin, based on the BioCentury database. These compounds are in different stages of clinical development and those in NDA stage or beyond are in bold

Cabazitaxel	Noscapine
Combretastatin A1	Obrabulin
CYT997	Ortataxel
Dehydelone	Paclitaxel
Dolastatin 10	Plinabulin
E7974 (hemiasterlin)	Poliglumex
Epothilone B	Sogopilone
Epothilone D	Taxoprexin
Eribulin	Tesetaxel
GRN-1005	Verubulin
Ixabepilone	Zybrestat

Although tubulin is a well-known and established target for anti-neoplastic therapies, the number of approved drugs targeting tubulin molecules is relatively low when compared to the number of compounds in clinical development. Table 1 lists compounds targeting tubulin in different stages of clinical development for investigational or clinical use based on information published in the BioCentury database (http://www.biocentury.com/Home).

Below, we briefly discuss a few examples of tubulin-targeting drugs in the taxane family that are in development. Paclitaxel (Taxol) is a chemotherapeutic agent formulated as an injection that is administered as an I.V. infusion over a period of 1-24 hours. The formulation is done with a conjugation to Cremophor in order to increase the solubility of (water-insoluble) taxol within the body. Certain toxicities arise from the use of the drug including hypersensitivity reactions such as face/skin rash or shortness of breath. Some damage to the bone marrow occurs during treatment, leaving the body susceptible to infections, anemia and bruising. Other side effects occur in the limbs causing pain or numbness. Other toxicities include nausea, vomiting, diarrhea, burning or tingling sensations and hair loss. Paclitaxel has a long residence time within the body and can stay trapped in cancer cells for over a week. It is also highly bound to CrEL micelles, plasma proteins, platelets, and red blood cells.

Many taxane compounds exist that closely resemble taxol which has been derivatized to form the precise compounds to be used therapeutically to fight cancer. The most common derivatives seem to be the ones that work with the C7 and C10 carbons of the parental ring structure. Different methods are being tried such as inserting alkyl chains, ring structures or even halides to change the efficacy, binding, or polarity of the structure to make it more effective or tolerable in humans. Tesetaxel is an oral synthetic taxane derivative developed by Daichii Sankyo. The development of Tesetaxel was placed on clinical hold by the FDA after severe neutropenia led to fatal outcomes in several patients with advanced cancer. Tesetaxel is being developed by Genta Inc. for five oncological uses (gastric cancer, melanoma, prostate, breast and bladder cancers, all in advanced stage). There are four currently open clinical trials in Phase II with the prostate cancer trial in the planning stage and one Phase I trial on Tesetaxel pharmacokinetics. Ortataxel is a synthetic taxane developed by Indena (Italy) and the initial clinical development was funded by Bayer. It is a third-generation taxane that has shown oral bioavailability. At this point, Ortataxel has completed Phase II studies in several taxane-refractory solid tumors. Two Phase II trials are still active (lymphoma and kidney cancer). Sanofi-Aventis in 2010 discontinued development of larotaxel. The compound was in Phase III testing for advanced pancreatic and bladder cancers. Negative outcomes were reported in the breast and pancreatic studies; together with the fact that the dose of larotaxel in combination with cisplatin had to be reduced owing to safety concerns.

The data from the international Phase III trial with cabazitaxel (marketed as Jevtana by Sanofi-Aventis) led to fast-track approval by the FDA in 2010 to treat second-line metastatic hormone-refractory prostate cancer in combination with prednisone. Cabazitaxel combined with prednisone extends survival by more than two months for men with advanced multidrug-resistant prostate cancer. Cabazitaxel is claimed to be the first drug to show a survival benefit in patients whose disease has progressed after standard chemotherapy with docetaxel and for whom there are currently no approved treatment options.

Conclusion

A fundamental question in the field of molecular biophysics is the increasingly complex and multifunctional behavior of the cellular cytoskeleton. The cytoskeleton is a complex network of filamentous protein polymers that organize the interior of eukaryotic cells. Their impairments give rise to a host of diseases, chief among which are neurological disorders and various types of cancer. Consequently, the building blocks of the cytoskeleton - actin, tubulin and proteins interacting with them - are excellent targets for drug discovery and development.

Nanomechanical cytoskeletal structures within neurons are fundamentally impaired in multiple nervous system disorders and nanotechnology is instrumental to the development of novel drug and gene therapies as well as prosthetic nanodevices. A striking number of neurodevelopmental, neurological, and neuropsychiatric disorders exhibit disruption of the nanomechanical properties of the cytoskeleton, affecting subunit proteins, binding proteins, related signal transduction molecules, or indirectly impairing transport mechanisms. A number of neurodevelopmental disorders are associated with abnormalities to dendrites and spines, indicating underlying cytoskeletal involvement. Motor neuron diseases and degenerative neurological disorders often present with profound disruption of the neuronal cytoskeleton, as well as compromised axonal transport. There is also evidence of cytoskeletal abnormalities in neuropsychiatric disorders. The genetic basis for many neurodevelopmental, neurological, and neuropsychiatric disorders remains largely undetermined; however, in those sporadic cases that have a gene locus specified, a deficit in cytoskeleton-related proteins or impaired transport is often noted.

Tubulin is the target for numerous small molecule ligands, which result in the alteration of microtubule dynamics and ultimately lead to cell cycle arrest and cell death. Many of these ligands are currently used clinically for the treatment of several types of cancer and include, but are not limited to, the drugs paclitaxel, colchicine and vinblastine. These drugs bind to one of three distinct binding sites within β tubulin, all of which have conveniently been identified through crystallographic determination. The drawback of all of these drugs is that when they are given systemically, they bind to tubulin indiscriminately, leading to the death of both cancerous and healthy cells. However, the existence and distribution of divergent tubulin isoforms provides a platform upon which to build novel chemotherapeutic drugs that can differentiate between different cell types, and therefore reduce undesirable side effects.

Acknowledgments

This research was funded by the Alberta Cancer Foundation, the Allard Foundation, NSERC, the Canadian Breast Cancer Foundation and Alberta Advanced Education and Technology.

References

Alaerts, M. *et al.* (2009) Support for NRG1 as a susceptibility factor for schizophrenia in a northern Swedish isolated population. *Archives of General Psychiatry*, 66, pp. 828-837.

Argyriou, A. A. (2005) Peripheral neuropathy induced by administration of cisplatin- and paclitaxel-based chemotherapy. Could it be predicted?. *Supportive Care in Cancer*, 13, pp. 647-651.

Armstrong, D. D. (2005) Can we relate MeCP2 deficiency to the structural and chemical abnormalities in the Rett brain?. *Brain and Development*, 27[Suppl 1], pp. 72-76.

Bartus, R. T. *et al.* (2011) Bioactivity of AAV2-neurturin gene therapy (CERE-120): differences between Parkinson's disease and nonhuman primate brains. *Movement Disorders*, 26, pp. 27-36.

Bishop, K. M. *et al.* (2008) Therapeutic potential of CERE-110 (AAV2-NGF): targeted, stable, and sustained NGF delivery and trophic activity on rodent basal forebrain cholinergic neurons. *Experimental Neurology*, 211, pp. 574-584.

Bollag, D. M. *et al.* (1995) Epothilones, a new class of microtubule-stabilizing agents with a taxol-like mechanism of action. *Cancer Research*, 55, pp. 2325-2333.

Buzdar, A. U. (2008) Clinical experience with epothilones in patients with breast cancer. *Clinical Breast Cancer*, 8[Suppl 2], pp. 71-78.

Calaghan, S. C. *et al.* (2004) Cytoskeletal modulation of electrical and mechanical activity in cardiac myocytes. *Progress in Biophysics and Molecular Biology*, 84, pp. 29-59.

Cash, A. D. *et al.* (2003) Microtubule reduction in Alzheimer's disease and aging is independent of tau filament formation. *American Journal of Pathology*, 162, pp. 1623-1627.

Castets, M. *et al* (2005) FMRP interferes with the Rac1 pathway and controls actin cytoskeleton dynamics in murine fibroblasts. *Human Molecular Genetics*, 14, pp. 835-844.

Cooper, G. 4th (2006) Cytoskeletal networks and the regulation of cardiac contractility: microtubules, hypertrophy, and cardiac dysfunction. *American Journal of Physiology - Heart and Circulatory Physiology*, 291, pp. 1003-1014.

Costa E Silva, J. A. (2004) From restoration of neuroplasticity to the treatment of depression: clinical experience. *European Neuropsychopharmacology*, 14[Suppl 5], pp. 511-521.

Cutter, W. J. *et al.* (2006) Influence of X chromosome and hormones on human brain development: a magnetic resonance imaging and proton magnetic resonance spectroscopy study of Turner syndrome. *Biological Psychiatry*, 59, pp. 273-283.

de Bree, E. *et al.* (2006) Intraperitoneal chemotherapy with taxanes for ovarian cancer with peritoneal dissemination. *European Journal of Surgical Oncology*, 32, pp. 666-670.

Devillard, L. *et al.* (2008) Involvement of microtubules in the tolerance of cardiomyocytes to cold ischemia-reperfusion. *Molecular and Cellular Biochemistry*, 307, pp. 149-157.

Dotan, A. and Avivi, L. (1986) Increased spindle resistance to antimicrotubule agents in women of high risk for meiotic nondisjunction. *Human Genetics*, 73, pp. 199-204.

Dumontet, C. *et al.* (2009) Ixabepilone: targeting betaIII-tubulin expression in taxane-resistant malignancies. *Molecular Cancer Therapeutics*, 8, pp. 17-25.

Dustin, P. (1984) *Microtubules*. Berlin: Springer.

Feng, J. (2006) Microtubule: a common target for parkin and Parkinson's disease toxins. *The Neuroscientist*, 12, pp. 469-476.

Gasser, T. (2009) Mendelian forms of Parkinson's disease. *Biochimica et Biophysica Acta*, 1792, pp. 587-96.

Gauthier, L. R. *et al.* (2004) Huntingtin controls neurotrophic support and survival of neurons by enhancing BDNF vesicular transport along microtubules. *Cell*, 118, pp. 127-138.

Gigant, B. *et al.* (2005) Structural basis for the regulation of tubulin by vinblastine. *Nature*, 435, pp. 519-522.

Hall, A. (2009) The cytoskeleton and cancer. Cancer Metastasis Review, 28, pp. 5-14.

Goes, F. S. *et al.* (2008) The genetics of psychotic bipolar disorder. *Current Psychiatry Reports*, 10, pp. 178-189.

Hein, S. *et al.* (2000) The role of the cytoskeleton in heart failure. *Cardiovascular Research*, 45, pp. 273-278.

Hennah, W. and Porteous, D. (2009) The DISC1 pathway modulates expression of neurodevelopmental, synaptogenic and sensory perception genes. PLoS One, 4, doi: 10.1371/journal.pone.0004906

Hoogenraad, C. C. *et al.* (2004) LIMK1 and CLIP-115: linking cytoskeletal defects to Williams syndrome. *Bioessays*, 2, pp. 141-150.

Jaaro-Peled, H. *et al.* (2009) Neurodevelopmental mechanisms of schizophrenia: understanding disturbed postnatal brain maturation through neuregulin-1-ErbB4 and DISC1. *Trends in Neurosciences*, 32, pp. 485-495.

Jordan, M. And Wilson, L. (2004) Microtubules as a target for anticancer drugs. *Nature Reviews - Cancer*, 4, pp. 253-265.

Katsetos, C. D. *et al.* (2009a) Tubulin targets in the pathobiology and therapy of glioblastoma multiforme. II. gamma-tubulin. *Journal of Cellular Physiology*, 221, pp. 514-520.

Katsetos, C. D. *et al.* (2009b) Tubulin targets in the pathobiology and therapy of glioblastoma multiforme. I. class III beta-tubulin. *Journal of Cellular Physiology*, 221, pp. 505-513.

Klein, L. E. *et al.* (2005) The microtubule stabilizing agent discodermolide is a potent inducer of accelerated cell senescence. *Cell Cycle*, 4, pp. 501-507.

Kloner, R. A. (2006) Natural and unnatural triggers of myocardial infarction. *Progress in Cardiovascular Diseases*, 48, pp. 285-300.

Kremer, H. *et al.* (2006) Usher syndrome: molecular links of pathogenesis, proteins and pathways. *Human Molecular Genetics*, 15, pp. 262-270.

Lee, J. *et al.* (2008) Rho plays a key role in TGF-beta1-induced cytoskeletal rearrangement in human retinal pigment epithelium. *Journal of Cellular Physiology*, 216, pp. 520-526.

Li, H. *et al.* (2004) Correlation of expression of the actin filament-bundling protein espin with stereociliary bundle formation in the developing inner ear. *The Journal of Comparative Neurology*, 468, pp. 125-134.

Lingwood, B. E. *et al.* (2008) MAP2 provides reliable early assessment of neural injury in the newborn piglet model of birth asphyxia. *Journal of Neuroscience Methods*, 171, pp. 140-146.

Lowe, J. *et al.* (2001) Refined structure of alpha beta-tubulin at 3.5 A resolution. *Journal of Molecular Biology*, 313, pp. 1045-1057.

Lu, R. *et al.* (2004) The fragile X protein controls microtubule-associated protein 1B translation and microtubule stability in brain neuron development. *Proceedings of the National Academy of Sciences of the United States of America*, 101, pp. 15201-15206.

Mandel, R. J. (2010) CERE-110, an adeno-associated virus-based gene delivery vector expressing human nerve growth factor for the treatment of Alzheimer's disease. *Current Opinion in Molecular Therapeutics*, 12, pp. 240-247.

Margolis, R. L. and Wilson, L. (1981) Microtubule treadmills-possible molecular machinery. *Nature*, 293, pp. 705-711.

Mathew, P. and Dipaola, R. (2007) Taxane refractory prostate cancer. *The Journal of Urology*, 178[Suppl], pp. 36-41.

Maussion, G. *et al.* (2008) Convergent evidence identifying MAP/microtubule affinity-regulating kinase 1 (MARK1) as a susceptibility gene for autism. *Human Molecular Genetics*, 17, pp. 2541-2551.

McDevitt, C. (2009) *The Big Money: Depression and the Recession* [www] The Washington Post. Available from: http://www.washingtonpost.com/wp-dyn/content/article/2009/08/28/AR2009082804069.html [Accessed 8/ 30/09].

Melki, R. *et al.* (1989) Cold depolymerization of microtubules to double rings: geometric stabilization of assemblies. *Biochemistry*, 28, pp. 9143-9152.

Mizuno, Y. *et al.* (2001) Familial Parkinson's disease. Alpha-synuclein and parkin. *Advances in Neurology*, 86, pp. 13-21.

Mogensen, M. M. *et al.* (2007) The deaf mouse mutant whirler suggests a role for whirlin in actin filament dynamics and stereocilia development. *Cell Motility and the Cytoskeleton*, 64, pp. 496-508.

Myers, K. A. *et al.* (2007) Osteoblast-like cells and fluid flow: cytoskeleton-dependent shear sensitivity. *Biochemical and Biophysical Research Communications*, 364, pp. 214-219.

Nettles, J. H. *et al.* (2004) The binding mode of epothilone A on alpha,beta-tubulin by electron crystallography. *Science*, 305, pp. 866-869.

Nogales, E. *et al.* (1998) Structure of the alpha beta tubulin dimer by electron crystallography. *Nature*, 391, pp. 199-203.

O'keefe, J. H. *et al.* (2009) Primary and secondary prevention of cardiovascular diseases: a practical evidence-based approach. *Mayo Clinic Proceedings*, 84, 741-757.

Paz-Ares, L. (2008) Phase III trial comparing paclitaxel poliglumex vs docetaxel in the second-line treatment of non-small-cell lung cancer. *British Journal of Cancer*, 98, pp. 1608-1613.

Pei, J. J. *et al.* (2008) Neurofibrillary degeneration in Alzheimer's disease: from molecular mechanisms to identification of drug targets. *Current Opinion in Psychiatry*, 21, pp. 555-561.

Piontkewitz, Y. *et al.* (2009) Clozapine administration in adolescence prevents postpubertal emergence of brain structural pathology in an animal model of schizophrenia. *Biological Psychiatry*, 66, pp. 1038-1046.

Pollak, D. *et al.* (2003) Cytoskeleton derangement in brain of patients with Down syndrome, Alzheimer's disease and Pick's disease. *Journal of Neural Transmission-Supplementum*, 67, pp. 149-158.

Ravelli, R. B. *et al.* (2004) Insight into tubulin regulation from a complex with colchicine and a stathmin-like domain. *Nature*, 428, pp. 198-202.

Rowinsky, E. K. *et al* (1989) Phase I and pharmacodynamic study of taxol in refractory acute leukemias. *Cancer Research*, 49, pp. 4640-4647.

Sánchez, C. *et al.* (2001) Microtubule-associated protein 2 phosphorylation is decreased in the human epileptic temporal lobe cortex. *Neuroscience*, 107, pp. 25-33.

Saussede-Aim, J. *et al.* (2009) Beta3-tubulin is induced by estradiol in human breast carcinoma cells through an estrogen-receptor dependent pathway. *Cell Motility and the Cytoskeleton*, 66, pp. 378-388.

Schiff, P.B. and Horwitz, S. B. (1980) Taxol stabilizes microtubules in mouse fibroblast cells. *Proceedings of the National Academy of Sciences of the United States of America*, 77, pp. 1561-1565.

Sigurdsson, E.M. (2009) Tau-Focused Immunotherapy for Alzheimer's disease and related tauopathies. *Current Alzheimer Research*, 6, pp. 446-450.

Souter, S. and Lee, G. (2009) Microtubule-associated protein tau in human prostate cancer cells: Isoforms, phosphorylation, and interactions. *Journal of Cellular Biochemistry*, 108, pp. 555-564.

Sugars, K. L. and Rubinsztein, D. C. (2003) Transcriptional abnormalities in Huntington disease. *Trends in Genetics*, 19, pp. 233-238.

Tanabe, K. and Takei, K. (2009) Dynamic instability of microtubules requires dynamin 2 and is impaired in a Charcot-Marie-Tooth mutant. *The Journal of Cell Biology*, 185, pp. 939-948.

Toso, R. J. *et al.* (1993) Kinetic stabilization of microtubule dynamic instability *in vitro* by vinblastine. *Biochemistry*, 32, pp. 1285-1293.

Tsutsui, H. *et al.* (1993) Cytoskeletal role in the contractile dysfunction of hypertrophied myocardium. *Science*, 260, pp. 682-687.

Tuszynski, J. A. (2008) *Molecular and Cellular Biophysics*. Boca Raton: Chapman and Hall/CRC.

Vickers, J. C. *et al.* (2009) Axonopathy and cytoskeletal disruption in degenerative diseases of the central nervous system. *Brain Research Bulletin*, 80, pp. 217-223

Walker, R. A. *et al.* (1991) Dilution of individual microtubules observed in real time *in vitro*: evidence that cap size is small and independent of elongation rate. *The Journal of Cell Biology*, 114, pp. 73-81

Wang, H. W. and Nogales, E. (2005) Nucleotide-dependent bending flexibility of tubulin regulates microtubule assembly. *Nature*, 435, pp. 911-915.

Woolf, N. J. *et al.* (2009) *Nanoneuroscience: Structural and Functional Roles of the Cytoskeleton in Health and Disease*. Berlin: Springer-Verlag.

Woolf, N. J. (2009) Bionic microtubules: potential applications to multiple neurological and neuropsychiatric diseases. *Journal of Nanoneuroscience*, 1, pp. 85-94.

Xiao, H. *et al.* (2006) Insights into the mechanism of microtubule stabilization by Taxol. *Proceedings of the National Academy of Sciences of the United States of America*, 103, pp. 10166-10173.

Yilmaz, M. and Christofori, G. (2009) EMT, the cytoskeleton, and cancer cell invasion. *Cancer Metastasis Reviews*, 28, pp. 15-33.

Yuen, E. Y. *et al.* (2005) Serotonin 5-HT1A receptors regulate NMDA receptor channels through a microtubule-dependent mechanism. *The Journal of Neuroscience*, 25, pp. 5488-5501.

Zhao, Y. *et al.* (2009) Microtubule stabilising agents for cancer chemotherapy. *Expert Opinion on Therapeutic Patents*. 19, pp. 607-622.

Zheng, Y. *et al.* (1995) Nucleation of microtubule assembly by a gamma-tubulin-containing ring complex. *Nature*, 378, pp. 578-583.

In: Hypotheses in Clinical Medicine
Editors: M.M. Shoja, P.S. Agutter et al.

ISBN: 978-1-62257-276-2

Chapter 16

Why Do We Yawn? Past and Current Hypotheses

Olivier Walusinski* [*]
Brou, France

Abstract

Yawning can be regarded as a prototype of stereotypical behaviors that has been recycled through evolution for different purposes. These purposes are combined with the increasing complexity of the central nervous system during evolution, and correlated with the richness of social interactions. In this chapter, past and current hypotheses concerning the generation and usefulness of yawning are discussed.

Introduction

Cognition, emotion, behavior and memory are all brain functions. However, this was not accepted to be true until the end of the 18th century. While eating, drinking, urination, sight and walking seem easy to understand, the purposes of other functions that originate in the brain, such as sleep, dreaming, hiccups and laughter, remain mysterious. Yawning belongs to this second group of functions, which appear more difficult to understand than the other functions of the brain. This might explain the vast array of beliefs and hypotheses, as varied as they are strange in certain cases, associated with what, for a human being, is a daily behavior. As we shall see, several diverse hypotheses exist in 2011, but for the moment none can be scientifically verified.

[*] E-mail: walusinski@baillement.com. Dr Olivier Walusinski, 20 rue de Chartres, F 28160 Brou, France.

What Is a Yawn?

Yawning is a stereotyped, and often repetitive, motor action characterised by gaping of the mouth accompanied by a long inspiration of breath, a brief acme, and then a short expiration of breath. Stretching and yawning simultaneously is known as pandiculation, which is not merely a simple opening of the mouth but a complex, coordinated movement bringing together a flexion followed by an extension of the neck and a wide dilatation of the pharyngolarynx with strong stretching of the diaphragm and anti-gravity muscles. Yawning is involuntary and only humans seem capable of altering its occurrence for cultural or social reasons. It is highly stereotypical because no environmental input changes the sequence of movements. Yawning is observed in cold-blooded and warm-blooded vertebrates, from reptiles with rudimentary "archaic" brains to human primates, in water, air and land environments. Ethologists agree that almost all vertebrates yawn. Yawning is morphologically similar in reptiles, birds, mammals and fish (Deputte 1994; Fraser 1989; Walusinski and Deputte 2004). These behaviors may be ancestral vestiges maintained throughout evolution with little variation (phylogenetically old origins). Correlatively, yawning can be viewed as early as 12 weeks during fetal development, and is considered an ontogenetically primitive behavior (Walusinski 2010).

Different Types of Yawns

The triune brain hypothesis is a model of the evolution of the vertebrate forebrain and behavior proposed by the American neuroscientist Paul D. MacLean (1913-2007). MacLean originally formulated his model in the 1960s, and propounded it at length in his 1990 book *The Triune Brain in Evolution*. The triune brain consists of the reptilian complex (archaic brain), the paleomammalian complex (limbic system), and the neomammalian complex (neocortex), viewed as structures sequentially added to the forebrain in the course of evolution (McLean 1990). Although the model never won wide acceptance among comparative neurobiologists, it helps to explain the different types of yawns:

1. “Universal yawning”, which is seen in nearly all vertebrates, is associated with sleep and arousal or with hunger and satiety, and appears to be generated by the reptilian brain (Giganti et al. 2010; Giganti and Salzarulo 2010);
2. What ethologists describe as “emotional yawning”, which is only seen in some mammals (but data are still being collected), and is generated by the paleomammalian brain. This is the yawn that helps to pacify after stress. Dogs in veterinary situations or caged chimpanzees yawn more frequently than during non-stressful times. Ethologists call this type of behavior a displacement activity. In humans, athletes yawn repeatedly before competitions, as do parachutists before jumping, and actors before making their entrance. In these cases, yawning has a calming, anti-stress effect. This might explain why yoga teachers use yawning to relax their students. A related type of yawning is that associated with sexuality in dominant male macaques, who yawn repeatedly before mating, as if to make their status within the group known. This sort of yawn disappears following castration and

reappears if testosterone is injected (Aureli and de Waal 1997; Beckmann and Zimmer 1981; Deputte 1994; Deputte et al. 1994; Maestripieri et al. 1992; Zucker et al. 1998);

3. "Contagious yawning", which is observed only in great apes and humans who display a theory of mind. This ability to respond to yawning in others is absent in autistic people. Functional imaging shows activation of the same brain structures as those used to decode empathy. As a neocortical activity (frontal and parietal lobes, insula and amygdala), communicative yawning is a sign of involuntary empathy (Helt et al. 2010; Senju 2010). One can conclude that, through evolution, a behavior can be recycled for different purposes according to the increasing complexity of the central nervous system, correlated with the richness of social interactions.

Neuropharmacology of Yawning

Most of the significant advances towards our understanding of the neuropharmacological regulation of yawning have been made during the past 50 years. We now know that a variety of neurotransmitters and neurohormones are involved in the induction and regulation of yawning, including acetylcholine, dopamine, glutamate, serotonin, oxytocin, gamma-aminobutyric acid (GABA), opioids, adrenergics and nitric oxide, as well as the pro-opio-melanocortic-derived peptides, e.g., adrenocorticotropic and alpha-melanocyte stimulating hormones (ACTH and alpha-MSH, respectively). Most yawning is mediated by at least three distinct pathways, all of which appear to converge on cholinergic neurons within the hippocampus, despite the diverse set of neurotransmitters involved. In addition, the importance of the hypothalamus (parvocellular nucleus, PVN) in regulating yawning has been demonstrated, as many of these neurotransmitters appear to affect yawning through their interactions with oxytocinergic neurons within the PVN. For instance, activation of these oxytocinergic neurons by dopamine, glutamate, nitric oxide and oxytocin is known to induce yawning, whereas inhibition of these neurons by μ-opioids and GABA has been shown to reduce the frequency of yawning. It is important to note that although the effects of ACTH and alpha-MSH are also mediated by the hypothalamus, the induction of yawning by these peptides does not involve oxytocinergic neurons. Similarly, the induction of yawning by serotonin is known to occur independently of oxytocinergic neurons within the PVN; however, the brain regions responsible for serotonergic yawning are currently unknown.

Despite the great advances made towards our understanding of the neuropharmacological regulation of yawning, further studies are needed to elucidate fully how these neuro-transmitter systems interact with each other, as well as the specific receptor subtypes and brain regions involved in the induction and inhibition of yawning. Such an understanding would not only advance the use of yawning as a tool for the pharmacological characterization of receptor subtype-selective agonists, partial-agonists and antagonists, but also further our knowledge of how a variety of environmental and pharmacological manipulations (such as dietary conditions or chronic drug treatments) affect the receptor systems involved in mediating yawning. In addition, a more complete understanding of the neuropharmacological regulation of yawning could also provide insight into the specific roles of different neurotransmitter systems and/or receptor subtypes in the occurrence of yawning under a variety of physiological conditions and disease states in which changes in the frequency of yawning are known to occur (Collins and Eguibar 2010).

Old Theories Now Considered False

Life, in all its aspects, has always given rise to thought and questioning. Explanations of physiological phenomena have always provided us with reassurance. As noted by Henry Louis Mencken (1880-1956): "Explanations exist and have always existed, because there is always a simple solution to each human problem, a clear solution that is plausible and false" (Mencken 1934). The history of knowledge about yawning is a perfect example of this precept. The causes and consequences of this intriguing phenomenon have defied the human mind for centuries. The most ancient theory on yawning was described in *De flatibus liber*, "a treatise on wind" written by Hippocrates in 400 BC. He observed: "Yawning precedes a fever, because the large quantity of air that has accumulated ascends all at once, lifting with the action of a lever and opening the mouth; in this manner the air can exit with ease. Like the large quantities of steam that escape from cauldrons when water boils, the accumulated air in the body is violently expelled through the mouth when the body temperature rises". This idea persisted until the 17th century (de Mercy 1831).

Santori Santorio (1561–1636), or Sanctorius of Padua, was a physician in Venice and a student and friend of Galileo. He may be considered as one of the founders of experimental physiology. He tried to quantify physiological and pathological phenomena with measuring devices such as the scale, the thermometer and the metronome. With a scale of his own invention, he measured and compared weight gain and loss in humans, particularly by perspiration. He built an entire medical theory based on weight differences related to nutrition and releases via the emunctories and perspiration, calling it static medicine. He mentioned yawning in his aphorisms: "Yawning and limb extension after sleep show that the body perspires abundantly, similar to the rooster that flaps its wings before it starts to sing. The urge to yawn and stretch the limbs upon waking stems from the abundance of perspirable matter, creating an inclination to perspire. Through yawning and limb extension, we perspire more in one half hour than we would during other times in three hours" (Santori 1634).

Johannes de Gorter (1689–1762), a prolific Dutch author in all areas of medicine in the early 18th century, holds a key place in the history of the knowledge on yawning. In his book, *De Perspiratione insensibili* in 1755, he attributed yawning "to a need for faster blood circulation and to cerebral anemia" (de Gorter 1725). This marks the birth of an idea that would persist for two centuries, repeated by almost all authors: yawning improves brain oxygenation. This hypothesis seems to predict that yawning is triggered when blood or brain oxygenation is insufficient, i.e. when oxygen (O_2) levels drop and carbon dioxide (CO_2) concentration rises. Provine *et al.* demonstrated, in 1987, that healthy subjects who are exposed to gas mixtures with high levels of CO_2, or to physical exercise, do not yawn more frequently. Similarly, high levels of O_2 had no influence on the yawning rate (Provine *et al.* 1987). Although hypoxia is frequent in patients with heart or lung disease, no increased yawning is usually observed in these patients. Yawning in the human fetus and in fish also rules out this hypothesis. During periods of low blood oxygenation, yawning does not increase and thus cannot improve brain oxygenation.

Hypotheses That Have not Been Experimentally Tested

A number of other hypotheses have arisen over time. Cahill (1978) argued that yawning prevents lung atelectasis; Pellatt *et al.* (1981) suggested that the thyroid gland may be compressed during yawning, with the resultant liberation of thyroid hormones; Forrester (1988) presumed that yawning renews the surfactant film in the lungs; McKenzie (1994) thought that yawning may enhance the evacuation of the tonsilar fossae. Because yawning opens the Eustachian tubes and therefore ventilates the tympanal cavities, Laskiewicz, in 1953, proposed that yawning may be a "defence reflex" to equalise air pressures in the ear, triggered by altitude changes or other conditions leading to air trapping in the middle ear.

Matikainen *et al.* (2008) argued that yawning causes movements and compressions that may affect the carotid body, which is situated strategically at the bifurcation of the common carotid artery. Thus, yawning may stimulate the carotid body by compression. The carotid body is a chemosensory organ that monitors blood chemicals and initiates compensatory reflex adjustments to maintain homeostasis. The 'afferent' sensory discharge induced by changes in blood chemicals, e.g. low PO_2 (hypoxia), is relayed by carotid sinus nerve fibers. A parallel autonomic (parasympathetic) 'efferent' pathway that is the source of carotid body inhibition is less well known. These autonomic neurons are embedded in 'paraganglia' within the glossopharyngeal and carotid sinus nerves. While the phylogeny of the carotid arteries is well established, the phylogeny of the carotid body is not. Peripheral respiratory O_2 chemoreceptors are found in multiple, dispersed sites in fish and amphibia; this is reduced to a single dominant receptor site in birds and mammals. In the process, the cells in the fish gill associated with O_2 chemosensing have been replaced by the glomus cells of the mammalian carotid body. Despite this, all these vertebrates, with or without carotid bodies, yawn widely (Campanucci and Nurse 2007; Milsom and Burleson 2007).

None of these hypotheses explains the association of yawning with arousal and sleepiness. None of these proposals have been experimentally tested, and there is currently no evidence for such mechanisms.

Why a Fetal Yawn?

The advent of ultrasound technology in the 1970s enabled live, unobtrusive observations of fetal behaviors in humans, vastly increasing our knowledge of many types of subtle motor activity (swallowing, respiratory movements, smiling, and yawning), and thus of human fetal development. Yawning is a phylogenetically old, and thus ontologically precocious, behavior. Ultrasound investigation reveals its onset at between 11 and 15 weeks of gestation. The fact that yawning has survived without evolutionary variation suggests its importance in terms of developmental need. The strong muscular contraction involved in yawning has a metabolically expensive cost. If we agree with the terms of Darwin's evolutionary propositions, the cost in brain activity must be outweighed by the advantages gained in terms of developmental fitness. Thus, a structural hypothesis suggests an activating role in neurotrophin synthesis, leading to a cascade of new synapse formation or recruitment and activation throughout the diencephalon, brainstem and spinal cord. The phenomenon of activity-dependent development has clearly been shown to be one mechanism by which early sensory or motor experience can affect the course of neural development. Activity-dependent development may be a ubiquitous process in brain maturation by which activity in one brain region can influence development in other regions. These suggestions are difficult to prove, however, because human research on prenatal programming of behavior is intrinsically correlational, never manipulatively experimental, and frequently based upon homologies with other vertebrates (Almli *et al.* 2001; Petrikovsky *et al.* 1999; van Woerden *et al.* 2008; Walusinski 2010).

Current Theories under Scientific Discussion

In this section, we will only discuss universal vertebrate yawning, i.e. the oldest yawning in phylogenetic terms, which is generated by the reptilian brain. So far, sereval theories are currently under consideration, as follows:

The Arousal-sleepiness Hypothesis

Each individual, from his or her own experience, is aware of the link that exists between fatigue, sleepiness and yawning. Monotonous circumstances lead to yawning, such as idle waiting, public transportation and long periods of motorway driving. A correlation exists between the degree of sleepiness and increased yawning frequency. Furthermore, yawning exhibits a circadian rhythm. Following sleep, it is more frequent and associated with stretching (the term pandiculation is used, referring to yawning together with generalized stretching of anti-gravity muscles). It is also more frequent during the drowsiness that precedes sleep (Giganti *et al.* 2010). Herbivores, which sleep less and have shorter periods of paradoxical sleep than carnivores or frugivores, yawn less often. Yawning and pandiculation lead to the maximal opening of the upper respiratory tract and increased muscle tone in anti-gravity muscles.

All motor activity results in adaptive feedback. The strong muscular contraction involved in yawning and pandiculation initiates sensory feedback, via the somatosensory tract (posterior funiculus), with projection to the locus ceruleus (trigeminal-cervical-spinal sensorimotor loops), the ascending reticular activating system in the brainstem, and the lateral hypothalamus. According to the most developed theory at this time, the physiological function of yawning is to stimulate vigilance rather than arousal, together with muscle tone, through feedback to the above-mentioned structures, which play a role in arousal, vigilance and muscle tone. One of the main arguments for this arousal enhancement derives from the observation that yawns are followed by a significant increase in motor activity. Notwithstanding, sleepy individuals trying to stay awake change their body position and move their limbs. These movements have an arousing effect measurable by EEG, just as yawning has (Walusinski 2006).

According to Guggisberg *et al.* (2007) “the increased motor activity observed after yawns is probably not an indicator of an arousing effect of yawning, but an effective countermeasure against the underlying drowsiness”. They analyzed spectral EEG changes after yawns in humans and the results were negative. Yawning activates the autonomic system but Guggisberg *et al.* suggested that this is non-specific and related to the associated movements and respiration. These researchers noticed no specific increase in skin conductance (indicating increased arousal level) after yawning (Guggisberg *et al.* 2007). Note that the hypothesis explored was that yawning induces arousal, whereas the initial theory was to interpret yawning as a means of stimulating vigilance, and not specifically arousal.

Pandiculation in Interoception and the Body Schema

Given the demonstration that yawning does not impact arousal, the theory that vigilance rather than arousal is stimulated can be reformulated. In the Aristotelian tradition, school children learn that we have five senses. But we receive information from a sixth sense, interoception, which includes proprioception, i.e. the ability to perceive sensory stimuli inside our bodies. The term interoception, related to somaesthesia, was proposed by Sherrington, as was the term proprioception (Sherrington 1906). Arousal is essential to consciousness, and requires the ability to integrate sensory information about the outside world as well as our sensations concerning our internal physical state, modulated by emotion and memory.

Afferent sensations from the musculoskeletal system converge, via the spinothalamic and spinoreticular tracts, on the thalamus and raphe nuclei and from there, on the thalamocortical tract to the postcentral gyrus in the parietal lobe. The thalamus and the paraventricular nucleus in the hypothalamus are part of a circuit that sends and receives signals from the locus ceruleus and the mammillary bodies; all of these structures are involved in autonomic reflexes. The cranial trigeminal (V), facial (VII) and vagus (X) nerves and the motor and/or sensory cervical nerves C1-C4 also convey somaesthetic information that converges on the nucleus of the solitary tract (NTS). The NTS is an interface for the peripheral information needed to stimulate the ascending reticular activating system in the brain stem, particularly the locus ceruleus, which activates arousal systems (adrenergic system at the pons, dopaminergic system at the peduncles, histaminergic system at the hypothalamus and cholinergic system at the nucleus basalis of Meynert). The neurons of the NTS project to the parabrachial nucleus, which in turn projects to various brain stem, diencephalic and thalamic sites. These structures also project to the visceral sensory area of the insula, amygdala and lateral frontal cortex, especially the right lateral frontal cortex. These circuits enable a subcortical homeostatic activity that is unconscious and automatic to result in a conscious representation. Autonomic, somatic and limbic integration make it possible to extract bodily perception, which may in turn lead to a sensation of pleasure (Cameron 2002; Craig 2003; Critchley *et al.* 2004). Thus, muscle tone variations in peripheral anti-gravity muscles, transmitted by these pathways, may trigger yawning and pandiculation which, through the powerful muscular contractions that accompany them, may activate vigilance systems.

Our perception of musculoskeletal activity, therefore, brings a feeling of well-being and a more acute bodily reflectivity of the self, for example during arousal, as proposed by the James-Lange theory of emotion or by Damasio's somatic marker hypothesis of consciousness (James 1884; Lange 1885; Damasio 1999).

Auto-regulation of the Locomotor System

For Bertolucci (2011), "pandiculation seems to be elicited by a complex array or sequence of stimuli, which might include both exteroceptive signals (e.g. light-darkness) and interoceptive ones (e.g. circadian endocrine cycles and somatic interoception). Yawning is a series of coordinated actions that unfold sequentially, building up soft tissue contractile tension to a peak, at which point the joints of the limbs and trunk are maximally extended or, alternatively, the trunk is arched in flexion. After the peak, the soft tissue tension level plummets, yielding a sense of pleasure and well-being. The actions can be regional or involve the whole body, and are often bilaterally symmetrical". The musculoskeletal system is constantly being reshaped by the mechanical constraints to which it is exposed. For example, prolonged immobilization leads to muscle loss and skeletal demineralisation.

Bertolucci (2011) argues that "pandiculation with its specific and vigorous muscle activity, might be a means to compensate for the mechanical signals delivered by rest periods and sub-optimal movements". Yawning might be considered a feedback mechanism resulting from stiffness, and possibly be triggered by extended periods of immobility in asymmetrical positions. If the body tends to stiffen, pandiculation "can serve to restore the limb (and related musculature) to an original (homeostatic) state".

Pandiculation "might be a biological compensation for periods of immobility and/or vicious body positions, restoring the animal's mobility by breaking up abnormal muscle metabolism cross-links formed by inactivity or suboptimal activity". "Perhaps the vigorous co-contractions of pandiculation systematically reshape the structural linkage among segments and simultaneously signal the cells (via mechanotransduction) to synthesize the cellular muscle components required to maintain the appropriate environment. If so, pandiculation might help restore optimal musculoskeletal arrangements, and thus optimize motor capabilities" (Bertolucci 2011).

The Thermoregulation Hypothesis

The existence of yawning across almost all vertebrate species suggests important basic functions, and the spontaneous and involuntary nature of a yawn lends support for it having adaptive significance. Recent research by Andrew C. Gallup (2010, 2011) suggests that one biological function of yawning among homeotherms is central thermoregulation. Comparative research from birds, rats and humans suggests, for them, that yawning reduces brain and body temperature, and is influenced by the range and direction of ambient temperature change. According to this model, the increased facial and brain circulation that follows yawning acts like a radiator, by eliminating calories from the blood in the brain via the face and head, and by introducing cooler blood from the extremities and lungs into the brain. In one of the experiments developed by this team, subjects wore refrigerated packs on their foreheads. Under these conditions, they were less susceptible to contagious yawning than with no forehead refrigeration. It should be noted that cold temperatures have an arousing effect and can, by themselves, modify the outcome. Other experiments on birds in various temperature conditions showed an increased frequency in the number of yawns with increasing temperature. However, no other parameters that could interfere with this finding were taken into consideration, which significantly limits the scientific value of this study (Gallup 2010,

2011). Until direct, intraparenchymal measurements can be performed, this theory will not be acceptable.

Furthermore, according to calculations by Hannu Elo, this hypothesis is physically impossible. It is impossible to lower body temperature through yawning, unless the yawns result in heavy perspiration. Similarly, yawning cannot lower brain temperature, which would require water evaporation (lungs and respiratory tract), loss by conduction, thermal radiation, and a slowdown in metabolism (Elo 2010, 2011). In addition, this explanation overlooks the existence of fetal yawning and yawning in poikilotherms such as reptiles. For these reasons, the hypothesis of brain cooling through yawning obviously requires further analysis, with due consideration given to anatomy and physiology as well as the actual need, if any, to cool the brain.

Yawning and the Cerebrospinal Fluid System

Domenico Cotugno was the first, in 1764, to describe the circulation of cerebrospinal fluid (CSF) (Cotugno 1988). The beating of the heart and the movements associated with breathing cause pressure variations in the ventricular system. Each deep inhalation is followed be an increase in CSF flow rate in the fourth ventricle (Schroth and Klose 1992).

Jaw kinematics, together with inhalation, have been shown to alter intracranial circulation. Lepp (1982) describes jaw kinematics as follows. Jaw movements activate the pterygoid musculovenous pump, located in the upper part of the anterior parapharyngeal space, known as the prestyloid parapharyngeal space. As a result, this pump, also known as the paratubal pump, can impact the mechanism of venous blood flow out of the endocranium, mainly via the plexus venosus foraminis ovalis. The pterygoid cistern, a component of this pump, corresponds to the cavernous part of the pterygoid plexus. It is an extracranial extension of the cavernous sinus and passes through the foramen ovale. It plays an important role as an intermediary station of acceleration for return blood flow from the brain (Bouyssou and Tricoire 1985; Patra *et al.* 1988). Lepp notes that it would be reasonable to consider jaw kinematics together with the lateral pterygoid muscle as a venous trigger, given that they act as the starter for the alternating musculovenous pumping action that takes place in the cavernous part of the pterygoid plexus. This pumping action is particularly efficient during isolated yawning, especially when the mouth reaches its maximum opening. However, Lepp emphasizes that yawning itself is often merely the initiation of a musculovenous motor chain reaction, which extends to the limbs and the entire skeletal musculature as tonic waves propagated in the rostrocaudal direction, and ends at the tips of the fingers and toes (Lepp 1982).

It would thus appear that the large inhalation and maximal opening of the mouth accelerate the circulation of CSF. Already, in 1912, Legendre and Piéron had demonstrated the presence of a hypnogenic factor in the CSF, which accumulates during the waking state (Legendre and Pieron 1912). Almost a hundred years of research into the hormonal, non-neuronal factors that induce sleep has identified over 50 molecules. Of current interest is prostaglandin PGD2, a hormone that acts locally and is produced by the meninges. When it binds to a specific receptor, transduction occurs from the leptomeninges to brain parenchyma through the activation of adenosine production, which induces sleep in the ventrolateral preoptic (VLPO) nucleus of the anterior hypothalamus (Huang *et al.* 2007, 2011). Yawning and pandiculation may accelerate clearance of PGD2, thus reducing sleepiness. They may also act on other neuromediators that are currently unknown.

Conclusion

We close this survey of the different functional theories on yawning, none of which have been scientifically demonstrated, by proposing that yawning appears to be a homeostatic process involving circadian variations in vigilance and emotion. Yawning externalizes a parasympathetic stimulation during the balancing of adrenergic and cholinergic homeostasis of the autonomic nervous system. Thus, it seems closer to a behavioral stereotypy than to a reflex. This is, indeed, a curious behavioral display, and is a beautiful example of an involuntary expression that is pleasurable and that we, as humans, use voluntarily to communicate boredom deliberately.

References

Almli, C. R. *et al.* (2001) Human fetal and neonatal movement patterns: Gender differences and fetal-to-neonatal continuity. *Developmental Psychobiology*, 38, pp. 252-273.

Aureli, F. and de Waal, F. B. (1997) Inhibition of social behavior in chimpanzees under high-density conditions. *American Journal of Primatology*, 41, pp. 213-228.

Beckmann, H. and Zimmer, R. (1981) An ethological interpretation of stereotypy induced by environmental stimulus. *Archiv fur Psychiatrie und Nervenkrankheiten*, 230, pp. 81-89.

Bertolucci, L.F. (2011) Pandiculation: Nature's way of maintaining the functional integrity of the myofascial system? *Journal of Bodywork and Movement Therapies*, 15, pp. 268-280.

Bouyssou, M. and Tricoire, J. (1985) Experimental detection of a cervical arousal mechanism of yawning, enhancing intracerebral (CSF) fluid pressure. *Journal of Dental Research*, 64, p. 721.

Cahill, C. A. (1978) Yawn maneuver to prevent atelectasis. *AORN Journal*, 27, pp.1000-1004.

Cameron, O.G. (2002) *Visceral Sensory Neuroscience*. New York: Oxford University Press. p. 359.

Campanucci, V. A. and Nurse, C. A. (2007) Autonomic innervation of the carotid body: role in efferent inhibition. *Respiratory Physiology and Neurobiology*, 157, pp. 83-92.

Collins, G. T. and Eguibar, J. R. (2010) Neurophamacology of yawning. *Frontiers of Neurology and Neuroscience*, 28, pp. 90-106.

Cotugno, D. (1988) The first description of the spinal fluid. By Domenico Cotugno, 1775. *Clinical Orthopaedics and Related Research*, 227, pp. 6-9.

Craig, A. D. (2003) Interoception: the sense of the physiological condition of the body. *Current Opinions in Neurobiology*, 13, pp. 500-505.

Critchley, H. D. *et al* (2004) Neural systems supporting interoceptive awareness. *Nature Neuroscience*, 7, pp. 189-195.

Damasio, A. R. (1999) *The feeling of What Happens: Body and Emotion in the Making of Consciousness*. New York: Harcourt Brace. p. 396.

de Gorter, J. (1725) *De Perspiratione Insensibili Sanctoriana-Batava: Tractatus Experimentis Proprii In Hollandia.* Lugduni Batavorum: Sumptibus Auctoris & Prostant Janssonois Vander, p. 246.

de Mercy, F. C. (1831) *Oeuvres d'Hippocrate. Traité de la Maladie Sacrée, des Vents ou des Fluxions.* Paris: Béchet Jeune, p. 359.

Deputte, B. L. (1994) Ethological study of yawning in primates. *Ethology*, 98, pp. 221-245.

Deputte, B. L. *et al.* (1994) Behavioral effects of an antiandrogen in adult male rhesus macaques (Macaca mulatta). *Hormones and Behavior*, 28, pp. 155-164.

Elo, H. (2010) Yawning and thermoregulation. *Sleep and Breathing*, 14, pp. 391-392.

Elo, H. (2011) Yawning cannot cause significant temperature decreases in humans. *Sleep Medicine*, 12, p. 102.

Forrester, J. M. (1988) Is yawning a brainstem phenomenon? *The Lancet*, 331, p. 596.

Fraser, A. F. (1989) Pandiculation: the comparative phenomenon of systematic stretching. *Applied Animal Behavioural Science*, 23, pp. 263-268.

Gallup, A. C. (2010) A thermoregulatory behavior. *Frontiers of Neurology and Neuroscience*, 28, pp. 84-89.

Gallup, A. C. (2011) Why do we yawn? Primitive versus derived features. *Neuroscience and Biobehavioral Reviews*, 35, pp. 765-769.

Giganti, F. *et al.* (2010) Sleep, sleepiness and yawning. *Frontiers of Neurology and Neuroscience*, 28, pp. 42-46.

Giganti, F. and Salzarulo, P. (2010) Yawning throughout life. *Frontiers of Neurology and Neuroscience,* 28, pp. 26-31.

Guggisberg, A. G. *et al.*(2007) The functional relationship between yawning and vigilance. *Behavioural Brain Research*, 179, pp. 159-166.

Helt, M. S. *et al.* (2010) Contagious yawning in autistic and typical development. *Child Development*, 81, pp. 1620-1631.

Huang, Z. L. *et al.* (2007) Prostaglandins and adenosine in the regulation of sleep and wakefulness. *Current Opinions in Pharmacology*, 7, pp. 33-8.

Huang, Z. L. *et al.* (2011) The role of adenosine in the regulation of sleep. *Current Topics in Medical Chemistry*, 11, pp. 1047-57.

James, W. (1884) What is an emotion? *Mind*, 9, pp. 188-205.

Lange, K. G. (1885) *Om Sindsbevægelser et Psyko-Fysiologisk Studie*. Denmark: Kjøbenhavn, p. 91.

Laskiewicz, A. (1953) Yawning with regard to the respiratory organs and the ear. *Practical Otorhinolaryngology (Basel)*, 15, pp. 105-122.

Legendre, R. and Pieron, H. (1912) De la propriété hypnotoxique des humeurs développée au cours d'une veille prolongée. *C.R. Société de Biologie de Paris*, 72, pp. 210-212.

Lepp, F. H. (1982) Remarques sur la signification physiologique du bâillement. *Bulletin du Groupement International pour la Recherche Scientifique en Stomatologie et Odontologie*, 25, pp. 251-90.

Maestripieri, D. *et al.* (1992) A modest proposal: displacement activities as an indicator of emotions in primates. *Animal Behaviour*, 44, pp. 967-979.

Matikainen, J. and Elo, H. (2008) Does yawning increase arousal through mechanical stimulation of the carotid body? *Medical Hypotheses*, 70, pp. 488-492.

McKenzie, A. A. (1994) The tonsillar evacuation hypothesis of yawning behavior. *South African Journal of Science*, 90, pp. 64-66.

McLean, P. D. (1990) *The Triune Brain in Evolution: Role in Paleocerebral*. New York: Plenum Press, p. 672.

Mencken, H. L.(1934) *Treatrise on Right and Wrong*. New York: Knopf., p. 331.

Milsom, W. K. and Burleson, M. L. (2007) Peripheral arterial chemoreceptors and the evolution of the carotid body. *Respiratory Physiology and Neurobiology*, 157, pp. 4-11.

Nahab, F. B. (2010) Exploring yawning with neuroimaging. *Frontiers in Neurology and Neuroscience*, 28, pp.128-133.

Patra, P. *et al.* (1988) Physiologic variations of the internal jugular vein surface, role of the omohyoid muscle, a preliminary echographic study. *Surgical and Radiological Anatomy*, 10, pp. 107-112.

Pellatt, A. *et al.* (1981) Yawning and the Thyroid Gland. *South African Journal of Science*, 77, pp. 391-394.

Petrikovsky, B. *et al.*(1999) Fetal yawning activity in normal and high-risk fetuses: a preliminary observation. *Ultrasound in Obstetrics and Gynecology*, 13, pp. 127-130.

Provine, R. R. *et al.*(1987) Yawning: no effect of 3-5% CO2, 100% O2, and exercise. *Behavioral and Neural Biology*, 48, pp. 382-393.

Santori, S. (1634) *De Statica Medicina et de Responsione ad Staticomasticem. Aphorismorum Sectionibus Septem Comprehensa.* Italy: MA Brogiollo, p.71.

Schroth, G. and Klose, U. (1992) Cerebrospinal fluid flow; Physiology of respiration-related pulsations. *Neuroradiology*, 35, pp. 10-15.

Senju, A. (2010) Developmental and comparative perspectives of contagious yawning. *Frontiers in Neurology and Neuroscience*, 28, pp. 113-119.

Sherrington, C. S. (1906) *The Integrative Action of the Nervous System*. New Haven: Yale University Press, p. 412

van Woerden, E. E. *et al.* (1988) Fetal mouth movements during behavioral states 1F and 2F. European Journal of Obstetrics. *Gynecology and Reproductive Biology*, 29, pp. 97-105.

Walusinski, O. and Deputte, B. L. (2004) The phylogeny, ethology and nosology of yawning. *Reviews in Neurology (Paris)*, 160, pp. 1011-1021.

Walusinski, O. (2006) Yawning: unsuspected avenue for a better understanding of arousal and interoception. *Medical Hypotheses*, 67, pp. 6-14.

Walusinski, O. (2010) Fetal yawning. *Frontiers in Neurology and Neuroscience*, 28, pp. 32-41.

Woodbury, R. and Abretj, B. (1944) Influence of dying gasps, yawns and sighs on blood pressure and blood flow. *American Journal of Physiology*, 142, pp. 721-726.

Zucker, E. L. *et al.* (1998) Frequencies and contexts of gape yawn displays of free-ranging Patas Monkeys. *American Journal of Primatology*, 45, p. 215.

In: Hypotheses in Clinical Medicine
Editors: M.M. Shoja, P.S. Agutter et al.
ISBN: 978-1-62257-276-2

Chapter 17

Regressive Autism and Defective Evolution of Cerebral Laterality

Matteo Chiappedi*
Don Carlo Gnocchi ONLUS Foundation, Milan, Italy
University of Pavia, Pavia, Italy

Abstract

Autism spectrum disorders (ASDs) are the phenotypic manifestation of a neurodevelopmental syndrome, thought to be associated with brain abnormalities. This paper focuses on a specific subgroup of these disorders, known as "regressive autism". The aetiology of this disorder is still unclear. It is hypothesized that, in children affected by regressive autism, the initial normal developmental period is the result of good right hemisphere function, and regressive symptoms could be the result of a failure of the inter-regulation between the two brain hemispheres, leading to an alteration of the physiological neural networks, and to a blockade (or even loss) of acquired skills. According to the present hypothesis, regressive autism is the final stage of a process beginning in early stages of development, involving multiple genetic and/or environmental mechanisms that control cerebral lateralization, with a failure of the functional right to left hemisphere switch. This represents a significant development of the original hypothesis by Geschwin and Galaburda (1985a-c), in the light of recent findings in neuroscience.

Introduction

Autism spectrum disorders (ASDs) are the phenotypic manifestation of a neurodevelopmental syndrome, thought to be associated with brain abnormalities (Amaral *et al.* 2008) and generally characterized by an early onset in childhood. DSM-IV-TR classification (American Psychiatric Association 2000) employs the term pervasive

* E-mail: mchiappedi@gmail.com.

developmental disorders to indicate this group of disorders, which profoundly alter child neurodevelopment, and are clinically related to autistic disorders. These include autistic disorder, Asperger's syndrome, Rett's syndrome, childhood disintegrative disorder (CDD), and pervasive developmental disorders not otherwise specified (PDD-NOS). The incidence of ASDs has dramatically risen by tenfold (from 2-5/10000 to 15-60/10000 live born children) during the past two decades; broader diagnostic criteria and increased medical awareness have likely to have contributed to determine this trend (Rutter 2005; Persico and Bourgeron 2006). The aetiology of ASDs is still unclear; nevertheless both genetic and non-genetic causes have been suggested to account for this condition (Hughes 2009). Still, existing classification systems are thought to be insufficient to fully discriminate different aetiologies and phenotypes (Chiappedi *et al.* 2010), and other factors have been proposed by examining the problem of ASDs from a different theoretical position (Bonaccorsi 2007).

When a careful history is taken, one can find a group of parents of ASD children who describe a period of normal development, lasting from birth to around 18 months of age, followed by a period characterized by arrest or regression of language development, communicative, and social skills. Approximately 25-30% of children with ASDs stop speaking after beginning to say words, often before the age of two (Johnson and Myers 2007). Even with the possibility that these reported data are somewhat incorrect due to recall problems (Andrews *et al.* 2002), the term "regressive autism" has been used to describe the clinical conditions in which a child appears to have a normal development, but then starts to lose speech and/or social skills, typically between 15 and 30 months, and is subsequently diagnosed as affected by ASDs (Stefanatos 2008; Ozonoff *et al.* 2008).

While there is increasing evidence of the existence of a subtype of ASDs with the typical features of "regressive autism" (Werner and Dawson 2005), its aetiology is far from clear. It has been proposed that a wide spectrum of environmental factors could potentially be involved in this regression (mainly toxic agents and vaccine injuries) (Stefanatos 2008). However, although the controversy has escalated since the earliest reports of a possible link with vaccines began to surface in the 1980s, data on this are not conclusive (Richler *et al.* 2006). There are further studies being carried out to test if a subgroup of children with regressive autism has an autoimmune dysfunction (Rogers 2004).

Physiological Brain Asymmetries and Development of Cerebral Hemispheres

A fundamental property of brain organization, which was identified more than forty years ago (Milner 1971) and has been continuously confirmed since, is the presence of structural and functional asymmetries between the hemispheres (Toga and Thompson 2003). Normal children and adults have an asymmetry of the temporal lobes, already detectable in the fetal brain, where the left temporal lobe is larger than the right one (Galaburda *et al.* 1978). Recent data suggest that multiple genetic or environmental mechanisms control cerebral lateralization, involving asymmetric gene expression patterns in multiple forebrain structures during early human fetal development (Liu *et al.* 2009).

The left and right hemispheres develop at different rates, and with different postnatal onset times. During the first period of life, there is a physiological hyperactivity of the right cerebral hemisphere compared to the left one; the left seems to evolve later through a sort of "reciprocal regulation". This is evident in the parieto-temporal region, with the right hemisphere dominating the left one, before there is a switch from right to left dominance during the third year of life (Thatcher *et al.* 1987). This is also the time of a shift from right to left dominance of the sensorimotor region (Chiron *et al.* 1997).

In 2-to-3 month old infants, functional asymmetry with left-hemispheric dominance has been observed for language processing (Dehaene-Lambertz *et al.* 2002). However, the right hemisphere is involved in language development as well. Perani *et al.* (2010) demonstrated that, ontogenetically, infants' first steps into language are based on prosodic information, and that musical communication in early childhood (such as maternal language) plays a major role for emotional, cognitive, and social development in children; in this process, the contribution of the right hemisphere is predominant. A hemispheric functional asymmetry for music is also present at birth, with clear right hemisphere predominance in the primary, secondary, and higher order auditory cortices. Grossmann *et al.* (2010) showed that, in 7-month-old infants, hearing emotional prosody resulted in increased responses in a voice-sensitive region in the right hemisphere. Moreover, a region in the right inferior frontal cortex, believed to serve evaluative functions in the adult brain, showed particular sensitivity to prosodic specificities induced by a state of happiness in the speaker.

ASDs, Attention Deficit Hyperactivity Disorder (ADHD) and Cerebral Asymmetry

In ASDs, an altered cerebral asymmetry has been consistently shown: a loss of the language-related frontal cortex asymmetry (De Fossé *et al.* 2004); reduced left lateralization of cerebral dominance (Boddaert *et al.* 2003); reduced left hemisphere activation (Gendry Meresse *et al.* 2005) with apparent compensatory right hemisphere hyperactivation (Flagg *et al.* 2005); reduced Broca's area activation when listening to language or trying to speak (Müller *et al.* 1998); and increased right frontal activation compared to healthy controls during a language task requiring mental state attribution (Takeuchi *et al.* 2004). Moreover, an increased prevalence of left-handedness has been reported (Dane and Balci 2007) in ASD children with early detected language deficiency (Escalante-Mead *et al.* 2003). In short, a pattern of left hemisphere hypoactivity and right hemisphere hyperactivity has been consistently shown in patients with ASDs. Geschwind and Galaburda (2005a-c) advanced a theory of the development of anomalous dominance and its biological associations; this theory is based on the argument that increased fetal testosterone levels modify neural development, and can explain many aspects of cerebral lateralization and its relation to some neuro-psychiatric disorders, including autism and ASDs in general.

The importance of cerebral asymmetry has also been considered for other neuro-psychiatric conditions. A recent study showed BAIAP2 (Ribasés *et al.* 2009), a gene asymmetrically expressed in the two cerebral hemispheres (Sun *et al.* 2005), is involved in attention deficit hyperactivity disorder (ADHD), a neuropsychiatric condition which highly overlaps ASDs in both clinical and epidemiological terms (Murray 2010; Rommelse *et al.* 2010). Moreover, maternal depressive symptoms during pregnancy and critical life events are associated with an increased risk of child non-right-handedness and mixed handedness

(Rodriguez and Waldenström 2008). Mixed-handedness, in turn, is associated with atypical cerebral lateralization, but also with neuropsychiatric problems, including ADHD symptoms and difficulties with language and scholastic performance (Rodriguez *et al.* 2010). It is also worth mentioning that, from a clinical and rehabilitative point of view, it has been suggested that ASD children may show some improvement before the age of 5 (Bonaccorsi 1984). This phenomenon has been theoretically linked to the acquisition of definitive hemispheric dominance (Bonaccorsi 2008).

Hypothesis: Defective Evolution of Cerebral Laterality in Regressive Autism

As mentioned above, regressive autism is generally considered to be caused by environmental factors occurring in infancy and inducing a significant alteration in the brains developmental trajectory. An alternative explanation of regressive autism can be proposed, involving altered cerebral asymmetry. According to the present hypothesis, during the first months of life children with ASDs are able to reach a basic language and social development, due to good right hemisphere development (which is supposed to be fundamental for child neurological and psychological development in the first 12-18 months of life). When the left hemisphere should become functionally dominant in language development, however, the neuroanatomical and functional deficits of language-related fronto-temporal areas found in ASDs subjects become evident, and block the normal development of communicative and social functioning. As has already been shown in the case of congenital agenesis of the corpus callosum (a disorder of prosencephalic development for which an association with ASDs has been identified (Chiappedi and Bejor 2010)), the interaction between the two hemispheres is fundamental for higher order neuropsychological functions (Turk *et al.* 2010), which are possible only if a sufficiently and efficiently developed connectivity is present (Paul *et al.* 2007). In ASDs, the inadequate communication and interaction between the two hemispheres could explain the loss of already acquired skills, since the left hemisphere would not acquire its "physiological" role, the right hemisphere would not lose its functional dominance, and "normal" neural connectivity and circuitry would not develop. This is consistent with the peculiar cortical activation patterns seen in children with ASDs (Minshew and Keller 2010), who have a reliance on visual mediation even for neuropsychological tasks usually performed using different strategies, especially in children with higher global cognitive functioning (Sahyoun *et al.* 2010).

Conclusion and Future Directions

The present hypothesis predicts that an alteration in the normal development of the functional balance between the two hemispheres should be present in ASD children: brain studies with neurophysiological and/or functional imaging techniques could be used to investigate this, assuming that operational criteria to separate "regressive autism" from other ASDs could be defined and applied (to prevent confusion with findings already obtained in ASDs subjects such as those by Lazarev *et al.* (2010)). Moreover, the basic dysfunction supporting right-left hemisphere unbalancing should be evaluated. This unbalancing could be due to hypoactivity of the left hemisphere, hyperactivity of the right hemisphere, a lack of reciprocal modulation, or a mix of the three. According to this hypothesis, regressive autism can be conceptualized as the ultimate phenotypic result of a process beginning at an early stage of brain development, and involving multiple genetic or environmental mechanisms that control cerebral lateralization.

References

Amaral, D.G. *et al.* (2008) Neuroanatomy of autism. *Trends in Neurosciences*, 31, pp. 137-145.

American Psychiatric Association (2000) *Diagnostic and Statistical Manual of Mental Disorders, 4th Edition, Text Revised.* Washington DC: American Psychiatric Association.

Andrews, N. *et al.* (2002) Recall bias, MMR, and autism. *Archives of Disease in Childhood*, 87, pp. 493-494.

Boddaert, N. *et al.* (2003) Perception of complex sounds: abnormal pattern of cortical activation in autism. *American Journal of Psychiatry*, 160, pp. 2057-2060.

Bonaccorsi, M.T. (1984) Catamnesi critica dell'approccio all'autismo infantile. *Giornale di Neuropsichiatria dell'Età Evolutiva*, 3, pp. 511-527.

Bonaccorsi, M.T. (2007) Il trattamento del bambino psicotico. In: Fava, A. (ed) *Il Trattamento del Bambino Psicotico e Altre Esperienze di Psicoterapia*. Milan: Edizioni Anfora, pp. 9-30.

Bonaccorsi, M.T. (2008) *La Psicoterapia Analitica del Bambino Organico, Edizione Riveduta e Ampliata*. Milan: Edizioni Anfora.

Chiappedi, M. and Bejor, M. (2010) Corpus callosum agenesis and rehabilitative treatment. *Italian Journal of Pediatrics*, 36, doi: 10.1186/1824-7288-36-64.

Chiappedi, M. *et al.* (2010) Autism and classification systems: a study of 84 children. *Italian Journal of Pediatrics*, 36, doi: 10.1186/1824-7288-36-10.

Chiron, C. *et al.* (1997) The right brain hemisphere is dominant in human infants. *Brain*, 120, pp. 1057-1065.

Dane, S. and Balci, N. (2007) Handedness, eyedness and nasal cycle in children with autism. *International Journal of Developmental Neuroscience*, 25, pp. 223-226.

De Fossé, L. *et al.* (2004) Language-association cortex asymmetry in autism and specific language impairment. *Annals of Neurology*, 56, pp. 757-766.

Dehaene-Lambertz, G. *et al.* (2002) Functional neuroimaging of speech perception in infants. *Science*, 298, pp. 2013- 2015.

Escalante-Mead, P.R. *et al.* (2003) Abnormal brain lateralization in high-functioning autism. *Journal of Autism and Developmental Disorders*, 33, pp. 539-543.

Flagg, E.J. *et al.* (2005) Language lateralization development in children with autism: insights from the late field magnetoencephalogram. *Neuroscience Letters*, 386, pp. 82-87.

Galaburda, A.M. *et al.* (1978) Right-left asymmetrics in the brain. *Science*, 199, pp. 852–856.

Gendry Meresse, I. *et al.* (2005) Autism severity and temporal lobe functional abnormalities. *Annals of Neurology*, 58, pp. 466-469.

Geschwind, N. and Galaburda, A.M. (1985a) Cerebral lateralization. Biological mechanisms, associations, and pathology: I. A hypothesis and a program for research. *Archives of Neurology*, 42, pp. 428-459.

Geschwind, N. and Galaburda, A.M. (1985b) Cerebral lateralization. Biological mechanisms, associations, and pathology: II. A hypothesis and a program for research. *Archives of Neurology*, 42, pp. 521-552.

Geschwind, N. and Galaburda, A.M. (1985c) Cerebral lateralization. Biological mechanisms, associations, and pathology: III. A hypothesis and a program for research. *Archives of Neurology*, 42, pp. 634-654.

Grossmann, T. *et al.* (2010) The developmental origins of voice processing in the human brain. *Neuron*, 65, pp. 852-858.

Hughes, J.R. (2009) Update on autism: a review of 1300 reports published in 2008. *Epilepsy and Behavior*, 16, pp. 569-589.

Johnson, C.P. and Myers, S.M. (2007) Identification and evaluation of children with autism spectrum disorders. *Pediatrics*, 120, pp. 1183-1215.

Lazarev, V.V. *et al.* (2010) Interhemispheric asymmetry in EEG photic driving coherence in childhood autism. *Clinical Neurophysiology,* 121, pp. 145-152.

Liu, H. *et al.* (2009) Evidence from intrinsic activity that asymmetry of the human brain is controlled by multiple factors. *Proceedings of the National Academy of Sciences*, 106, pp. 20499-20503.

Milner, B. (1971) Interhemispheric differences in the localization of psychological processes in man. *British Medical Bulletin*, 27, pp. 272-277.

Minshew, N.J. and Keller, T.A. (2010) The nature of brain dysfunction in autism: functional brain imaging studies. *Current Opinions in Neurology*, 23, pp. 124-130.

Müller, R.A. *et al.* (1998) Impairment of dentato-thalamo-cortical pathway in autistic men: language activation data from positron emission tomography. *Neuroscience Letters*, 245, pp. 1-4.

Murray, M.J. (2010) Attention-deficit/hyperactivity disorder in the context of autism spectrum disorders. *Current Psychiatry Reports*, 12, pp. 382-388.

Ozonoff, S. *et al.* (2008) The onset of autism: patterns of symptom emergence in the first years of life. *Autism Research*, 1, pp. 320-328.

Paul, L.K. *et al.* (2007) Agenesis of the corpus callosum: genetic, developmental and functional aspects of connectivity. *Nature Reviews Neuroscience*, 8, pp. 287 -299.

Perani, D. *et al.* (2010) Functional specializations for music processing in the human newborn brain. *Proceedings of the National Academy of Sciences of the United States of America*, 107, pp. 4758-4763.

Persico, A.M. and Bourgeron, T. (2006) Searching for ways out of the autism maze: genetic, epigenetic and environmental clues. *Trends in Neurosciences*, 29, pp. 349-358.

Ribasés, M. *et al.* (2009) Case-control study of six genes asymmetrically expressed in the two cerebral hemispheres: association of BAIAP2 with attention-deficit/hyperactivity disorder. *Biological Psychiatry*, 66, pp. 926-934.

Richler, J. *et al.* (2006) Is there a regressive phenotype of Autism Spectrum Disorder associated with the measles-mumps-rubella vaccine? A CPEA study. *Journal of Autism and Developmental Disorders*, 36, pp. 299-316.

Rodriguez, A. *et al.* (2010) Mixed-Handedness is linked to mental health problems in children and adolescents. *Pediatrics*, 125, pp. 340-348.

Rodriguez, A. and Waldenström, U. (2008) Fetal origins of child non-right-handedness and mental health. *Journal of Child Psychology and Psychiatry*, 49, pp. 967-976.

Rogers, S.J. (2004) Developmental regression in autism spectrum disorders. *Mental Retardation and Developmental Disabilities Research Reviews*, 10, pp. 139-143.

Rommelse, N.N. *et al.* (2010) Shared heritability of attention-deficit/hyperactivity disorder and autism spectrum disorder. *European Child and Adolescent Psychiatry*, 19, pp. 281-295.

Rutter, M. (2005) Incidence of autism spectrum disorders: changes over time and their meaning. *Acta Paediatrica*, 94, pp. 2-15.

Sahyoun, C.P. *et al.* (2010) Neuroimaging of the functional and structural networks underlying visuospatial vs. linguistic reasoning in high-functioning autism. *Neuropsychologia*, 48, pp. 86-95.

Stefanatos, G.A. (2008) Regression in autistic spectrum disorders. *Neuropsychology Review*, 18, pp. 305-319.

Sun, T. *et al.* (2005) Early asymmetry of gene transcription in embryonic human left and right cerebral cortex. *Science*, 308, pp. 1794-1798.

Takeuchi, M. *et al.* (2004) Difference of signal change by a language task on autistic patients using functional MRI. *Journal of Investigative Medicine*, 51, pp. 59-62.

Thatcher, R. W. *et al.* (1987) Human cerebral hemispheres develop at different rates and ages. *Science*, 236, pp. 1110-1113.

Toga, A.W. and Thompson, P.M. (2003) Mapping brain asymmetry. *Nature Reviews - Neuroscience*, 4, pp. 37-48.

Turk, A.A. *et al.* (2010) Social narratives in agenesis of the corpus callosum: linguistic analysis of the Thematic Apperception Test. *Neuropsychologia*, 48, pp. 43-50.

Werner, E. and Dawson, G. (2005) Validation of the phenomenon of autistic regression using home videotapes. *Archives of General Psychiatry*, 62, pp. 889-895.

In: Hypotheses in Clinical Medicine
Editors: M.M. Shoja, P.S. Agutter et al.

ISBN: 978-1-62257-276-2

Chapter 18

The Human Sensory Processing Sensitivity: Biological Implications for Introversion, Submission and Creativity

Carlos V. Rizzo-Sierra*
SVYASA, Yoga University, Division of Yoga and Physical Sciences,
ICMR Center for Advanced Research in Yoga & Neurophysiology, Bangalore, India
Neuronikas Research Group, Advanced Biomedical Research Center,
Bogota, Colombia

Abstract

High sensitivity (HS) is a recently proposed psychological trait characterizing approximately 15-20% of the human population; it is also present in higher animals. HS individuals are described as processing information deeply and also reflecting on it deeply. Having such an active nervous system makes the HS person (HSP) prone to a more responsive arousal system in the brain. On the other hand, having an active nervous system allows larger amounts of sensory information to be processed simultaneously by the brain, making the HSP excellent at picking up subtle environmental details and cues. The hypothesis presented in this chapter concerns how the brain of the HSP is configured; it is important to develop appreciation and empathy for the minority of humans who present this HS trait, which, it is suggested, is correlated with qualities such as higher perception, consciousness, inventiveness, imagination and creativity. In addition, it is important to realize that the HS trait presents enormous but unexploited potential for developments within society. Hence, this trait should be better understood and should be scientifically studied in detail without social prejudice.

---

* E-mail: rizzo.sierra.c.v@gmail.com.

Introduction

High sensitivity (HS) is a recently proposed psychological trait characterizing approximately 15-20% of the human population; it is also present in higher animals (Aron 2003). HS persons (HSPs) are described as processing information deeply and also reflecting on it deeply (Ketay *et al.* 2007). Having such an active nervous system makes the HSP prone to a more responsive arousal system in the brain, especially after exposure to bright lights, dense and chaotic environments, loud noise or just strong smells (Aron 2003). On the other hand, having an active nervous system allows higher amounts of sensory information to be processed simultaneously by the brain, making HSPs excellent at picking up subtle environmental details and cues. This heightened sensitivity leads to sensory overloads, maximizing brain activity and making HSPs feel easily worn out, overwhelmed and exhausted, since they seem to sense every single detail in their interactions with the environment (Aron 1997; Aron *et al.* 2004). In order to recover from this sensory overload they require more quiet time alone daily than individuals who do not show this trait, suggesting a greater requirement for sleeping recovery hours (Aron 1997, 1999; Aron *et al.* 2004). On the other hand, it is suggested that HS is correlated to qualities such as higher perception, consciousness, inventiveness, imagination and creativity (Aron 2003). HSPs readily perceive and experience the external moods of people around them, so they tend to avoid encountering negative situations and emotions. Internal cognitive processes such as thoughts, fantasies or just ideas stimulate the HSP nervous system much more than the non-HSP system. Certain situations such as talking to strangers, hunger, worry, anxiety, lack of sleep, and especially anger (from outside or inside), elicit a high nervous response from people with the trait.

Aron (2010) and Jagiellowicz *et al.* (2011) have shown the connection between HS trait and higher sensory processing sensitivity. These papers (Aron 2010; Jagiellowicz *et al.* 2011) demonstrated that the brains of those with higher sensory processing sensitivity (SPS) behave differently from those who do not present higher SPS. Specifically, different neural responses occurred for cultural difference neuroimaging tasks (Aron 2010), and for neural responses to changes in visual scenes (Jagiellowicz *et al.* 2011); the latter also during neuroimaging tasks. However, none of these studies has proposed formal mechanisms for the purpose of characterizing the brains of those with higher SPS. Therefore, this chapter describes an attempt to propose in terms of current neuroscience how the brain of the HSP is configured. Studies of animal behavior are introduced in order to support some of the ideas presented. Moreover, the biological and behavioral implications for the HS trait such as creativity are briefly discussed.

Hypothesis

I. HSP Connectivity Pattern, Synthesis and Neurotransmission

It is proposed that a more complex pattern of connectivity present in HSP brains is responsible for increased sensory information input and deeper sensory processing. At the same time, the storage and retrieval of information (working memory) works synthetically, ensuring deep and slow evaluation of the sensory and cognitive processes on the basis of past experience, identifying a common pattern, difference or novelty. This higher connectivity pattern is mediated by different concentrations of the HSP brain's neurotransmitters (acetylcholine, norepinephrine, dopamine, and serotonin) from those in non-HSP brains. These neurotransmitters are responsible for modulating arousal in the HSP while promoting more detailed information processing by connecting the relevant brain areas in a more complex and holistic way than in the non-HSP. In addition, it is reasonable to suppose that the more complex connectivity pattern between the HSP's sensory information input and memory interferes somewhat with higher cognitive processes, making these processes slower as the cost of heightened sensory function.

II. HSP Pain, Sensory Thresholds and Mirror Neurons

It is proposed that the overall HSP nervous system presents smaller rheobase values than the non-HSP, which means the transmembrane voltage threshold for HSP is smaller than non-HSP. Hence, there is less tolerance to pain and stimulation, since evoked potentials are present with minimal sensory or nerve excitation. In this regard, the ability of (for instance) an autistic person in reading minds and intentions will show impaired functioning of the mirror neuron system compared to that of an HSP. The heightened activity in this mirror neuron system in the HSP accounts for the higher levels of social empathy, reading minds, and intentions.

III. HSP Decision-making Process, Frontal Lobe Interaction and Amygdala

It is suggested here that during decision-making processes in HSPs, the frontal lobe is more active than in a non-HSP, while the amygdala activity is relatively low. In this regard, it is expected that the HSP would be biologically less likely to inflict significant pain and suffering on other human beings since he would feel it strongly himself. In contrast, humans who present low levels of social empathy are more likely to be involved in aggressive or antisocial behavior without noticing it, since they would not be strongly disturbed by experiencing deep emotions and feelings as the HSP experiences them. Furthermore, the fact that the HSP is highly aware of the needs of others could explain his/her highly conscious and thoughtful behavioral tendencies towards society. The HSP is most likely to be a natural-born healer, artisan, advisor, guardian and scientist.

IV. HSP Genetics

It is proposed that the HS trait is inherited, and it is displayed from infancy as highly reactive (irritable) babies that grow into inhibited children (Kagan *et al.* 2004) who develop into highly sensitive teenagers and adults.

Validation

Many different techniques and procedures will be proposed for validating the hypothesis, but it is understood that testing all the procedures would require a long time. However, carrying out just few of the following procedures is expected to validate the current hypothesis in part.

I. The first part of the hypothesis, regarding the HSP connectivity pattern, synthesis and neurotransmission, could be corroborated by implementing recent functional neuroimaging techniques to make comparative functional connectivity analyses between the brains of healthy HS and non-HS subjects. The tasks to be presented must include sufficient sensory stimulation, auditory and visual, mixed with cognitive functions to be performed by the subjects. These tasks are carried out inside functional imaging machines to assess the above-mentioned differences in brain activation (performance). One option is to employ functional magnetic resonance imaging (fMRI) for those studies. More activity, for a longer time, and greater connectivity, are expected for the HSP than the non-HSP, in regions involved in sensory perception, processing and memory connected to regions involved in higher cognitive functions. According to the hypothesis, the higher cognitive function regions are less connected to brain regions related to sensory information perception, processing and memory in the non-HSP than the HSP. In addition, differences in the concentrations of neurotransmitters - acetylcholine, norepinephrine, dopamine, and serotonin - between HSP and non-HSP brains could be assessed by a combination of magnetic resonance and recent infrared spectroscopy techniques. This spectroscopic assessment would be performed while the HSP and non-HSP carry out the above-mentioned tasks.

II. The second part of the hypothesis, concerning HSP pain, sensory thresholds and mirror neurons, could be corroborated by a study comparing physical pain tolerance and sensory evoked potentials between HSPs and non–HSPs; the prediction is that the former will show lower thresholds. The transmembrane voltage threshold is smaller for HSPs; hence, there is less tolerance to pain and stimulation given that evoked potentials are present with minimal sensory or nerve excitation. This also explains the natural tendency of HSPs to be easily over-stimulated. An additional sensitivity assessment involving functional brain studies of human responses to visual and auditory stimuli of deep emotions is possible. This assessment includes videos portraying extreme emotions such as pain and anger presented to an HSP and a non-HSP inside the fMRI machine (Rizzo-Sierra *et al.* 2008) through a projector. Different and more active patterns of brain activation are expected for the HSP during such tasks. This difference is expected in the emotional processing region of the brain, thus explaining the strong empathetic effect that deep emotions from others have on an HSP. As discussed in the previous section, an autistic person (for example) is expected to show less activation than the normal non-HSP, in contrast to the HSP. The HSP's excessive activity in this mirror neuron system accounts for higher levels of social empathy, reading minds, and intentions. In addition, videos inside fMRI (Rizzo-Sierra *et al.* 2008) presenting sensory system stimulation - for example, a person being knocked down by a heavy object - will elicit more activity in the corresponding mirror neuron system (premotor and sensorimotor cortices) of an HSP than in an autistic person.

III. The third part of the hypothesis, concerning decision making processes, frontal lobe interaction and amygdala, could be corroborated by employing (functional) cognitive neuroimaging experiments targeting decision-making brain areas. Higher frontal lobe activation and lower amygdala activation in the HSP than in the non-HSP is related to less impulsive decision-making by the former. In addition, physiological arousal responses, such as heart rate and sweating, should be recorded during this experiment.

IV. The last part of the hypothesis, concerning HSP genetics, could be tested by extending the experiments described above to babies, children, teenagers and adults.

Discussion

Empirical findings in more than 100 species, ranging from insects to mammals, suggest that personalities are a widespread phenomenon in the animal kingdom. Individuals differ profoundly from each other in their behavior, and these differences are often consistent over time and extend to various contexts. In birds, fish, and rodents, for example, some individuals are consistently more aggressive than others, and aggressive individuals differ from non-aggressive individuals in many other respects such as foraging behavior or the exploration of novel environments. In this regard, the defining trait for dominance in all animal species is lack of fear or greater confidence, and for submissiveness it is fear or lower confidence (Kagan *et al.* 2004).

It is clearly seen that aggressive and non-aggressive male mice react distinctly to a changing social environment. Aggressive males fulfill their task fairly, in a routine-like fashion, and do not react to any change; this contrasts to the behavior displayed by non-aggressive ones. Specifically, in both mice and rats (Benus *et al.* 1987; Rizzo-Sierra *et al.* 2011c), individuals differ substantially in their responsiveness to environmental changes in a maze task. Some individuals quickly form a routine, are not influenced by minor environmental changes, and perform relatively badly when confronted with a changing maze configuration. Others do not form a routine, are strongly influenced by minor changes, and perform relatively well when confronted with changing maze configurations (Wolf *et al.* 2008). The finding that humans and other primates differ in their susceptibilities to environmental influences (Aron 1997; Belsky *et al.* 2007; Sih *et al.* 2004) might also be interpreted along these lines.

For instance, in rodents, after many hours of not receiving food and when the location of the food is changed in a maze, the dominant male mouse goes impulsively though the maze for the food without reacting to any change or novelty; whereas the submissive one goes slowly through the maze to the new food location, watching this new location carefully for few minutes before attempting to approach it. In this regard, the submissive mouse seems more cautious but much less impulsive (Koolhaas *et al.* 2010). Therefore, it is suggested that the behavior of aggressive males is mainly controlled by intrinsic factors, whereas in non-aggressive males it is more dependent on external factors (Benus *et al.* 1987; Koolhaas *et al.* 2010; Proppe *et al.* 2011).

For example, male mice born in unstable, unpredictable environments would develop submissiveness at an early age as an energy-saving strategy, displaying special adaptative characteristics such as smaller and less mature body frames. Further, the development of secondary male characteristics would be delayed (Rizzo-Sierra 2011a). Similar behavior would be expected in rats (Benus *et al.* 2011). In this context, unstable and unpredictable environments are those where food supplies are scarce and fluctuating and where the social order is also changing, sometimes characterized by war, conflict and violent changes. In human terms, it is closely related to catastrophes and war-times and great social changes. It is plausible that more submissive than dominant animals are born under these conditions, since the sperm and ovum conditions at the time of conception, the condition within the uterus, the food and lifestyle of the mother during pregnancy and the nature of the elements constituting the fetus would be such that submissive traits would prevail, guaranteeing much easier adaptation to a rapidly changing environment (Rizzo-Sierra *et al.* 2011c).

Furthermore, submissive animals must display the high degree of creativity needed to survive in such unstable and unpredictable environments. In this case we relate such environments to the ones found in some newly-developing rural areas under conflict; in contrast, in more stable environments such as those found in developed urban areas with no conflicts foreseen, it would be more profitable to be born as a dominant animal since the environment barely changes, supporting the less adaptive nature of the dominant animal (Benus *et al.* 1987). Furthermore, for this last condition, the dominant animal cannot properly sense subtle changes whereas the submissive animal can and does, allowing the latter to adapt more easily to rapidly changing environments (Benus *et al.* 1987; Proppe *et al.* 2011; Verbeek *et al.* 1994).

I point out that under these extreme environmental conditions, both dominant and submissive animals are born. However, it is suggested that the probability of being born dominant or submissive does depend on the environment. Finally, such dominant or submissive adaptation might also support subsequent genetic changes. As stable environments with fewer conflicts increase in the world, dominant individuals with very low sensory processing sensitivity may experience selective advantages over their submissive creative counterparts, while also increasing the reproduction rate, given that more dominant males are available. Some evidence for such directional selection is provided by recent studies reporting that only approximately 20% of the population nowadays is HS, non-aggressive or submissive, with heightened sensory processing sensitivity and higher creativity (Aron 2003).

The fact that behavioral measures, metabolic rate, immunological function and response to stressful environments differ between submissive and dominant animals supports our view (Audet *et al.* 2009; Constantini *et al.* 2008). For instance, Henry and Stephens (Koolhaas *et al.* 2010) were the first to suggest that individual variations in aggression might express ways of actively coping with environmental challenges in general. The consistency of aggression as an expression of coping style across situations can best be demonstrated in tests that allow the animal a choice of different response patterns (Koolhaas *et al.* 2010). For example, in the defensive burying paradigm (Koolhaas *et al.* 2010), animals are confronted with an electrified probe inserted into their home cage. In response to a brief contact with the shock probe, the animal can either actively bury the probe under the bedding of their cage (dominant type) or show immobility and passively avoid the electrified probe (submissive type). Both response patterns can be considered as successful coping, because in neither case will the animal ever touch the probe again. More importantly, the above-described characteristics and behaviors of animals resemble findings reported in humans (Kagan *et al.* 2004; Aron *et al.* 2010; Herbener *et al.* 1989) and are referred to as ectomorphic body type or somatotype for the submissive animal (Rizzo-Sierra 2011a; Sheldon 1940, 1970).

In detail, highly reactive human babies show higher heart rates than others from the time they are in utero (Kagan *et al.* 2004). Moreover, after the fourth month of age, these babies display stronger motor responses to sensory perceptions such as objects, noise and odors (Kagan *et al.* 2004). When they are placed in an unknown environment they tend to cry more than other babies. After their first year of age they continue to show a higher than average heart rate when confronted with new situations (Kagan *et al.* 2004). At the same time, brain studies show more activity in the right hemisphere and the vegetative nervous system for these babies (Kagan *et al.* 2004). It is known that the amygdala in such babies is over–active; in this sense the amygdala is responsible for their hyperarousal (Kagan *et al.* 2004). In line with this, it is already known that highly reactive and irritable babies become inhibited children (Kagan *et al.* 2004) harboring the HS trait that is displayed in teenage and adult years (Rizzo-Sierra 2011a), which suggests that this trait is also inherited and displayed at a later stage in life. Moreover, higher levels of salivary cortisol have been found in inhibited children both at home and in the laboratory (Herbener *et al.* 1989). This profile implies a lower threshold of reactivity to unfamiliarity in limbic sites, especially the amygdala and its projections to the hypothalamus (Herbener *et al.* 1989). One possible basis for the lower thresholds in the amygdala is a higher level of central norepinephrine (NE). In sensory areas, NE enhances the signal to noise ratio and should lower sensory thresholds (Herbener *et al.* 1989).

Now, considering the five main trait dimensions in humans (big five), trait characteristics in animals are likely to be multidimensional as well. Research in this area is still relatively young and underdeveloped. In an extensive review of the available animal literature, five trait characteristics have been suggested (Koolhaas *et al.* 2010), some of which seem to be in line with the two dimensions suggested here: dominant and submissive. Clearly, this issue requires further experimental study using multidimensional scaling methods on animals tested under a wide range of situations (Koolhaas *et al.* 2010).

It should be remembered that the concept of uninhibited-low reactive and inhibited-high reactive somatotypes (Aron 2003; Kagan *et al.* 2004; Rizzo-Sierra 2011a) came from William H. Sheldon (Sheldon 1940, 1970). He proposed that the human physique is classified according to the relative contribution of three fundamental elements or somatotypes according to the widely-known three germ layers of embryonic development, the *endoderm*, which develops into the digestive tract, the *mesoderm* that becomes muscle, heart, and blood vessels, and the *ectoderm* that forms the skin and nervous system (Sheldon 1940, 1970). Specifically, the ectomorphic somatotype found in people with long and thin muscles/limbs and low fat storage is usually referred to as slim. These people tend to be artistic, sensitive, apprehensive and introverted (Sheldon 1940, 1970). They also require more sleep hours than other body types to get energetically recharged. Owing to their physical frame they are not suitable for heavy physical work or exhausting long exercises (Rizzo-Sierra 2011a; Frawley *et al.* 2001). If in balance, they are vibrant, enthusiastic, clear and alert of mind, flexible, imaginative, sensitive, talkative, and quick to respond (Rizzo-Sierra 2011a; Frawley *et al.* 2001); however, if out of balance, they tend to display excessive worry, fear and anxiety behavior, to be depressed, with restless mind, light sleep, tendency to overexert, fatigued, constipated and underweight, among other characteristics.

Interestingly, the traditional medicine of India comments on the so-called Vata somatotype (Rizzo-Sierra 2011a; Frawley *et al.* 2001), which shares similar characteristics with the ectomorphic type described by western medicine: higher processing sensitivity, introversion and creativity (Sheldon 1940, 1970). This ectomorphic or submissive, cautious trait is the one I correlate with higher prevalence, or in other words, greater frequency at birth, in developing rural areas under conflict, since other (dominant) males being born in unstable and rapidly changing environments would additionally imply a stronger need for reproduction, a very expensive task in an uncertain context such as the developing rural area under conflict. In contrast, the predictable environment or developed urban area with a stable source of food, energy required for growth, reproduction, and raising offspring could be sustained from the environment itself; this would make the mesomorphic trait, described as the pitta somatotype, which is correlated with dominance (Rizzo-Sierra 2011a; Frawley *et al.* 2001), more common and suitable in such geographical areas.

Creativity is a trait that has recently gained attention in human research. It has been associated with low testosterone levels in humans (Hassler 1991). In addition, creativity has been related to heightened sensory perception, and it has been especially linked with low latent inhibition when combined with above average intelligence (Carson *et al.* 2003; Rizzo-Sierra 2011b). Therefore, strong correlations among ectomorphic body types, higher immune system reactivity, heightened sensory perception, higher sensitivity trait and creativity are very likely (Rizzo-Sierra 2011a, 2011b).

In humans, the ectomorphic type (Rizzo-Sierra 2011a, 2011b) resembles a younger body frame, not fully developed and more delicate than the mesomorphic type. This ectomorphic body type (vata) displays more cautious and submissive behavior; it is more sensitive and perceptive to the environment, and more likely to develop allergies and introversion (Herbener *et al.* 1989). However, it seems more agile and creative than the other two types, described as mesomorphic and endomorphic. It is reasonable to suggest that nature would not allow this body type to display aggressive tendencies, since the small and delicate body frame could not sustain fighting and winning most of the time; nature would allow a more appropriate biological response, to fly or escape, but certainly not to fight. The characteristics just described for this body type resemble the psychological aspects displayed by HSPs, high-reactive babies and inhibited children. From an evolutionary biology perspective, this type of human would at most times be the provider and caretaker and the one who raises children, but not often the male biologically chosen by females for mating and generation of those children. Furthermore, the ectomorphic type seems more suitable for living in warm environments, whereas the endomorphic type is more suitable for colder climates.

Moreover, specific nervous system configurations within the human body accounting for different temperaments and behaviors have been proposed (Kagan *et al.* 2004). Interestingly, inhibited children or high-reactive babies are more likely to possess a tall, lean body mass, narrow face and light blue eyes than uninhibited children (Aron *et al.* 2010; Herbener *et al.* 1989; Kagan *et al.* 2004); the latter are considered to be low-reactive. This striking similarity with the ectomorphic constitution might also suggest the most likely phenotype for HSPs (Aggarwal *et al.* 2010; Frawley *et al.* 2001; Sheldon 1940, 1970; Rizzo-Sierra 2011a, 2011b); in other words, the most common phenotype for humans with HS processing sensitivity and creativity.

Conclusion

It is very important to start taking into consideration the clear differences in human brain physiology among subjects when discussing human psychological traits such as introversion and higher sensory processing sensitivity. Understanding how the HSP brain operates could help elucidate proper treatment and therapy for low self-esteem maladies, depression and mental disorders that tend to be found especially in the male HS population (Liss *et al.* 2005). Finally, it is also appropriate and reasonable for any society to modify its biased perception of this HS trait, which is wrongly associated with weakness.

References

Aggarwal, S. *et al.* (2010). EGLN1 involvement in high-altitude adaptation revealed through genetic analysis of extreme constitution types defined in Ayurveda. *Proceedings of the National Academy of Sciences of the United States of America*, 107, pp. 18961-18966.

Aron, E. N. (1999) High sensitivity as one source of fearfulness and shyness. In Schmidt, L. A. and Schulkin, J. (eds) *Preliminary Research and Clinical Implications in Extreme Fear, Shyness and Social Phobia: Origins, Biological Mechanisms, and Clinical Outcomes*. New York: Oxford University Press. pp. 251-272.

Aron, E. N. (2003) *The Highly Sensitive Person (HSP): How to Thrive When the World Overwhelms You*. London: Element, An Imprint of Harper Collins Publishers.

Aron, E. N. (2004) Revisiting Jung's concept of innate sensitiveness. *Journal of Analytical Psychology*, 49, pp. 337-367.

Aron, E. N. and Aron, A. (1997) Sensory-Processing Sensitivity and Its Relation to Introversion and Emotionality. *Journal of Personality and Social Psychology*, 73, pp. 345-368.

Aron, A. *et al.* (2010) Temperament trait of sensory processing sensitivity moderates cultural differences in neural response. *Social, Cognitive and Affective Neuroscience*, 5, pp. 219-226.

Audet, M. C. and Anisman, H. (2009) Neuroendocrine and neurochemical impact of aggressive social interactions in submissive and dominant mice: implications for stress-related disorders. *International Journal of Neuropharmacology*, 23, pp. 1-12.

Belsky, J. *et al.* (2007) For better and for worse: Differential susceptibility to environmental influences. *Current Directions in Psychological Sciences*, 16, pp. 300-304.

Benus, R. F. *et al.* (1987) Individual differences in behavioural reaction to a changing environment in mice. *Behaviour*, 100, pp. 105-122.

Carson, S. H. *et al.* (2003) Decreased latent inhibition is associated with increased creative achievement in high-functioning individuals. *Journal of Personality and Social Psychology*, 85, pp. 499-506.

Costantini, D. *et al.* (2008) Aggressive and non-aggressive personalities differ in oxidative statusin selected lines of mice (Mus musculus). *Biology Letters* 4, pp. 119-122.

Frawley, D. and Ranade, S. (2001) *Ayurveda, Nature's Medicine*. New York: Lotus Press.

Hassler, M. (1991) Testosterone and musical talent. *Experimental and Clinical Endocrinology*, 98, pp. 89-98.

Herbener, E. S. *et al.* (1989) Shyness and olfactory threshold. *Personality and Individual Differences*, 10, pp. 1159-1163.

Jagiellowicz, J. *et al.* (2011) The trait of sensory processing sensitivity and neural responses to changes in visual scenes. *Social, Cognitive and Affective Neuroscience,* 6, pp. 38-47.

Kagan, J. and Snidman, N. (2004) *The Long Shadow of Temperament.* Cambridge, MA: Belknap Press.

Ketay, S. *et al.* (2007) The personality/temperament trait of high sensitivity: fMRI evidence for independence of cultural context in attentional processing. In: *Posters Presented at the 8th Annual Meeting of the Society for Personality and Social Psychology, Memphis, TN.*

Koolhaas, J. M. *et al.* (2010) Neuroendocrinology of coping styles: towards understanding the biology of individual variation. *Frontiers of Neuroendocrinology*, 31, pp. 307-321.

Liss, M. *et al.* (2005) Sensory processing sensitivity and its relation to parental bonding, anxiety, and depression. *Personality and Individual Differences,* 39, pp. 1429-1439.

Proppe, D. S. *et al.* (2011) Flexibility in animal signals facilitates adaptation to rapidly changing environments. *PLoS One*, 6, doi: 10.1371/journal.pone.0025413.

Rizzo-Sierra, C. V. *et al.* (2008) Acoustic fMRI noise: linear time-invariant model. *IEEE Transactions of Biomedical Engineering*, 55, pp. 2115-2123.

Rizzo-Sierra, C. V. (2011a) Ayurvedic genomics, constitutional psychology and endocrinology: the missing connection. *Journal of Alternative and Complementary Medicine*, 17, pp. 465-468.

Rizzo-Sierra, C. V. *et al.* (2011b) Highly sensitive trait and ectomorphism: another link on creativity and psychopathology. *Canadian Journal of Psychiatry*, 56, pp. 702-703.

Rizzo-Sierra C. V. *et al.* (2011c) Higher sensory processing sensitivity, introversion and ectomorphism: New biomarkers for human creativity in developing rural areas under conflict? *Journal of Neurosciences in Rural Practice*, in press.

Sheldon, W. H. (1940) *The Varieties of Human Physique: an Introduction to Constitutional Psychology*. New York: Harper.

Sheldon, W. H. (1970) *Atlas of Men*. New York: Macmillan.

Sih, A. *et al.* (2004) Behavioral syndromes: an integrative overview. *Quarterly Review of Biology*, 79, pp. 241-277.

Verbeek, M. E. M. *et al.* (1994) Consistent individual differences in early exploratory behavior of male great tits. *Animal Behavior*, 48, pp. 1113–1121.

Wolf, M. *et al.* (2008) Evolutionary emergence of responsive and unresponsive personalities. *Proceedings of the National Academy of Sciences of the United States of America*, 105, pp. 15825-15830.

In: Hypotheses in Clinical Medicine
Editors: M.M. Shoja, P.S. Agutter et al.

ISBN: 978-1-62257-276-2

Chapter 19

Are the Systemic Arterial Blood, Intracranial and Intraocular Pressures Co-regulated?

Mohammadali M. Shoja[1*], Alon Harris[2], Yochai Shoshani[2], R. Shane Tubbs[3], Brent Siesky[2], Christoph J. Griessenauer[1], Marios Loukas[4], Paul S. Agutter[5], Barbara M. Wirostko[6] and Aaron A. Cohen-Gadol[7]

[1]Division of Neurological Surgery, Department of Surgery, University of Alabama at Birmingham, Birmingham, Alabama, US, and Medical Philosophy and History Research Center, Tabriz University of Medical Sciences, Tabriz, Iran
[2]Department of Ophthalmology, Indiana University School of Medicine, Indianapolis, Indiana, US
[3]Pediatric Neurosurgery, Children's Hospital, Birmingham, Alabama, US
[4]Department of Anatomical Sciences, St. George's University, Grenada, West Indies
[5]Theoretical Medicine and Biology Group, Glossop, Derbyshire, UK
[6]Department of Ophthalmology, Moran Eye Center, University of Utah, Salt Lake City, Utah, US
[7]Goodman Campbell Brain and Spine, Department of Neurological Surgery, Indiana University, Indianapolis, Indiana, US

Abstract

In this chapter, the physiological maintenance of intracranial pressure (ICP) and intraocular pressure (IOP) and their pathophysiological aspects are presented with emphasis on glaucoma and head trauma as two conditions associated respectively with

* E-mail: shoja.m@gmail.com.

elavated IOP and ICP. At the end, emphasis is placed on the hypothesis that systemic arterial blood, intracranial, and intraocular pressures are co-regulated. It is known that the cerebral and ocular blood flows are autoregulated over a range of systemic blood pressures. When this autoregulation is impaired under pathological circumstances, ICP and IOP become functions of systemic blood pressure (SBP). Recent evidence indicates that a common vascular mechanism controls ICP, IOP and systemic arterial blood pressure even in healthy individuals. An improved understanding of the co-regulatory mechanism could help to elucidate various ocular and neurological pathologies and their relationship with the systemic vasculopathies. To what extent and under which circumstances SBP, ICP and IOP can affect each other should be explored in detail.

Introduction

In normal healthy individuals, intracranial pressure (ICP) is maintained by autoregulation of the cerebral vasculature, which helps control the balance between production and reabsorption of cerebrospinal fluid (CSF). A number of clinical conditions are associated with significant increases, or more rarely decreases, in ICP. It is therefore important to understand how ICP is regulated and to be able to measure it reliably; different measurement techniques have significant advantages and disadvantages. Analogously, intraocular pressure (IOP) is maintained by a balance between the secretion and drainage of aqueous humor, and abnormal values are associated with various pathological conditions, notably certain forms of glaucoma and/or ocular hypotony. Therefore, reliable measurement is clinically important, and several measurement techniques are available.

There is a close relationship between IOP and ICP, which has been explored only incidentally in the literature. Changes in ICP can affect ocular blood flow and consequently IOP because the CSF is separated from the intraocular fluid by a porous membrane, the lamina cribrosa. Changes in ICP due to excessive CSF production can also be directly visualized and assessed from within the ocular system. For example, a swollen optic nerve is a reliable sign of intracranial hypertension. An improved understanding of the relationship between IOP and ICP could elucidate the pathophysiology of both and potentially lead to improved treatment(s) for various conditions. This chapter focuses on the normal physiological maintenance and pathophysiological aspects of IOP and ICP and their relationships with the systemic arterial blood pressure. Emphasis is placed on the hypothesis that systemic arterial blood pressure, IOP and ICP are co-regulated. The potential implication of this co-regulatory mechanism is briefly discussed.

Intraocular Pressure (IOP)

IOP ranges between 10 and 20 mm Hg in normal individuals and is a function of aqueous humor dynamics and of episcleral venous pressure (Funk *et al.* 1985; Shiose and Kawase 1986; Bárány 1963; Green and Pederson 1972; Pederson and Green 1973; Pederson 1986; Bill 1973; Toris *et al.* 2002). Numerous systemic conditions, ocular conditions, and various external factors can affect "normal" IOP. IOP changes with a change in posture (Wuthrich 1976; Jorge *et al.* 2010; Prata *et al.* 2010) and exercise (Marcus 1970; Qureshi 1995;

Dickerman *et al.* 1999; Price *et al.* 2003; Risner *et al.* 2009). It decreases after walking (Leighton 1972) and various forms of exercise (Risner *et al.* 2009), though it is increased during weightlifting (Vieira *et al.* 2006). Physically fit subjects present with a lower IOP than less fit individuals (Qureshi 1996; Qureshi 1997; Risner *et al.* 2009). IOP can also be increased and/or decreased by ocular venous malformations, inflammatory disorders, genetic/hereditary factors, myopia, various ocular diseases such as uveitis and iritis, corotid insufficiency, certain drugs, and aging (Bhattacherjee 1980; Craig and Mackey 1999; Kaufman *et al.* 2007; Qureshi 1995; Potter and Rowland 1978; Wolfs *et al.* 1998).

Elevated IOP is one of the most important risk factors for glaucoma, a slowly progressive optic neuropathy. Other risk factors may include increased age, family history, and thinner central corneal thickness (Coleman and Miglior 2008) and low ocular perfusion pressure (Gugleta *et al.* 2012). Theoretical models have demonstrated that large eyes with greater axial length (i.e., myopia) are more vulnerable to the deleterious effects of IOP elevation (Cahane and Bartov 1992; Mark 2007). This is in agreement with a prior study of Leighton (1974) who, in a series of glaucoma cases, observed a tendency towards low-tension glaucoma and lower maximum IOP in patients with larger globes. Notably, the vitreous length was greater in eyes with low-tension glaucoma than in those with open angle glaucoma (Tomlinson and Leighton 1972). Moreover, larger globes could demonstrate evidence of glaucomatous optic neuropathy at relatively lower IOP.

Measurement of IOP and Inter-method Agreement

Following the introduction of hand-held transpalpebral and transcorneal impression tonometers by Graefe in 1862 and Weber in 1867 (see Knecht *et al.* 2011), Maklakoff invented a device to estimate IOP by applying a series of fixed weights on the cornea and measuring the size of the applanated, flattened area (as cited in Goldmann and Schmidt 1957). The Imbert-Fick law was later proposed to provide an explanation for this applanation tonometry (Goldmann and Schmidt 1957). Assuming that the liquid sphere is surrounded by an infinitely thin membrane, is flexible and has no inherent stiffness, and that no other forces act upon the sphere (e.g., surface tension), the Imbert-Fick law states that the pressure within the sphere (Ps) times the area flattened by an external force (Af) equals the applied external force (W), thus $W = Ps \times Af$ (Goldmann and Schmidt 1957; Harvey 2003). However, such assumptions are not fulfilled in the case of the eyeball. As Goldmann and Schmidt (1957) indicated, the cornea is of finite thickness and stiffness, and "the capillary force" created by the tear film violates the assumptions of the Imbert-Fick law. In an attempt to resolve these shortcomings, Goldmann and Schmidt (1957) proved that with a flattened area of 3 to 3.5 mm, the capillary and elastic forces balance each other in the normal cornea with a presumed thickness of 0.5 mm, and the changes in IOP secondary to the displacement of intraocular fluid become negligible. IOP measurements on 94 eyes by Goldman applanation tonometry (GAT), Maklakoff applanation tonometry, and indentation tonometry by the Schioetz method revealed that the mean GAT reading was higher than Schioetz or Maklakoff; the low coefficient of variation meant that GAT was the most accurate method, while the high coefficient of variation in the Maklakoff method made it less reliable (Atanassov and Konareva 2002).

So far, three main types of tonometry have been developed: applanation, indentation, and contour matching tonometry or dynamic contour tomometry (DCT) (Stamper 2010). DCT does not depend on the corneal thickness (Loewen and Tanna 2010) and mechanistically is not based on corneal applanation or indentation (Kanngiesser *et al.* 2005). Unlike Goldman and Schioetz, the IOP measured by DCT is not subject to bias owing to corneal physics and abnormalities (Stamper 2010). The different methods of tonometry have been reviewed by Garway-Heath *et al.* (2007), Kniestedt *et al.* (2008), ElMallah and Asrani (2008), Stamper (2010) and Loewen and Tanna (2010).

In a study carried out on enucleated human cadaver eyes, DCT readings were considerably closer, albeit slightly higher, to the real manometric pressure over a wide range of IOP (5 to 58 mmHg); GAT and pneumatonometry yielded consistently lower values (Kniestedt *et al.* 2004). Notably, within the IOP range of 10-25 mmHg, DCT had a mean deviation of +0.33 mmHg from real manometric pressure, GAT a mean deviation of -3.43 mmHg, and pneumatonometry a mean deviation of -2.97 mmHg. Examining 100 non-glaucomatous eyes, Schneider and Grehn (2006) reported a median difference of +1.8 between DCT and GTA readings, which could be related to the confounding effect of central corneal thickness on GTA measurements. However, in 100 eyes with glaucoma/ocular hypertension, Halkiadakis *et al.* (2009) found no significant association between measurement differences and central corneal thickness. They also found a mean difference of +2.1 mmHg between the GAT and DCT readings (Halkiadakis *et al.* 2009). Davies *et al.* (2006) measured IOP in normal, healthy subjects using the ICare rebound tonometer and GAT. They demonstrated that the former produced an insignificant positive bias of ~0.5 mmHg compared with GAT and a higher coefficient of variation on repeated measurements. Sahin *et al.* (2007) found a strong correlation between the readings of GAT and rebound tonometer in 61 glaucomatous eyes; however, the results of rebound tonometery were influenced by central corneal thickness considerably more than those of GAT (Sahin *et al.* 2007).

Compared to GAT, IOP readings from the ocular blood flow pneumotonometer and non-contact tonometer are more subject to the confounding effect of central corneal thickness (Gupta *et al.* 2006). Gupta *et al.* (2006) concluded that the non-contact tonometer and ocular blood flow pneumotonometer could be as reliable as the GAT over different IOP ranges in glaucomatous eyes, provided appropriate corrections were made for corneal thickness. A comparison of GAT with Pascal DCT, the Reichert ocular response analyzer (ORA), and the TonoPen XL tonometer in 118 normal and 76 keratoconic eyes by Mollan *et al.* (2008) demonstrated that the DCT and the ORA are the most appropriate tonometers for measuring IOP in cases of keratoconia. Corneal hysteresis and corneal resistance (calculated using ORA) were more likely to confound the results of applanation tonometry (such as GAT). In an elegant study on 62 healthy individuals, Hsu *et al.* (2009) revealed that IOP measured by GAT is confounded by mean keratometric power, central corneal thickness, and ocular pulse amplitude, DCT by lens thickness and mean keratometric power, and Tono-Pen by central corneal thickness and ocular pulse amplitude. Ultimately, in a consensus on IOP established by the World Glaucoma Association, it was stated that IOP measured by DCT and ORA is less affected by central corneal thickness than, sequentially, GAT measurements, non-contact tonometry, and rebound tonometry readings (Garway-Heath *et al.* 2007). Ultimately, although

GAT is still the method of choice for IOP measurement, DCT is emerging as a more plausible measure; the IOP readings obtained from DCT only slightly overestimate the actual IOP.

The Aqueous Humor

Aqueous humor is secreted by the epithelium of the ciliary body and is drained through the trabecular meshwork (TM) and uveoscleral outflow pathway (Alm and Nilsson 2009; Bill 1975; Do *et al.* 2008; Joseph and Grierson 1994; Nilsson 1997). Numerous vascular mediators, electrolytes and proteins are actively involved in regulating this dynamic (see Civan 2008). Aqueous humor contains various proteins and glycosaminoglycans. In a recent proteome analysis, 676 proteins were identified in human aqueous humor, most with concentrations between 0.1 and 2.5 ng/ml (Roy Chowdhury *et al.* 2010). Johnson *et al.* (1986) and Sit *et al.* (1997) opined that the proteins, or at least certain proteins, could contribute to the flow resistance of the aqueous outflow tract. Notably, Prata *et al.* (2007) demonstrated a two-fold higher protein concentration of the aqueous humor in patients with primary open angle glaucoma than in non-glaucomatous individuals. Various growth factors are also present in the aqueous humor (Tripathi *et al.* 1991); elevated levels of transforming growth factor-beta-2 (TGFβ2) and endothelin-1 have been reported in the aqueous humor of glaucomatous eyes (Picht *et al.* 2001; Ochiai and Ochiai 2002; Stefan *et al.* 2008; Shoshani *et al.* 2012). *In vitro*, TGFβ2 increases the secretion of fibronectin and plasminogen activator inhibitor-1 from human TM cells, which in turn could contribute to the outflow resistance and increased IOP as shown in an *ex vivo* anterior segment model (Fleenor *et al.* 2006). TM cells secret myocilin, a glycoprotein with the ability to polymerize (Tamm 2002); increased TM myocilin in some cases of primary open-angle glaucoma can enhance outflow resistance (Konz *et al.* 2009). Mutant myocilin may accumulate within TM cells leading to TM dysfunction and outflow obstruction (Tamm 2002; Liu and Vollrath 2004). Glycosaminoglycans further contribute to the formation of a pressure gradient across the TM (Knepper and McLone 1985-6). TM depletion of hyaluronic acid and accumulation of chondroitin sulfates have been reported in primary open angle glaucoma (Knepper *et al.* 1996). Lower concentrations of hyaluronic acid have been detected in the aqueous humor of patients with primary open angle glaucoma (Navajas *et al.* 2005).

The Aqueous Humor in Relation to IOP, Blood Pressure, and Ciliary Blood Flow

Several studies have investigated the relationship between IOP and aqueous humor production and drainage. Bill (1968) noted that the reduction in the aqueous humor production as a result of increased IOP produced an overestimation in the measured aqueous outflow facility, the so-called pseudofacility. In primates, this pseudofacility varied from subject to subject (Bill 1968) and increased with decreasing blood pressure (Bill and Bárány 1966). Based on his studies, Bill (1968) came to the conclusion that in subjects with high pseudofacility, a rise in outflow resistance could be easily balanced by a fall in aqueous humor production. However, in the context of low pseudofacility, aqueous humor production was affected the least, so a higher IOP was required to ensure aqueous humor drainage (Bill 1968). A further study revealed that at a fixed IOP and following stepwise reduction of arterial blood pressure, the decrease in aqueous humor production only became significant when systolic blood pressure fell below a critical level (70 mmHg in primates), an effect that was independent of the function of the sympathetic nervous system (Bill 1970). In his next seminal work, Bill (1971) noted that increasing IOP had a biphasic effect on aqueous humor production. The first phase, which was more pronounced but transient, was to some degree related to the immediate ocular tissue dehydration. This was followed by a second phase of long-lasting reduction in aqueous humor production. In primates, this reduction averaged 0.024 μL/min per 1 mmHg rise in IOP over the range 10 to 25 mmHg (Bill 1971). Moreover, with increasing IOP, the TM undergoes morphological changes, which reduce the aqueous outflow facility (Battista *et al.* 2008).

Bill's concept of pseudofacility was re-emphasized in the more recent studies of Reitsamer and Kiel (2003) and Kiel and Reitsamer (2006). They further revealed that the association between aqueous humor production and ciliary blood flow as well as the association between ciliary blood flow and ocular perfusion pressure are non-linear. In an animal model, aqueous humor production only declined when ciliary blood flow fell below a critical level; above that level, the aqueous production was blood flow-independent (Reitsamer and Kiel, 2003). On the other hand, above a certain level of ocular perfusion pressure, the so-called critical pressure, the ciliary blood flow reaches a plateau and further increase in the ocular perfusion pressure has a negligible effect on the actual ciliary blood flow (Reitsamer and Kiel 2003). Hence, the relationship between blood pressure and aqueous production is more complex than previously perceived.

Aqueous production is particularly vulnerable to reductions below critical levels in the ciliary blood flow and perfusion pressure. Within a middle range of ocular perfusion pressure, ciliary blood flow is maintained. However, when ciliary blood flow is diminished, the aqueous production is further maintained until a critical flow level is reached. Taken together, in response to a decrease in the arterial pressure and ocular perfusion, aqueous humor production remains relatively unchanged by the mediation of two autoregulatory mechanisms, one controlling ciliary blood flow and the other controlling aqueous production itself. When these autoregulatory mechanisms are overwhelmed, the aqueous production is diminished by decreasing ciliary perfusion and blood flow. This regulatory phenomenon has been well demonstrated and accepted clinically; carotid insufficiency and secondarily impaired ocular perfusion manifest with lower IOP in the ischemic eye (Knox 1973). However, the molecular basis of ciliary blood flow and aqueous inflow autoregulation has not been fully elucidated. It has been demonstrated that inhibition of nitric oxide production causes ciliary vaso-constriction, decreasing the rate of aqueous secretion and leading to a marked decrease in IOP (Kiel *et al.* 2001). Further studies are desirable to address whether nitric oxide synthase gene polymorphisms and indigenous levels of nitric oxide production confer susceptibility to glaucoma or its progression.

The relationship between IOP and blood pressure has been subject to extensive debates. In a study on 573 individuals over 60 years of age, Bulpitt *et al.* (1975) found that systolic blood pressure and obesity were directly and independently related to IOP. Hypertensive patients have an impaired control of IOP, marked by a greater rise in IOP than normotensive individuals with change in posture from sitting to lying down for 15 minutes (Williams *et al.* 1980); the magnitude of IOP elevation does not correlate with the changes in blood pressure

(Williams *et al.* 1980). In a longitudinal cohort of an African-origin population, systemic hypertension was independently associated with the rise of IOP during a four-year follow-up (Hennis *et al.* 2003). Dielemans *et al.* (1995) demonstrated that isolated systolic hypertension was associated with a mean of 0.65 mmHg higher than control IOP. In the Egna-Neumarkt study, 10 mmHg increases in systolic and diastolic blood pressures were associated with 0.4 mmHg and 0.24 mmHg rises in IOP, respectively (Bonomi *et al.* 2000). The prevalence of glaucoma decreased with increasing ocular diastolic perfusion pressure, but it was independent of mean and systolic ocular perfusion pressures (Bonomi *et al.* 2000). On the other hand, up to 73% of patients with primary open angle glaucoma suffer from systemic hypertension (Salim and Shields 2010). In an animal model, the rate of aqueous secretion correlated strongly with the ocular perfusion pressure (Macri 1982). In healthy individuals, IOP rises with the same kinetic and in parallel with increased systemic blood pressure during isometric exercise (Bakke *et al.* 2009). Castejon *et al.* (2010) further revealed that IOP increased markedly, rapidly, and linearly with increasing blood pressure during hand gripping and squatting exercises in humans. To what degree this observed effect was related to episcleral venous pressure remains to be fully understood.

Taken together, it appears that IOP and systemic blood pressure are related and that, aside from ocular autoregulatory mechanisms, the pathways for systemic control of blood pressure may share some common features with those of IOP. Although these pathways still remain to be elucidated fully, the renin-angiotensin system and endothelium-derived nitric oxide and endothelin could provide a basis for further studies as elements of this system are involved in the regulation of both systemic arterial pressure and IOP (Vaajanen *et al.* 2008; Shoshani *et al.* 2012).

The Role of Systemic Blood Pressure in Ocular Hemodynamic Response to IOP Changes

Maintaining blood flow and preventing episodes of ischemia and/or hypoxia to the optic nerve head during IOP elevation is essential for preserving the function and structural integrity of the optic nerve. The systemic blood pressure plays an important role in this maintenance. Furthermore, the autoregulatory capacity of the ocular circulation ceases during acute, large elevations in IOP (Joos *et al.* 1999); it has been demonstrated that short posterior ciliary artery flow velocities diminish substantially and linearly with acute elevation in IOP up to 50 mmHg (Joos *et al.* 1999). There is also a critical level of IOP (40 mmHg in primates) above which the optic disc blood flow ceases rapidly (Ernest 1976). The autoregulation is effective in restoring retinal circulation in IOP as low as 6-7 mmHg (Grunwald *et al.* 1982) and is impaired by hypoxia and hypercapnia (Ernest, 1974).

Nocturnal hypotension and reduced ocular perfusion pressure are two risk factors for *progression of glaucomatous* optic neuropathy (Graham and Drance 1999; Stefánsson *et al.* 2005; Werne *et al.* 2008). In non-human primates, Liang *et al.* (2009) showed that over a range of systemic blood pressures, increasing IOP was associated with dramatic reductions in the optic nerve head blood flow in the context of low-to-medium range blood pressure, an effect that was absent in higher levels of systemic blood pressure. Furthermore, following IOP reduction to the basal value, animals with medium-range blood pressure demonstrated a greater increase in the optic nerve head blood flow, an "overshoot" from the baseline. The results indicated that under low systemic blood pressure, autoregulatory mechanisms are less effective in maintaining optic nerve head blood flow in response to IOP changes. Notably, markedly lower nocturnal and diurnal systolic blood pressures have been observed in patients with progressive open angle glaucoma despite adequate IOP control as well as in patients with normal tension glaucoma (Kaiser *et al.* 1993). In another study, nocturnal reduction in diastolic blood pressure was associated with visual loss in normal tension glaucoma patients (Hayreh *et al.* 1999). Several other studies have supported this view (Liu *et al.* 2003; Collignon *et al.* 1998; Graham and Drance 1999).

Intracranial Pressure (ICP) and CSF Dynamics

ICP, a function of the extensibility and compressibility as well as the volumes of the intrcranial cavity and its contents (March and Madden 2009), is directly related to the rate of CSF production and is indirectly related to the rate of CSF drainage (Razumovsky and Hanley 1992). The CSF is secreted by the choroidal plexus (CP), an endothelium-lined highly vasculature structure, and brain parenchyma and capillaries (Hammock and Milhorat 1976; Lenke 2003; McComb 1983; Milhorat *et al.* 1971; Oresković *et al.* 1991; Speake *et al.* 2001; Welch 1967). The CSF circulates through the ventricular and subarachnoid spaces (Coxon 1968). Caprihan *et al.* (1999) investigated the effects of head-down tilt on cranial and ocular fluid distributions using T2-magnetic resonance imaging. They noted that increased transmural pressure led to a loss of water from the cranial CSF and ocular compartments via the spinal CSF compartment or the venous circulation. As suggested by Quincke in 1872 and Key and Retzius in 1875 (see Pollay 2010), CSF is essentially absorbed into the superior sagittal venous sinus. However, this view was questioned in the light of radionuclide cisternography and phantom flow study findings of maximum distribution of contrast over the cerebral convexities and techal sac (Greitz and Hannerz 1996). Thus, it has been advocated that the CSF is predominantly absorbed through the brain and spinal cord parenchyma into the capillaries (Greitz and Hannerz 1996). In a rat model, Koh *et al.* (2007) traced a contrast agent from the subarachnoid space into the lymphatic vessels in the olfactory submucosa and deep cervical lymph nodes. Koh and colleagues stated that CSF-derived water, which enters the lymphatic vessels on the olfactory turbinates, drains into the regional capillaries to balance the Starling forces at the lymph-blood interface (Koh *et al.* 2007).

The relationship between intracranial volume and pressure is non-linear; thus, above a critical level of ICP, further increase in the volume of intracranial contents substantially increases ICP (Tans and Poortvliet 1983). Normally, ICP is higher in supine (up to 15-20 mm Hg) than in upright position (Steiner and Andrews 2006; Roquefeuil 1983). It is interesting to note that positional changes have the same effect on both ICP and IOP. Changes in posture are clinically important in managing patients with elevated ICP (Porchet *et al.* 1998; Ng *et al.* 2004). Ng *et al.* (2004) noted a significant and consistent reduction of ICP and slight increase in cerebral perfusion pressure (CPP) at a 30 degree head elevation in patients with severe head injury. Iencean and Ciurea (2008) distinguished four categories of intracranial hypertension in terms of pathogenesis: (1) brain parenchymal diseases, (2) cerebrovascular disorders, (3) disorders of CSF circulation, and (4) idiopathic intracranial hypertension.

They opined that the interaction between the rate of ICP elevation and its peak value and duration of elevation determines the state of decompensation in a symptomatic patient (Iencean and Ciurea 2008).

Methods of Measuring ICP

Several invasive (direct) and non-invasive (indirect) measures are available for assessing ICP. Lundberg's method of continuous ICP recording via a ventricular cannula is popular but invasive (Lundberg 1960; Lundberg *et al.* 1965; North and Reilly 1986; North 1997; Ravi and Morgan 2003). Non-invasive and indirect methods for estimating ICP by measuring various parameters have been utilized, including optic nerve sheath diameter (Blaivas *et al.* 2003; Geeraerts, *et al.* 2008; Kimberly *et al.* 2008), calculating the pulsatility index of the middle cerebral artery (Bellner *et al.* 2004), measuring otoacoustic emissions (Frank *et al.* 2000), measuring outflow pressure in the central retinal vein, the Glosing pulsatility index of the ophthalmic artery or central retinal artery (Querfurth *et al.* 2004) and measuring tympanic membrane displacement upon stapedial reflex contraction (Reid *et al.* 1990). A review of different methods of ICP measurement and their advantages versus disadvantages has been given by Ravi and Morgan (2003).

The relationship between IOP and ICP and the question of whether or not IOP can be used to estimate ICP is still controversial. Sajjadi et al. (2006) reported a strong positive correlation between IOP and ICP, measured by lumbar puncture (LP), among patients with variable underlying pathologies (pseudotumor cerebri, meningitis, multiple sclerosis, etc.). On the other hand, Han et al. (2008) failed to find such an association in a group of patients with pseudotumor cerebri as the most common clinical diagnosis. In another study of 32 patients who underwent LP in emergency departments, ICP did not correlate with LP opening pressure (Muchnok et al. 2010). In the latter study, only nine patients had elevated IOP and five of them had concomitantly elevated opening pressures. These results should be interpreted cautiously as (1) there might be a time lag in the equilibration of ICP and IOP and thus, in the settings of acute decompensation, ICP alterations may not be reflected by changes in IOP; (2) the underlying pathology could potentially confound the relationship between ICP and IOP; (3) ICP surrogated by lumbar opening pressure may not represent the CSF pressure on the back of LC, particularly in an acute setting; and (4) the relationship between IOP and ICP could depend on the absolute value of ICP. This last point was demonstrated in the study of Spentzas *et al.* (2010), which noted that in children with traumatic brain injury, the relationship is quadratic. That is, above a certain level of ICP (20 cm H_2O), the regression slope becomes steeper and ICP and IOP become more closely related. They opined that "studies where many patients with normal ICP are included will find a nonsignificant relationship between ICP and IOP" (Spentzas *et al.* 2010).

The absence of a spontaneous retinal venous pulse (SRVP) is sometimes used as a clinical sign of increased ICP (Hedges *et al.* 1994). Jacks and Miller (2003) argued that SRVP is caused by "variation in the pressure gradient along the retinal vein as it traverses the lamina cribrosa". SRVP ceases with an increase in ICP when the intracranial pulse pressure and intraocular pulse pressure become equalized. Donnelly and Subramanian (2009) suggested that with an intraocular pulse pressure of at least 1.2 mm Hg, the absence of a spontaneous venous pulse predicts an elevated ICP. In nutshell, the available data imply that ICP and IOP may are related under certain conditions. IOP measurement thus represents a potentially useful, indirect estimate of ICP. The validity of this indirect estimate in various clinical conditions (e.g., acute versus chronic intracranial pathologies) and how the ocular morphology affects it remain to be fully understood.

Cerebral Blood Flow (CBF), Cerebral Perfusion Pressure (CPP), and ICP

In the 1930s, Mogens Fog noted that an increase or decrease in systemic blood pressure resulted in the constriction or dilation of the pial arteries, respectively, providing early evidence for the systemic control of cerebral circulation and autoregulation (Fog 1939). CBF is a product of cerebral perfusion pressure (CPP) and cerebrovascular resistance. Over a wide range of CPP, CBF is maintained by changes in the vascular resistance to ensure adequate brain oxygenation. As CBF is difficult to measure clinically and is stable over a wide range of cerebrovascular hemodynamic variations, CPP is often preferred for clinical assessments (Booth *et al.* 2003). A CPP less than 60 mmHg is associated with a higher risk of brain tissue hypoxia in patients presenting with severe head injuries (Marín-Caballos *et al.* 2005). CPP is the difference between the mean arterial pressure (MAP) at the point of its entry into the brain and the venous pressure on exiting the skull, and this represents the gradient of blood pressure along the cerebral vasculature (Roper *et al.*, 2004). It is calculated as CPP = MAP – ICP (Cottrell *et al.* 1978; Steiner and Andrews 2006). Controlling CBF and CPP is important in the management of head-injured patients (Lang and Chesnut 1994). In the seminal work of Robertson *et al.* (1999), a CBF-targeted protocol (MAP > 90 mmHg and CPP > 70 mmHg) was compared to an ICP-targeted protocol (MAP > 70 mmHg and CPP > 50 mmHg) in patients with severe head trauma. Although the mean ICP did not differ with either protocol, the CBF-targeted protocol ensured a higher MAP and CPP and decreased the episodes and duration of critical jugular venous desaturation, primarily as a result of reduction in the frequencies of hypotension and hypocapnia (Robertson *et al.* 1999). In a study of brain trauma patients, Johnston *et al.* (2005) demonstrated that increasing CPP from 70 to 90 mmHg resulted in a significant increase in the brain oxygen tension and a decrease, though to a lesser degree, in the oxygen extraction fraction. Based on various studies conducted in head trauma victims, the overall impressions are that (1) CPP represents a favorable estimate of cerebral hemodynamic and oxygen supply by embracing the elements of system circulation (e.g., MAP) and cranial vault mechanics (e.g., ICP) and (2) changes in CPP despite a controlled ICP (< 20 mmHg), as in the study of Robertson *et al.* (1999), can alter the brain oxygen balance. However, this by no means indicates that controlling CPP alone is sufficient, as Juul *et al.* (2000) revealed that regardless of CPP, an ICP greater than 20 mmHg was associated with high mortality and poor neurological outcome in patients with severe head injury. In a study of patients with severe head injuries, Gasco *et al.* (2005) noted that reduction of ICP by mannitol therapy substantially improved peri-contusional brain tissue oxygen tension in a linear fashion, and the relationship was stronger among patients with initial ICP < 20 mmHg than among those with ICP > 20 mmHg (Gasco *et al.* 2005). Thus, carefully managing both ICP and CPP are desirable in patients with an intracranial pathology.

Notably, Carter *et al.* (2008) revealed that ICP $\geq$ 40 mmHg and CPP $\leq$ 49 mmHg well predicted poor outcome in children with severe brain injury.

Direct, invasive measurement of ICP and CPP is often recommended in clinical practice, but intracranial placement of a transducer for measuring ICP is sometimes impractical, and the value obtained may be subject to bias from drift of the pressure transducer or the interhemispheric pressure gradient (Schmidt *et al.* 2001). Thrombocytopenia, prior anticoagulant therapy, immunosuppression, cerebral edema, presence of midline shift, and CNS or scalp infection represent some challenges to invasive ICP monitoring (Bekar *et al.* 2009; Hertelendy *et al.* 2009). Non-invasive techniques have been developed and tested by several groups (Belfort *et al.* 2000; Czosnyka *et al.* 1998; Edouard *et al.* 2005; Schmidt *et al.* 2001;). Having measured transcranial Doppler middle cerebral artery (MCA) mean and diastolic flow velocities in patients with head injuries with a mean Glasgow Coma Scale score of 6, Czosnyka *et al.* (1998) developed the following formula:

eCPP = (time-averaged arterial blood pressure) x (diastolic MCA velocity/mean MCA flow velocity) + 14

They found a good agreement between the measured and estimated values, with 71% of the estimations having < 10 mm Hg difference from the measured CPP. Belfort *et al.* (2000) measured MCA systolic, diastolic, and mean velocities with a transcranial Doppler in pregnant women. They found that CPP estimated from the following formula (eCPP) strongly correlated with the directly measured CPP (mCPP) (r = 0.92). The obtained the following formula:

eCPP = [mean MCA velocity/(mean MCA velocity – diastolic MCA velocity)] x (MAP – diastolic blood pressure)

The utility of various non-invasive methods could be case-specific; thus, the accuracy of a given equation should be tested before being implemented in another context. Furthermore, the characteristics of cranial vault mechanics may confound the association between real CPP and CPP estimated by the systemic arterial pressure and cerebral artery flow rates.

CSF pressure and Lamina Cribrosa

Lamina cribrosa is a connective tissue membrane through which the optic nerve fibers enter the globe (Jonas *et al.* 1991; Jonas and Holbach 2005; Kotecha *et al.* 2006). Radius and Gonzales (1981) revealed that on histological examination of specimens from human eyes, the density of connective tissue in the lamina cribrosa is higher at the nasal or temporal side. Focal densities were also reported. However, the most consistent finding was that the density of trabecular elements was higher at the level of the sclera than at the choroidal and retrobulbar levels (Radius and Gonzales 1981). As a partition of small surface area, the lamina cribrosa is continually under tension on its ocular and intracranial sides. In a mathematical model, Cahane and Bartov (1992) demonstrated that with an axial length of

0.014 m and sclera thickness of 2 mm, lamina cribrosa could withstand the tension created by an IOP as high as ~75 mmHg.

Under normal circumstances, IOP is ~4 mmHg greater than ICP (Berdahl and Allingham 2010). Increase in the ICP-IOP difference destabilizes the LC. Patients with primary open-angle glaucoma have low CSF pressures (Berdahl *et al.* 2008a), and are believed to have an unstable lamina cribrosa; thus, an increase in IOP results in a significantly more optic disc structural damage or cupping than in healthy individuals (Astakhov and Akopov 2005). Notably, the translaminar pressure difference predicts glaucomatous optic nerve injury better than IOP or CPP alone (Ren *et al.* 2010). Applying the *elastic mechanics theory on a thin plate* to estimate the behavior of the lamina cribrosa under pressure, Dongqi and Zeqin (1999) proposed that lamina cribrosa thickness and diameter are two major determinants of its deformation and retrodisplacement; the thinner the lamina cribrosa and the greater the radius, the larger the displacement.

In this context, the hypothesis of “optic nerve compartment syndrome” and retrograde optic nerve atrophy, as suggested by Killer *et al.* (2008), is worth mentioning. In their early study, Killer *et al.* (2007) noted an abnormal flow and diminished distribution of intracranial contrast-loaded CSF into the perioptic subarachnoid space in two patients with normal tension glaucoma, suggesting a phenomenon of perioptic CSF compartmentalization and low CSF turnover. They later hypothesized that such impaired CSF recycling could in turn lead to accumulation in the perioptic space of biologically active substances and inflammatory mediators with potentially neurotoxic effects, ultimately resulting in optic nerve fiber damage and subsequent retinal ganglion cell loss. The hypothesis of Killer *et al.* (2008) mentions that any intracranial pathology, which can reduce CSF recycling between perioptic and intra-cranial spaces, may potentially contribute to the pathogenesis of some forms of glaucoma.

The Relationship between ICP, IOP and Systemic Arterial Blood Pressure in Health and Diseases and Its Implication

In a study of 71 healthy individuals and 43 patients with open-angle glaucoma, Ren *et al.* (2010) found significant correlations between the CSF pressure, IOP, and systolic and mean arterial blood pressures among the healthy individuals, but not among the glaucoma patients. They suggested the presence of a common, systemic mechanism for controlling the CSF and intraocular and systemic blood pressures. Such a mechanism could ensure a stable translaminar pressure difference in patients with elevated IOP and MAP (Ren *et al.* 2010). Interestingly, in the Framingham Eye Study, the frequency distribution of IOP was found to be analogous to the frequency distribution of systemic blood pressure, with both showing a unimodal pattern with rightward skewness (Colton and Ederer 1980). Jonas (2011) obtained insights into the role of CSF pressure in the pathogenesis of normal-pressure glaucoma. He maintained that the optic nerve heads in cases of normal-pressure glaucoma and high-IOP glaucoma share common morphological features characterized by loss of neuroretinal rim and enlarged parapapillary atrophy, features that are absent from most other vascular optic neuropathies. Consulting the works of Berdahl *et al.* (2008b) and Ren *et al.* (2010), Jonas

(2011) emphasized that the biomechanics of the lamina cribrosa and the translaminar pressure difference, not IOP, determine the pathophysiology of the optic nerve head.

Assuming that the MAP at the levels of the ophthalmic artery and circle of Willis are approximate, the IOP-ICP difference may become directly related to the difference between the ocular perfusion pressure (OPP) and CPP. This implies that under physiological conditions, maintaining a stable lamina cribrosa requires a balance between the local and systemic factors controlling ocular and cerebral hemodynamics. Any disturbance in either of these could alter the status of lamina cribrosa, optic nerve axonal transport and blood supply, and thus may affect the susceptibility of the optic nerve to injury. Notably, studies have demonstrated impaired cerebral autoregulation and a cerebral perfusion defect in glaucoma. Tutaj *et al.* (2004) found that oscillations in the cerebral blood flow velocity in response to changes in the arterial pressure were enhanced in patients with normal pressure glaucoma and primary open angle glaucoma compared with healthy individuals. Compared with healthy, age-matched controls, the baseline MCA blood flow velocities were lower and the cerebral vasoconstrictive response to hyperoxia was blunted in normal tension and high tension open angle glaucoma, implying impaired brain perfusion (Harris *et al.* 2003). In a study of 31 patients with normal tension glaucoma, Sugiyama *et al.* (2006) noted a perfusion abnormality in 19 patients; the regional cerebral perfusion in the territory of the left MCA as estimated by single photon emission computed tomography was defective in glaucoma patients compared to age-matched controls (Sugiyama *et al.* 2006). As migraines are also associated with cerebral vasospasm and reduced cerebral blood flow, one may expect to see a relatively higher rate of glaucoma in patients with migraines and vice versa. Notably, Comoğlu *et al.* (2003) found glaucomatous-like visual field defects in ~62% of migraine patients with otherwise normal IOP. Phelps and Corbett (1985) noted a high rate of migraine in elderly low-tension glaucoma patients. These data imply that cerebral perfusion abnormality and autoregulatory dysfunction may play a key role in the pathogenesis of glaucoma. It is very possible that the cerebral vascular autoregulatory dysfunction may be a consequence of more diffuse endothelial state of dysfunction with altered nitric oxide and endothelin levels. Evidence of systemic endothelial dysfunction in open angle glaucoma has been suspected and demonstrated in the literature. Su *et al.* (2008) revealed that brachial artery flow-mediated vasodilatation, an indirect measure of endothelial nitric oxide activity, is significantly lower in normal tension glaucoma than in high tension open angle glaucoma and healthy controls. The authors suggested that an endogenous nitric oxide defect could contribute to the pathogenesis of glaucoma. However, the mechanisms by which a defect in systemic endothelial function affects cerebral hemodynamic and optic nerve head physiology in various pathologies remains to be explored fully.

In cases of glaucoma, the role of systemic vascular dysfunction, which can manifest as systemic hypertension, is suspected as mentioned above. A similar consideration should be taken into account in evaluating the disorders associated with an elevated ICP and/or impaired brain perfusion. Systemic hypertension is associated with a variety of neurological conditions including seizure, head trauma, idiopathic intracranial hypertension, brain tumors, migraine and Alzheimer disease (Flynn and Woroniecki 2004; Power *et al.* 2011; Wang *et al.* 2010). The association of hypertension with glaucoma and intracranial/neurological disorders may be related to dysfunction of a common regulatory mechanism, which controls systemic arterial blood pressure, IOP, ICP and CPP. This hypothesis is worth consideration, and the mediators and components of the co-regulatory mechanism need to be explored in detail.

Conclusion

ICP and IOP can be affected by various physiological and pathological conditions. The latter include head trauma and glaucoma as prototypes. Understanding the relationship between systemic arterial blood pressure, ICP and IOP is of the utmost importance in managing these conditions. The recent evidence that a common vascular mechanism controls the ICP, IOP and central MAP suggests a program of research that could further elucidate the pathophysiologies of ICP and IOP, with implications for the treatment of a number of clinical conditions as mentioned above. As for glaucoma, the proposed mechanism presumably ensures a stable lamina cribrosa in patients with elevated IOP and MAP, as suggested by Ren *et al.* (2010); it is now clear that the pressure gradient across the lamina cribrosa has important implications for optic nerve pathology. Further research concerning the drainage of CSF and *ipso facto* the maintenance of CSF pressure may also be indicated.

References

Alm, A. and Nilsson, S. F. (2009) Uveoscleral outflow-a review. *Experimental Eye Research*, 88, pp. 760-768.

Astakhov, Y. S. and Akopov, E. L. (2005) Evaluation of lamina cribrosa tolerance to the increase of intraocular pressure in healthy people and primary open angle glaucoma patients. *Proceedings of the International Society for Optical Engineering (Society of Photo-optical Instrumentation Engineers)*, 5630, DOI: 10.1117/12.570590.

Atanassov, M. A. and Konareva, M. I. (2002) Reproducibility and agreement between three methods of intraocular pressure measurement. *Folia Medica (Plovdiv),* 44, pp. 19-22.

Bakke, E. F. *et al.* (2009) Intraocular pressure increases in parallel with systemic blood pressure during isometric exercise. *Investigative Ophthalmology and Visual Science*, 50, pp. 760-764.

Battista, S. A. *et al.* (2008) Reduction of the available area for aqueous humor outflow and increase in meshwork herniations into collector channels following acute IOP elevation in bovine eyes. *Investigative Ophthalmology and Visual Science*, 49, pp. 5346-5352.

Bárány, E. H. (1963) A mathematical formulation of intraocular pressure as dependent on secretion, ultrafiltration, bulk outflow, and osmotic reabsorption of fluid. *Investigative Ophthalmology*, 2, pp. 584-90.

Bekar, A. *et al.* (2009) Risk factors and complications of intracranial pressure monitoring with a fiberoptic device. *Journal of Clinical Neuroscience*, 16, pp. 236-240.

Belfort, M. A. *et al.* (2000) Evaluation of a noninvasive transcranial Doppler and blood pressure-based method for the assessment of cerebral perfusion pressure in pregnant women. *Hypertension in Pregnancy*, 19, pp. 331-340.

Bellner, J. *et al.* (2004) Transcranial Doppler sonography pulsatility index (PI) reflects intracranial pressure (ICP). *Surgical Neurology*, 62, pp. 45-51.

Berdahl, J. P. *et al.* (2008a) Cerebrospinal fluid pressure is decreased in primary open-angle glaucoma. *Ophthalmology*, 115, pp. 763-768.

Berdahl, J. P. *et al.* (2008b) Intracranial pressure in primary open angle glaucoma, normal tension glaucoma, and ocular hypertension: a case-control study. *Investigative Ophthalmology and Visual Science*, 49, pp. 5412-5418.

Berdahl, J. P. and Allingham, R. R. (2010) Intracranial pressure and glaucoma. Current *Opinion in Ophthalmology*, 21, pp. 106-111.

Bhattacherjee, P. (1980) Prostaglandins and inflammatory reactions *Methods and Findings in Experimental and Clinical Pharmacology*, 2, pp. 17-31.

Bill, A. (1968) The effect of ocular hypertension caused by red cells on the rate of formation of aqueous humor. *Investigative Ophthalmology*, 7, pp. 162-168.

Bill, A. (1970) The effect of changes in arterial blood pressure on the rate of aqueous humour formation in a primate (Cercopithecus ethiops). *Ophthalmic Research*, 1, pp. 193-200.

Bill, A. (1971) Effects of longstanding stepwise increments in eye pressure on the rate of aqueous humor formation in a primate (Cercopithecus ethiops). *Experimental Eye Research*, 12, pp. 184-193.

Bill, A. (1973) The role of ciliary blood flow and ultrafiltration in aqueous humor formation. *Experimental Eye Research*, 16, pp. 287-298.

Bill, A. (1975) Blood circulation and fluid dynamics in the eye. *Physiological Reviews*, 55, pp. 383-417.

Bill, A. and Bárány, E. H. (1966) Gross facility, facility of conventional routes, and pseudofacility of aqueous humor outflow in the cynomolgus monkey. The reduction in aqueous humor formation rate caused by moderate increments in intraocular pressure. *Archives of Ophthalmology*, 75, pp. 665-673.

Blaivas, M. *et al.* (2003) Elevated intracranial pressure detected by bedside emergency ultrasonography of the optic nerve sheath. *Academic Emergency Medicine*, 10, pp. 376-381.

Bonomi, L. *et al.* (2000) Vascular risk factors for primary open angle glaucoma: the Egna-Neumarkt Study. *Ophthalmology,* 107, pp. 1287-1293.

Booth, P. W. *et al.* (eds) (2003) *Maxillofacial Trauma and Esthetic Facial Reconstruction.* Edinburgh: Churchill Livingstone, p. 71.

Brown, P. *et al.* (2004) Molecular mechanisms of cerebrospinal fluid production. *Neuroscience*, 129, pp. 957-970.

Bulpitt, C. J. *et al.* (1975) Intraocular pressure and systemic blood pressure in the elderly. *British Journal of Ophthalmology*, 59, pp. 717-720.

Cahane, M. and Bartov, E. (1992) Axial length and scleral thickness effect on susceptibility to glaucomatous damage: a theoretical model implementing Laplace's law. *Ophthalmic Research*, 24, pp. 280-284.

Caprihan, A. et al. (1999) Effect of head-down tilt on brain water distribution. *European Journal of Applied Physiology and Occupational Physiology*, 79, pp. 367-373.

Carter, B. G. *et al.* (2008) ICP and CPP: excellent predictors of long term outcome in severely brain injured children. *Child's Nervous System*, 24, pp. 245-251.

Castejon, H. *et al.* (2010) Effect of acute increase in blood pressure on intraocular pressure in pigs and humans. *Investigative Ophthalmology and Visual Science*, 51, pp. 1599-1605.

Civan, M. (ed) (2008) *The Eyes's Aqueous Humor, Edition 2*. San Diego: Academic Press.

Coleman, A. L. and Miglior, S. (2008) Risk factors for glaucoma onset and progression. *Survey of Ophthalmology*, 53[Suppl1], pp. 3-10.

Collignon, N. *et al.* (1998) Ambulatory blood pressure monitoring in glaucoma patients. The nocturnal systolic dip and its relationship with disease progression. *International Ophthalmology*, 22, pp. 19-25.

Colton, T. and Ederer, F. (1980) The distribution of intraocular pressures in the general population. *Survey of Ophthalmology*, 25, pp. 123-129.

Comoğlu, S. *et al.* (2003) Glaucomatous visual field defects in patients with migraine. *Journal of Neurology*, 250, pp. 201-206.

Cottrell, J. E. *et al.* (1978) Intracranial pressure changes induced by sodium nitroprusside in patients with intracranial mass lesions. *Journal of Neurosurgery*, 48, pp. 329-331.

Coxon, R. V. (1968) Cerebrospinal fluid *Progress in Brain Research*, 29, pp. 135-146.

Craig, J. E. and Mackey, D. A. (1999) Glaucoma genetics *Current Opinion in Ophthalmology*, 10, pp. 126-134.

Czosnyka, M. *et al.* (1998) Cerebral perfusion pressure in head-injured patients: a noninvasive assessment using transcranial Doppler ultrasonography. *Journal of Neurosurgery*, 88, pp. 802-808.

Davies, L. N. *et al.* (2006) Clinical evaluation of rebound tonometer. *Acta Ophthalmologica Scandinavica*, 84, Pp. 206-209.

Dickerman, R. D. *et al.* (1999) Intra-ocular pressure changes during maximal isometric contraction: does this reflect intra-cranial pressure or retinal venous pressure? *Neurological Research*, 21, pp. 243-246.

Dielemans, I. *et al.* (1995) Primary open-angle glaucoma, intraocular pressure, and systemic blood pressure in the general elderly population. The Rotterdam Study. *Ophthalmology*, 102, pp. 54-60.

Do, C. *et al.* (2008) Mechanisms of aqueous humor formation. In: Tombran-Tink, J. and Barnstable, C. J. (eds) *Ocular Transporters in Ophthalmic Diseases and Drug Delivery.* Totowa, NJ: Humana Press, pp. 61-88.

Dongqi, H. and Zeqin, R. (1999) A biomathematical model for pressure-dependent lamina cribrosa behavior. *Journal of Biomechanics*, 32, pp. 579-584.

Donnelly, S. J. and Subramanian, P. S. (2009) Relationship of intraocular pulse pressure and spontaneous venous pulsations. *American Journal of Ophthalmology,* 147, pp. 51-55.

Edouard, A. R. *et al.* (2005) Non-invasive assessment of cerebral perfusion pressure in brain injured patients with moderate intracranial hypertension. *British Journal of Anaesthesia*, 94, pp. 216-221.

Elmallah, M. K. and Asrani, S. G. (2008) New ways to measure intraocular pressure. *Current Opinion in Ophthalmology*, 19, pp. 122-126.

Ernest, J. T. (1974) Autoregulation of optic-disk oxygen tension. *Investigative ophthalmology*, 13, pp. 101-106.

Ernest, J. T. (1976) Optic disc blood flow. *Transactions of the Ophthalmological Societies of the United Kingdom*, 96, pp. 348-351.

Fleenor, D. L. *et al.* (2006) TGFbeta2-induced changes in human trabecular meshwork: implications for intraocular pressure. *Investigative Ophthalmology and Visual Science*, 47, pp. 226-234.

Flynn, J. T. and Woroniecki, R. P. (2004) Phathophysiology of hypertension. In: Avner, E. D. *et al.* (eds.) *Pediatric Nephrology*. Philadelphia: Lippincott Williams & Wilkins, pp. 1153-1178.

Fog, M. (1939) Cerebral circulation: II. Reaction of pial arteries to increase in blood pressure. *Archives of Neurology and Psychiatry*, 41, pp. 260-268.

Frank, A. M. *et al.* (2000) Non-invasive measurement of intracranial pressure changes by otoacoustic emissions (OAEs)-a report of preliminary data. *Zentralblatt für Neurochirurgie*, 61, pp. 177-180.

Funk, R. *et al.* (1985) Intraocular pressure and systemic blood pressure after administration of vasoactive substances in hypertensive and normal rats. *Graefe's Archive for Clinical and Experimental Ophthalmology*, 223, pp. 145-149.

Garway-Heath, T. *et al.* (2007) Measurement of intraocular pressure. In: Weinreb, R. N. *et al.* (eds) *Intraocular Pressure, Consensus Series 4*. Amsterdam, Kugler Publications, pp. 17-58.

Gasco, J. *et al.* (2005) Linear correlation between stable intracranial pressure decrease and regional cerebral oxygenation improvement following mannitol administration in severe acute head injury patients. *Acta Neurochirurgica Supplementum*, 95, pp. 73-77.

Geeraerts, T. *et al.* (2008) Non-invasive assessment of intracranial pressure using ocular sonography in neurocritical care patients. *Intensive Care Medicine*, 34, pp. 2062-2067.

Goldmann, H. and Schmidt, T. (1957) über Applanationstonometrie. *Ophthalmologica*, 134, pp. 221-242.

Green, K. and Pederson, J. E. (1972) Contribution of secretion and filtration to aqueous humor formation. *American Journal Physiology*, 222, pp. 1218-1226.

Greitz, D. and Hannerz, J. (1996) A proposed model of cerebrospinal fluid circulation: observations with radionuclide cisternography. *American Journal Of Neuroradiology*, 17, pp. 431-438.

Graham, S. L. and Drance, S. M. (1999) Nocturnal hypotension: role in glaucoma progression. *Survey of Ophthalmology*, 43[Suppl 1], pp. 10-16.

Grunwald, J. E. *et al.* (1982) Autoregulation of the retinal circulation in response to decrease of intraocular pressure below normal. *Investigative Ophthalmology and Visual Science*, 23, pp. 124-127.

Gugleta, K. *et al.* (2012) Association between risk factors and glaucomatous damage in untreated primary open-angle glaucoma. *Journal of Glaucoma*, doi: 10.1097/IJG.0b013e3182447d9b.

Gupta, V. *et al.* (2006) Inter-instrument agreement and influence of central corneal thickness on measurements with Goldmann, pneumotonometer and noncontact tonometer in glaucomatous eyes. *Indian Journal of Ophthalmology*, 54, pp. 261-265.

Halkiadakis, I. *et al.* (2009) Comparison of dynamic contour tonometry with Goldmann applanation tonometry in glaucoma practice. *Acta Ophthalmologica*, 87, pp. 323-328.

Hammock, M. K. and Milhorat, T. H. (1976) The cerebrospinal fluid: current concepts of its formation. *Annals of Clinical and Laboratory Science*, 6, pp. 22-26.

Han, Y. *et al.* (2008) No correlation between intraocular pressure and intracranial pressure. *Annals of Neurology*, 64, pp. 221-224.

Harris, A. *et al.* (2003) Reduced cerebrovascular blood flow velocities and vasoreactivity in open-angle glaucoma. *American Journal of Ophthalmology*, 135, pp. 144-147.

Harvey, B. (2003) Examination of intraocular pressure. In: Doshi, S. and Harvey, W. (eds.) *Investigative Techniques and Ocular Examination.* Edinburgh: Butterworth-Heinemann optician/Elsevier Science Limited, pp. 61-68.

Hayreh, S. S. *et al.* (1999) Role of nocturnal arterial hypotension in optic nerve head ischemic disorders. *Ophthalmologica*, 213, pp. 76-96.

Hedges Jr, T. R. *et al.* (1994) The retinal venous pulse. Its relation to optic disc characteristics and choroidal pulse. *Ophthalmology*, 101, pp. 542-547.

Hennis, A. *et al.* (2003) Hypertension, diabetes, and longitudinal changes in intraocular pressure. *Ophthalmology*, 110, pp. 908-914.

Hertelendy, A. J. *et al.* (2009) Neurologic emergencies. In: Pollak, A. N. *et al.* (eds.) *Critical Care Transport*. Sudbury: Jones and Bartlett Learning, pp. 364-441.

Hsu, S. Y. *et al.* (2009) Comparisons of intraocular pressure measurements: Goldmann applanation tonometry, noncontact tonometry, Tono-Pen tonometry, and dynamic contour tonometry. *Eye (Lond)*, 23, pp. 1582-1588.

Iencean, S. M. and Ciurea, A. V. (2008) Intracranial hypertension: classification and patterns of evolution. Journal of Medicine and Life, 1, pp. 101-107.

Jacks, A. S. and Miller, N. R. (2003) Spontaneous retinal venous pulsation: aetiology and significance. *Journal of Neurology, Neurosurgery, and Psychiatry*, 74, pp. 7-9.

Johnson, M. *et al.* (1986) The flow of aqueous humor through micro-porous filters. *Investigative Ophthalmology and Visual Science*, 27, pp. 92-97.

Johnston, A. J. *et al.* (2005) Effect of cerebral perfusion pressure augmentation on regional oxygenation and metabolism after head injury. *Critical Care Medicine*, 33, pp. 189-195.

Jonas, J. B. *et al.* (1991) Morphometry of the human lamina cribrosa surface. *Investigative Ophthalmology and Visual Science*, 32, pp. 401-405.

Jonas, J. B. and Holbach, L. (2005) Central corneal thickness and thickness of the lamina cribrosa in human eyes. *Investigative Ophthalmology and Visual Science*, 46, pp. 1275-1279.

Jonas, J. B. (2011) Role of cerebrospinal fluid pressure in the pathogenesis of glaucoma. *Acta Ophthalmologica*, 89, pp. 505-514.

Joos, K. M. *et al.* (1999) Effect of acute intraocular pressure changes on short posterior ciliary artery haemodynamics. *British Journal of Ophthalmology*, 83, pp. 33-38.

Jorge, J. *et al.* (2010) IOP variations in the sitting and supine positions. *Journal of Glaucoma*, 19, pp. 609-612.

Joseph, J. and Grierson, I. (1994) Anterior segment changes in glaucoma. In: Garner, A. and Klintworth, G. K. (eds.) *Pathobiology of Ocular Disease: A Dynamic Approach, 2nd edition*: *Part A*. New York: Marcel Dekker, pp 433-465.

Juul, N. *et al.* (2000) Intracranial hypertension and cerebral perfusion pressure: influence on neurological deterioration and outcome in severe head injury. The Executive Committee of the International Selfotel Trial. *Journal of Neurosurgery*, 92, pp. 1-6.

Kaiser, H. J. *et al.* (1993) Systemic blood pressure in glaucoma patients. *Graefe's Archive for Clinical and Experimental Ophthalmology*, 231, pp. 677-680.

Kanngiesser, H. E. *et al.* (2005) Dynamic contour tonometry: presentation of a new tonometer. *Journal of Glaucoma*, 14, pp. 344-350.

Kaufman, Y. *et al.* (2007) Intraorbital arteriovenous malformation *The Journal of Craniofacial Surgery*, 18, pp. 1091-1093.

Kellie, G. (1824) Appearances observed in the disection of two individuals; death from cold and congestion of the brain. *Transactions of Medical and Chirurgical Society of Edinburgh*, 1, pp. 84-169.

Kiel, J. W. and Reitsamer, H. A. (2006) Relationship between ciliary blood flow and aqueous production: does it play a role in glaucoma therapy? *Journal of Glaucoma*, 15, pp. 172-181.

Kiel, J. W. *et al.* (2001) Effects of nitric oxide synthase inhibition on ciliary blood flow, aqueous production and intraocular pressure. *Experimental Eye Research*, 73, pp. 355-364.

Killer, H. E. *et al.* (2008) Is open-angle glaucoma caused by impaired cerebrospinal fluid circulation: around the optic nerve? *Clinical and Experimental Ophthalmology*, 36, pp. 308-311.

Killer, H. E. *et al.* (2007) Cerebrospinal fluid dynamics between the intracranial and the subarachnoid space of the optic nerve. Is it always bidirectional? *Brain*, 130, pp. 514-520.

Kimberly, H. H. *et al.* (2008) Correlation of optic nerve sheath diameter with direct measurement of intracranial pressure. *Academic Emergency Medicine*, 15, pp. 201-204.

Kniestedt, C. *et al.* (2004) Dynamic contour tonometry: a comparative study on human cadaver eyes. *Archives of Ophthalmology*, 122, pp. 1287-1293.

Kniestedt, C. *et al.* (2008) Tonometry through the ages. *Survey of Ophthalmology*, 53, pp. 568-591.

Knox, D. L. (1973) Ocular pressure studies in the diagnosis of carotid artery disease. *Transactions of the American Ophthalmological Society*, 71, pp. 459-487.

Koh, L. *et al.* (2007) Properties of the lymphatic cerebrospinal fluid transport system in the rat: impact of elevated intracranial pressure. *Journal of Vascular Research*, 44, pp. 423-432.

Konz, D. D. *et al.* (2009) Myocilin in the trabecular meshwork of eyes with primary open-angle glaucoma. *Graefe's Archive for Clinical and Experimental Ophthalmology*, 247, pp. 1643-1649.

Kotecha, A. *et al.* (2006) Age-related changes in the thickness of the human lamina cribrosa. *British Journal of Ophthalmology*, 90, pp. 1531-1534.

Knepper, P. A. *et al.* (1996) Glycosaminoglycans of the human trabecular meshwork in primary open-angle glaucoma. *Investigative Ophthalmology and Visual Science*, 37, pp. 1360-1367.

Knepper, P. A. and Mclone, D. G. (1985-6) Glycosaminoglycans and outflow pathways of the eye and brain. *Pediatric Neuroscience*, 12, pp. 240-251.

Knecht, P. B. *et al.* (2011) Hand-held dynamic contour tonometry. *Acta Ophthalmologica*, 89, pp. 132-137.

Lam, W. W. *et al.* (2005) Early computed tomography features in extensive middle cerebral artery territory infarct: prediction of survival. *Journal of Neurology, Neurosurgery, and Psychiatry*, 76, pp. 354-357.

Lang, E. W. and Chesnut, R. M. (1994) Intracranial pressure. Monitoring and management. *Neurosurgery Clinics of North America*, 5, pp. 573-605.

Leighton, D. A. (1974) Modifying influence of the size of the eye-ball in glaucomas [German]. *Klinische Monatsblätter für Augenheilkunde*, 164, pp. 475-478.

Leighton, D. A. (1972) Effect of walking on the ocular tension in open-angle glaucoma. *British Journal of Ophthalmology*, 56, pp. 126-130.

Lenke, L. G. (2003) Cerebral spinal fluid physiology. In: DEWALD, R.L. (ed) *Spinal Deformities: The Comprehensive Text*. New York: Thieme, pp. 149-152.

Liang, Y. *et al.* (2009) Impact of systemic blood pressure on the relationship between intraocular pressure and blood flow in the optic nerve head of nonhuman primates. *Investigative Ophthalmology and Visual Science*, 50, pp. 2154-2160.

Liu, J. H. *et al.* (2003) Twenty-four-hour intraocular pressure pattern associated with early glaucomatous changes. *Investigative Ophthalmology and Visual Science*, 44, pp. 1586-1590.

Liu, Y. and Vollrath, D. (2004) Reversal of mutant myocilin non-secretion and cell killing: implications for glaucoma. *Human Molecular Genetics*, 13, pp. 1193-1204.

Loewen, N. A. and Tanna, A. P. (2010) Glaucoma risk factors: Intraocular pressure. In: Schacknow, P. N. and Samples, J. R. (eds.) *The Glaucoma Book: A Practical, Evidence-Based Approach to Patient Care*. New York, Springer, pp. 35-50.

Lundberg, N. (1960) Continuous recording and control of ventricular fluid pressure in neurosurgical practice. *Acta psychiatrica Scandinavica - Supplementum*, 36, pp. 1-193.

Lundberg, N. et al. (1965) Continuous recording of the ventricular-fluid pressure in patients with severe acute traumatic brain injury. A preliminary report. *Journal of Neurosurgery*, 22, pp. 581-590.

March, K. and Madden, L. (2009) Intracranial pressure management. In: *AACN-AANN Protocols for Practice: Monitoring Technologies in Critically Ill Neuroscience Patients*. Sudbury, M A: Jones & Bartlett Learning, pp 35-70.

Macri, F. J. (1982) The pressure dependency of aqueous humor formation in the anesthetized cat. *Ophthalmic Research*, 14, pp. 279-283.

Marcus, D. F. *et al.* (1970) The effect of exercise on intraocular pressure. I. Human beings. *Investigative Ophthalmology*, 9, pp. 749-752.

Marín-Caballos, A. J. *et al.* (2005) Cerebral perfusion pressure and risk of brain hypoxia in severe head injury: a prospective observational study. *Critical care (London, England)*, 9, pp. 670-676.

Mark, H. H. (2007) The role of eye size in its pressure and motility. *Clinical Ophthalmology*, 1, pp. 105-109.

McComb, J. G. (1983) Recent research into the nature of cerebrospinal fluid formation and absorption. *Journal of Neurosurgery*, 59, pp. 369-383.

Milhorat, T. H. *et al.* (1971) Cerebrospinal fluid production by the choroid plexus and brain. *Science*, 173, pp. 330-332.

Mollan, S. P. *et al.* (2008) Accuracy of Goldmann, ocular response analyzer, Pascal and TonoPen XL tonometry in keratoconic and normal eyes. *British Journal of Ophthalmology*, 92, pp. 1661-1665.

Muchnok T, *et al.* (2010) Can intraocular pressure measurements be used to screen for elevated intracranial pressure in emergency department patients? *The Journal of Emergency Medicine*, doi: 10. 1016 /j.jemermed. 2010. 04. 032.

Navajas, E. V. *et al.* (2005) Concentration of hyaluronic acid in primary open-angle glaucoma aqueous humor. *Experimental Eye Research*, 80, pp. 853-857.

NG, I. *et al.* (2004) Effects of head posture on cerebral hemodynamics: its influences on intracranial pressure, cerebral perfusion pressure, and cerebral oxygenation. *Neurosurgery*, 54, pp. 593-597.

Nilsson, S. F. (1997) The uveoscleral outflow routes. *Eye (Lond)*, 11, pp. 149-154.

North, B. and Reilly, P. (1986) Comparison among three methods of intracranial pressure recording. *Neurosurgery*, 18, pp. 730-732.

North, B. (1997) Intracranial pressure monitoring. In: Reilly, P. and Bullock, R. (eds.) *Head Injury*. London: Chapman & Hall, pp. 209-216.

Ochiai, Y. and Ochiai, H. (2002) Higher concentration of transforming growth factor-beta in aqueous humor of glaucomatous eyes and diabetic eyes. *Japanese Journal of Ophthalmology*, 46, pp. 249-253.

Oresković, D. *et al.* (1991) Effect of intracranial pressure on cerebrospinal fluid formation in isolated brain ventricles. *Neuroscience*, 41, pp. 773-777.

Pollay, M. (2010) The function and structure of the cerebrospinal fluid outflow system. *Cerebrospinal Fluid Research*. 2010, 7, doi: 10.1186/1743-8454-7-9.

Prata, T. S. *et al.* (2007) Aqueous humor protein concentration in patients with primary open-angle glaucoma under clinical treatment [Portuguese]. *Arquivos Brasileiros de Oftalmologia*, 70, pp. 217-220.

Prata, T. S. *et al.* (2010) Posture-induced intraocular pressure changes: considerations regarding body position in glaucoma patients. *Survey of Ophthalmology*, 55, pp. 445-453.

Pederson, J. E. (1986) Ocular hypotony. *Transactions of the Ophthalmological Societies of the United Kingdom*, 105, pp. 220-226.

Pederson, J. E. and Green, K. (1973) Aqueous humor dynamics: a mathematical approach to measurement of facility, pseudofacility, capillary pressure, active secretion and X c. *Experimental Eye Research*, 15, pp. 265-276.

Pena, J. D. *et al.* (1998) Elastosis of the lamina cribrosa in glaucomatous optic neuropathy. *Experimental Eye Research*, 67, pp. 517-524.

Phelps, C. D. and Corbett, J. J. (1985) Migraine and low-tension glaucoma. A case-control study. *Investigative Ophthalmology and Visual Science*, 26, pp. 1105-1108.

Picht, G. *et al.* (2001) Transforming growth factor beta 2 levels in the aqueous humor in different types of glaucoma and the relation to filtering bleb development. *Graefe's Archive for Clinical and Experimental Ophthalmology*, 239, pp. 199-207.

Porchet, F. *et al.* (1998) The effect of position on intracranial pressure [French]. *Annales Françaises d'Anesthèsie et de Rèanimation*, 17, pp. 149-156.

Potter, D. E. and Rowland, J. M. (1978) Adrenergic drugs and intraocular pressure: effects of selective beta-adrenergic agonists. *Experimental Eye Research*, 27, pp. 615-625.

Power, M. C. *et al.* (2011) The association between blood pressure and incident Alzheimer disease: a systematic review and meta-analysis. *Epidemiology*, 22, pp. 646-65.

Price, E. L. *et al.* (2003) Effect of exercise on intraocular pressure and pulsatile ocular blood flow in a young normal population. *Optometry and Vision Science*, 80, pp. 460-466.

Querfurth, H. W. *et al.* (2004) Prediction of intracranial pressure from noninvasive transocular venous and arterial hemodynamic measurements: a pilot study. *Neurocritical Care*, 1, pp. 183-194.

Qureshi, I. A. (1995) Effects of mild, moderate and severe exercise on intraocular pressure of sedentary subjects. *Annals of Human Biology*, 22, pp. 545-553.

Qureshi, I. A. (1995) Age and intraocular pressure: how are they correlated? *Journal of the Pakistan Medical Association*, 45, pp. 150-152.

Qureshi, I. A. (1996) Effects of exercise on intraocular pressure in physically fit subjects. *Clinical and Experimental Pharmacology and Physiology*, 23, pp. 648-652.

Qureshi, I. (1997) Does physical fitness influence intraocular pressure? *Journal of the Pakistan Medical Association*, 47, pp. 81-84.

Radius, R. L. and Gonzales, M. (1981) Anatomy of the lamina cribrosa in human eyes. *Archives of Ophthalmology*, 99, pp. 2159-2162.

Ravi, R. and Morgan, R. J. (2003) Intracranial pressure monitoring. Current Anaesthesia and Critical Care, 14, pp. 229-235.

Razumovsky, A. Y. and Hanley, D.F. (1992) Intracranial pressure measurement/cranial vault mechanics: clinical and experimental observations. *Current Opinion in Neurology and Neurosurgery*, 5, pp. 818-825.

Reid, A. *et al.* (1990) The relationship between intracranial pressure and tympanic membrane displacement. *British Journal of Audiology*, 24, pp. 123-129.

Reitsamer, H. A. and Kiel, J. W. (2003) Relationship between ciliary blood flow and aqueous production in rabbits. *Investigative Ophthalmology and Visual Science*, 44, pp. 3967-3971.

Ren, R. *et al.* (2010) Cerebrospinal fluid pressure in glaucoma: a prospective study. *Ophthalmology*, 117, pp. 259-266.

Risner, D. *et al.* (2009) Effects of exercise *Journal of Glaucoma*, 18, pp. 429-436.

Robertson, C. S. *et al.* (1999) Prevention of secondary ischemic insults after severe head injury. *Critical Care Medicine*, 27, pp. 2086-2095.

Roper, A. H. *et al.* (2004) *Neurological and Neurosurgical Intensive Care, 4th edition.* Philadelphia: Lippincott Williams & Wilkins, pp. 12-25.

Roquefeuil, B. (1983) Posture and cerebral perfusion pressure [French]. Agressologie, 24, pp. 395-401.

Roy Chowdhury, U. *et al.* (2010) Proteome analysis of human aqueous humor. *Investigative Ophthalmology and Visual Science*, 51, pp. 4921-4931.

Sahin, A. *et al.* (2007) Comparison of the rebound tonometer with the Goldmann applanation tonometer in glaucoma patients. *Clinical and Experimental Ophthalmology*, 35, pp. 335-339.

Sajjadi, S. A. *et al.* (2006) The relation between intracranial and intraocular pressures: study of 50 patients. *Annals of Neurology*, 59, pp. 867-870.

Salim, S. and Shields, M. B. (2010) Glaucoma and systemic diseases. *Survey of Ophthalmology*, 55, pp. 64-77.

Schmidt, E. A. et al. (2001) Preliminary experience of the estimation of cerebral perfusion pressure using transcranial Doppler ultrasonography. Journal of Neurology, Neurosurgery, and Psychiatry, 70, pp. 198-204.

Schneider, E. and Grehn, F. (2006) Intraocular pressure measurement-comparison of dynamic contour tonometry and goldmann applanation tonometry. Journal of Glaucoma, 15, pp. 2-6.

Shiose, Y. and Kawase, Y. (1989) A new approach to stratified normal intraocular pressure in a general population. *American Journal of Ophthalmology*, 101, pp. 714-721.

Shoshani, Y. Z. et al. (2012) Endothelin and its suspected role in the pathogenesis and possible treatment of glaucoma. *Current Eye Research*, 37, pp. 1-11.

Sit, A. J. *et al.* (1997) The role of soluble proteins in generating aqueous outflow resistance in the bovine and human eye. *Experimental Eye Research*, 64, pp. 813-821.

Speake, T. *et al.* (2001) Mechanisms of CSF secretion by the choroid plexus. *Microscopy Research and Technique*, 52, pp. 49-59.

Spentzas, T. *et al.* (2010) Correlation of intraocular pressure with intracranial pressure in children with severe head injuries. *Pediatric Critical Care Medicine*, 11, pp. 593-598.

Stamper, R. (2010) IOP: Instruments to measure IOP. In: GIACONI, A.A. *et al.* (eds.) *Pearls of Glaucoma Management*. New York: Springer, pp. 79-86.

Stefan, C. *et al.* (2008) TGF-beta2 involvements in open angle glaucoma [Romanian]. *Oftalmologia*, 52, pp. 110-112.

Stefánsson, E. *et al.* (2005) Optic nerve oxygenation. *Progress in Retinal and Eye Research*, 24, pp. 307-332.

Steiner, L. A. and Andrews, P.J. (2006) Monitoring the injured brain: ICP and CBF. *British Journal of Anaesthesia*, 97, pp. 26-38.

Su, W. W. *et al.* (2008) Glaucoma is associated with peripheral vascular endothelial dysfunction. *Ophthalmology*, 115, doi: 10. 1016/j. ophtha. 2007.10.026.

Sugiyama, T. *et al.* (2006) Comparative study of cerebral blood flow in patients with normal-tension glaucoma and control subjects. *American Journal of Ophthalmology*, 141, pp. 394-396.

Tamm, E. R. (2002) Myocilin and glaucoma: facts and ideas. *Progress in Retinal and Eye Research*, 21, pp. 395-342.

Tans, J. T. and Poortvliet, D. C. (1983) Intracranial volume-pressure relationship in man. Part 2: Clinical significance of the pressure-volume index. *Journal of Neurosurgery*, 59, pp. 810-816.

Tiznado, E. *et al.* (1986) The effects of acute high dose fentanyl administration on experimental brain edema: analysis of intracranial pressure, systemic arterial pressure, central venous pressure and brain water content. *Pharmacology, Biochemistry, and Behavior*, 24, pp. 785-789.

To, C. H. *et al.* (2002) The mechanism of aqueous humour formation. *Clinical and Experimental Optometry*, 85, pp. 335-349.

Tomlinson, A. and Leighton, D. A. (1972) Ocular dimensions in low tension glaucoma compared with open-angle glaucoma and the normal. *British Journal of Ophthalmology*, 56, pp. 97-105.

Toris, C. B. *et al.* (2002) Aqueous humor dynamics in ocular hypertensive patients. *Journal of Glaucoma*, 11, pp. 253-258.

Tripathi, R. C. *et al.* (1991) Growth factors in the aqueous humor and their therapeutic implications in glaucoma and anterior segment disorders of the human eye. *Drug Development Research*, 22, pp. 1-23.

Tutaj, M. *et al.* (2004) Dynamic cerebral autoregulation is impaired in glaucoma. *Journal of the Neurological Sciences*, 220, pp. 49-54.

Vaajanen, A. *et al.* (2008) Does the renin-angiotensin system also regulate intra-ocular pressure? *Annals of Medicine*, 40, pp. 418-427.

Vieira, G. M. *et al.* (2006) Intraocular pressure variation during weight lifting. *Archives of Ophthalmology*, 124, pp. 1251-1254.

Wang, S. J. *et al.* (2010) Comorbidities of migraine. *Frontiers in Neurology*, 1, doi: 10.3389/fneur.2010.00016

Welch, K. (1967) The secretion *Monographs in the Surgical Sciences*, 4, pp. 155-192.

Werne, A. *et al.* (2008) The circadian variations in systemic blood pressure, ocular perfusion pressure, and ocular blood flow: risk factors for glaucoma? *Survey of Ophthalmology*, 53, pp. 559-567.

Williams, B. I. *et al.* (1980) Abnormal intraocular pressure control in systemic hypertension and diabetic mellitus. *British Journal of Ophthalmology*, 64, pp. 845-851.

Wolfs, R. C. et al. (1998) Genetic risk of primary open-angle glaucoma. Population-based familial aggregation study. *Archives of Ophthalmology*, 116, pp. 1640-1645.

Wuthrich, U. W. (1976) Postural changes and intraocular pressure in glaucomatous eyes. *British Journal of Ophthalmology*, 60, pp. 111-114.

Zakharov, A. *et al.* (2003) Lymphatic CSF absorption pathways in neonatal sheep revealed by subarachnoid injection of Microfil. *Neuropathology and Applied Neurobiology*, 29, pp. 563-573.

In: Hypotheses in Clinical Medicine
Editors: M.M. Shoja, P.S. Agutter et al.

ISBN: 978-1-62257-276-2

Chapter 20

Pathophysiological Basis for Anti-hypertensive Effects of Antioxidants and the Role of Oxidative Stress in Essential Hypertension

Ramón Rodrigo**, *Andrés Miranda-Merchak and Jaime González
Molecular and Clinical Pharmacology Program, Institute of Biomedical Sciences, Faculty of Medicine, University of Chile, Santiago, Chile

Abstract

Hypertension is considered the most important risk factor in the development of cardiovascular disease. An increasing body of evidence suggests that oxidative stress, which results in an excessive generation of reactive oxygen species (ROS), plays a key role in the pathogenesis of hypertension. The modulation of the vasomotor system involves ROS as mediators of vasoconstriction induced by angiotensin II, endothelin-1 and urotensin-II, among other factors. The bioavailability of nitric oxide (NO), a major vasodilator, is modulated by the cellular redox status. Under physiological conditions, low concentrations of intracellular ROS are important in normal redox signaling to maintain vascular function and integrity. However, under pathological conditions, ROS contribute to vascular dysfunction and remodeling through oxidative injury. Increased production of superoxide anion and hydrogen peroxide, decreased NO synthesis and diminished antioxidant capacity have been found in patients with essential hypertension. Antioxidants are reducing agents that can neutralize these oxidative compounds, which otherwise damage biomolecules and thereby cause functional and even structural impairment of the end-organs. The use of antioxidant vitamins such as vitamins C and E for protection against vascular endothelial injury has gained considerable interest. Available data support the role of these vitamins as effective antioxidants to counteract the effects of ROS. In this chapter, the following core hypothesis is evaluated: essential hypertension is a manifestation of subtle vascular inflammation brought about by heightened oxidative stress. For this purpose, the mechanisms involved in the generation

* E-mail: rrodrigo@med.uchile.cl.

of vascular ROS are discussed, as well as the role of oxidative stress in the pathogenesis of hypertension. Possible therapeutic strategies to overcome the heightened oxidative stress in essential hypertension are suggested.

Introduction

Hypertension is considered the most important risk factor for the occurrence of cardiovascular disease (Yusuf *et al.* 2004). Essential hypertension (EH) is by far the most common form of systemic hypertension. Recently, oxidative stress has gained attention as one of the fundamental mechanisms responsible for the development of hypertension. Reactive oxygen species (ROS) have an important role in homeostasis within the vascular wall; hence they could contribute to this mechanism (Paravicini and Touyz 2006; Rodrigo *et al.* 2003; Lassègue and Griendling 2004). Indeed, increased ROS production and reduced bio-availability of nitric oxide (NO) and antioxidants have been demonstrated in experimental and clinical hypertension. Vascular superoxide is derived primarily from NADPH (reduced nicotinamide adenine dinucleotide phosphate) oxidase when stimulated by hormones such as angiotensin II (AT-II), endothelin-1 (ET-1) and urotensin II (U-II), among others. In addition, ROS production may be increased by mechanical forces, which increase with hypertension. ROS-induced vasoconstriction results from increased intracellular calcium concentration (Paravicini and Touyz 2006). Vasomotor tone is dependent upon a delicate balance between vasoconstrictor and vasodilator forces resulting from the interaction of vascular wall components with the blood, and both sets of forces can be altered by oxidative stress. These findings have stimulated interest in antihypertensive therapies targeted at decreasing ROS generation and/or increasing NO bioavailability.

This chapter discusses the available evidence pointing to the role of oxidative stress in the mechanisms underlying increased blood pressure. A pilot study was conducted to examine the utility of antioxidants in the prevention or treatment of EH.

Pathophysiology OF Hypertension

Endothelial Dysfunction

Endothelial dysfunction has been implicated in the pathogenesis of different forms of cardiovascular disease including hypertension. It is characterized by a shift of the actions of the endothelium toward reduced vasodilatation and proinflammatory or prothrombotic states. These events lead to vascular inflammation, which may be mediated, partly, by ROS generated by activated mononuclear cells.

Vascular Oxidative Stress

Oxidative stress constitutes a unifying mechanism of injury among many disease processes. It occurs when there is an imbalance between the generation of ROS and the antioxidant defense systems in the body. The ROS family comprises several molecules that have divergent effects on cellular function. Many of these actions are associated with pathological changes observed in the cardiovascular system. The effects of ROS are mediated through the redox-sensitive regulation of multiple signaling molecules and second messengers (Kimura *et al.* 2005; Hool and Corry 2007; Yoshioka *et al.* 2006). Several studies have demonstrated that excessive amount of ROS are produced in patients with EH and in various animal models of hypertension (Lacy *et al.* 2000; Stojilkovic *et al.* 2002; Redon *et al.* 2003; Tanito *et al.* 2004; Touyz 2004), where antioxidant levels are abnormal (Briones and Touyz 2010; Zhou *et al.* 2006). These findings contribute to the accumulating evidence that increased vascular oxidative stress could be involved in the pathogenesis of EH (Paravicini and Touyz 2006; Rodrigo *et al.* 2003; Bengtsson *et al.* 2003).

Recently, a strong association between blood pressure and some oxidative stress-related parameters has been demonstrated (Rodrigo *et al.* 2007a-c). Mouse models with genetic deficits in ROS-generating enzymes have lower blood pressure than wild type animals (Landmesser *et al.* 2003; Gavazzi *et al.* 2006). In addition, in cultured vascular smooth muscle cells (VSMC) and in arteries isolated from hypertensive rats and humans, ROS production is enhanced, redox-dependent signaling is amplified, and antioxidant bioactivity is reduced (Touyz and Schiffrin 2001). The action of classical antihypertensive agents such as β-adrenergic blockers, angiotensin converting enzyme (ACE) inhibitors, angiotensin receptor antagonists and calcium channel blockers may be mediated, in part, by decreasing vascular oxidative stress (Ghiandoni *et al.* 2003; Yoshida *et al.* 2004).

Sources of ROS in the Vascular Wall

A variety of enzymatic and non-enzymatic sources of ROS exist in the vasculature. The best-characterized source of ROS is NADPH oxidase. Several other enzymes may also contribute to the generation of ROS including xanthine oxidase and NO synthase. The mitochondrion also adds to the intracellular pool of ROS.

NADPH Oxidase

NADPH oxidase is the primary biochemical source of ROS in the vasculature, particularly of superoxide. The kidney and vasculature are rich sources of NADPH oxidase-derived ROS, which under pathological conditions play an important role in renal dysfunction and vascular injury (Touyz 2004; Feairheller *et al.* 2009). This enzyme catalyzes the reduction of molecular oxygen by NADPH, thus generating superoxide. NADPH oxidase is up-regulated in hypertension by both humoral and mechanical signals. Angiotensin II (AT-II) is the most extensively studied of these, but ET-1 and urotensin II (U-II) also participate in the activation of NADPH oxidase, thereby resulting in increased ROS. A well-known function of NADPH oxidase-derived superoxide is inactivation of NO to form peroxynitrite, which then leads to impaired endothelium-dependent vasodilatation and uncoupling of eNOS to produce additional superoxide (Landmesser *et al.* 2003; Zou *et al.* 2004). Vascular NADPH oxidase activation has been strongly associated with hypertension (Lassègue and Clempus 2003).

Uncoupling of Endothelial Nitric Oxide Synthase (eNOS)

The primary function of eNOS is to generate the vasodilator, NO. Lack of L-arginine or tetrahydrobiopterin, the substrate and essential cofactor of eNOS, is associated with uncoupling of the L-arginine-NO pathway. This uncoupling results in a decreased formation of NO and increased eNOS-mediated generation of superoxide. NADPH oxidase becomes the initial source of ROS. The superoxide anion combines with NO synthesized by eNOS to form peroxynitrite (Kuzkaya *et al.* 2003). In turn, peroxynitrite oxidizes and destabilizes eNOS to produce more superoxide (Zou *et al.* 2004; Laursen *et al.* 2001). Superoxide also oxidizes tetrahydrobiopterin (which is highly sensitive to oxidation), further promoting eNOS uncoupling and ROS production.

Xanthine Oxidase

Xanthine oxidase is an important source of oxygen free radicals present in the vascular endothelium (Lassègue and Clempus 2003; Viel *et al.* 2008). It catalyzes the last two steps in purine catabolism in primates, during which oxygen is reduced to superoxide anion. There is evidence suggesting that this enzyme is involved in the pathogenesis of hypertension. Spontaneously hypertensive rats demonstrate elevated levels of endothelial xanthine oxidase and increased ROS production, which is itself associated with increased arteriolar tone (Fearheller *et al.* 2009). In addition to its effects on the vasculature, xanthine oxidase may play a role in end-organ injury in hypertension (Laakso *et al.* 2004).

Mitochondrion

The mitochondrion is a major source and target of ROS. A proportion of the superoxide anions produced in the intermembrane space may be carried to the cytoplasm (Han *et al.* 2004). Ubiquinol or coenzyme Q is a source of superoxide when it is partially reduced (semiquinone form) and an antioxidant when fully reduced (Eto *et al.* 1992). Complex I produces most of the superoxide anions generated in mammalian mitochondria *in vitro*. Complexes II and IV do not contribute significantly to ROS generation under normal conditions. Mild uncoupling effectively decreases the generation of superoxide anion by complex I (Rodrigo *et al.* 2007a-c).

The Role of the Vessel Wall

The endothelium senses mechanical stimuli as well as local and humoral mediators. In response, it releases agents that alter vasomotor function. There is no doubt that the endothelium plays a regulatory and protective role by generating vasorelaxing substances. Under some pathophysiological circumstances, endothelium-derived vasoconstricting factors such as ET-1, AT-II, U-II, superoxide anions, vasoconstrictor prostaglandins and thromboxane A_2 can be released and contribute to paradoxical vasoconstrictor effects. Vascular smooth muscle cells (VSMC) are responsible not only for short-term regulation of the blood vessel diameter and therefore of blood pressure, but also for long-term adaptation via structural remodeling. ROS mediate many of these pathophysiological processes.

The Role of Local and Humoral Mediators

Nitric Oxide (NO)

Nitric oxide is a key paracrine regulator of vascular tone. Physiologically, it inhibits leukocyte-endothelial cell adhesion, VSMC proliferation and migration, and platelet aggregation to maintain the integrity of the vascular endothelium. Therefore, it has multiple beneficial effects. A decrease in bioactivity of NO in the vasculature reduces the vasodilatory signals and contributes to hypertension. The enzyme that catalyzes the formation of NO from oxygen and arginine is NO synthase (NOS), which in fact is a whole family of enzymes. Endothelial NOS (eNOS) is the predominant isoform in the vessel wall. Shear stress and allosteric effectors are important modulators of eNOS activity (Michel *et al.* 1997). In addition to its vasorelaxing and antiproliferative properties *per se*, NO plays an important role in antagonizing the effects of AT-II, endothelin and ROS. It diffuses to the adjacent smooth muscle where it interacts with different receptor molecules such as those linked to soluble guanylyl cyclase.

It is accepted that normal production of NO is crucial for maintaining physiological conditions within the cardiovascular system. L-arginine, a substrate for eNOS, is necessary for NO production. Pre-treatment with L-NAME (methyl ester of N-nitro-L-arginine), an inhibitor of eNOS, blocks the anti-hypertensive effect of L-arginine (Simko et al. 2005). The angiotensin converting enzyme (ACE) inhibitor captopril completely prevented hypertension in NO-deficient animal models, yet without improving NOS activity (Pechánová *et al.* 2007). Nitric oxide reduces the activity of ACE. Thiols protect NO from oxidation by scavenging oxygen-free radicals and by forming nitrosothiols, prolonging the half-life and duration of action of NO (Zhang and Hogg 2005; Sládková *et al.* 2007). Elevated ROS is associated with a reduction in NO level. As mentioned earlier, the superoxide anion combines with NO to form peroxynitrite, which oxidizes tetrahydrobiopterin and destabilizes eNOS to produce more superoxide (Zou *et al.* 2004; Kuzkaya *et al.* 2003; Laursen *et al.* 2001), thus further enhancing the development of oxidative stress. The balance between NO and AT-II in the vasomotor centers seems to be important for the regulation of sympathetic tone (Hitomi *et al.* 2007).

Renin-angiotensin System

The renin-angiotensin system plays a key role in the development of cardiovascular disease. AT-II is a potent vasoactive peptide that can be formed in vascular beds rich in ACE. When AT-II production increases above normal levels, it results in hypertension and induces vascular remodeling and endothelial dysfunction. As a potent activator of NADPH oxidase, AT-II contributes to the production of ROS (Touyz 2004; Hitomi *et al.* 2007). In rats and mice made hypertensive by AT-II infusion, expression of NADPH oxidase subunits, oxidase activity, and generation of ROS are all increased (Landmesser *et al.* 2002). AT-II not only increases NADPH oxidase activity but also enhances superoxide dismutase (SOD) activity, possibly to compensate for the increased ROS. In situations where this compensatory effect is efficient, ROS levels may appear normal even in the face of prooxidants. However, when ROS production becomes overwhelming, the compensatory mechanism becomes exhausted and pathophysiological consequences ensue (Taniyama and Griendling 2003).

Captopril and enalapril decreased blood pressure in young spontaneously hypertensive rats; captopril had a greater hypotensive effect than enalapril, probably because its thiol group acted as an antioxidant (Bitar *et al.* 2005). NO not only antagonizes the effects of AT-II on vascular tone, cell growth and renal sodium excretion, but also down-regulates the synthesis of ACE and AT-I receptors. On the other hand, ACE inhibition up-regulates eNOS expression. The ability of AT-II to induce endothelial dysfunction is also due to its ability to down-regulate soluble guanylyl cyclase, thereby leading to impaired NO/cGMP signaling.

Acetylcholine

In the vasculature, acetylcholine (ACh) induces vasodilatation via production of endothelium-driven factors, mainly NO. NO then diffuses to the underlying VSMC, where it induces relaxation. A diminution in NO bioactivity reduces ACh-mediated vasodilatation (Pechánová 2007; Bitar *et al.* 2005). As discussed earlier, a decrease in the NO level is a direct and indirect consequence of heightened vascular oxidative stress.

Endothelins

Endothelins are potent vasoconstrictor isopeptides produced by different parts of a blood vessel, including the vascular endothelium. Endothelin-1 (ET-1) is the main endothelin generated by the endothelium and the most important in the cardiovascular system. When ET-1 is administered in high concentrations, it acts as a potent vasoconstrictor capable of exerting an array of physiological effects, including the potential to alter arterial pressure. ET-1 mediates its effects through two receptors, endothelin-1 type A (ET_A) and type B (ET_B) receptors. Some effects of ET_A stimulation are mediated by the activation of NADPH oxidase, xanthine oxidase, lipoxygenase, uncoupling of NO synthase, and mitochondrial respiratory chain enzymes. ET_B induces vasorelaxation by acting on endothelial cells (Gomez-Alamillo *et al.* 2003). Many factors that normally stimulate ET-1 synthesis (e.g. thrombin, AT-II) also cause the release of vasodilators such as prostacyclin (PGI_2) and/or NO, which oppose the vasoconstricting action of ET-1. It has been reported that EH is associated with an increased vasoreactivity (vasoconstrictor response) to ET-1, an effect that seems to be related to decreased endothelial ET_B-mediated NO production (Verhaar *et al.* 1998).

Urotensin-II

Urotensin-II (UT-II) is a potent vasoactive peptide (Djordjevic *et al.* 2005), indeed the most potent vasoconstrictor so far identified. It also activates NADPH oxidase. Its role in vascular disease is not clear. The constrictor response to UT-II appears to be variable and highly dependent on the vascular bed examined. Vasoconstriction is not its only effect, because UT receptors have been found in other organs as well (Matsushita *et al.* 2001; Jegou *et al.* 2006). UT-II has also been shown to act as a potent vasodilator in some isolated vessels (Stirrat *et al.* 2001).

Prostaglandins

Prostacyclin (PGI_2) is another endothelium-derived vasodilator. This mediator is released in greater amount in response to thrombin, arachidonic acid, histamine, or serotonin. The enzyme prostaglandin H_2 synthase utilizes arachidonic acid as a substrate, forming prostaglandin H_2. Prostaglandin H_2 is converted to vasoactive molecules such as PGI_2. The isoform prostaglandin H_2 synthase-2 may mediate vascular dysfunction under conditions characterized by oxidative stress. Thus, oxidative stress, induced through the production of peroxynitrite from the reaction between superoxide and NO, inhibits the activity of prostacyclin synthase, thereby impairing PGI_2-mediated vasodilatation (Vaziri 2008).

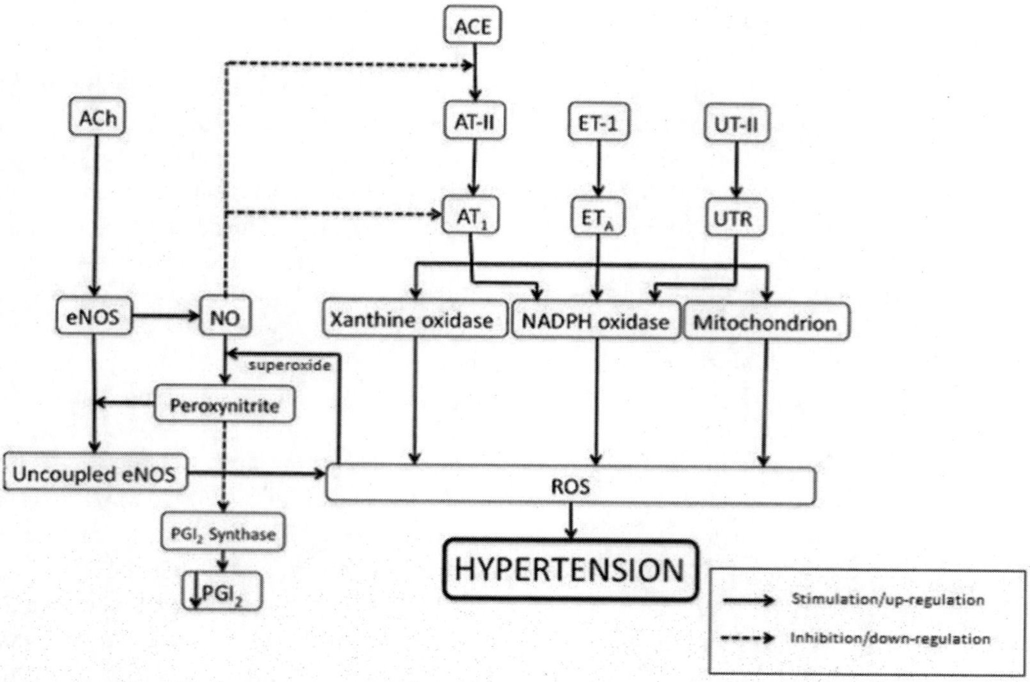

Figure 20.1. A schematic summary of the role of vascular oxidative stress in the pathogenesis of hypertension. ACE, angiotensin converting enzyme; AT-II, angiotensin II; AT1, type 1 angiotensin II receptor; ET-1, endothelin-1; ETA, endothelin-1 type A receptor; UT-II, urotensin II; UTR, urotensin-II receptor; Ach, acetylcholine; NO, nitric oxide; eNOS, nitric oxide synthase; PGI2, prostacyclin; ROS, reactive oxygen species (from Rodrigo et al. 2011 – reproduced with permission from Nature Publishing Group).

The core hypothesis concerning the role of vascular oxidative stress in hypertension is depicted in Figure 20.1. The role of ROS in the vasculature and its relation to hypertension have already been discussed. It is necessary to mention that hypertensive stimuli such as high salt and AT-II promote the generation of ROS not only in the vasculature, but also in the kidney and the central nervous system (Harrison and Gongora 2009). The following section refers to the antihypertensive effects of endogenous and exogenous antioxidants, which have been shown to alter vascular function and to participate in the main redox reactions involved in the pathophysiology of hypertension.

Endogenous Antioxidants

The main endogenous antioxidant enzymes are glutathione peroxidase (GSH-Px), catalase (CAT) and superoxide dismutase (SOD). Glutathione peroxidase reduces hydrogen peroxide and organic hydroperoxides into water and alcohols, respectively (Andreoli 1991; Meister and Anderson 1983). Catalase catalyzes the breakdown of hydrogen peroxide into water and molecular oxygen. Superoxide dismutase is a major superoxide scavenger. It converts the superoxide anion to hydrogen peroxide, which is a substrate for GSH-Px and CAT (Rubanyi and Vanhoutte 1986). Decreased enzymatic antioxidant activity in human and animal models of hypertension has been widely reported (Lee *et al.* 2010; De Cavanagh *et al.* 2010; Zhou *et al.* 2006; Kashyap *et al.* 2005; Kedziora-Kornatowska *et al.* 2004; Zhan *et al.* 2004). These findings indicate a state of reduced antioxidant defense capacity in systemic hypertension.

The reduced form of glutathione (GSH), endogenously generated, is the substrate for GSH-Px and the hydrogens of its sulfhydryl groups serve as reductants (Wernerman and Hammarqvist, 1999). Patients with hypertension have an impaired glutathione system (Da Silva et al. 2010; Joules et al. 2010). The thioredoxin system also plays a role in maintaining the redox state (Ebrahimian and Touyz 2008; Xu et al. 2009). In spontaneously hypertensive rats, thioredoxin expression is altered (Tanito et al. 2004). Thus, thioredoxin could be a potential therapeutic target for the prevention and treatment of hypertension (Widder et al. 2009; Maulik and Das 2008; World et *al.* 2006).

Finally, uric acid exhibits antioxidant properties and is the most abundant scavenger of free radicals in humans. High concentrations are associated with increased serum antioxidant capacity and reduced oxidative stress (Waring *et al.* 2001; Waring *et al.* 2003). However, there is evidence for the potential association of high plasma uric acid concentrations with hypertension and cardiovascular risk (Feig *et al.* 2008; Mazzali *et al.* 2001; Mazzali *et al.* 2010; Baker and Schumacher 2010; Nagahama *et al.* 2004). To explain this apparently paradoxical association, it should be assumed that the elevation of plasma uric acid concentrations in hypertension is due to the hyperactivity of vascular xanthine oxidase (Feairheller *et al.* 2009; Zou *et al.* 2004; Lassègue and Clempus 2003; Kuzkaya *et al.* 2003; Laursen *et al.* 2001; Viel *et al.* 2008; Laakso *et al.* 2004). This enzyme, as discussed earlier, is known to increase oxidative stress in the vasculature.

Exogenous Antioxidants

Vitamin C

Vitamin C (ascorbic acid) is a potent water-soluble antioxidant. It up-regulates eNOS and down-regulates NADPH oxidase (Ulker *et al.* 2003). Vitamin C favors vasodilatation, possibly through its effects on NO (Vita *et al.* 1998; Jackson *et al.* 1998; Duffy *et al.* 2001). Most studies have demonstrated an inverse relationship between plasma ascorbate levels and blood pressure in both normotensive and hypertensive individuals (Redrigo *et al.* 2007). It has been shown that treatment with vitamin antioxidants including ascorbic acid reduces blood pressure in animal models (Nishikawa *et al.* 2003; Reckelhoff *et al.* 1998) and improves hypertension in human (Chen *et al.* 2001; Atarashi *et al.* 1997).

Several short-term clinical trials to study the effect of vitamin C supplements on blood pressure have yielded inconsistent findings (Duffy *et al.* 1999; Fotherby *et al.* 2000; Block *et al.* 2001; Ghosh *et al.* 1994; Duffy *et al.* 2004; Galley *et al.* 1997; Mullan *et al.* 2002). In this connection, the lack of antihypertensive efficacy observed in some studies using supplementation with vitamin C alone could be related to the impairment of NO bioavailability by heightened oxidative stress (Steinbrenner and Sied 2009). In addition, the pharmacokinetic properties of vitamin C should be taken into account. Experimentally, it has been determined that vitamin C exerts an antihypertensive effect at 10 mmol/L (Jackson *et al.* 1998), a plasma level unobtainable in humans through oral administration but necessary to compete efficiently with the reaction of NO with superoxide. The renal ascorbic acid reabsorption threshold is reached by a daily vitamin C dose of 60 to 100 mg. The plasma is completely saturated with a 400 mg daily dose, producing a steady-state plasma concentration of approximately 80 μM (Padayatty *et al.* 2003). Thus, the antihypertensive effect of vitamin C may only be achievable if high doses are infused.

Vitamin E

This major lipid-soluble vitamin has received considerable attention for its antioxidant potential. Epidemiological data support a role of high dietary vitamin E intake in reducing the incidence of cardiovascular disease (Malyszko 2010). Vitamin E is capable of dose-dependently decreasing the mitochondrial generation of superoxide and hydrogen peroxide (Venditti *et al.* 2007).

The results of trials have not been satisfactory, with a number of studies demonstrating no beneficial effect of vitamin E on cardiovascular disease outcomes (Rapola et al. 1999; Lonn et al. 2005; Lee et al. 2005). Moreover, a study using supplementation with vitamin E, either as α-tocopherol or as mixed tocopherols, showed a significant increase in blood pressure, pulse pressure and heart rate in individuals with type 2 diabetes (Ward et al. 2007). This may be secondary to vitamin-E-induced oxidative stress and the oxidation of α-tocopherol to α-tocopheroxyl in a lipophilic environment, particularly in plasma membranes (Münzel and Keaney 2001; Clarke et al. 2008).

Reciprocal Relationship between Vitamins C and E

Ascorbic acid reduces the α-tocopheroxyl radical (an intermediate in the antioxidative reaction of vitamin E) and is required for the beneficial vascular effects of α-tocopherol (Heller *et al.* 2006). The effect of α-tocopherol seems to be dependent on tissue saturation with vitamin C, and the two vitamins may act synergistically to provide optimal conditions for endothelial NO formation (Heller *et al.* 2004). Thus, a combination of vitamins C and E is expected to exert a greater antihypertensive effect, because this combined therapy reinforces their individual properties (Bilodeau and Hubel 2003).

Although short-term clinical trials have shown that intake of supplemental antioxidant vitamins lowers blood pressure (Fotherby *et al.* 2000; Mullan *et al.* 2002; Galley *et al.* 1997; Plantinga *et al.* 2007), most long-term trials have failed to reveal a significant antihypertensive effect. However, most of those studies lacked rigorous exclusion criteria in the selection of subjects to avoid the influence of potential confounders (Rodrigo *et al.* 2007a-c). It is worth mentioning that the anti-hypertensive effects of antioxidant vitamins are likely to obtainable early in the course of hypertension when there is no end-organ injury. A study involving newly-diagnosed hypertensive patients without end-organ injury demonstrated an association between oxidative-stress-related parameters and blood pressure (Rodrigo *et al.* 2008; Rodrigo *et al.* 2010). These data support the view that the antihypertensive effect of vitamins C and E is achieved if they are administered during the endothelial dysfunction phase, which precedes the irreversible vascular changes that result from remodeling. Thus, the antihypertensive effect of antioxidant vitamins is not expected to be observed in patients with advanced cardiovascular disease in whom the chronic and irreversible effects of oxidative stress on the vasculature are already established. It seems that ROS may be more important in the induction than in the maintenance of hypertension.

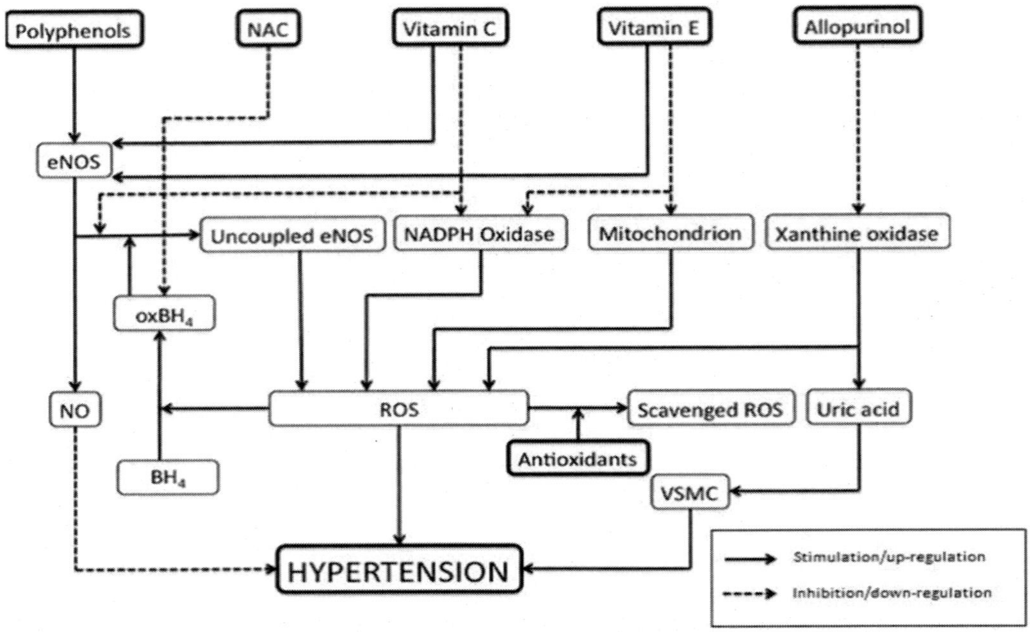

Figure 20.2. A schematic summary accounting for the potential anti-hypertensive effects of the exogenous antioxidants. BH4, tetrahydrobiopterin; eNOS, nitric oxide synthase; NAC, N-acetylcysteine; NO, nitric oxide; oxBH4, oxidized tetrahydrobiopterin; ROS, reactive oxygen species; VSMC, vascular smooth muscle cells (from Rodrigo et al. 2011 – reproduced with permission from Nature Publishing Group).

Allopurinol

Xanthine oxidase is an important source of ROS in the vascular endothelium (George and Struthers 2009). Xanthine oxidase activity is associated with an increasing arteriolar tone and therefore hypertension (Suzuki *et al.* 1998; Delano *et al.* 2006). Xanthine oxidase inhibitors such as allopurinol cause a marked improvement in endothelial function in various cohorts of patients at risk of cardiovascular events. Treatment with allopurinol reduces blood pressure in adolescents (Feig *et al.* 2008) and in patients with chronic kidney disease (Goicoechea *et al.* 2010). Nevertheless, most of the evidence to date has come from small studies, and the few large randomized controlled trials have shown no significant mortality benefit from these agents (George and Struthers 2009).

N-Acetylcysteine

The antioxidant N-acetylcysteine, which contains a sulfhydryl group, protects against lipid peroxidation and scavenges ROS (De la Fuente and Victor 2001; Penugonda *et al.* 2005). It improves renal function and decreases arterial pressure and renal injury in salt-sensitive hypertension (Tian *et al.* 2006). The inhibition of oxidative stress in hypertensive states probably contributes to the therapeutic value of N-acetylcysteine, an effect probably mediated by an NO-dependent mechanism (Pechánová *et al.* 2006a). This protective mechanism involves the prevention of tetrahydrobiopterin oxidation by the increased superoxide anion level (Zembowicz *et al.* 1993).

Polyphenols

Polyphenols are the most abundant antioxidants in the diet. They can act as ROS scavengers and iron chelators (Rodrigo and Bosco, 2006; Pietta *et al.* 1998), and possibly enhance the production of NO (Duarte *et al.* 2004; Zenebe *et al.* 2003). In humans, circulating NO concentrations are increased after the consumption of polyphenols (Pechánová *et al.* 2006b). However, some studies have shown that blood pressure is increased when polyphenols are combined with vitamin C (Ward *et al.* 2005).

A Trial to Assess the Efficacy of Antioxidant Vitamins in Treating EH

A summary of the mechanisms underlying the antihypertensive effects of exogenous antioxidants is shown in Figure 20.2. In order to test the hypothesis that co-supplementation with vitamins C and E could reduce blood pressure in patients with EH, a double-blind, randomized, placebo-controlled clinical trial was conducted (Rodrigo *et al.* 2008). The study was also aimed at evaluating the relationship between the oxidative stress and blood pressure.

Materials and Methods

Study Population and the Diagnosis of EH

The study included 110 previously-untreated male patients with EH (mean age, 46 years (range, 35–60 years)) recruited from among newly-diagnosed patients at the Cardiovascular Center, University of Chile Clinical Hospital, Santiago, Chile between March 2004 and December 2006. During each patient visit, blood pressure was measured with a standard mercury sphygmomanometer. Secondary hypertension was excluded by clinical history, physical examination and appropriate tests. Inclusion criteria were: men, age between 35 and 60 years, hypertension (defined as a mean daytime systolic blood pressure (SBP) between 135 and 154 mmHg or diastolic blood pressure (DBP) between 85 and 94 mmHg on ambulatory blood pressure monitoring (ABPM)) (Myers *et al.* 2005), no diabetes or impaired glucose tolerance (American Diabetes Association 2004), absence of semiquantitative proteinuria, body mass index between 23 and 29.9 kg/m^2, total serum cholesterol less than 5.4 mmol/l, and serum triacyglycerol (triglyceride) less than 2.3 mmol/l. Exclusion criteria included smoking, consumption of alcoholic beverages (> 40 g/week), concomitant systemic diseases, vigorous physical exercise, use of medication (including mineral or vitamin supplements, antihypertensive drugs or statins) and/or the high consumption of fruits and vegetables. Grade I EH was diagnosed according to the European Society of Hypertension and Cardiology criteria (European Society of Hypertension-European Society of Cardiology Guidelines Committee 2003). Dietary food and nutrient intake was assessed using a 3-day food record, and physical activity levels were controlled with a modified Baecke questionnaire (Baecke *et al.* 1982) at baseline and at the end of the study. Recruited patients were asked not to change their physical activity habits or dietary intake during the study.

One hundred and ten normotensive individuals were recruited from the same clinic as the subjects with hypertension. This group served as a normotensive reference to determine control values for the studied parameters. The inclusion and exclusion criteria for this group were the same as the patients with EH. The study was conducted according to the Helsinki Declaration of the World Medical Association (2000), and written informed consent was obtained from all individuals prior to participation in the trial.

Table 1. The baseline characteristics of patients with EH and healthy normotensive controls

Characteristic	Controls	Patients	*P* value
Number	110	110	
Age (years)	44.1 ± 0.9	45.6 ± 1.1	0.29
Body mass index (kg/m^2)	25.1 ± 0.3	25.5 ± 0.2	0.26
Heart rate (beats/min)	72.2 ± 1.1	73.6 ± 1.4	0.43
Serum glucose (mmol/L)	4.96 ± 0.04	5.07 ± 0.08	0.22
Creatinine (μmol/L)	77.4 ± 1.3	79.2 ± 1.9	0.43
Total cholesterol (mmol/L)	4.62 ± 0.17	4.72 ± 0.22	0.71
HDL-cholesterol (mmol/L)	1.26 ± 0.02	1.20 ± 0.05	0.26
LDL-cholesterol (mmol/L)	2.62 ± 0.20	2.82 ± 0.14	0.41
Serum triacylglycerols (mmol/L)	1.44 ± 0.06	1.50 ± 0.02	0.34
Renin (pmol x l^{-1} x h^{-1})	24.1 ± 2.1	21.1 ± 1.9	0.29
Aldosterone (nmol/L)	0.22 ± 0.02	0.24 ± 0.01	0.37
Endothelin-I (pmol/L)	2.67 ± 0.18	2.71 ± 0.14	0.86
Homocysteine (μmol/L)	8.62 ± 0.21	9.11 ± 0.33	0.21
Folic acid (nmol/L)	44.9 ± 1.2	46.1 ± 1.2	0.47
Vitamin B_{12} (pmol/L)	226 ± 6	226 ± 6	1.00
Systolic blood pressure (mmHg)	119 ± 0	139 ± 0	**<0.001**
Diastolic blood pressure (mmHg)	77.4 ± 0.3	96.3 ± 0.7	**<0.001**
Mean arterial pressure (mmHg)	92 ± 1	107 ± 1	**<0.001**

Note values are means ± SEM. HDL, high-density lipoprotein; LDL, low-density lipoprotein. The *P* values were determined using an unpaired Student's t-test.

Blood pressure was measured by ABPM on a normal workday (over 24 h from 08:30 AM) using an oscillometric monitor (SpaceLabs 90207). This device fulfils the validation criteria of the British Hypertension Society protocol (O'Brien *et al.* 1991) and satisfies the criteria of the AAMI (Association for the Advancement of Medical Instrumentation) for studies in ambulatory conditions (Groppelli *et al.* 1992). The adult cuff and the large adult cuff were used for arm circumferences of 24-31 cm and 32-42 cm, respectively.

Group Design and Measurements

A randomized, double-blind, placebo-controlled clinical trial was conducted. The hypertensive patients were randomly allocated to daily treatment with either placebo (n = 55) or vitamins C plus E (n = 55; 1 g of vitamin C as L-ascorbic acid plus 400 IU (international unit) of vitamin E as RRR-α-tocopheryl acetate) once a day for eight weeks. Both medications were given in encapsulated forms to ensure that the placebo and vitamins were indistinguishable, and were provided by Procaps and Gynopharm CFR Laboratories. All patients were asked to take the assigned medication 30 min before breakfast once a day. At baseline and at the end of the study, subjects underwent 24-h blood monitoring (ABPM) to check for blood pressure changes, and blood samples were collected for the determination of lipid, glucose profile, plasma levels of blood pressure modulators (renin, aldosterone, ET-1 (endothelin-1), homocysteine, folic acid and vitamin B_{12}), plasma and erythrocyte oxidative-stress-related parameters and antioxidant status. All blood samples were collected at the same time of day to minimize circadian variations. Adverse events, clinic blood pressure measurements and compliance with the study medication were recorded during each follow-up visit and through weekly direct communications with the patients (by telephone or email). The methods of measuring blood pressure followed the Joint National Committee guidelines (Chobanian *et al.* 2003). All study personnel and participants remained blinded to the treatment assigned for the duration of the study.

Table 2. The baseline parameters related to the plasma and erythrocyte antioxidant system and oxidative stress in patients with essential hypertension versus healthy normotensive individuals

Parameter	Normotensive individuals	Patients with EH	P value
Number	110	110	
FRAP (μmol/L)	426 ± 14	311 ± 8	**<0.01**
Vitamin C (μmol/L)	44.2 ± 1.7	37.5 ± 1.8	**<0.01**
Vitamin E (μmol/L)	16.1 ± 1.2	16.4 ± 1.1	0.84
8-Isoprostane (pmol/L)	76.7 ± 3.6	105 ± 3	**<0.01**
CAT (K/g of Hb)	290 ± 6	220 ± 8	**<0.01**
SOD (units/g of Hb)	1472 ± 21	1157 ± 26	**<0.01**
GSH-Px (units/g of Hb)	6.11 ± 0.11	5.48 ± 0.14	**<0.01**
GSH/GSSG ratio	5.98 ± 0.14	5.20 ± 0.13	**<0.01**
MDA (nmol/g of Hb)	311 ± 8	383 ± 11	**<0.01**

Blood samples from the antecubital vein were collected in chilled Vacutainers containing EDTA (1.5 mg/mL) and were centrifuged at 3000 g for 10 min to obtain plasma. Erythrocytes were subjected to hypotonic haemolysis by dilution with distilled water. Plasma samples and erythrocyte lysates were stored at −70°C. For the measurement of 8-isoprostane, blood was collected in plastic tubes treated with the antioxidant butylated hydroxytoluene (final concentration 1 mmol/L).

Assays for Oxidative Stress-related Parameters

FRAP (Ferric Reducing Ability of Plasma)

Plasma antioxidant status was assessed by measuring its ability to reduce ferric to ferrous iron, with a detection limit of 10 μmol/L (Benzie and Strain 1996).

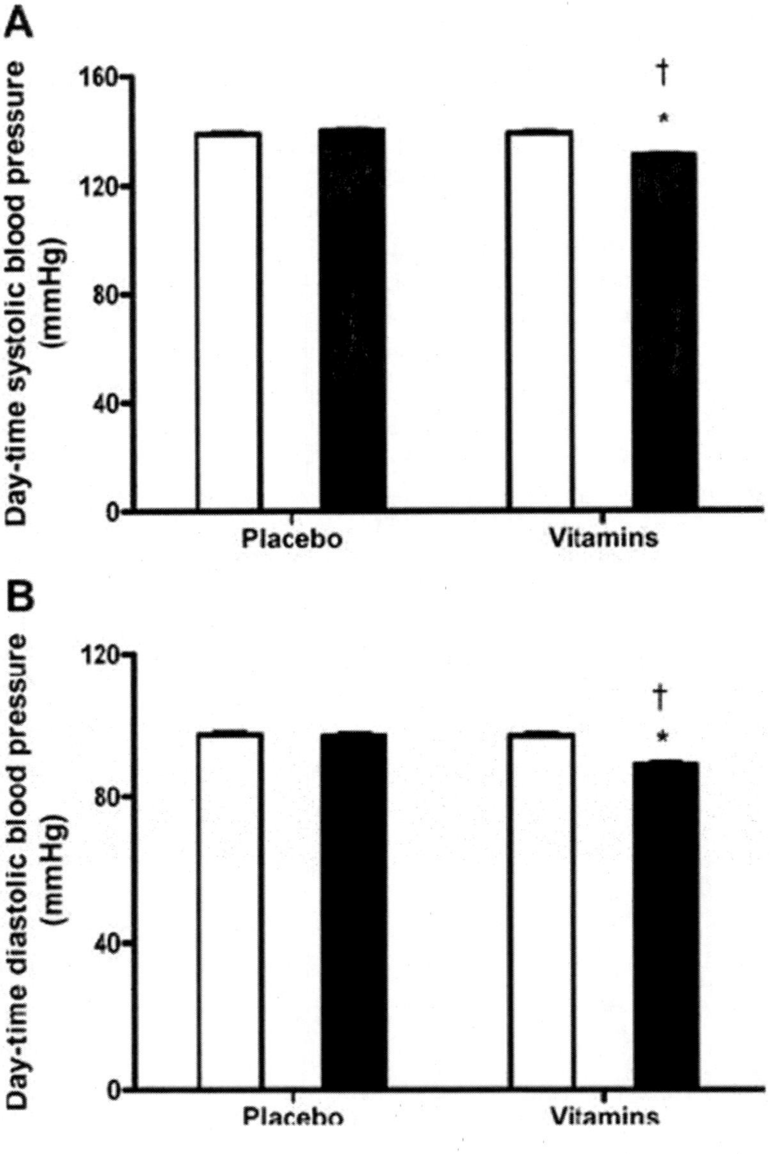

Figure 20.3. Daytime SBP (A) and DBP (B) in hypertensive patients before (open bars) and after (closed bars) treatment with vitamins C plus E or placebo. The sources of variation were assessed by one-way ANOVA followed by Bonferroni's multiple comparison test as the post-hoc test. $^{*}P < 0.001$ compared with basal; $^{\dagger}P < 0.001$ compared with placebo-treated patients with essential hypertension (from Rodrigo et al. 2008 – reproduced with permission from Nature Publishing Group).

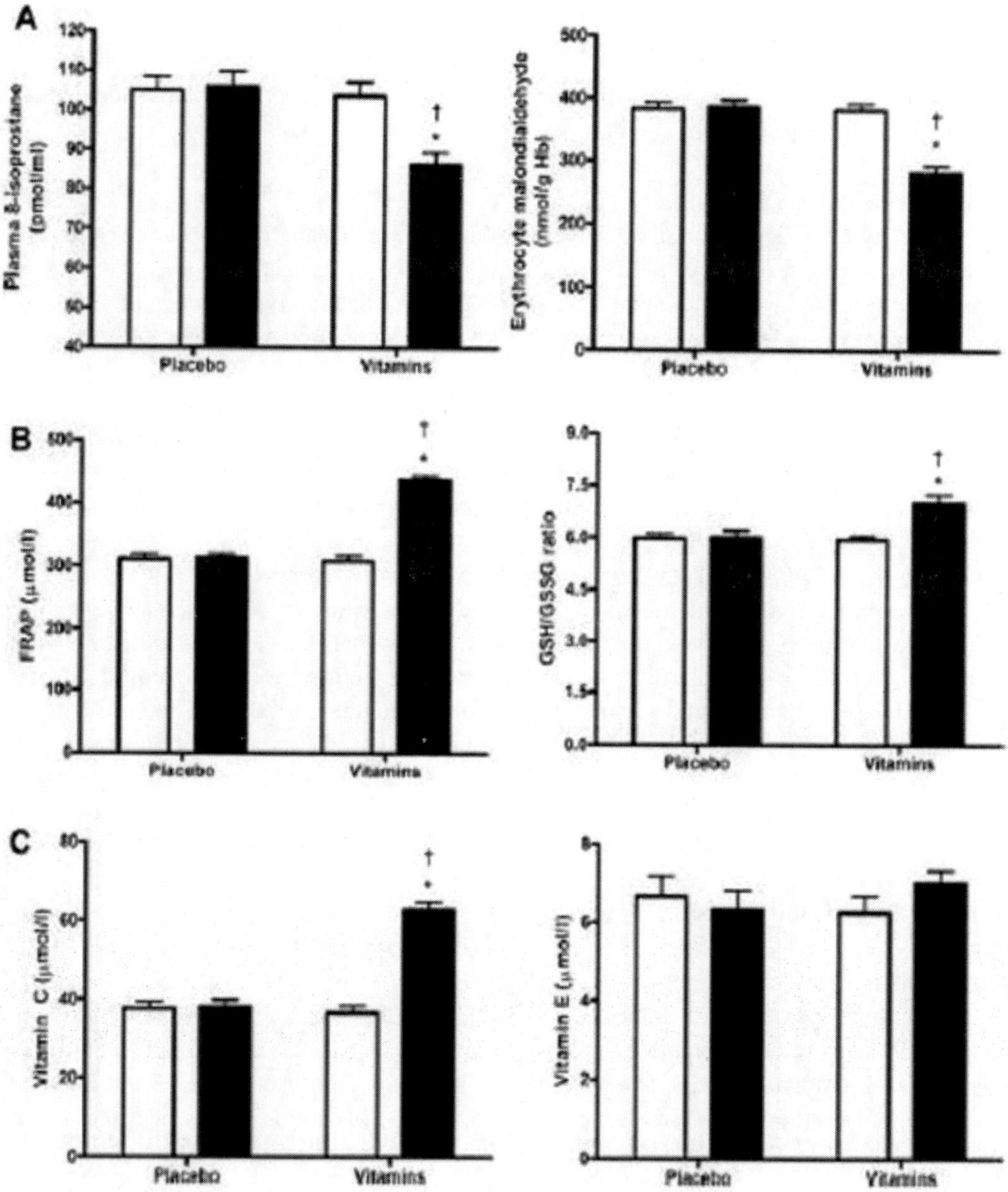

Figure 20.4. Lipid peroxidation and antioxidant status in patients with EH before (open bars) and after (closed bars) treatment with vitamins C plus E or placebo. The lipid peroxidation was estimated from plasma 8-isoprostane and erythrocyte malondialdehyde concentrations (A). The antioxidant status was assessed by plasma FRAP and the erythrocyte GSH/GSSG ratio (B) and plasma vitamin C and E concentrations (C). The sources of variation were assessed by one-way ANOVA followed by Bonferroni's multiple comparison test as the post-hoc test. $^{*}P < 0.001$ compared with the baseline values; $^{\dagger}P < 0.001$ compared with placebo-treated hypertensive patients (from Rodrigo et al. 2008 – reproduced with permission from Nature Publishing Group).

Glutathione

The levels of reduced and oxidized forms of glutathione (GSH and GSSG, respectively) were assayed by fluorimetry in erythrocytes, and the GSH/GSSG ratio was calculated and considered an indicator of intracellular redox status (Hissin and Hilf 1976).

Malondialdehyde (MDA)

Erythrocyte lipid peroxidation was assayed spectrophotometrically at 532 nm by the thiobarbituric acid reaction at pH 3.5 followed by solvent extraction with a mixture of n-butanol:pyridine (15:1, v/v) (Ohkawa *et al.* 1979). Tetramethoxypropane was used as the external standard, and the levels of lipid peroxides were expressed as nmol of MDA/g Hb.

8-Isoprostane

Plasma 8-isoprostane concentration (in pmol/ml), recognized as a reliable biomarker of lipid peroxidation *in vivo* (Milne *et al.* 2005), was determined by an enzyme-linked immunosorbent assay (ELISA) kit (Cayman) (Pradelles *et al.* 1985).

Assessment of Plasma Vitamin C and E Concentrations

Plasma vitamin C levels were assessed by a colorimetric FRASC (ferric reducing/ antioxidant and ascorbate concentration) assay no later than 2 h after blood samples were collected. FRASC is a fast and reliable alternative to high-performance liquid chromatography (HPLC), with a detection limit of 3.0 μmol/l (Chung *et al.* 2001). The intra- and inter-assay CVs were 2.7% and 4.9%, respectively. Plasma vitamin E concentration was measured by HPLC, and the inter- and intra-assay CVs were 6.4% and 4.5%, respectively (Morena *et al.* 2002). Blood samples were centrifuged for 5 min. A hexane extract of the supernatant was evaporated to dryness. The dry residue was dissolved in methanol and used for reverse-phase HPLC using a NovaPack 15033.9 mm column (4 mm particle size) and a UV detector at 292 nm (Lambda max 480; Millipore-Waters).

Antioxidant Enzymes

Erythrocyte lysates were homogenized in 0.25 mol/L sucrose for the determination of Cu-Zn SOD (superoxide dismutase) activity, or in 1.15%KCl/10 mmol/l Tris/HCl buffer (pH 7.4) for CAT (catalase) and GSH-Px (glutathione peroxidase) activities. The Cu-Zn SOD assay is based on the SOD-mediated increase in the rate of autooxidation of catechols in an aqueous alkaline solution to yield a chromophore with a maximum absorbance at 525 nm (Nebot *et al.* 1993). One Cu-Zn SOD unit is defined as the activity that doubles the auto-oxidation background, and results are expressed as units/g Hb. The CAT activity was assayed by the kinetics of hydrogen peroxide breakdown at 240 nm by an aliquot of the 2400 g supernatant and are expressed as the first-order reaction rate constant (k)/g Hb (Aebi 1974). Soluble GSH-Px activity was measured spectrophotometrically in the cytosolic fraction (100,000 g supernatant) by the reduction of glutathione disulfide coupled to NADPH oxidation by glutathione reductase (Flohé and Günzler 1984). One GSH-Px unit is defined as the activity that oxidizes 1 μmol of NADPH/min; activity was expressed as units/g Hb.

Other Measurements

Plasma levels of renin and aldosterone were measured by radioimmunoassay (RIA), and ET-1, homocysteine, folic acid and vitamin B12 by ELISA kits.

Statistical Analysis

The required sample size was calculated by using blood pressure as the primary endpoint; 45 patients in each group provided us with 80% power to detect a 5 mmHg difference between the mean arterial blood pressures (MAP) of the two treatment groups. This calculation was also applied to the biochemical parameters of the study. Descriptive statistics of variables are presented as means ± standard error of the mean (SEM). Baseline differences between the normotensive control group and patients with EH and between the clinical characteristics of the groups receiving vitamins C plus E and placebo were assessed using Student's t-test. Biochemical parameters, and SBP, DBP and MAP of patients with EH at baseline and following treatment with the placebo or vitamin combination, were compared by one-way analysis of variance (ANOVA) using Bonferroni's multiple comparison test as the post-hoc test. A P value less than 0.05 was considered statistically significant. In view of their Gaussian distribution, the association of variables was studied by Pearson correlation test. All statistical analyses were calculated using GraphPad PrismTM version 2.0.

Results

The baseline characteristics of the normotensive control group (n = 110) and patients with EH (n = 110) are shown in Table 1. The two groups were comparable with respect to age, body mass index, lipid panel, and serum glucose and creatinine concentrations. The mean daytime SBP, DBP and MAP in the group with EH were significantly higher ($P < 0.001$). In addition, the plasma concentrations of renin, aldosterone, ET-1, homocysteine, folic acid and vitamin B_{12} were comparable between the two groups.

Antioxidant Status and Oxidative Stress-related Parameters at Baseline: Hypertensive versus Normotensive Individuals

As described earlier, the normotensive individuals were recruited to serve as a reference group to determine the normal values of the biochemical parameters studied. The parameters related to plasma and erythrocyte oxidative stress and antioxidant status are shown in Table 2. Patients with EH had a lower antioxidant capacity; FRAP, vitamin C levels and erythrocyte GSH/GSSG ratios were significantly lower by 27%, 15% and 15%, respectively ($P < 0.01$) (Table 2). The activities of erythrocytic CAT, SOD and GSH-Px in EH patients were 24%, 21% and 10% lower, respectively, than the corresponding values in the normotensive individuals ($P < 0.01$). Furthermore, patients with EH had 37% higher plasma 8-isoprostane levels and 23% higher erythrocyte MDA or lipid peroxidation levels than the normotensive individuals ($P < 0.001$).

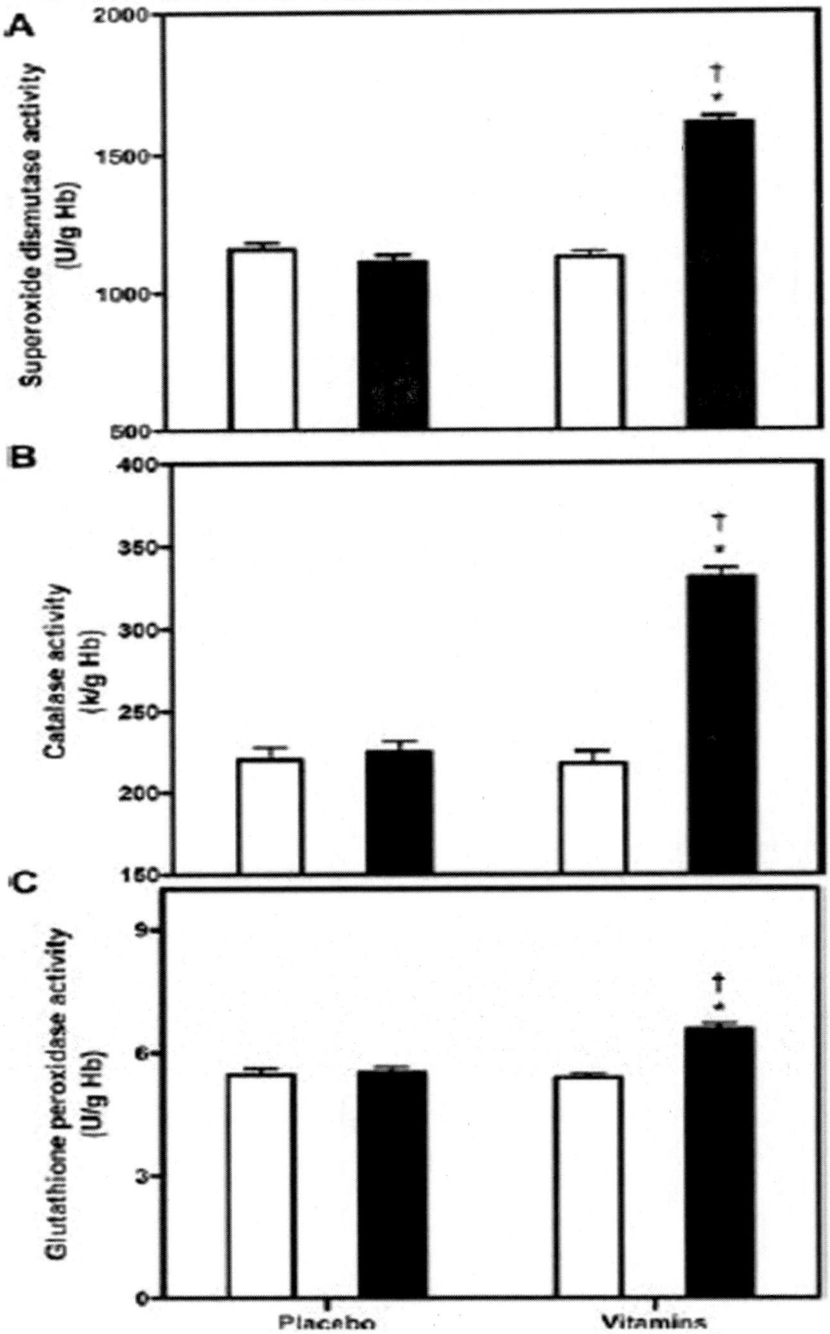

Figure 20.5. The activities of erythrocytic glutathione peroxidase, catalase and superoxide dismutase in hypertensive patients before (open bars) and after (closed bars) treatment with vitamins C plus E or placebo. The sources of variation were assessed by one-way ANOVA followed by Bonferroni's multiple comparison test as the post-hoc test. $^{*}P < 0.001$ compared with the baseline values; $^{\dagger}P < 0.001$ compared with the placebo-treated hypertensive patients (from Rodrigo et al. 2008 – reproduced with permission from Nature Publishing Group).

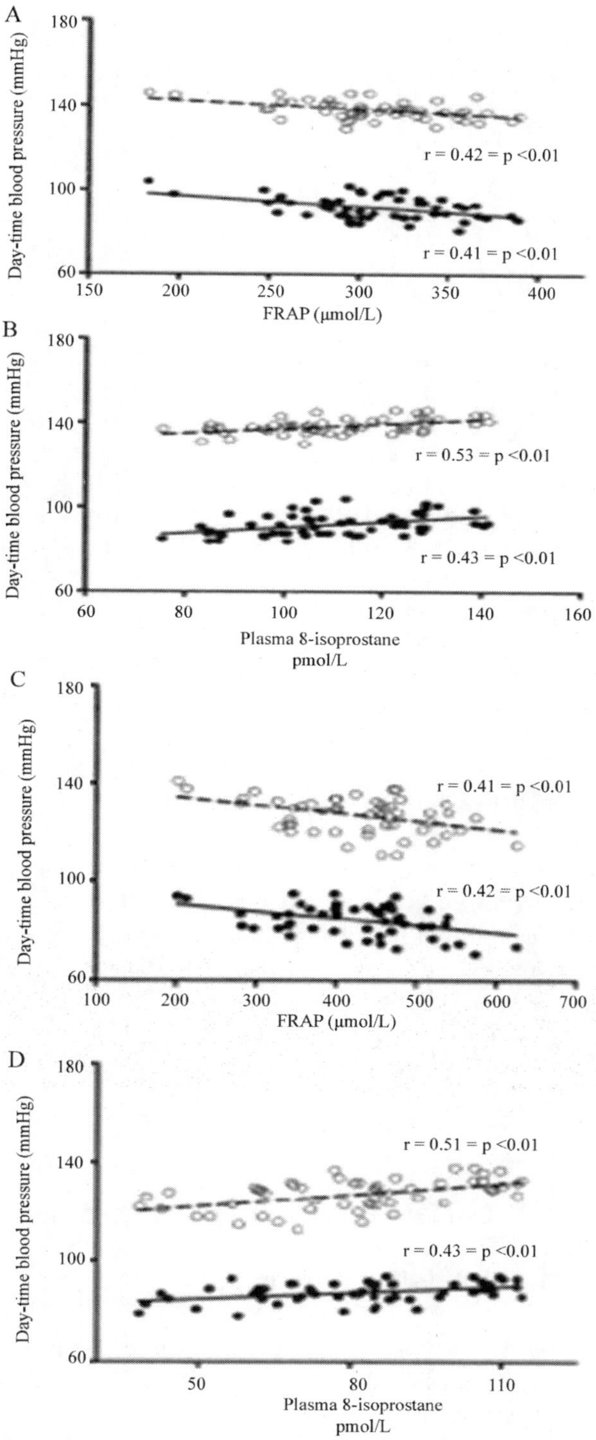

Figure 20.6. The associations among blood pressure, antioxidant status and oxidative stress in the placebo-treated (A-B) and vitamin-treated (C-D) hypertensive patients. Pearson correlations of systolic blood pressure (white circles) and diastolic blood pressure (black circles) with plasma antioxidant capacity (FRAP) and plasma 8-isoprostane levels are shown (from Rodrigo et al. 2008 – reproduced with permission from Nature Publishing Group).

Table 3. Effects of treatment with vitamins C plus E or placebo on clinical and laboratory characteristics in patients with essential hypertension

Characteristic	Placebo	Vitamins C plus E	*P* value
Number	55	55	
Age (years)	45.6 ± 1.5	45.4 ± 1.1	0.91
BMI (kg/m^2)	25.3 ± 0.3	25.6 ± 0.7	0.69
Heart rate (beats/min)	72.1 ± 1.1	74.4 ± 1.7	0.25
Serum glucose (mmol/L)	4.96 ± 0.12	5.16 ± 0.16	0.31
Creatinine (µmol/L)	80.1 ± 1.2	79.1 ± 2.1	0.68
Total cholesterol (mmol/L)	4.64 ± 0.18	4.76 ± 0.23	0.49
HDL-cholesterol (mmol/L)	1.21 ± 0.03	1.18 ± 0.02	0.40
LDL-cholesterol (mmol/L)	2.79 ± 0.09	2.83 ± 0.10	0.76
Serum triacylglycerols (mmol/L)	1.49 ± 0.11	1.52 ± 0.09	0.83
Renin (pmol/L/h)	19.1 ± 2.0	22.2 ± 2.2	0.30
Aldosterone (nmol/L)	0.25 ± 0.01	0.24 ± 0.03	0.75
ET-I (pmol/L)	2.73 ± 0.15	2.70 ± 0.23	0.91
Homocysteine (µmol/L)	9.30 ± 0.39	9.11 ± 0.41	0.73
Folic acid (nmol/L)	47.3 ± 1.3	45.6 ± 1.1	0.32
Vitamin B_{12} (pmol/L)	221 ± 7	231 ± 7	0.31

Note values are means ± SEM. HDL, high-density lipoprotein; LDL, low-density lipoprotein. The *P* values were determined using an unpaired Student's t-test.

Treatment with Vitamins C Plus E versus Placebo

Fifty-five patients with EH completed the eight-week treatment period with vitamins C plus E. No side effects were observed or reported throughout the trial. Dietary and physical activity habits and body weight did not change during the study. No significant differences were observed among hypertensive patients treated with placebo or vitamins C plus E with respect to the plasma concentrations of renin, aldosterone, ET-1, homocysteine, folic acid or vitamin B_{12} (Table 3). Hypertensive patients treated with vitamins C plus E had significantly lower SBP, DBP and MAP than either the placebo-treated patients (n = 55) or the entire patient group prior to treatment (n = 110) (Figure 20.3).

Antioxidant Status and Oxidative Stress-related Parameters Following Treatment with Vitamins C Plus E or Placebo: Hypertensive versus Normotensive Individuals

Following treatment with vitamins C plus E, a statistically significant decrease in lipid peroxidation, as estimated by plasma 8-isoprostane and erythrocytic MDA concentrations, was noted among the hypertensive patients compared with the baseline or the placebo-treated hypertensive patients (Figure 20.4A). Plasma and erythrocyte antioxidant capacity, as measured by FRAP, GSH/GSSH ratio and plasma vitamin C levels, were significantly higher in EH patients treated with vitamins C plus E than the baseline or the placebo-treated hypertensive patients (Figure 20.4). However, no statistically significant differences were observed in the plasma vitamin E concentrations between the placebo- and vitamin-treated groups (Figure 20.4C). The activities of the antioxidant enzymes SOD, CAT and GSH-Px were higher among EH patients treated with vitamins C plus E than the baseline or the placebo-treated patients (Figure 20.5).

The Associations among Blood Pressure, Antioxidant Status and Oxidative Stress

In both the placebo-treated and vitamin-treated groups of EH patients, negative correlations were observed between the total plasma antioxidant capacity (i.e. FRAP) and SBP and DBP (Figure 20.6). The plasma level of lipid peroxidation correlated positively with SBP and DBP in both groups (Figure 20.6).

Discussion

The present study provides evidence that oral administration of vitamins C+E to patients with mild-to-moderate EH results in a significant decrease in blood pressure by enhancing their blood antioxidant status. Previous studies have reported decreased (Galley *et al.* 1997), unchanged (Kim *et al.* 2002; Plantinga *et al.* 2007; Hercberg *et al.* 204) or increased (Ward *et al.* 2007, Ward *et al.* 2005) blood pressure after oral administration of antioxidant vitamins. The results of the present study show a decrease in blood pressure following antioxidant vitamin administration, and are in agreement with others using a similar protocol design and vitamin treatment (Galley *et al.* 1997).

The findings of different studies could have conflicted because the inclusion criteria for participant selection and the pharmacokinetic properties of antioxidant vitamins were not considered. Also, there could be difficulties in making comparisons among the studies owing to various associations of antioxidants, the stage of the disease, and incomplete information on the oxidative stress status, which should be considered a necessary component of the clinical history of the patients enrolled (Rodrigo *et al.* 2007a-c). Moreover, most previous studies on the administration of antioxidant vitamins have focused on the prevention of cardiovascular events as the end point (Yusuf *et al.* 2005; Lonn *et al.* 2005; Salonen *et al.* 2003; Miller *et al.* 2005), and only a few have examined their potential antihypertensive effects (Hercberg *et al.* 2004). In the present study, patient inclusion criteria were more rigorous and the confounding effects of other factors likely to interfere with oxidative-stress/antioxidant-status-related parameters were avoided. The lack of antihypertensive efficacy observed in studies using supplementation with vitamin C alone could be due to the pharmacokinetics of vitamin C and/or the decreased bioavailability of NO under conditions of oxidative stress. Indeed, in our present study, plasma vitamin C concentrations did not exceed 70 μmol/l (Figure 20.4 C). Recent pharmacokinetic modeling indicates that, with oral administration of vitamin C, even at very large and frequent doses, plasma concentrations will be increased only modestly, from 70 μmol/l to a maximum of 220 μmol/l, whereas intravenous administration can increase it to as high as 15 mmol/l (Padayatty *et al.* 2004). The antihypertensive effect may only occur in plasma following infusion of high vitamin C doses.

Intra-arterial administration of vitamin C has been shown to cause a decrease in blood pressure in subjects with EH (Schneider *et al.* 2005).

The dosage of vitamin E supplementation used in the present study was based on previous trials to assess its clinical effect on the risk of cardiovascular events. These studies demonstrated that doses higher than 400 IU/day may increase all-cause mortality and should be avoided (Miller *et al.* 2005). Because of the distribution of vitamin E in various lipophilic environments, its plasma levels are not necessarily related to its oral dosage (Rodrigo *et al.* 2005). Our present results show no significant differences in plasma vitamin E levels between patients with EH treated with vitamins C+E and either placebo-treated patients with EH or patients with EH at baseline prior to treatment. This could be explained by the distribution of the administered vitamin E, implying that plasma levels are a poor index of vitamin E status (Rodrigo *et al.* 2005). The abundance of polyunsaturated fatty acids in biological membranes, which are particularly sensitive to oxidative damage, accounts for the increase in lipid peroxidation, probably caused by either ROS and/or α-tocopheroxyl. Vitamin C can reduce the α-tocopheroxyl radical, thereby abrogating lipid peroxidation (Heller *et al.* 2006). The association of vitamins C and E used in the present study, as well as in others (Galley *et al.* 1997), has an antihypertensive effect, probably because this combined therapy is expected to reinforce the individual properties of the two vitamins through a complementary effect in improving endothelial dysfunction (Bilodeau and Hubel 2003).

Vitamins C and E not only scavenge ROS but also induce the down-regulation of NADPH oxidase and the up-regulation of eNOS (Attia *et al.* 2001), thereby enhancing their antihypertensive effect. The greater oxidative stress and lower antioxidant capacity in patients with EH at baseline compared with normotensive subjects is in agreement with previous studies (Russo *et al.* 1998; Rodrigo *et al.* 2007a-c). The present study showed a significant decrease in SBP, DBP and MAP following supplementation with vitamins C+E in patients with EH compared with either placebo-treated patients with EH (Figure 20.3) or the patients with EH at baseline, which is in agreement with other studies (Galley *et al.* 1997; Duffy *et al.* 1999). The slight decrease in blood pressure induced by antioxidant vitamin administration was expected in view of the mild-to-moderate baseline blood pressure levels included in the protocol. These changes are associated with a decrease in lipid peroxidation parameters, plasma 8-isoprostane and erythrocyte MDA, but not with changes in plasma concentrations of blood pressure modulators including renin, aldosterone, ET-1 and homocysteine. In addition, an improved antioxidant status is shown by the increase in FRAP levels and the GSH/GSSG ratio, and the increased activity of antioxidant enzymes in erythrocytes.

Moreover, the strong association of plasma 8-isoprostane and FRAP levels with SBP and DBP, together with the results mentioned above, is consistent with the involvement of oxidative stress in the mechanism of EH. To our knowledge, the present study is the first to report this association following antioxidant vitamin supplementation to patients with EH and is in agreement with previous studies on untreated subjects with hypertension (Rodrigo *et al.* 2007a-c; Simic *et al.* 2006; Laffer *et al.* 2006). In contrast, a lack of association between oxidative stress and blood pressure was reported by Plantinga *et al.* (Plantinga *et al.* 2007), even though they used the same doses and time of exposure to supplementation with vitamins C+E; however, these authors used a cross-over study design. In addition, they did not consider the possible influence of other modulators that could contribute to the regulation of blood pressure, in contrast to the present study.

In summary, the results reported in the present study show for the first time a specific association between oxidative-stress-related parameters and blood pressure, thus suggesting the role of oxidative stress in the pathogenesis of EH. Moreover, the concomitant decrease in blood pressure and oxidative stress raises the possibility that oxidative stress may be considered a therapeutic target against the development of hypertension. Therefore oral administration of vitamins C plus E in patients with EH is suggested as an adjunct therapy for hypertension.

Conclusion and Perspectives

There is considerable evidence supporting the view that oxidative stress is involved in the pathophysiology of hypertension. ROS are mediators of the major physiological vasoconstrictors, increasing intracellular calcium concentration. In addition, superoxide reduces the bioavailability of NO and enhances its own production via uncoupled eNOS, further enhancing oxidative stress, a major factor in hypertension.

Antioxidant therapy can curtail the development of hypertension in animal models, but remains controversial in humans. Possible confounding factors in patients include co-existing pathologies and treatments, and lack of selection of treatments according to ROS levels, among others. However, the dietary intake of antioxidants and polyphenols could be effective in the primary prevention or reduction of hypertension. In this regard, our results showed that supplementation with vitamins C and E in patients with EH attenuates oxidative damage and also reduces blood pressure values. Thus, the combined use of antioxidant vitamins may be a useful alternative for treating EH in patients without target-organ injury. Although the role of antioxidant therapy remains an open question, it could be suggested that these interventions should be more efficient in preventing than in reducing established hypertension.

References

Aebi, H. (1974) Catalase. In: Bergmeyer, H. U. (ed.) *Methods in Enzymatic Analysis*. New York: Academic Press, pp. 673-677.

American Diabetes Association (2004) Diagnosis and classification of diabetes mellitus. *Diabetes Care,* 27[Suppl 1], pp. 5-10.

Andreoli, S. P. (1991) Reactive oxygen molecules, oxidant injury and renal disease. *Pediatric Nephrology*, 5, pp. 733-742.

Atarashi, K. *et al.* (1997) Vitamin E ameliorates the renal injury of Dahl Salt-sensitive rats. *American Journal of Hypertension*, 10, pp. 116-119.

Attia, D. M. *et al.* (2001) Vitamin E alleviates renal injury, but not hypertension, during chronic nitric oxide synthase inhibition in rats. *Journal of the American Society of Nephrology*, 12, pp. 2585-2593.

Baecke, J. A. *et al.* (1982) A short questionnaire for the measurement of habitual physical activity in epidemiological studies. *The American Journal of Clinical Nutrition*, 36, pp. 936-942.

Baker, J. F. and Schumacher, H. R. (2010) Update on gout and hyperuricemia. *International Journal of Clinical Practice*, 64, pp. 371-377.

Bengtsson, S. H. *et al.* (2003) Novel isoforms of NADPH oxidase in vascular physiology and pathophysiology. *Clinical and Experimental Pharmacology and Physiology*, 30, pp. 849-854.

Benzie, I. F. and Strain, J. J. (1996) The ferric reducing ability of plasma (FRAP) as a measure of 'antioxidant power': the FRAP assay. *Analytical Biochemistry*, 239, pp. 70-76.

Bilodeau, J. F. and Hubel, C. A. (2003) Current concepts in the use of antioxidants for the treatment of preeclampsia. *Journal of Obstetrics and Gynaecology Canada*, 25, pp. 742-750.

Bitar, M. S. *et al.* (2005) Nitric oxide dynamics and endothelial dysfunction in type II model of genetic diabetes. *European Journal of Pharmacology*, 511, pp. 53-64.

Block, G. *et al.* (2001) Ascorbic acid status and subsequent diastolic and systolic blood pressure. *Hypertension*, 37, pp. 261-267.

Briones, A. M. and Touyz, R. M. (2010) Oxidative stress and hypertension: current concepts. *Current Hypertension Reports*, 12, pp. 135-142.

Chen, X. *et al.* (2001) Antioxidant effects of vitamins C and E are associated with altered activation of vascular NADPH oxidase and superoxide dismutase in stroke-prone SHR. *Hypertension*, 38, pp. 606-611.

Chobanian, A. V. *et al.* (2003) Seventh report of the joint national committee on prevention, detection, evaluation, and treatment of high blood pressure. *Hypertension*, 289, pp. 2560-2572.

Chung, W. Y. *et al.* (2001) Plasma ascorbic acid: measurement, stability and clinical utility revisited. *Clinical Biochemistry*, 34, pp. 623-627.

Clarke, M. W. *et al.* (2008) Vitamin E in human health and disease. *Critical Reviews in Clinical Laboratory Sciences*, 45, pp. 417-450.

Da Silva, A. P. *et al.* (2010) Decreased erythrocyte activity of methemoglobin and glutathione reductases may explain age-related high blood pressure. *Revista Portuguesa de Cardiologia*, 29, pp. 403-412.

De Cavanagh, E. M. *et al.* (2010) Vascular Structure and Oxidative Stress in Salt-Loaded Spontaneously Hypertensive Rats: Effects of Losartan and Atenolol. *American Journal of Hypertension*, 23, pp. 1318-1325.

De la Fuente, M. and Victor, V. M. (2001) Ascorbic acid and N-acetylcysteine improve *in vitro* the function of lymphocytes from mice with endotoxin-induced oxidative stress. *Free Radical Research*, 35, pp. 73-84.

Delano, F. A. *et al.* (2006) Microvascular display of xanthine oxidase and NADPH oxidase in the spontaneously hypertensive rat. *Microcirculation*, 13, pp. 551-566.

Djordjevic, T. *et al.* (2005) Human urotensin II is a novel activator of NADPH oxidase in human pulmonary artery smooth muscle cells. *Arteriosclerosis, Thrombosis, and Vascular Biology*, 25, pp. 519-525.

Duarte, J. *et al.* (2004) Wine polyphenols stimulate superoxide anion production to promote calcium signaling and endothelialdependent vasodilatation. *Physiological Research*, 53, pp. 595-602.

Duffy, S. J. *et al.* (1999) Treatment of hypertension with ascorbic acid. *Lancet*, 354, pp. 2048-2049

Duffy, S. J. *et al.* (2001) Effect of ascorbic acid treatment on conduit vessel endothelial dysfunction in patients with hypertension. *American Journal of Physiology - Heart and Circulatory Physiology*, 280, pp. 528–534.

Duffy, S. J. *et al.* (2004) Treatment of hypertension with ascorbic acid. *Lancet*, 354, pp. 2048-2049.

Ebrahimian, T. and Touyz, R. M. (2008) Thioredoxin in vascular biology: role in hypertension. *Antioxidants and Redox Signaling*, 10, pp.1127-1136.

Eto, Y. *et al.* (1992) Succinate-dependent lipid peroxidation and its prevention by reduced ubiquinone in beef heart submitochondrial particles. *Archives of Biochemistry and Biophysics*, 295, pp. 101-106.

European Society Of Hypertension-European Society Of Cardiology Guidelines Committee (2003) European Society of Hypertension-European Society of Cardiology guidelines for the management of arterial hypertension. *Journal of Hypertension*, 21, pp. 1011-1053.

Feairheller, D. L. *et al.* (2009) Exercise training, NADPH oxidase p22phox gene polymorphisms, and hypertension. *Medicine and Science in Sports and Exercise*, 41, pp. 1421-1428.

Feig, D. I. *et al.* (2008) Effect of allopurinol on blood pressure of adolescents with newly diagnosed essential hypertension: a randomized trial. J*ournal of the American Medical Association*, 300, pp. 924-932.

Flohé, L. and Günzler, W. A. (1984) Assays of glutathione peroxidase. *Methods in Enzymology*, 105, pp. 114-121.

Fotherby, M. D. *et al.* (2000) Effect of vitamin C on ambulatory blood pressure and plasma lipids in older persons. *Journal of Hypertension*, 18, pp. 411-415.

Galley, H. F. *et al.* (1997) Combination oral antioxidant supplementation reduces blood pressure. *Clinical Science*, 92, pp. 361-365.

Gavazzi, G. *et al.* (2006) Decreased blood pressure in NOX1-deficient mice. *FEBS Letters*, 580, pp. 497-504.

George, J. and Struthers, A. (2009) The role of urate and xanthine oxidase in vascular oxidative stress: future directions. *Journal of Therapeutics and Clinical Risk Management*, 5, pp. 799-803.

Ghiadoni, L. *et al.* (2003) Different effect of antihypertensive drugs on conduit artery endothelial function. *Hypertension*, 41, pp. 1281-1286.

Ghosh, S. K. *et al.* (1994) A double-blind, placebo-controlled parallel trial of vitamin C treatment in elderly patients with hypertension. *Gerontology*, 40, pp. 268-272.

Goicoechea, M. *et al.* (2010) Effect of allopurinol in chronic kidney disease progression and cardiovascular risk. *Clinical Journal of the American Society of Nephrology*, 5, 1388-1393. Gomez-Alamillo, C. *et al.* (2003) Interactions between vasoconstrictors and vasodilators in regulating hemodynamics of distinct vascular beds. *Hypertension*, 42, pp. 831-836.

Groppelli, A. *et al.* (1992) Evaluation of noninvasive blood pressure monitoring devices Spacelabs 90202 and 90207 versus resting and ambulatory 24-hour intra-arterial blood pressure. *Hypertension*, 20, pp. 227-232.

Han, D. *et al.* (2003) Voltage-dependent anion channels control the release of the superoxide anion from mitochondria to cytosol. *Journal of Biological Chemistry*, 278, pp. 5557-5563.

Harrison, D. G. and Gongora, M. C. (2009) Oxidative stress and hypertension. *Medical Clinics of North America*, 93, pp. 621-635.

Heller, R. *et al.* (2004) Alpha-tocopherol and endothelial nitric oxide synthesis. *Annals of the New York Academy of Sciences*, 1031, pp. 74-85.

Heller, R. *et al.* (2006) Antioxidants and endothelial nitric oxide synthesis. *European Journal of Clinical Pharmacology*, 62[Suppl 13], pp. 21-28.

Hercberg, S. *et al.* (2004) A randomized, placebo-controlled trial of the health effects of antioxidant vitamins and minerals. *Archives of Internal Medicine*, 164, pp. 2335-2342.

Hissin, P. J. and Hilf, R. (1976) A fluorometric method for determination of oxidized and reduced glutathione in tissues. *Analytical Biochemistry*, 74, pp. 214-226.

Hitomi, H. *et al.* (2007) Angiotensin II and oxidative stress. *Current Opinion in Cardiology*, 22, pp. 311-315.

Hool, L. C. and Corry, B. (2007) Redox control of calcium channels: from mechanisms to therapeutic opportunities. *Antioxidants and Redox Signaling*, 9, pp. 409-435.

Jackson, T. S. *et al.* (1998) Ascorbate prevents the interaction of superoxide and nitric oxide only at very high physiological concentrations. *Circulation Research*, 83, pp. 916-922.

Jegou, S. *et al.* (2006) Localization of the urotensin II receptor in the rat central nervous system. *Journal of Comparative Neurology*, 495, pp. 21-36.

Joles, J. A. *et al.* (2010) Renal glutathione S-transferase mu type 1 expression is already reduced in new-born spontaneously hypertensive rats. *Journal of Hypertension*, 28, pp. 633-634.

Kashyap, M. K. *et al.* (2005) Different antioxidants status, total antioxidant power and free radicals in essential hypertension. *Molecular and Cellular Biochemistry*, 277, pp. 89-99.

Kedziora-Kornatowska, K. *et al.* (2004) The markers of oxidative stress and activity of the antioxidant system in the blood of elderly patients with essential arterial hypertension. *Cellular and Molecular Biology Letters*, 9, pp. 635-641.

Kim, M. K. *et al.* (2002) Lack of long-term effect of vitamin C supplementation on blood pressure. *Hypertension*, 40, pp. 797-803.

Kimura, S. *et al.* (2005) Mitochondria-derived reactive oxygen species and vascular MAP kinases: comparison of angiotensin II and diazoxide. *Hypertension*, 45, pp. 438-444.

Kuzkaya, N. *et al.* (2003) Interactions of peroxynitrite, tetrahydrobiopterin, ascorbic acid, and thiols: implications for uncoupling endothelial nitric-oxide synthase. Jo*urnal of Biological Chemistry*, 278, pp. 22546-22554.

Laakso, J. T. *et al.* (2004) Renal xanthine oxidoreductase activity during development of hypertension in spontaneously hypertensive rats. *Journal of Hypertension*, 22, pp. 1333-1340.

Lacy, F. *et al.* (2000) Plasma hydrogen peroxide production in human essential hypertension: role of heredity, gender, and ethnicity. *Hypertension*, 36, pp. 878-884.

Laffer, C. L. *et al.* (2006) Effect of salt on isoprostanes in salt-sensitive essential hypertension. *Hypertension*, 47, pp. 434-444.

Landmesser, U. *et al.* (2003) Oxidation of tetrahydrobiopterin leads to uncoupling of endothelial cell nitric oxide synthase in hypertension. *Journal of Clinical Investigation*, 111, pp. 1201-1209.

Landmesser, U. *et al.* (2002) Role of p47(phox) in vascular oxidative stress and hypertension caused by angiotensin II. *Hypertension*, 40, pp. 511-515.

Lassègue, B. and Clempus, R. E. (2003) Vascular NAD(P)H oxidases: specific features, expression, and regulation. *American Journal of Physiology - Regulatory Integrative and Comparative Physiology*, 285, pp. 277-297.

Lassègue, B. and Griendling, K (2004) Reactive oxygen species in hypertension, an update. *American Journal of Hypertension*, 17, pp. 852-860.

Laursen, J. B. *et al.* (2001) Endothelial regulation of vasomotion in apoE-deficient mice: implications for interactions between peroxynitrite and tetrahydrobiopterin. *Circulation*, 103, pp. 1282-1288.

Lee, I. M. *et al.* (2005) Vitamin E in the primary prevention of cardiovascular disease and cancer: the Women's Health Study: a randomized controlled trial. *Journal of American Medical Association*, 294, pp. 56-65.

Lee, S. K. *et al.* (2010) Glutathione system in young spontaneously hypertensive rats. *Journal of Physiology and Biochemistry*, 66, 321-327.

Lonn, E. *et al.* (2005) Effects of long-term vitamin E supplementation on cardiovascular events and cancer: a randomized controlled trial. *Journal of American Medical Association*, 293, pp. 1338-1347.

Malyszko, J. (2010) Mechanism of endothelial dysfunction in chronic kidney disease. *Clinica Chimica Acta*, 411, pp. 1412-1420.

Matsushita, M. *et al.* (2001) Co-expression of urotensin II and its receptor (GPR14) in human cardiovascular and renal tissues. *Journal of Hypertension*, 19, pp. 2185-2190.

Maulik, N. and Das, D. K. (2008) Emerging potential of thioredoxin and thioredoxin interacting proteins in various disease conditions. *Biochimica et Biophysica Acta*, 1780, pp. 1368-1382.

Mazzali, M. *et al.* (2001) Elevated Uric Acid Increases Blood Pressure in the Rat by a Novel Crystal-Independent Mechanism. *Hypertension*, 38, pp. 1101-1106.

Mazzali, M. *et al.* (2010) Uric acid and hypertension: cause or effect? Current Rheumatology Reports, 12, pp. 108-117.

Meister, A. and Anderson, M. E. (1983) Glutathione. *Annual Review of Biochemistry*, 52, pp. 711-760.

Michel, J. B. *et al.* (1997) Caveolin versus calmodulin. Counterbalancing allosteric modulators of endothelial nitric oxide synthase. *Journal of Biological Chemistry*, 272, pp. 25907-25912.

Miller, E. R. *et al.* (2005) Meta-analysis: high-dosage vitamin E supplementation may increase all-cause mortality. *Annals of Internal Medicine*, 142, pp. 1-11.

Milne, G. L. *et al.* (2005) F2-isoprostanes as markers of oxidative stress *in vivo*: an overview. *Biomarkers*, 10[Suppl 1], pp.10-23.

Morena, M. *et al.* (2002) Convective and diffusive losses of vitamin C during haemodiafiltration session: a contributive factor to oxidative stress in haemodialysis patients. *Nephrology Dialysis Transplantation*, 17, pp. 422-427.

Münzel, T. and Keaney, J. F. Jr. (2001) Are ACE inhibitors a “magic bullet” against oxidative stress? *Circulation*, 104, pp. 1571-1574.

Mullan, B. *et al.* (2002) Ascorbic acid reduces blood pressure and arterial stiffness in type 2 diabetes. *Hypertension*, 40, pp. 804-809.

Myers, *et al* (2005) New algorithm for the diagnosis of hypertension. *American Journal of Hypertension*, 18, pp. 369-1374.

Nebot, C. *et al.* (1993) Spectrophotometric assay of superoxide dismutase activity based on the activated autoxidation of a tetracyclic catechol. *Analytical Biochemistry*, 14, pp. 442-451.

Nishikawa, Y. *et al.* (2003) Effects of vitamin C on high blood pressure induced by salt in spontaneously hypertensive rats. *Journal of Nutritional Science and Vitaminology (Tokyo)*, 49, pp. 301-309.

O'Brien, E. *et al.* (1991) Accuracy of the Spacelabs 90207 determined by the British Hypertension Society Protocol. *Journal of Hypertension*, 9, 573-574.

Ohkawa, H. *et al.* (1979) Assay for lipid peroxides in animal tissues by thiobarbituric acid reaction. *Analytical Biochemistry*, 95, pp. 351-358.

Padayatty, S. J. *et al.* (2004) Vitamin C pharmacokinetics: implications for oral and intravenous use. *Annals of Internal Medicine*, 140, pp. 533-537.

Paravicini, T. M. and Touyz, R. M. (2006) Redox signalling in hypertension. *Cardiovascular Research*, 71, pp. 247-258.

Pechánová, O. (2007) Contribution of captopril thiol group to the prevention of spontaneous hypertension. *Physiological Research*, 56, pp. 41-48.

Pechánová, O. *et al.* (2006a) Effect of chronic N-acetylcysteine treatment on the development of spontaneous hypertension. *Clinical Science (London)*, 110, pp. 235-242. PECHÁNOVÁ, O. *et al.* (2006b) Beneficial effects of Provinols: cardiovascular system and kidney. *Physiological Research*, 55, pp. 17-30.

Penugonda, S. *et al.* (2005) Effects of N-acetylcysteine amide (NACA), a novel thiol antioxidant against glutamate-induced cytotoxicity in neuronal cell line PC12. *Brain Research*, 1056, pp. 132-138.

Pietta, P. *et al.* (1998) Relationship between rate and extent of catechin absorption and plasma antioxidant status. *Biochemistry and Molecular Biology International*, 46, pp. 895-903.

Plantinga, Y. *et al.* (2007) Suplementation with vitamins C and E improves arterial stiffness and endothelial function in essential hypertensive patients. *American Journal of Hypertension*, 20, pp. 392-397.

Pradelles, P. *et al.* (1985) Enzyme immunoassays of eicosanoids using AchE as label: an alternative to radioimmunoassay. *Analytical Chemistry*, 57, pp.1170-1173

Rapola, J. M. *et al.* (1999) Randomised trial of α-tocopherol and β-carotene supplements on incidence of major coronary events in men with previous myocardial infarction. *Lancet*, 349, pp. 1715-1720.

Reckelhoff, J. F. *et al.* (1998) Vitamin E ameliorates enhanced renal lipid peroxidation and accumulation of F2-isoprostanes in aging kidneys. *American Journal of Physiology*, 274, pp. 767-774.

Redon, J. *et al.* (2003) Antioxidant activities and oxidative stress byproducts in human hypertension. *Hypertension*, 41, pp. 1096-1101.

Rodrigo, R. and Bosco, C. (2006) Oxidative stress and protective effects of polyphenols: comparative studies in human and rodent kidney. A review. *Comparative Biochemistry and Physiology Part C: Toxicology and Pharmacology*, 142, pp. 317-327.

Rodrigo, R. *et al.* (2003) Implications of oxidative stress and homocysteine in the pathophysiology of essential hypertension. *Journal of Cardiovascular Pharmacology*, 42, pp. 453-461.

Rodrigo, R. *et al.* (2005) Pathophysiological basis for the prophylaxis of preeclampsia through early supplementation with antioxidant vitamins. *Pharmacology and Therapeutics*, 107, 177-197.

Rodrigo, R. *et al.* (2007a) Clinical pharmacology and therapeutic use of antioxidant vitamins. *Fundamental and Clinical Pharmacology*, 21, pp. 111-127.

Rodrigo, R. *et al.* (2007b) Relationship between oxidative stress and essential hypertension. *Hypertension Research*, 30, pp. 1159-1167.

Rodrigo, R. *et al.* (2007c) Relationship between (Na+K)-ATPase activity, lipid peroxidation and fatty acid profile in erythrocytes of hypertensive and normotensive subjects. *Molecular and Cellular Biochemistry*, 303, pp. 73-81.

Rodrigo, R. *et al.* (2008) Decrease in oxidative stress through supplementation of vitamins C and E is associated with a reduction in blood pressure in patients with essential hypertension. *Clinical Science (London)*, 114, pp. 625-634.

Rodrigo, R. *et al.* (2010) Use of vitamins C and E as a prophylactic therapy to prevent postoperative atrial fibrillation. *International Journal of Cardiology*, 138, pp. 221-228.

Rodrigo, R. *et al.* (2011) The role of oxidative stress in the pathophysiology of hypertension. *Hypertension Research*, 34, pp. 431-440.

Rubanyi, G. M. and Vanhoutte, P. M. (1986) Superoxide anions and hyperoxia inactivate endothelium-derived relaxing factor. *American Journal of Physiology*, 250, pp. 822-827.

Russo, C. *et al.* (1998) Anti-oxidant status and lipid peroxidation in patients with essential hypertension. *Journal of Hypertension*, 16, pp. 1267-1271.

Salonen, R. M. *et al.* (2003) Six-year effect of combined vitamin C and E supplementation on atherosclerotic progression: the Antioxidant Supplementation in Atherosclerosis Prevention (ASAP) Study. *Circulation*, 107, pp. 947-953.

Schneider, M. P. *et al.* (2005) Superoxide scavenging effects of N-acetylcysteine and vitamin C in subjects with essential hypertension. *American Journal of Hypertension*, 18, pp. 1111–1117.

Simic, D. V. *et al.* (2006) Byproducts of oxidative protein damage and antioxidant enzyme activities in plasma of patients with different degrees of essential hypertension. *Journal of Human Hypertension*, 20, pp. 149-155.

Simko, F. *et al.* (2005) L-arginine fails to protect against myocardial remodelling in L-NAME-induced hypertension. *European Journal of Clinical Investigatio*n, 35, pp. 362-368.

Sládková, M. *et al.* (2007) Chronic and acute effects of different antihypertensive drugs on femoral artery relaxation of L-Name hypertensive rats. *Physiological Research*, 56, pp. 85-91.

Steinbrenner, H. and Sied, H. (2009) Protection against reactive oxygen species by selenoproteins. *Biochimica et Biophysica Acta*, 1790, pp. 1478-1485.

Stirrat, A. *et al.* (2001) Potent vasodilator responses to human urotensin-II in human pulmonary and abdominal resistance arteries. *American Journal of Physiology - Heart and Circulatory Physiology*, 280, pp. 925-928.

Stojiljkovic, M. P. *et al.* (2002) Increasing plasma fatty acids elevates F2-isoprostanes in humans: implications for the cardiovascular risk factor cluster. *Journal of Hypertension*, 201, pp. 1215-1221.

Suzuki, H. *et al.* (1998) Xanthine oxidase activity associated with arterial blood pressure in spontaneously hypertensive rats. *Proceedings of the National Academy of Sciences of United States of America*, 95, pp. 4754-4759.

Tanito, M. *et al.* (2004) Enhanced oxidative stress and impaired thioredoxin expression in spontaneously hypertensive rats. *Antioxidants and Redox Signaling*, 6, pp. 89-97.

Taniyama, Y. and Griendling, K. (2003) Reactive Oxygen Species in the Vasculature: Molecular and Cellular Mechanisms. Hypertension, 42, pp. 1075-1081.

Tian, N. *et al.* (2006) N-Acetylcysteine improves renal dysfunction, ameliorates kidney damage and decreases blood pressure in salt-sensitive hypertension. *Journal of Hypertension*, 24, pp. 2263-2270.

Touyz, R. M. (2004) Reactive oxygen species and angiotensin II signaling in vascular cells - implications in cardiovascular disease. *Brazilian Journal of Medical Research*, 37, pp. 1263-1273.

Touyz, R. M. (2004) Reactive oxygen species, vascular oxidative stress, and redox signaling in hypertension: what is the clinical significance? *Hypertension*, 44, pp. 248-252.

Touyz, R. M. and Schiffrin, E. L. (2001) Increased generation of superoxide by angiotensin II in smooth muscle cells from resistance arteries of hypertensive patients: role of phospholipase D-dependent NAD(P)H oxidase-sensitive pathways. *Journal of Hypertension*, 19, pp. 1245-1254.

Ulker, S. *et al.* (2003) Vitamins reverse endothelial dysfunction through regulation of eNOS and NAD(P)H oxidase activities. *Hypertension*, 41, pp. 534-539.

Vaziri, N. D. (2008) Mechanisms of lead-induced hypertension and cardiovascular disease. *American Journal of Physiology - Heart and Circulation Physiology*, 295, pp. 454-465.

Venditti, P. *et al.* (2007). Vitamin E attenuates cold-induced rat liver oxidative damage reducing H_2O_2 mitochondrial release. *The International Journal of Biochemistry and Cell Biology*, 39, pp. 1731-1742.

Verhaar, M. C. *et al.* (1998). Endothelin-A receptor antagonist-mediated vasodilatation is attenuated by inhibition of nitric oxide synthesis and by endothelin-B receptor blockade. *Circulation*, 97, pp, 752-756.

Viel, E. C. *et al.* (2008) Xanthine oxidase and mitochondria contribute to vascular superoxide anion generation in DOCA-salt hypertensive rats. *American Journal of Physiology - Heart and Circulatory Physiology*, 295, pp. 281-288.

Vita, J. A. *et al.* (1998) L-2-Oxothiazolidine-4-carboxylic acid reverses endothelial dysfunction in patients with coronary artery disease. *Journal of Clinical Investigation*, 101, pp. 1408-1414.

Ward, N. C. *et al.* (2005) The combination of vitamin C and grape-seed polyphenols increases blood pressure: a randomized, double-blind, placebo-controlled trial. *Journal of Hypertension*, 23, pp. 427-434.

Ward, N. C. *et al.* (2007) The effect of vitamin E on blood pressure in individuals with type 2 diabetes: a randomized, double-blind, placebo-controlled trial. *Journal of Hypertension*, 25, pp. 227-234.

Waring, W. S. *et al.* (2001) Systemic uric acid administration increases serum antioxidant capacity in healthy volunteers. *Journal of Cardiovascular Pharmacology*, 38, pp. 365-371.

Waring, W. S. *et al.* (2003) Uric acid reduces exercise-induced oxidative stress in healthy adults. *Clinical Science (London)*, 105, pp. 425-430.

Wernerman, J. and Hammarqvist, F. (1999) Modulation of endogenous glutathione availability. *Current Opinion in Clinical Nutrition and Metabolic Care*, 2, pp. 487-492.

Widder, J. D. *et al.* (2009) Attenuation of angiotensin II-induced vascular dysfunction and hypertension by overexpression of thioredoxin 2. *Hypertension*, 54, pp. 338-344.

World, C. J. *et al.* (2006) Thioredoxin in the cardiovascular system. J*ournal of Molecular Medicine*, 84, pp. 997-1003.

Xu, S. *et al.* (2009) Endothelial cells negatively modulate reactive oxygen species generation in vascular smooth muscle cells: role of thioredoxin. *Hypertension*, 54, pp. 427-433.

Yoshida, J. *et al.* (2004) AT1 receptor blocker added to ACE inhibitor provides benefits at advanced stage of hypertensive diastolic heart failure. *Hypertension*, 43, pp. 686-691.

Yoshioka, J. *et al.* (2006) Role of thioredoxin in cell growth through interactions with signaling molecules. *Antioxidants and Redox Signaling*, 8, pp. 2143-2145.

Yusuf, S. *et al.* (2004) Effect of potentially modifiable risk factors associated with myocardial infarction in 52 countries (the INTERHEART Study): case control study. *Lancet*, 364, pp. 937-952.

Yusuf, S. et al. (2005) Vitamin E supplementation and cardiovascular events in high-risk patients. The Heart Outcomes Prevention Evaluation Study Investigators. *New England Journal of Medicine*, 342, pp. 154-160.

Zembowicz, A. *et al.* (1993) Inhibition of endothelial nitric oxide synthase by ebselen. Prevention by thiols suggests the inactivation by ebselen of a critical thiol essential for the catalytic activity of nitric oxide synthase. *Journal of Pharmacology and Experimental Therapeutics*, 267, pp. 1112-1118.

Zenebe, W. *et al.* (2003) Red wine polyphenols induce vasorelaxation by increased nitric oxide bioactivity. *Physiological Research*, 52, pp. 425–432.

Zhan, C. D. *et al.* (2004) Superoxide dismutase, catalase and glutathione peroxidase in the spontaneously hypertensive rat kidney: effect of antioxidant-rich diet. *Journal of Hypertension*, 22, pp. 2025-2033.

Zhang, Y. and HOGG, N. (2005) S-Nitrosothiols: cellular formation and transport. *Free Radical Biology and Medicine*, 38, pp. 831-838.

Zhou, L. *et al.* (2006) Reduction in extracellular superoxide dismutase activity in African-American patients with hypertension. *Free Radical Biology and Medicine*, 41, pp. 1384-1391.

Zou, M. H. *et al.* (2004) Peroxynitrite and vascular endothelial dysfunction in diabetes mellitus. *Endothelium*, 11, pp. 89-97.

In: Hypotheses in Clinical Medicine
Editors: M.M. Shoja, P.S. Agutter et al.

ISBN: 978-1-62257-276-2

Chapter 21

Deep Venous Thrombosis: Etiology and Prophylaxis

Mark P. Henderson**[*]**
Editorial Officer, Theoretical Medicine and Biology Group,
Glossop, United Kingdom

Abstract

A critical analysis based on a historical review shows that Virchow's triad is imprecise and could, in its modern-day interpretation, lead to misunderstanding of the mechanism by which deep venous thrombosis (DVT) is initiated. However, when due account is taken of these criticisms, a hypothesis about the etiological process emerges. This hypothesis has significant implications for prophylaxis against DVT and a fortiori its sequelae such as pulmonary embolism and chronic venous insufficiency. Exploration of this hypothesis and its implications supports the view that far from being multifactorial, as is often supposed, DVT results from a single pathogenic process, though it is potentiated by various risk factors. This exploration also raises the question: is it helpful to regard DVT as a hematological disorder? Differences between medical and scientific research in the formulation and testing of hypotheses are indicated.

Introduction

The motive for medical research is to improve the prevention and treatment of diseases. The motive for scientific research is to establish reliable knowledge. The two are broadly compatible; medicine benefits from a scientific underpinning. However, while the best scientific research is characterized by experiments or empirical studies designed to falsify hypotheses (Popper 1964), the best medical research can be methodologically different. The

[*] E-mail: mark.p.henderson1946@googlemail.com.

difference has implications for both clinical practice and the pursuit of knowledge, as the study of deep venous thrombosis (DVT) illustrates.

DVT is a common condition and its sequelae can be fatal (pulmonary embolism, PE) or debilitating (chronic venous insufficiency, CVI), so it is medically important (Peterson 1986). Research into its etiology has generated controversies during the past two centuries, providing abundant evidence for this chapter (Browse *et al.* 1988). Although the morphological and pathogenic features shared by all deep venous thrombi could imply a single etiology, many different risk factors have been identified (Geerts *et al.* 2004). It is therefore germane to ask whether the etiology of DVT is best explained by a single, overarching hypothesis or whether the workers in the field who consider it 'multifactorial' are correct (Rosendaal 2005; Lippi and Franchini 2008). Scientists may opt for the former alternative, clinicians the latter.

This chapter is organized as follows. First, the status, value and provenance of Virchow's triad are examined. Second, the three facets of the triad as currently interpreted are scrutinized in the light of historical evidence. Third, a unifying hypothesis of the etiology of DVT is discussed and related to Virchow's triad. Fourth, the implications for prophylaxis against venous thromboembolism are considered.

Virchow's Triad

Status

It is obvious that intravascular coagula such as venous thrombi are formed because of abnormalities in either the vessel wall, or the composition and behavior of the circulating blood, or the dynamics of blood flow; or some combination of these. Nothing else can plausibly be involved. During the late 1950s, after the historical study by Anning (1957) was published, this truism came to be labeled 'Virchow's triad'. Since then, it has become well-nigh impossible to publish anything about the causation of DVT without mentioning Virchow's triad, which is regarded as the *sine qua non* for understanding the condition. The modern reading of the triad is 'vessel injury, hypercoagulability, stasis' (Peterson 1986; Rosendaal 2005; Esmon 2009; Kyrle and Eichinger 2009; Meetoo 2010). Many authors have questioned whether the vessel-injury facet of the triad is significant (Comerota *et al.* 1985; Kyrle and Eichinger 2009), and most emphasis has been placed on abnormal tendencies of the blood to coagulate (Thiangarajan 2002; Bulger *et al.* 2004). Retarded blood flow or 'stasis' has been viewed as a potentiating factor because - so it is conjectured - it allows coagulation factors to accumulate locally (Thomas 1988; Mammen 1992; Hamby 2005).

Overall, this interpretation portrays DVT as a hematological disorder. Many workers today would consider that designation 'obvious', but it is challengeable. Until the early 1960s, thrombosis was hardly mentioned in hematology publications, which were concerned with the coagulation mechanism and defects such as hemophilia. For example, in the third edition of their classic text, Biggs and MacFarlane (1962) mentioned 'thrombosis' on only six out of some 350 pages of text. Earlier research into what we now call DVT, extending back to the late 18th century, had no connection at all with hematology; and that history, of course, includes the work of Virchow. Interestingly, the invention of 'Virchow's triad', and the concomitant interpretation of DVT as a hematological disorder, coincided with the acceptance of anticoagulant therapy and prophylaxis by the FDA (Cundiff *et al.* 2010). Some connection might be suspected.

Value

Virchow's triad is not a hypothesis because it is not empirically falsifiable, and it specifies no particular etiology. It is a general perspective through which the causation of DVT can be viewed. Its inherent imprecision (e.g. exactly what does 'stasis' entail?), and its failure to indicate how the three facets are supposed to cooperate or synergize in venous thrombogenesis, seriously limit its explanatory value from a scientific standpoint. Clinically, however, it is held to be useful (Brotman *et al.* 2004; Bagot and Arya 2008). It is taken as a guide for both prophylaxis and treatment: deal appropriately with injured veins, administer anticoagulants, and maintain a reasonably high venous blood flow rate (especially in the lower limbs, where DVT most often occurs).

That seems unexceptionable, but it underscores the point made in earlier: the motivational and methodological differences between medicine and science make Virchow's triad appear valuable in the former context but virtually useless in the latter.

Provenance

An intriguing point about 'Virchow's triad' is that Virchow never conceived it. The phrase was not used until a century after his seminal works were published. In both *Thrombose und Embolie* (Virchow 1856) and *Die Cellularpathologie in ihrer Begründung auf physiologische und pathologische Gewebelehre* (Virchow 1858), the focus was pulmonary embolism, not thrombosis. The only relevant passage in *Thrombose und Embolie* (pp. 293-4 of the Matzdorff-Bell translation) states that '*the sequence of the possible stages and consequences of blockage may be classified and studied under three headings: (1) phenomena associated with irritation of the vessel and its vicinity;(2) phenomena of blood-coagulation; and (3) phenomena of interrupted blood-flow*'. But this refers to the 'blockage' of the pulmonary artery by a metastasized thrombus, not to the formation of that thrombus in a distal vein. Virchow's name has been attached to the triad only because the quoted passage has been misread. Several authors have made this point (Brinkhous 1969; Owen 2001; Brotman *et al.* 2004; Dickson 2004; Malone and Agutter 2006; Bagot and Arya 2008), but historical veracity has not corrected the error.

This misuse of his name would doubtless have displeased the irascible Virchow, since he never so much as implied the notion of 'hypercoagulability', and he explicitly rejected the 'doctrine' (*die Lehre*) that stasis has any causal role in thrombosis or embolism.

The Three Facets of the Triad

For convenience of presentation, I will consider the modern interpretation of the triad in the sequence: hypercoagulability, endothelial injury, stasis.

Hypercoagulability

Strictly speaking, 'hypercoagulability' denotes an abnormally low clotting time *in vitro*; the corresponding *in vivo* condition is a 'thrombophilia'. The confusion of *in vitro* with *in vivo* coagulation is commonplace, though Virchow warned against it; for instance, he told us that a venous thrombus is in many ways like an *in vitro* clot, but it is not the same as a clot. On pp. 514-5 of *Gessamelte Abhandlungen* (Virchow 1862), we are reminded that (1) a thrombus has a layered structure (the Lines of Zahn), unlike a clot; (2) the fibrin content is denser; (3) the white cell content is vastly greater. This tripartite distinction between 'venous thrombus' and 'clot' has a better claim to the label 'Virchow's triad' than the stasis-hypercoagulability-injury perspective, since Virchow actually wrote it. Moreover, it encapsulates common clinical knowledge; anyone who has seen a thrombus extracted during a venectomy or an embolism removed at post-mortem has seen the white 'tail' of the structure, well described by Welch (1899) and Aschoff (1924). The commonplace elision of 'venous thrombus' with 'clot' is therefore surprising. It may be another effect of viewing DVT through hematological spectacles.

Nevertheless, thrombophilias definitely increase the risk for DVT. Since hereditary antithrombin III deficiency was described almost half a century ago (Egeberg 1965), a number of inherited and acquired thrombophilias have been identified, and the molecular bases of many of the inherited ones are now known. There are many reviews of the field, e.g. Mazza (2004), Rosendaal (2005), Hassouna (2009), Anderson and Weitz (2010). Inherited thrombophilias are generally associated with a family history of predisposition to DVT and PE, occurrence of a first DVT before the age of 40 years, and frequent recurrences. The most common ones are defects in the protein C pathway (Lane *et al.* 1996). Acquired thrombophilias are many and varied; the most common is antiphospholipid syndrome (Asherton and Hughes 1989).

However, a difficulty arises. If the condition is hematological, then thrombophilias are causal; they explain the etiology. Since a patient with an identifiable thrombophilia might not develop DVT, various other risk factors must be present to carry the patient over the imagined thrombogenic threshold (Mammen 1992; Lippi and Franchini 2008; Anderson and Weitz 2010). This is one reason why DVT is described as 'multifactorial'. The fact that some patients with normally coagulable blood fall victim to DVT and PE could be fatal to the supposition that a thrombophilia is a prerequisite for venous thrombogenesis, so a 'multifactorial etiology' is again invoked. This is hand-waving; scientifically, it explains nothing. Experts on thrombophilia such as the aforementioned reviewers make a good case for their position, with plentiful clinical and laboratory evidence, but the flaws in the hematological perspective remain too wide and deep for repair. The inference to be drawn from this literature is clear: thrombophilias increase the likelihood that DVT will become clinically significant, but they are not causal. In other words, DVT is *not* a hematological condition.

That inference could have been drawn 150 years ago from Lister's Croonian lecture (Lister 1863), which showed that blood coagulates *only* when it comes into contact with a 'foreign' surface, i.e. with something other than normal vascular endothelium. This is true irrespective of the presence or absence of thrombophilia. But Lister's exposition begs the question: what 'foreign' surface does the blood encounter in an apparently uninjured vein (almost all DVT cases in clinical practice have apparently uninjured veins) so that coagulation is induced?

Endothelial Injury

The obvious answer is that subtle changes in some part of the venous endothelium must be instrumental in causing DVT. What can injure endothelial tissue in an intact, functioning vein? A hypothesis was proposed by Drinker (1938) and van Ottingen (1941), who found that thrombus-like coagula formed in the veins of victims of carbon monoxide poisoning, associated with endothelial alterations; so hypoxemia could cause the endothelial injury associated with DVT. Studies by O'Neill (1947) and Samuels and Webster (1952) supported this proposal. Interestingly, Samuels and Webster (1952) showed that heparin does not prevent the development of a nascent thrombus on a hypoxically injured endothelium.

In these mid-20th century papers, there was a debate about whether oxygen was supplied to the venous endothelium from the luminal blood or the vasa venarum. Presumably, hypoxia sufficiently severe to cause endothelial injury would require impaired oxygenation from both sources. It is well established that the venous endothelium can survive moderately prolonged hypoxia (Jackson *et al.* 1988), using anaerobic glycolysis to provide ATP (Berna *et al.* 2001). During the period 1980-2000, studies in a number of laboratories established that hypoxia in cultured venous endothelial cells induced the expression of the early growth response-1 (egr-1) gene, and this unleashed a cascade of gene-expression and phenotypic changes that would, *in vivo,* promote local coagulation and leukocyte accumulation (Pinsky *et al.* 1995; Yan *et al.* 1999a,b; Karimova and Pinsky 2001; Ten and Pinsky 2002).

Extrapolation of these findings to the *in vivo* situation seems reasonable, arguing against the view that endothelial injury has no significant role in the etiology of DVT. However, it leads to a further question: what part(s) of the venous endothelium is/are susceptible to hypoxic injury, and under what circumstances?

Stasis

By the late 19th century, it was clear that paralyzed patients were susceptible to DVT and PE (Malpother 1880), and by the middle of the 20th century it was known that prolonged bed rest e.g. in spinal injury patients had the same consequence (Wright and Osborn 1952; Gibbs 1957). The association between restricted mobility and DVT was attributed to slow venous return flow (Ochsner *et al.* 1950; Wright and Osborn 1952). Thus, 'venous stasis' was established as a cause of DVT by the early 1960s (Zweifach 1963); it was imagined to promote local coagulation (Mammen 1992). In view of the endothelial hypoxia hypothesis, this notion could be plausible. If blood flows slowly enough to injure some part of the endothelium by hypoxemia, local coagulation could be promoted through the molecular mechanisms discovered by Pinsky and his colleagues.

Unfortunately, the idea seemed inconsistent with the results of an experiment conducted two centuries earlier. Hewson (1771) doubly-ligated part of a dog's jugular vein, causing no noticeable injury to the vessel, and the (stationary) blood between the ligatures failed to coagulate after more than an hour; even after three hours, coagulation was only partial. Zero flow, as in Hewson's experiment - i.e. *literal* stasis - is the lowest possible venous return rate and should therefore be most likely to promote coagulation. Hewson's finding was so counter-intuitive that the experiment was repeated by Lister (1863) and Baumgarten (1876); the results were the same. We therefore have an apparent paradox: under conditions of prolonged bed rest, when venous return is slow, the likelihood of DVT is increased; but under conditions of zero venous flow, the blood does not coagulate in less than an hour and a half. As often happens in science, the seeming paradox was resolved by a new hypothesis.

A Unifying Hypothesis

Most if not all venous thrombi form in valve pockets (Virchow 1858; McLachlin and Paterson 1951; Sevitt 1974). Thrombi that arise at vein junctions probably arise in the ostial valves controlling those junctions, as illustrated by Virchow (1858). This well-known observation, combined with the foregoing arguments, led to the articulation of a valve cusp hypoxia hypothesis (VCHH) of the etiology of DVT. The VCHH was conceived around 1970 but not articulated in full until recently (Malone and Agutter 2006, 2008), several years after definitive experimental corroboration had been published (see below).

According to the VCHH, DVT may occur if there is sustained non-pulsatile (streamline) venous blood flow, irrespective of the overall flow rate. Non-pulsatile flow leads to suffocating hypoxemia in a valve pocket, resulting in hypoxic injury to the inner (parietalis) endothelium of the cusp leaflet, which is not supplied by the vasa venarum (Franklin 1937; Saphir and Lev 1950; Sevitt 1974). This injury activates the egr-1 pathway within the endothelial cells, which in turn activates a number of chemoattractant and procoagulant factors (see above). When normal pulsatile blood flow is restored, even transiently, leukocytes and platelets swarm at the site of injury, attracted by those factors. Local blood coagulation may be initiated, though not immediately; leukocytes attack the injured and possibly necrotic parietalis endothelial cells before coagulation ensues (Aschoff 1924; Saphir and Lev 1952), explaining the white *Kopfteil* of venous thrombi and emboli. This could be consistent with the failure of heparin to prevent the formation of nascent thrombi (Samuels and Webster 1952).

A further period of non-pulsatile flow kills the accumulated leukocytes in the valve pocket. These dead cells may then form the core of a nascent thrombus. If periods of non-pulsatile and pulsatile flow continue to alternate, serial deposition of white cells and fibrin may ensue, resulting in the characteristic Lines of Zahn morphology of a venous thrombus. Because the thrombus is attached to a (partially) necrotic layer of endothelial cells, it is readily detached when venous flow resumes, explaining the tendency of venous thrombi to embolize.

The VCHH leads to two obvious testable predictions: (1) sustained non-pulsatile flow causes extreme hypoxemia in the valve pockets and hypoxia (verging on anoxia) of the endothelial cells in the depths of the pocket; (2) sustained non-pulsatile flow alternating with brief episodes of pulsatile flow will generate coagula indistinguishable from autochthonous venous thrombi in experimental animals. Each of these predictions was corroborated experimentally in the 1980s. An hour of non-pulsatile flow in anesthetized patients sufficed to lower the PO_2 in the depths of the valve pockets to below the detection threshold of an oxygen electrode (Hamer *et al.* 1981); and thrombi morphologically indistinguishable from those encountered clinically were formed in the leg veins of anesthetized dogs when brief episodes of pulsatile flow interrupted prolonged periods of immobility in the leg muscles (Hamer and Malone 1984).

These studies confirmed the VCHH, so it is now legitimate to assert that the cause of DVT is valve cusp hypoxia induced by sustained non-pulsatile venous blood flow interspersed with short episodes of pulsatile flow. However, alternating pulsatile and non-pulsatile flow in the deep limb veins is probably a daily consequence of many modern lifestyles, so why is DVT not even more common than it is? The finding of Brooks *et al.*

(2009) that the parietalis endothelium is more resistant than the luminal endothelium to the induction of coagulation could provide an answer.

The valve cusp hypoxia etiology can be viewed in terms of Virchow's triad: stasis (in the valve pockets) leads to local hypoxemia and hypoxic injury to the endothelium (of the valve cusp parietalis), leading to leukocyte infiltration and, potentially, subsequent coagulation; coagulation would be expected to be more rapid and intense in cases of thrombophilia. This is not an especially helpful interpretation, but it demonstrates the compatibility between the unifying, overarching etiological hypothesis and the consensus perspective on DVT. The valve cusp hypoxia mechanism can accommodate and explain the known risk factors for DVT (Malone and Agutter 2008), but it denies the 'multifactorial' view of the condition; it envisages a single etiological process for all cases of venous thrombosis, including those that are conventionally deemed 'idiopathic' (because they occur when no known risk factor can be demonstrated).

The significance of the experimental findings was acknowledged by Hume (1985), but the discovery has exerted strangely little impact on the DVT field, despite the outstanding scholarship of the Malone-Agutter book (Malone and Agutter 2008). It has been extended to a plausible explanation of the progression of CVI (Malone and Agutter 2009), but it is seldom cited. López and Chen (2009) recognized that events at the vessel wall precede coagulation, and a comprehensive review by Bovill and van der Vliet (2011) emphasized the critical significance of valve pocket hypoxaemia, but these are among the few publications consistent with the VCHH. One characteristic that science and medicine share is the resistance of entrenched ideas to change (cf. Kuhn 1970).

The valve cusp hypoxia account is probably incomplete. For example, although valves (including the ostial valves at vein junctions) are the predominant sites of thrombus formation, they might not be the only sites. Can this account of etiology be extended or modified to account for thrombogenesis the cerebral sinus and splanchnic veins, where flow conditions are different and valves are much less frequent than in the deep leg veins (Kyrle and Eichinger 2009)? Moreover, some of the clinical implications considered by the authors of the VCHH and its corroboration are questionable and need to be investigated further.

Conclusion and Implications for Prophylaxis

One clear implication of the VCHH is that anticoagulants do not prevent the *initiation* of DVT; they prevent the growth of already-formed venous thrombi to clinically significant size. From the point of view of patient care, that hardly matters; what is important for the patient is to prevent the potential morbidity and mortality associated with DVT, so it is as useful to prevent thrombus growth as thrombus initiation. From the point of view of etiological understanding, however, it is highly significant. It makes the control of coagulation less of a priority than the hematological perspective insists and suggests that alternatives to anticoagulant prophylaxis should be reconsidered, i.e. mechanical prophylaxis.

Malone and Agutter (2008) argue that the objective of mechanical prophylaxis should be to ensure that blood in the valve pockets is exchanged at regular intervals; the venous blood flow rate is less important. Therefore, regular but *infrequent* artificial pulses (e.g. once per hour) would preclude thrombogenesis. That would be more comfortable for the patient than current methods of mechanical prophylaxis. Another proposal, for patients confined to prolonged bed-rest, is alternate end-to-end Trendelenberg/ anti-Trendelenberg tilting of the bed, through a 5-10 degree angle, every hour or so. That would empty the valve pockets in the upper and lower parts of the body by gravity, allowing them to refill passively with fresh venous blood and prevent injurious hypoxemia.

These proposals need to be tested on animals. If successful, the tests would provide further corroboration of the VCHH. The experimental design used by Hamer and Malone (1984) would suffice. At least three matched groups of animals would be required, each subjected to prolonged non-pulsatile blood flow in the leg veins, with brief alternating pulsatile episodes: (a) controls, given no treatment; (b) given standard anticoagulant prophylaxis; (c) given mechanical prophylaxis by one or other of the methods proposed by Malone and Agutter (2008). At the end of the experiment, valves from deep limb veins would be examined microscopically. The VCHH and its prophylactic implications predict: group (a) will show the formation of autochthonous thrombi, as in Hamer and Malone (1984); group (b) will show incipient thrombi on the parietalis endothelia; and group (c) will show normal endothelia with no incipient thrombi. To date, such experiments have not been performed.

A proposal for dietary prophylaxis has also been advanced on the basis of the valve cusp hypoxia thesis (Cundiff *et al.* 2010). Using mostly epidemiological evidence, these authors suggested that a vegan diet is likely to decrease the likelihood of DVT. Although their argument was accompanied by a thorough study of the literature, it scarcely seems plausible, and a very large patient population would be required for the necessary randomized controlled trial. The Cundiff *et al.* (2010) paper seems to have been motivated by a desire to find alternatives to anticoagulant prophylaxis because of the associated bleeding risk, which is real and worrying. However, it seems unlikely to lead to a further critical test of the thesis, or to a significant improvement in patient care. The proposals for mechanical prophylaxis are another matter. There is a strong argument for an experimental test of these proposals, such as the one outlined above, to be followed - if the test is successful - by controlled clinical trials.

References

Anderson, J. A. and Weitz, J. I. (2010) Hypercoagulable states. *Clinics in Chest Medicine*, 31, pp. 659-673.

Anning, S. T. (1957) The historical aspects of venous thrombosis. *Medical History*, 1, pp. 28-37.

Aschoff, L. (1924) *Lectures in General Pathology*. New York: Hueber, p. 254.

Asherton, R. A. and Hughes, G. R. (1989) Recurrent deep vein thrombosis and Addison's disease in 'primary' antiphospholipid syndrome. *Journal of Rheumatology*, 16, pp. 378-380.

Bagot, C. N. and Arya, R. (2008) Virchow and his triad: a question of attribution. *British Journal of Haematology*, 143, pp. 180-190.

Baumgarten, P. (1876) Űber die sog. organisation des thrombus. *Zentralblatt für den Wissenschaft*, 14, pp. 593-597.

Berna, N. *et al.* (2001) Hypoxia-induced increase in calcium concentration in endothelial cells: role of the Na^+-glucose cotransporter. *Journal of Cellular Biochemistry*, 84, pp. 115-131.

Biggs, R. and Macfarlane, R. G. (1962) *Human Blood Coagulation and its Disorders, 3rd edition*. Oxford: Blackwell.

Bovill, E. G. and van Der Vliet, A. (2011) Venous valvular stasis-associated hypoxia and thrombosis: what is the link? *Annual Review of Physiology*, 73, pp. 527-545.

Brinkhous, K. M. (1969) The problem in perspective. In: SHERRY, S. (ed) *Thrombosis*. Washington: National Academy of Sciences, pp. 37-48.

Brooks, E. G. *et al.* (2009) Valves of the deep venous system: an overlooked risk factor. *Blood*, 114, pp. 1276-1279.

Brotman, D. J. *et al.* (2004) Virchow's triad revisited. *Southern Medical Journal*, 97, pp. 213-214.

Browse, N. L. *et al.* (1988) Aetiology of DVT. In: BROWSE, N.L. (ed) *Diseases of the Veins*. London: Edward Arnold, pp. 447-460.

Comerota, A. J. *et al.* (1985) Combined dihydroergotamine and heparin prophylaxis of postoperative deep vein thrombosis: proposed mechanism of action. *American Journal of Surgery*, 150, pp. 39-44.

Cundiff, D. K. *et al.* (2010) Diet as prophylaxis and treatment for venous thromboembolism? *Theoretical Biology and Medical Modelling*, 7, doi: 10.1186/1742-4682-7-31.

Dickson, B. C. (2004) Venous thrombosis: on the history of Virchow's triad. *University of Toronto Medical Journal*, 81, pp. 166-171.

Drinker, C. K. (1938) *Carbon Monoxide Asphyxia*. New York: Oxford University Press; see especially pp. 124 ff.

Egeberg, O. (1965) Inherited antithrombin III deficiency causing thrombophilia. *Thrombosis et Diathesis Haemorrhagica*, 13, pp. 516-530.

Esmon, C. T. (2009) Basic mechanisms and pathogenesis of venous thrombosis. *Blood Review*, 23, pp. 225-229.

Franklin, K. J. (1937) *A Monograph on Veins*. Springfield, IL: Charles Thomas, chapter 5.

Geerts, W. H. *et al.* (2004) Prevention of venous thromboembolism: the seventh ACCP Conference on antithrombotic and thrombolytic therapy. *Chest*, 126[Suppl 3], pp. 338-400.

Gibbs, N. M. (1957) Venous thrombosis in the lower limbs with particular reference to bed rest. *British Journal of Surgery*, 45, pp. 209-236.

Hamby, R. I. (2005) [www] Heart Center Online Website. Available from: www.heartcenter online.com [Accessed 3/14/08].

Hamer, J. D. *et al.* (1981) The PO_2 in venous valve pockets: its possible bearing on thrombogenesis. *British Journal of Surgery*, 68, pp. 166-170.

Hamer, J. D. and Malone, P. C. (1984) Experimental deep venous thrombogenesis by a non-invasive method. *Annals of the Royal College of Surgeons of England*, 66, pp. 416-419.

Hassouna, H. I. (2009) Thrombophilia and hypercoagulability. *Medical Principles and Practice (Kuwait)*, 18, pp. 429-440.

Hewson, W. (1771) *An Experimental Enquiry into the Properties of Blood*. London: T. Cadell, p. 20.

Jackson, R. M. *et al.* (1988) Hypoxia-induced oxygen tolerance: maintenance of endothelial metabolic function. *Experimental Lung Research*, 14[Suppl], pp. 887-896.

Karimova, A. and Pinsky, D. J. (2001) The endothelial response to oxygen deprivation: biology and clinical implications. *Intensive Care Medicine*, 27, pp. 19-31.

Kuhn, T. S. (1970) *The Structure of Scientific Revolutions*. 2nd edition. Chicago: University of Chicago Press.

Kyrle, P. A. and Eichinger, S. (2009) Is Virchow's triad complete? *Blood*, 114, pp. 1138-1139.

Lane, D. A. *et al.* (1996) Inherited thrombophilia. *Thrombosis and Haemostasis*, 76, pp. 651-662, 824-834.

Lippi, G. and Franchini, M. (2008) Pathogenesis of venous thromboembolism: when the cup runneth over. *Seminars in Thrombosis and Hemostasis*, 34, pp. 747-761.

Lister, J. L. (1863) Croonian Lecture: On the coagulation of the blood. *Proceedings of the Royal Society*, 13, pp. 355-364.

López, J. A. and Chen, J. (2009) Pathophysiology of venous thrombosis. *Thrombosis Research*, 123[Suppl 4], pp. 30-34.

Malone, P. C. and Agutter, P. S. (2006) The aetiology of deep venous thrombosis. *Quarterly Journal of Medicine*, 99, pp. 581-593.

Malone, P. C. and Agutter, P. S. (2008) *The Aetiology of Deep Venous Thrombosis*. Dordrecht: Springer.

Malone, P. C. and Agutter, P. S. (2009) To what extent might deep venous thrombosis and chronic venous insufficiency share a common aetiology?. *International Angiology*, 28, pp. 254-268.

Malpother, E. D. (1880) Phlebitis of the lower extremities: a secondary complication of injuries to the head. *British Medical Journal*, 1, p. 483.

Mammen, E. F. (1992) Pathogenesis of venous thrombosis. *Chest*, 102[Suppl], pp. 640-644.

Mazza, J. J. (2004) Hypercoagulability and venous thromboembolism: a review. *Wisconsin Medical Journal*, 103, pp. 41-49.

McLachlin, J. and Paterson, J. C. (1951) Some basic observations on venous thrombosis and pulmonary embolism. *Surgery, Gynecology and Obstetrics*, 93, pp. 1-8.

Meetoo, D. (2010) In too deep: understanding, detecting and managing DVT. *British Journal of Nursing*, 19, pp. 1021-1027.

Ochsner, A. *et al.* (1950) Venous thrombosis. Analysis of 580 cases. *Surgery*, 29, pp. 24-43.

O'Neill, J. F. (1947) The effect on venous endothelium of alterations in blood flow through vessels in vein walls and the possible relation to thrombosis. *Annals of Surgery*, 126, pp. 270-288.

Owen, C. (2001) *A History of Blood Coagulation*. Rochester: Mayo Foundation for Medical Education and Research.

Peterson, C. (1986) Venous thrombosis: an overview. *Pharmacotherapy*, 6[Suppl], pp. 12-17.

Pinsky, D. J. *et al.* (1995) Hypoxia and modification of the endothelium: implications for regulation of vascular homeostatic properties. *Seminars in Cell Biology*, 6, pp. 283-294.

Popper, K. R. (1979) *The Logic of Scientific Discovery*. London: Hutchinson.

Rosendaal, F. R. (2005) Venous thrombosis: the role of genes, environment, and behavior. *American Society of Hematology, Education Program*, pp. 1-12.

Samuels, P. B. and Webster, D. R. (1952) The role of venous endothelium in the inception of thrombosis. *Annals of Surgery*, 136, pp. 422-438.

Saphir, O. and Lev, M. (1952) Venous valvulitis. *Archives of Pathogy*, 53, pp. 456-469.

Sevitt, S. (1974) Organization of valve pocket thrombi and the anomalies of double thrombi and valve cusp involvement. *British Journal of Surgery*, 61, pp. 641-649.

Ten, V. S. and Pinsky, D. J. (2002) Endothelial response to hypoxia: physiologic adaptation and pathologic dysfunction. *Current Opinion in Critical Care*, 8, pp. 242-250.

Thiagarajan, P. (2002) New targets for antithrombotic drugs. *American Journal of Cardiovascular Drugs*, 2, pp. 227-235.

Thomas, D. P. (1988) Overview of venous thrombogenesis. *Seminars in Thrombosis and Hemostasis*, 14, pp. 1-8.

van Ottingen, W. F. (1941) *Studies on the Mechanism of Carbon Monoxide Poisoning as Observed in Dogs Anesthetized with Sodium Amytal*. Washington DC: United States Public Health Service.

Virchow, R. L. K. (1856) Thrombosis und Embolie. In: BARTH, J.A. (ed) *Klassiker der Medizin herausgegeben von Karl Sudhoff, Leipzig, 1910* (Translated by Matzdorff, A. C. and Bell, W. R. Canton: Science History Publications, 1998).

Virchow, R. L. K. (1858) *Die Cellularpathologie in ihrer Begründung auf Physiologische und Pathologische Gewebelehre*. Berlin: A. Hirschwald.

Virchow, R. L. K. (1862) *Gessamelte Abhandlungen zur Wissenschaftlichen Medizin von Rudolf Virchow*. Frankfurt am Main: Meidinger.

Welch, W. H. (1887) The structure of white thrombi. *Transactions of the Pathological Society of Philadelphia*, 13, pp. 281-300.

Wright, I. S. and Osborn, S. B. (1953) Venous velocity in bedridden medical patients. *Lancet*, 2, pp. 699-700.

Yan, S. F. *et al.* (1999a) Hypoxia/hypoxemia-induced activation of the procoagulant pathways and the pathogenesis of ischemia-associated thrombosis. *Atherosclerosis, Thrombosis and Vascular Biology*, 19, pp. 2029-2035.

Yan, S. F. *et al.* (1999b) Hypoxia-associated induction of early growth response-1 gene expression. *Journal of Biological Chemistry*, 274, pp. 15030-15040.

Zweifach, B. W. (1963) Peripheral vascular factors in the genesis of stasis and thrombosis. *Federation Proceedings*, 22, pp. 1351-1355.

In: Hypotheses in Clinical Medicine
Editors: M.M. Shoja, P.S. Agutter et al.
ISBN: 978-1-62257-276-2

Chapter 22

Pathogenesis of Preeclampsia and the Preventive Role of L-Arginine Supplementation

Ramón Rodrigo*[*], *Jaime González and Rodrigo Valenzuela
Oxidative Stress and Nephrotoxicity Laboratory,
Molecular and Clinical Pharmacology Program, Institute of Biomedical Sciences,
Faculty of Medicine, University of Chile, Santiago, Chile

Abstract

Preeclampsia (PE) is a syndrome expressing a highly prevalent pregnancy disorder associated with maternal-fetal morbidity and mortality. Although the etiology of PE remains elusive, oxidative stress and endothelial dysfunction have been implicated in the pathogenesis. Currently, there is no satisfactory measure to prevent the development of PE, except to follow certain measures to avoid or reduce complications, early delivery being the only successful treatment for severe PE. Recent studies have given clues about the importance of nitric oxide (NO) in the pathophysiology of PE. During pregnancy, NO is one of the most important relaxing factors of the myometrium and also plays a key role in the control of blood flow in the uterus and placenta. In PE, the bioavailability of NO is lower than in normal pregnancy. It is proposed that this alteration is due to a decreased NO half-life rather than to an impairment in endothelial nitric oxide synthase (eNOS) activity. Deficit of substrates and increased reactive oxygen species (ROS) might also contribute to the decrease in NO bioavailability. Accordingly, plasma L-arginine levels have been reported to be lower in women with PE than those in normal pregnancy. In this chapter, we provide evidence supporting the view that L-arginine supplementation in early pregnancy could reduce the occurrence of PE.

[*] E-mail: rrodrigo@med.uchile.cl.

Introduction

Preeclampsia (PE) is a multisystem disorder affecting about 5% of all pregnancies; about 20% of cases of early onset PE lead to delivery before 34 weeks (Rodgers *et al.* 1998). It is associated with substantial maternal and neonatal morbidity and mortality (Roberts and Cooper 2001; Davison *et al.* 2004; Ronsmans *et al.* 2006). It is widely accepted that the placenta plays a key role in the origin of PE (Redman *et al.* 1991; Scott *et al.* 1958; Hou *et al.* 2008). Preeclampsia develops in habitually normotensive women and is characterized by high blood pressure and proteinuria, both of which are resolved after delivery of the fetus (Davey *et al.* 1988).

At particular risk for this disease are (among others) primigravid women aged about 40, multiparous women who have changed partners, and those with increased body mass index (Trupin *et al.* 1996; Sibai *et al.* 1991; Duckitt and Harrington 2005). Preeclampsia is accompanied by low cardiac output and high peripheral resistance (Walker 2000), and proteinuria associated with a decrease in intravascular volume (Brown 1998). The disease can be associated with a low platelet count (Brown 1998), diminished renal function (Martin *et al.* 1999; Saphier and Repke 1998), liver injury and central nervous system dysfunction (Brown 1998; Martin *et al.* 1999; Saphier and Repke 1998; Leitch *et al.* 1997). There is no satisfactory way of preventing the development of the disease, except measures to avoid or reduce complications (Afifi and Churchill 2003; Meher and Duley 2005). Indeed, early delivery is the only successful treatment.

Deficient invasion of the endometrial spiral arteries wall by extravillous cytotrophoblast cells during the first trimester of pregnancy is the most widely recognized predisposing factor for preeclampsia (Khong *et al.* 1986; Hubel 1999; Mignini *et al.* 2006). The normal process consists of the physiological conversion of spiral arteries from highly tortuous and thick-walled vessels into flaccid conduits of low resistance but is impaired in PE, consequent on the failure of placental trophoblast invasion (Aquilina and Harrington 1996; Burton and Jauniaix 2004; Merviel *et al.* 2004). Thus, the spiral arteries display an abnormally high vascular resistance with reduced utero-placental perfusion. Maternal humoral influences lead to changes in vasomotor activity and to inadequate, intermittent placental perfusion; this is likely to result in oxidative stress (Burton and Jauniaux 2004; Sibai *et al.* 2005; Davidge 1998), giving rise to hypoxia-reoxygenation cycles. Also, the resulting activation of apoptotic pathways could lead to increased deportation of syncytiotrophoblast microvesicles into the maternal circulation. These microparticles have been directly linked to activation of maternal neutrophils and the development of the maternal syndrome (Raijmakers *et al.* 2004; Holthe *et al.* 2004). The primary event of PE remains largely unknown, but endothelial dysfunction plays a major role in the underlying pathophysiology of the disease. Most of the clinical attributes of PE, such as hypertension, proteinuria, and edema, are derived from pathological changes within the maternal vascular endothelium or involve oxidative stress and endothelial dysfunction.

Preeclampsia consists of two phases. The first is related to altered placentation and the second to generalized endothelial dysfunction attributed to the synthesis of an unknown factor by the hypoxic placenta. Nevertheless, less than half of all pregnancies with PE have altered placentation. Accordingly, new hypotheses have emerged proposing that PE is a condition determined by an exacerbated systemic inflammatory response, secondary to a major deportation of trophoblastic microparticles. This systemic inflammatory response is associated with endothelial dysfunction. The exacerbation of the inflammatory response could be mediated by two factors: (1) A placenta of greater than normal volume associated with a more susceptible vasculature ("maternal" PE); (2) an altered placentation associated with oxidative stress ("placental" PE) (Uzan *et al.* 2011). The cause and mechanisms of the latter have been widely studied in recent years. Various intrinsic and extrinsic mechanisms can alter the physiological process of placentation at the fetal-maternal interface. Among these, and related to hypoxia and reperfusion (or to hypoxia alone), is the increase in extra-villous trophoblast (EVT) apoptosis. This increased apoptosis is mediated, partly, by a diminished bioavailability of nitric oxide (NO) and increases in oxidative stress and pro-inflammatory factors. Additionally, hypoxia generates an anti-angiogenic state mediated by a local and systemic increase of sFlt-1, the soluble receptor of vascular endothelial growth factor (VEGF), which in turn lowers the bioavailability of the latter and of placental growth factor (PlGF), thus resulting in impaired placentation (Maynard and Karumanchi 2011).

In spite of growing knowledge about the pathophysiology of PE, successful prevention is still lacking. Several multicenter international studies have demonstrated the ineffectiveness of aspirin and antioxidant vitamins in preventing PE. Recent studies have shown the importance of NO in protecting the extra-villous trophoblast against pro-apoptotic mechanisms generated at the fetal-maternal interface. Nitric oxide is synthesized by nitric oxide synthase (NOS); this is in fact a group of enzymes, but the most important in pregnancy is the endothelial isoform. Endothelial nitric oxide synthase (eNOS) uses L-arginine as substrate and tetrahydrobiopterin (BH_4) as a cofactor, producing NO. Under pathological conditions, the bioavailability of NO is diminished owing to a deficit of substrate (mediated by decreased substrate availability and especially by increased arginase activity) and an increase of reactive oxygen species (ROS), which shifts the synthesis of NO by eNOS to synthesis of peroxynitrite, a powerful oxidant (Rodrigo *et al.* 2005). In view of this, several studies have used L-arginine supplementation in the treatment of PE, with very promising results (Vadillo-Ortega *et al.* 2011). The ability of L-arginine to prevent PE merits further investigation. This chapter is focused in the potential role of L-arginine for preventing PE, based on the role of NO bioavailability - a factor likely to be influenced by oxidative stress - in the pathogenesis of the disease.

Pathophysiology of Preeclampsia

Oxidative Stress in Normal Pregnancy

Pregnancy itself is a condition of increased susceptibility to oxidative stress, leading to potential oxidative injury to tissues (Sies 1991). Several organs in pregnant women show increased basal oxygen consumption and changes in substrate energy use. The production of ROS within the fetal-placental unit has special relevance because the unit is highly vascularized and the tissue is rich in mitochondria; there is also an abundance of macrophages. At pregnancy term, the human placenta is hemomonochorial, meaning that only one chorionic trophoblast cell layer exists between the maternal and fetal blood, which favors the exchange of gases, nutrients, and metabolic products. In turn, oxygen delivery is favored by the lower partial pressure of oxygen, which raises lactic acid production and lowers the pH within the placental cells and fetal circulation. In addition, as the hypoxic placenta matures, vascularization develops to create an oxygen-rich environment. Moreover, the increasing mitochondrial mass favors the production of ROS (Liochev and Fridovich 1997).

The placenta also produces NO (Dotsch *et al.* 2001), giving rise to another local source of free radicals, which are likely to contribute to endothelial dysfunction, as will be further discussed below. Finally, because the placenta is also rich in macrophages, local production of free radicals including reactive chlorine species might also contribute to the development of oxidative stress (Myatt and Cui 2004). Macrophages express both inducible nitric oxide synthase (iNOS) activity (Myatt *et al.* 1993) and NADPH oxidase activity (Matsubara 2001a), though studies on xanthine oxidase are still lacking. On the other hand, defense mechanisms against ROS damage are also enhanced in pregnancy. Thus, a progressive increase in free radical scavengers such as glutathione and bilirubin, as well as in the activity of antioxidant enzymes in the placenta, has been reported (Qanungo and Mukherjea 2000). The activities of glutathione peroxidase in erythrocytes and platelets and of extracellular superoxide dismutase (SOD) also increase progressively throughout gestation up to the third trimester (Tamura *et al.* 2001), which suggests an increased demand for protection against superoxide anions. In agreement with these observations, the induction of antioxidant enzymes after exposure to oxidative stress is well documented (Bae *et al.* 2004). Genes encoding these enzymes are often coordinately regulated through antioxidant responsive elements (ARE) in their gene regulatory regions (Lee and Johnson 2004). It has been reported that a transcription factor named nuclear factor erythroid-derived 2 related factor 2 (Nrf2) binds to these ARE sites, leading to the up-regulation of downstream genes that regulate a wide array of ARE-driven genes in various cell types. To compensate for these effects, lipid peroxidation becomes more attenuated with the progress of gestation, protecting the fetus against ROS toxicity (Qanungo and Mukherjea 2000). Adaptive mechanisms enhancing the maternal antioxidant defense system that counteract the effect of free radicals through enzymatic induction, as well as through nonenzymatic free radical protectors and scavengers, could prevent the occurrence of oxidative stress. However, pregnancy is a state in which this adaptation and equilibrium could easily be overwhelmed. Thus, oxidative injury has been implicated in the preterm premature rupture of membranes (Wood *et al.* 2001) and is associated with fetal growth restriction (Takagi *et al.* 2004).

Current Theories of PE

There are several hypotheses about the genesis of PE, but recently a consensus has emerged that PE is a syndrome and therefore has multiple causes. There is also agreement that PE has two phases. In this model, the first stage, associated with the histological and molecular changes described above, is the reduction of maternal blood flow to the intervillous space. The second stage is the transference of the reduced placental perfusion to systemic maternal pathophysiology (Roberts *et al.* 1995). This abnormal perfusion of the intervillous space may lead to the production of different molecules that ultimately affect endothelial function and reduce organ perfusion. The search for this factor has led to the identification of numerous candidate substances. An integrated model has been proposed (Redman and Sargent 2005), which assumes that the placenta plays a central role in the pathogenesis of PE but that abnormal placentation is unlikely to be the exclusive cause of this syndrome (Roberts *et al.* 1995). However, it is well known that abnormal placentation does not necessarily mean PE, so it is necessary to find the link between the placental and maternal disease.

First Phase: Placental Insufficiency

Alteration of Placentation

The primary objective of placentation is the transformation of the spiral arteries, terminal branches of the uterine artery, into vessels with high capacitance and low contractility. To achieve this goal, the process requires complex interactions among several tissues at the fetal-maternal interface. It is accepted today that during early pregnancy, normal placentation occurs in a relatively hypoxic environment (<2% oxygen) that is essential for development by preventing trophoblast differentiation to an invasive phenotype (Caniggia *et al.* 2000; Jauniaux *et al.* 2000; Jauniaux *et al.* 2003). Intervillous blood flow increases at around 10-12 weeks of gestation and results in exposure of the trophoblast to increased oxygen tension (PO_2) and increases in the activities and levels of the major antioxidant enzymes superoxide dismutase, catalase, and glutathione peroxidase in the villous tissues (Watson *et al.* 1998). Hypoxia inducible factor-1 (HIF-1), specifically its 1α subunit, and transforming growth factor β_3 (TGFβ_3), an inhibitor of early trophoblast differentiation, mediate the effects of low oxygen tension during the first trimester of pregnancy. The expression of both molecules is high in early pregnancy and falls at around 10-12 weeks of gestation when placental PO_2 levels are believed to increase owing to the unplugging of the uterine spiral arteries (Caniggia *et al.* 2000). In addition, there is also evidence that leptin, TGFβ_1 and PAI-2 are involved in physiological trophoblast invasion (Gonzalez *et al.* 2000; Irving and Lala 1995; Kruithof *et al.* 1995).

In normal pregnancy, endovascular trophoblast invasion progresses from the decidua into the inner third of the myometrium between 12 and 20 weeks of gestation (Lyall *et al.* 1995; Pijnenborg *et al.* 1996; Zho *et al.* 1997). These changes are characterized by spiral artery remodeling including the disintegration of the tunica media along with the internal elastic lamina, and replacement of the endothelium with extravillous trophoblast cells expressing an endothelial phenotype. The changes involve conversion of the narrow muscular arterial tubes into more flaccid and wider tubes, which facilitate the unimpeded placental perfusion with maternal blood flow required for adequate exchange of key molecules between the maternal and fetal circulations. In consequence of previous physiological changes, remodeling of the spiral arteries facilitates the ten-fold increase in uteroplacental blood flow that occurs between conception and term (Myatt and Webster 2009).

Histological studies have shown that the spiral arteries undergo only partial remodeling in pregnancies affected by PE or fetal growth restriction (Khong *et al.* 1986). Extravillous trophoblast invasion and spiral artery remodeling occur either very superficially or not at all in PE. This dysfunctional invasion and replacement of endothelial function results in both high resistance to flow in the maternal uterine arteries and relative placental hypoperfusion at a time when the first symptoms of PE may appear.

There is a molecular explanation for abnormal placentation: Caniggia *et al.* (1999) found that TGFβ_3 expression was greater in human PE placenta than in age-matched controls, and that inhibition of $TGF\beta_3$ by antibodies restored invasive ability to the trophoblast cells in PE explants. The authors speculated that if oxygen tension fails to increase, or the trophoblast does not detect this increase, expression of the two factors remains high, resulting in shallow trophoblast invasion and predisposing the pregnancy to PE. In brief, women with PE have a lower oxygen concentration, and this leads to a high concentration of HIF-1α and TGF-β3 in the trophoblast, inhibiting the trophoblast differentiation. Endoglin, which impairs the activation of NOS mediated by $TGB\text{-}\beta_3$, is also increased in PE pregnancies (Venkatesha *et al.* 2006). Initiation of apoptosis has two known pathways, intrinsic and extrinsic. Both pathways finally lead to the activation of caspases, the family of cysteine proteases responsible for apoptosis. The extra-villous trophoblast invades the spiral arteries, replacing the endothelium and the muscular wall. Recent studies suggest that this transformation of the spiral arteries is mediated by extra-villous trophoblast-induced apoptosis through activation of the Fas/FasL pathway. Additionally, the development of the placenta requires continual remodeling, which is mediated by apoptosis. The inflammatory response of normal pregnancies is partly due to a constant liberation of microparticles to the maternal circulation mediated by the apoptosis of trophoblastic cells. There is evidence that the apoptosis rate is higher in pregnancies with PE than in normal ones, suggesting that an alteration in the apoptotic process plays a role in the pathophysiology of PE.

Oxidative Stress

Although the cause of PE still remains uncertain, it has been proposed that enhanced oxidative stress is a basic component of this condition that could provide the connection between abnormal placentation and the maternal syndrome (Roberts and Hubel 1999; Moretti *et al.* 2004). The placenta appears to be the main source of ROS initiating the pathophysiological events in PE (Serdar *et al.* 2002), but maternal leukocytes and the maternal endothelium are also likely to contribute. In addition, it has been proposed that oxidative stress is a component of PE that could provide the link between decreased placental perfusion and the maternal syndrome (Moretti *et al.* 2004).

There is much evidence suggesting that PE is associated with oxidative status (Rodrigo *et al.* 2005). It has been observed that biomarkers for lipid peroxidation are increased in women with PE (Takacs *et al.* 2003; Aydin *et al.* 2004). Oxidative stress in PE is also related to a decrease of antioxidants, such as vitamin C and E and β-carotenes, and a diminished activity of antioxidant enzymes such as glutathione peroxidase and superoxide dismutase (SOD) (Rodrigo *et al.* 2005; Myatt and Cui 2004). This endorses the hypothesis that hypoxia/ ischemia of the placenta could be an important source of ROS.

The failure of placental perfusion, explained previously, is likely to result in hypoxia-reoxygenation cycles that lead to oxidative stress because maternal humoral and neural influences induce changes in vascular vasomotor activity (Burton and Jauniaux 2004). It has been suggested that the cause of PE is the associated abnormal oxidative insult, not the mRNA expression of antioxidant proteins that may be responsible for reduced antioxidant enzyme activity in the preeclamptic placenta (Vanderlelie *et al.* 2008).Other mechanisms of ROS production in PE pregnancies could include the activation of maternal neutrophils by syncytiotrophoblast microvesicles following deportation due to increased apoptotic or aponecrotic mechanisms locally activated during the passage of maternal blood through the placenta (Raijmakers *et al* 2004). Thus, isolated neutrophils from women with PE synthesize more superoxide than those from normotensive pregnant women (Lee *et al.* 2003a). Consecutively, activated neutrophils may lead to activation of the vascular endothelium, therefore contributing to the pathophysiology of PE (Cadden and Walsh 2008). It has been found that oxidative stress early in pregnancy influences maternal outcome; urinary F2-isoprostanes, biomarkers of lipid peroxidation, are associated with an increased risk of PE (Peter-Stein *et al.* 2008). Recent studies have suggested that this imbalance between oxidants and antioxidants is an effect of the disease and not the cause (Kaur *et al.* 2008).

Since maternal neutrophils may be activated during the passage of blood through the placenta (Lee *et al.* 2003b) as well as through the export of syncytiotrophoblast microvesicles into the maternal circulation, isolated neutrophils from women with PE synthesize more superoxide than those of normotensive pregnant women. In turn, the activated neutrophils may contribute to the activation of the vascular endothelium. Maternal blood leukocytes in preeclamptic women are activated and this supports the view that oxidative stress is a contributing factor in the pathophysiology of PE (Holthe *et al.* 2004).

Although the generation of the placental oxidative stress could be related to hypoxia due to reduced uteroplacental perfusion, hypoxia itself is not sufficient to account for all the morphological findings (Burton *et al.* 1999). In fact, an ischemia-reperfusion cycle associated with the uteroplacental blood flow may be more important for establishing placental oxidative stress (Hung *et al.* 2001). As a consequence, an increased capacity of placental as well as other cells to generate ROS has been found in PE (Many *et al.* 2000). Oxidative stress in this context is a consequence of an imbalance between excessive generation of ROS and reduced capacity of the antioxidant defenses, causing placental injury, which in turn could account for the increased rates of infarction and syncytial necrosis observed in this condition.

The most common ROS is the superoxide anion. Xanthine and NADPH oxidases have been identified as major vascular superoxide-forming enzyme systems, but the contribution of xanthine oxidase (XO) is generally minor (Poston and Raijmakers 2004). However, XO is abundantly expressed in cytotrophoblast and syncytiotrophoblast cells because ischemia-reperfusion is a potent stimulus of the conversion from xanthine dehydrogenase (Hassoun *et al.* 1994). In addition, NADPH oxidase activity, constitutive in the trophoblast of the human placenta, is highly stimulated in PE (Matsubara *et al.* 2001b). This enzyme consists mainly of five subunits and it has been observed that placentae from preeclamptic women show increased expression of the NADPH oxidase components p22, p47, and p67 (Dechend *et al.* 2003). Other forms of NADPH oxidase are also implicated in the pathophysiology of PE, such as those present in phagocytes (neutrophilic and eosinophilic granulocytes, monocytes, and macrophages) and vascular cells. NADPH oxidase mediates the increased production of superoxide by neutrophils isolated from women with PE (Lee *et al.* 2003a). It has been well established that vascular NADPH oxidase plays a major role in the development of hypertension (Touyz *et al.* 2005) and is a target for down-regulation by antioxidant vitamins. It is interesting to note that under oxidative stress conditions, eNOS could be uncoupled owing to the oxidation of BH_4, the coupling factor accounting for the dimerization of the enzyme subunits. Consequently, another source of superoxide anion production will arise, accounting for the exacerbation of oxidative injury. Figure 22.1 shows a summary of the role of oxidative stress in the pathophysiology of PE.

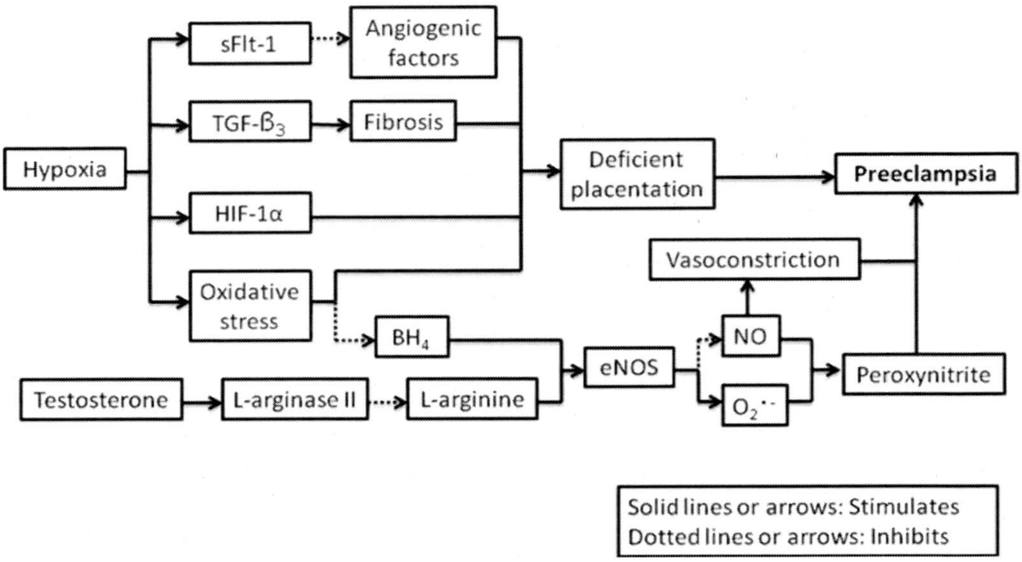

Figure 22.1. Summary of mechanisms by which oxidative stress could lead to development of preeclampsia. Abbreviations: sFlt-1, fms-like tyrosine kinase 1; HIF-1α, Hypoxia inducible factor-1; TGF-β3, transforming growth factor β3; BH4, tetrahydrobiopterin; eNOS, endothelial nitric oxide synthase; NO, nitric oxide; PE, preeclampsia; $O2^{*}$-, superoxide anion.

Second Phase: Maternal Expression

Maternal Syndrome

It has been long presumed that the generalized endothelial dysfunction in PE is mediated by an unknown factor generated by the placenta. Because the angiogenic/antiangiogenic balance could be impaired in PE, considerable attention has recently been focused on angiogenesis-related gene products; VEGF, PlGF, and soluble fms-like tyrosine kinase 1 (sFlt1). VEGF is an endothelial cell-specific mitogen that promotes placental vascularization. It regulates multiple endothelial cell functions including mitogenesis, permeability, vascular tone and vasoactive molecule production (Zachary 1998). The biological effects of the VEGF family receptors are mediated by members of the class III subfamily of tyrosine kinase receptors: fms-like tyrosine kinase (Flt-1) and kinase insert domain-containing receptor (KDR) (Zachary and Gliki 2001). VEGF is abundant in placental tissue and fetal membrane cells and its expression increases during gestation. Some studies have reported a decrease of this factor in PE (Lyall et al. 1997), while in other studies an unaltered (Oh *et al.* 2006) or an increased (Sgambati *et al.* 2004) expression have been observed**.** Recently, increased levels of two circulating antiangiogenic proteins - sFlt1 (Levine *et al.* 2004) and its splicing form (sFlt1-14) (Sela *et al.* 2008), both binding PlGF and VEGF - were suggested to predict the subsequent development of PE. PlGF is another member of the VEGF family that is predominantly produced in the placenta. sFlt1 is an endogenously secreted protein that captures free VEGF and PlGF, thus preventing these molecules from interacting with the respective endogenous receptors. An increased level of sFlt1 was suggested as a biomarker for the subsequent development of PE (Maynard *et al.* 2003). In PE, free VEGF and PlGF synthesis is reduced, whereas sFlt1 is up-regulated in the placenta from the second trimester of pregnancy (Ahmad and Ahmed 2004; Karumachi and Bdolah 2004). Decreased plasma levels of VEGF have been found to be associated with a diminution of NO. It has been suggested that this represents an impaired stimulus to vascular formation and endothelial regulation that induces placental disease and PE (Tranquilli *et al.* 2004). There is controversy about the importance of pro-inflammatory cytokines in the maternal syndrome.

Finally, another candidate that has been studied is the deportation of cellular, sub-cellular and molecular microparticles from the placenta during apoptosis (van der Post *et al.* 2011). The apoptosis rate is higher in PE. These microparticles could generate an exacerbated inflammatory response. Figure 22.2 shows a summary of the possible mechanisms that could explain the occurrence of the maternal syndrome in PE.

Endothelial Dysfunction

The endothelium participates in the modulation of vascular tone, control of hemostasis, host defense and inflammation, transport of nutrients and activation/inactivation of vasoactive hormones. Endothelial dysfunction is characterized by a shift of the actions of the endothelium toward reduced vasodilatation, a proinflammatory state and prothrombic properties (Endemann and Schiffrin 2004; Luscher and Barton 1997). Endothelial dysfunction seems to play a major role in the underlying pathophysiological mechanism of PE (Roberts 1998). Factors likely to play a role in the impairment of endothelial cell function in PE include placental ischemia, lipoprotein-induced toxicity, ROS, antiangiogenic effects and immune maladaptation, which result in the synthesis and release of proinflammatory cytokines. Factors released into the maternal blood stream by the abnormally developed placenta could lead to systemic endothelial dysfunction, and this could be responsible for the clinical aspects of the maternal syndrome of PE (Davison *et al.* 2004).

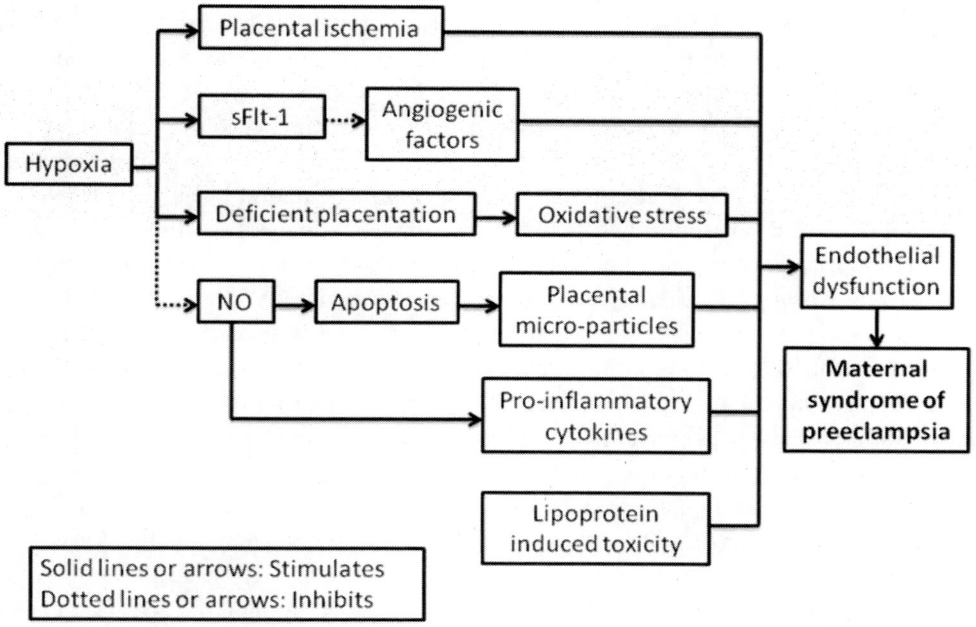

Figure 22.2. Summary of mechanisms that could explain the occurrence of the maternal syndrome in preeclampsia. Abbreviations: sFlt1, fms-like tyrosine kinase 1; NO, nitric oxide.

There is evidence of endothelial dysfunction in PE, such as high levels of von Willebrand factor (Bouchlariotou *et al.* 2008; Hulstein *et al.* 2006; Nadar *et al.* 2004), tissue plasminogen activator (TPA) and endothelial and placental plasminogen activator inhibitor (PAI 1 and 2). In normal pregnancies, the quotient PAI 1/PAI 2 is low owing to the high placental mass. In PE, this quotient is high owing to cellular activation and insufficient placental mass (Brown 2010; Ma *et al.* 2002; Akolekar *et al.* 2011; Reith *et al.* 1993).

Several vasoactive substances that could be altered because of endothelial dysfunction have been implicated. Among them are endothelin-1 (ET-1) and thromboxane A_2 (TXA_2), both potent vasoconstrictors found at high levels in PE (Davison *et al.* 2004). At the same time, the decrease of NO, a potent vasodilator, could also be involved in the pathogenesis of PE. Recently, an increase of asymmetric dimethylarginine, a competitive inhibitor of eNOS, has gained attention. The inactivation of dimethylarginine dimethylaminohydrolase (DDAH 1 and 2), which metabolizes asymmetric dimethylarginine, is partly responsible for the increase of ROS (Savvidou *et al.* 2003).

Nitric Oxide

Nitric oxide is a potent endothelium-derived vasodilator (Rees *et al.* 1989) and defective synthesis of it has been documented in PE pregnancies (Morris *et al.* 1996). During pregnancy, NO is one of the most important relaxants of the myometrium and it is no less important in the control of blood flow in the uterus and placenta. It is formed through a reaction catalyzed by endothelial NO synthase (eNOS) and plays a major role in maintaining vascular homeostasis. The availability of the cofactor tetrahydrobiopterin (BH_4) is crucial for the function of the enzyme. In normal placenta, adequate concentrations of L-arginine orient eNOS toward the synthesis of NO. However, in PE, a lower than normal L-arginine concentration caused by arginase II over-expression (Noris *et al.* 2004) or altered erythrocyte uptake of L-arginine (Da Costa *et al.* 2004) could redirect eNOS toward the synthesis of peroxynitrite. Also, placental hypoxia, which is associated with PE, does not induce up-regulation of eNOS (Orange *et al.* 2003). The eNOS inhibitor N(omega)-nitro-L-arginine methyl ester (L-NAME) generates a vasoconstrictor response through inhibition of NO synthesis. Interestingly, this response is significantly lower in women with PE. This fact can be interpreted as a reduced effect of functional NO in the circulation in PE, which proves that the NO pathway in the vascular bed is impaired in these women (Bisseling *et al.* 2004). L-NAME administration in pregnant rats induces PE, and the fetuses show endothelial dysfunction that disappears after birth (Martinez-Orgado *et al.* 2004).

Because the placenta lacks autonomic innervation, locally produced mediators such as NO are important for maintaining placental blood flow. In addition, NO regulates leukocyte adhesion to the endothelium (Kubes *et al.* 1991) and inhibits vascular smooth muscle cell proliferation and platelet aggregation (Moncada and Higgs 2006). All these functions could be impaired by the consumption of NO by superoxide anions produced during oxidative stress, thereby diminishing NO bioavailability. Consistent with this was the finding of a diminished concentration of NO in plasma (Var *et al.* 2003) or amniotic fluid (Luscher and Barton 1997) in preeclamptic women.

Despite the numerous studies of NO production, assessed by monitoring plasma levels of the stable NO degradation products nitrite and nitrate (NOx) in both normal pregnancy and PE, the status of NO is controversial. Elevation (Nobunaga *et al.* 1996), decrease (Choi *et al.* 2002) and no change (Diejomaoh *et al.* 2004) in NOx levels have been shown. This controversy may be partly due to the effects of potential confounders. In this regard, the relevance of the dietary intake of nitrate should be mentioned, since it can dramatically affect the plasma level and urinary excretion of NOx. In addition, the plasma levels of NOx are influenced by acute fluctuations in renal tubular reabsorption (Conrad *et al.* 1999). The authors previously used a reduced NOx diet to analyze the plasma and urinary levels of NOx and its second messenger cGMP (Conrad *et al.* 1999). Despite increases in both plasma and urinary cGMP during normal human pregnancy, NOx were either unchanged or reduced, suggesting that (1) another signal besides NO mediates augmented cGMP production and maternal vasodilation during pregnancy, or (2) body fluid NOx is an unreliable estimate of hemodynamically relevant NO. In turn, no unequivocal support for reduced NO production has been demonstrated in PE. Recently, it was reported that decreased eNOS expression and activity may be associated with increased endothelial permeability in PE (Wang *et al.* 2004). These authors suggested that IL-8, which is increased by oxidative stress (Scholz *et al.* 2003), could be a candidate mediator of this effect. The inhibition of eNOS made IL-8-induced endothelial monolayer permeability greater in preeclamptic endothelial cells than in those from normal pregnancies, probably because of greater susceptibility to proinflammatory cytokines in PE; however, these data need to be confirmed.

Finally, modulation of NOS isoforms by endothelin (ET)-1, as found in PE, suggests a functional relationship (Labonté *et al.* 2008). The trophoblastic cells in preeclamptic women show increased expression of eNOS, whereas expression of the inducible isoform (iNOS) - the main source of NO synthesis - is decreased (Napolitano *et al.* 2000). Although the trophoblast has eNOS activity, whether extra-villous trophoblast expresses this enzyme is controversial. In the cytotrophoblast, NO increases the expression and activity of both matrix metalloproteinases 2 and 9, which play a fundamental role in embryo implantation. Additionally, NO is important for trophoblastic migration and motility through angiopoietines (Ahmed *et al.* 2009). This effect is enhanced by the actions of VEGF, both binding to its receptor Flt1 and increasing expression of cadherins by the extra-villous trophoblast (Oh *et al.* 2006).

It is proposed that in PE the decrease of NO bioavailability is not due to a decrease in activity or expression of eNOS, but to decreased activity or half-life of NO, measured by the concentration of cGMP, its second messenger (Aydin *et al.* 2004; Szabo *et al.* 2003). An interesting explanation for the decrease in NO activity is related to the fact that eNOS also synthesizes superoxide anion and that the rate of NO vs. superoxide anion production depends on the intracellular concentrations of L-arginine and superoxide dismutase (SOD) among others (Rodrigo *et al.* 2005). The reaction between NO and superoxide anion generates peroxynitrite, a potent cytotoxic anion that lacks angiogenic properties. Peroxynitrite can alter cellular functions in many ways and nitrates many proteins, particularly on tyrosine residues. In addition, it diminishes NO bioavailability because it oxidizes BH_4, thereby leading to the degradation of eNOS (Szabo *et al.* 2003). The altered vascular reactivity in the preeclamptic placenta may be partly explained by the effect of peroxynitrite inducing vascular dysfunction via selective impairment of adrenoreceptors (Benkuski *et al.* 1999). It has been demonstrated that peroxynitrite also selectively inactivates the prostacyclin receptor (Zou *et al.* 1999) and decreases the amount of prostacyclin synthase through a mechanism mediated by NF-κB (Cooke and Davidge 2002). These peroxynitrite effects contribute to the development of hypertension in PE. Furthermore, cytotrophoblasts from preeclamptic women showed increased TXA_2 production, thereby causing an imbalance between TXA_2 and prostacyclin levels (Ding *et al.* 2002) and further contributing to the generally observed elevation of blood pressure. Several studies have shown that women with PE have higher levels of peroxynitrite and nitrotyrosine (a marker for peroxynitrite activity) in the placenta. In normal pregnancies, an L-arginine gradient between fetal and maternal plasma has been demonstrated, the concentration being higher in the fetus (Tsukahara *et al.* 2008). This indicates active transport of L-arginine into the fetus. In PE, this gradient is decreased (Braekke *et al.* 2009).

Assuming that the activity and expression of eNOS are conserved, and that the cationic amino acid transporter in the placenta is also conserved, the eventually diminished concentration of L-arginine in PE could be attributable to increased activity of arginase II, the enzyme responsible for degrading L-arginine into ornithine and urea. Several studies have shown that this enzyme is more active in the trophoblast of PE than in that of normal pregnancies (Sankaralingam *et al.* 2009; Sankaralingam *et al.* 2010). The mechanism explaining the increase of arginase II in PE is still unknown, but it has been suggested that an elevation of testosterone levels, as is observed in PE, could play an important role (Lowe 2000; Carlsen *et al.* 2005).

In summary, the changes in concentrations of vasoactive substance in PE could be understood as a consequence of the systemic inflammatory response in this disease, mediated by an exaggerated deportation of syncytiotrophoblast cells or generation of ROS, which activates the endothelium and the white blood cells.

Role of L-Arginine Supplementation

Many alternative methods for prophylaxis against PE have been tested during the past 20 years, unfortunately without success. In relation to the use of aspirin, a recent meta-analysis of 31 studies on 32,217 pregnant women who received aspirin in order to prevent PE found a significant reduction of only 10% in global and severe PE and also a 10% reduction in adverse pregnancy outcomes (Askie et al. 2007). However, despite these results, two groups recently showed that aspirin is not useful for preventing PE when administered to risk groups (Yo et al. 2003; Subtil et al. 2003).

A study of women at high risk for PE (Chappell et al. 1999) demonstrated the usefulness of antioxidant vitamins administered early in pregnancy in reducing oxidative stress and thus its effect on endothelial function. More recently, the use of antioxidant vitamins to prevent PE has been questioned following the results of three multicenter studies (Poston et al. 2006; Rumbold et al. 2006; Spinnato et al. 2007). All of these studies indicate that antioxidant vitamins are not useful for preventing PE and/or fetal growth restriction. Moreover, it has been reported that antioxidant vitamins may have undesirable effects on the fetus and newborn (Poston et al. 2006).

There is little evidence as to whether the manipulation of diet in pregnancy can prevent PE (Fraser 1998). L-arginine is considered a semi-essential amino acid because endogenous synthesis is not enough to meet the requirements under increased demands (Visek 1986). Furthermore, pregnancy has been described as a state of relative deficiency of this amino acid owing to increased demand for synthesis of NO for further strengthening the adaptive vasodilatation of pregnancy, and the increased use of L-arginine by the fetus (Conrad *et al.* 1993). For these reasons, it has been suggested that dietary supplementation with L-arginine may prevent the development of PE.

There are studies suggesting that L-arginine has direct effects on blood pressure in animal models and in normotensive humans, humans with hypertension, and women with PE or healthy pregnancy (Hishikawa *et al.* 1992; Campese *et al.*, 1997; Rosano *et al.* 1998; Creager *et al.* 1992; Adams *et al.* 1997; Rector *et al.* 1996; Bode-Boger *et al.* 1998; Facchinetti *et al.* 1996; Neri *et al.* 1996). Notably, L-arginine supplementation improves vascular function in patients with atherosclerosis and peripheral vascular disease (Creager *et al.* 1992; Adams *et al.* 1997; Rector *et al.* 1996; Bode-Boger *et al.* 1998). Oral administration of L-arginine to women with cardiovascular disease showed no adverse side effects (Facchinetti *et al.* 1996; Neri *et al.* 1996).

As mentioned earlier, the bioavailability of NO, one of the key elements in the pathophysiology of PE, is decreased. Approximately 1% of the daily intake of L-arginine is metabolized through the eNOS pathway (Castillo *et al.* 1995). NO diffuses from the endothelium to the underlying layer of smooth muscle cells, mediating vasodilatation and inhibition of platelet aggregation and adhesion. These processes are dependent on cyclic guanylyl monophosphate (cGMP).

There are several possible ways in which exogenous L-arginine may increase NO production. Some authors have demonstrated lower plasma L-arginine levels in PE women (D`Àniello *et al.* 2001). Theoretically, exogenous L-arginine could compensate for this shortage of endogenous substrate. Another possible mode of action of exogenous L-arginine could depend on the attenuation of the inhibition of NOS activity by methylated arginines. It has been demonstrated that plasma levels of endogenous inhibitors of NOS, asymmetric and symmetric dimethylarginines, are elevated in PE (Ellis *et al.* 2001; Savvidou *et al.* 2003). One could argue that an excess of L-arginine might restore NOS activity by competitively displacing endogenous inhibitors from the active site of the enzyme (Cooke 2000). However, neither the plasma concentrations of L-arginine nor levels of methylated arginines (asymmetric and symmetric dimethylarginine, L-NMMA) changed significantly in women treated with L-arginine. Although speculative, another line of explanation for the observed phenomena could depend on the ability of L-arginine to inhibit the formation and/or action of ROS within the vascular wall, a well-documented phenomenon in PE. L-arginine, as a substrate for NOS, might not only increase NO synthesis but also prevent NOS-dependent formation of ROS (Parra-Cordero *et al.* 2011) and improve NO bioavailability. Interestingly, L-arginine could also be an ROS scavenger (Davidge 1998). The proposal that the antihypertensive action of L-arginine depends on such mechanisms remains an attractive hypothesis to be tested. Table 1 shows a summary of the main mechanisms by which exogenous supplementation with L-arginine could be beneficial for PE prevention.

Table 1. A summary of potential mechanisms by which L-arginine may interfere with the sequence of events leading to the development of preeclampsia

Mechanism	Reference
Compensation for a shortage of endogenous substrate	D´Aniello *et al.* 2001
Restoration of NOS activity by competitively displacing endogenous inhibitors	Ellis *et al.* 2001; Savvidou *et al.* 2003
Prevention of NOS-dependent formation of ROS	Parra-Cordero *et al.* 2001
ROS scavenging	Davidge 1998

NOS, nitric oxide synthase; ROS, reactive oxygen species.

Finally, current evidence on the use of L-arginine in pregnant women with PE should be provided. There are few reports on the use of L-arginine as a method of preventing PE. In 2004, there was a study of 70 women at risk of developing PE who were supplemented with L-arginine from the first quarter of pregnancy. The results showed a decrease in the resistance of uterine arteries under average blood pressure conditions; also, only one patient developed late-onset PE (Germain et al. 2004). However, another study (Staff et al. 2004) demonstrated that oral L-arginine supplementation did not reduce diastolic blood pressure in PE women with gestational length varying from 28 to 36 weeks, but whether this treatment could be clinically beneficial for the mother or the fetus if started earlier in the disease process than for the women in this study remains to be investigated. Another study conducted on women with PE demonstrated that infusion with L-arginine was associated with reduced blood pressure, concomitant with an increase of L-citrulline (surrogate marker of NO production), both in women with PE and in normotensive women (Facchinetti *et al.* 1999). Similar results were obtained in a double blind, randomized study on women with PE and with a low nitrate diet (Rytlewski *et al.* 2005). Women who received oral L-arginine for three weeks showed a decrease in blood pressure and increased urinary excretion of nitrite/nitrate and L-citrulline. Interestingly, there is only one study evaluating the fetal condition and neonatal outcome after oral supplementation with L-arginine, on women with a diagnosis of PE. In this group, the women were supplemented until delivery. The authors showed that in the supplemented group, the fetal blood redistribution was normalized and the APGAR score at birth and duration of pregnancy were significantly increased compared to the group receiving placebo (Rytlewski *et al.* 2006). Concomitantly, another study showed that supplementation with L-arginine alone in pregnant women with mild chronic hypertension had no significant overall effect on BP but was associated with less need for antihypertensive medications and a trend toward fewer maternal and neonatal complications (Neri *et al.* 2010).

Recently, a study conducted an interesting protocol of L-arginine and antioxidant vitamins supplementation on a group of 672 pregnant women at high risk of PE development (Vadillo-Ortega *et al.* 2011). Two hundred and twenty-eight women were supplemented with diet containing L-arginine plus antioxidant vitamins, 222 with antioxidant vitamins alone and 222 with placebo. The results showed that the incidence of PE was reduced significantly in women randomized to L-arginine plus antioxidant vitamins. Thus, these authors proposed that co-supplementation during pregnancy with L-arginine and antioxidant vitamins could reduce the incidence of PE in populations at high risk of the condition.

The appropriate conditions for L-arginine supplementation should be taken into account, as in the face of oxidative stress it could lead to increased arginase expression. This, in turn, could induce uncoupling of NOS as a source of superoxide anion in the maternal vasculature in preeclampsia. Consequently, it could result in a further increase in peroxynitrite and its deleterious consequences (Sankaralingam *et al.* 2010). As explained above, and because of the role of L-arginine in increasing NO bioavailability, it is possible that oral supplementation with this compound in early pregnancy could reduce the occurrence of PE, but further studies will be needed for definite conclusions.

Conclusion and Perspectives

Preeclampsia is one of the most important complication of human pregnancy worldwide and a major contributor to maternal and fetal morbidity and mortality. It is a syndrome of two stages. The first stage concerns the relative failure of early trophoblastic invasion and remodeling of the spiral arteries, leading to a poor blood supply to the fetal-placental unit, exposing it to oxidative stress. The second stage is characterized by maternal endothelial dysfunction, leading to the clinically recognized symptoms of the syndrome, which include hypertension, proteinuria, thrombocytopenia and impaired liver function. Despite much work during the last decade, the causes that trigger PE remain uncertain and the predictive value of potential risk factors is poor. Increasing evidence suggests that placental and systemic oxidative stress plays a crucial role in its development.

Nitric oxide is a potent vasodilator produced by the vascular endothelium and synthesized by NOS from the semi-essential amino acid L-arginine. During pregnancy, NO is one of the most important relaxants of the myometrium and important for the control of blood flow in the uterus and placenta. A diminished concentration of NO has been reported in PE, which could be explained by the consumption of NO by superoxide anions produced during oxidative stress, thereby diminishing NO bioavailability. There is evidence consistent with the view that as L-arginine is the substrate for NO synthesis, its increased availability through supplementation in the presence of antioxidant vitamins prolongs the latency to development of PE in a high risk population of women.

On the basis of pathophysiological arguments and some finished and ongoing clinical trials, it is conceivable that oral supplementation with L-arginine in women with risk of PE development could increase NO bioavailability and thus reduce the consequences of its deficit such as the development of PE. Therefore, in view of previous evidence, it is essential to clarify the role and mechanisms of antioxidant vitamins and L-arginine actions in risk groups. It is also essential to achieve a greater understanding of the pathophysiological processes underlying the clinical manifestation of PE, and what effect antioxidant vitamins and L-arginine may have on them.

References

Adams, M. R. *et al.* (1997) Oral L-arginine improves endothelium-dependent dilatation and reduces monocyte adhesion to endothelial cells in young men with coronary artery disease. *Atherosclerosis*, 129, pp. 261-269.

Afifi, Y. and Churchill, D. (2003) Pharmacological treatment of hypertension in pregnancy. *Current Pharmaceutical Design*, 9, pp. 1745-1753.

Ahmad, S. and Ahmed, A. (2004) Elevated placental soluble vascular endothelial growth *Circulation Research*, 95, pp. 884-891.

Ahmed, A. *et al.* (2009) Angiopoietin-2 confers Atheroprotection in apoE-/- mice by inhibiting LDL oxidation via nitric oxide. *Circulation Research*, 104, pp. 1333-1336.

Akolekar, R. *et al.* (2011) Maternal plasma plasminogen *Hypertension in Pregnancy*, 30, pp. 311-321.

Aquilina, J. and Harrington, K. (1996) Pregnancy hypertension and uterine Doppler ultrasound. *Current Opinion in Obstetrics and Gynaecology*, 8, pp. 435-440.

Askieske, L.M. *et al.* (2007) Antiplatelets agents for prevention of pre-eclampsia: a meta-analysis of individual patient data. *Lancet*, 369, pp. 1791-1798.

Aydin, S. *et al.* (2004) Plasma malondialdehyde, superoxide dismutase, sE-selectin, fibronectin, endothelin-1 and nitric oxide levels in women with preeclampsia. *European Journal of Obstetrics, Gynecology and Reproductive Biology*, 113, pp. 21-25.

Bae, I. *et al.* (2004) BRCA1 induces antioxidant gene expression and resistance to oxidative stress. *Cancer Research*, 64, pp. 7893-7909.

Benkuski, N. A. *et al.* (1999) Peroxynitritemediated attenuation of alpha- and beta-adrenoreceptor against induced vascular responses in vivo. *European Journal Pharmacology*, 364, pp. 151-158.

Bisseling, T. M. *et al.* (2004) N-acetylcysteine restores nitric oxide-mediated effects in the fetoplacental circulation of preeclamptic patients. *American Journal of Obstetrics and Gynecology*, 191, pp. 328-333.

Bode-Beger, S. M. *et al.* (1998) L-arginine-induced vasodilatation in healthy humans: pharmacokinetic pharmacodynamic relationship. *British Journal of Clinical Pharmacology*, 46, pp. 489-497.

Bouchlariotou, S. *et al.* (2008) Nocturnal hypertension is associated with an exacerbation of the endothelial damage in preeclampsia. *American Journal of Nephrology*, 28, pp. 424-430.

Braekke, K. *et al.* (2009) Asymmetric dimethylarginine in the maternal and fetal circulation in preeclampsia. *Pediatric Research*, 66, pp. 411-415.

Brown, N. J. (2010) Therapeutic potential of plasminogen activator inhibitor-1 inhibitors. *Therapeutic Advances in Cardiovascular Disease*, 4, pp. 315-324.

Brown, M. A. (1998) Pregnancy-induced hypertension: current concepts. *Anaesthesia and Intensive Care*, 17, pp. 185-197.

Burton, G. J. and Jauniaux, E. (2004) Placental oxidative stress: from miscarriage to preeclampsia. *Journal of the Society of Gynecologic Investigation*, 11, pp. 342-352.

Burton, G. J. *et al.* (1999) Maternal arterial connections to the placental intervillous space during the first trimester of human pregnancy: the Boyd collection revisited. *American Journal of Obstetrics and Gynecology*, 181, pp. 718-724.

Cadden, K. A. and Walsh, S. W. (2008) Neutrophils, but not lymphocytes or monocytes, infiltrate maternal systemic vasculature in women with preeclampsia. *Hypertension in Pregnancy*, 27, pp. 396-405.

Campese, V. M. *et al.* (1997) Effects of L-arginine on systemic and renal haemodynamics in salt-sensitive patients with essential hypertension. *Journal of Human Hypertension*, 11, pp. 527-532.

Caniggia, I. *et al.* (2000) Oxygen and placental development during the first trimester: implications for the pathophysiology of pre-eclampsia. *Placenta*, 21, pp. 25-30.

Caniggia, I. *et al.* (1999) Inhibition of TGF-beta 3 restores the invasive capability of extravillous trophoblasts in preeclamptic pregnancies. *Journal of Clinical Investigation*, 103, pp. 1641-1650.

Carlsen, S. M. *et al.* (2005) Early second–trimester maternal hyperandrogenemia and subsequent preeclampsia: a prospective study. *Acta Obstetricia et Gynecologica Scandinavica*, 84, pp.117-121.

Castillo, L. *et al.* (1995) Plasma arginine, citrulline, and ornithine kinetics in adults, with observations on nitric oxide synthesis. *American Journal of Physiology*, 268, pp. e360-e367.

Chappell, L. C. *et al.* (1999) Effect of antioxidants on the occurrence of pre-eclampsia in women at increased risk: a randomised trial. *Lancet,* 354, pp. 810-816.

Choi, J. W. *et al.* (2002) Nitric Oxide Production Increases during Normal Pregnancy and Decreases in Preeclampsia. *Annals of Clinical and Laboratory Science*, 32, pp. 257-263.

Conrad, K. P. *et al.* (1999) Plasma and 24-h NOx and cGMP during normal pregnancy and preeclampsia in women on a reduced NOx diet. *American Journal of Physiology - Renal Physiology*, 277, pp. 48-57.

Conrad, K. P. *et al.* (1993) Identification of increased nitric oxide biosynthesis during pregnancy in rats. *FASEB Journal*, 7, pp. 566-571.

Cooke, J. P. (2000) Does ADMA Cause Endothelial Dysfunction? *Arteriosclerosis, Thrombosis and Vascular Biology*, 20, pp. 2032-2037.

Cooke, C. L. and Davidge, S. T. (2002) Peroxynitrite increases iNOS through NF-nB and decreases prostacyclin synthase in endothelial cells. *American Journal of Physiology - Cell Physiology*, 282, pp. 395-402.

Creager, M. A. *et al.* (1992) L-arginine improves endothelium-dependent vasodilation in hypercholesterolemic humans. *Journal of Clinical Investigation*, 90, pp. 1248-1253.

D´Aniello, G. *et al.* (2001) Plasma L-arginine is markedly reduced in pregnant women affected by preeclampsia. *Journal of Chromatography B: Biomedical Sciences and Applications*, 753, pp. 427-431.

da Costa, B. P. *et al.* (2004) L-arginine erythrocyte transport in normal pregnant and preeclamptic women. *American Journal of Obstetrics and Gynecology,* 190, pp. 468-471.

Davey, D. and Mac Gillivray, I. (1988) The classification and definition of the hypertensive disorders of pregnancy. *American Journal of Obstetrics and Gynecology*, 158, pp. 892-898.

Davidge, S. (1998) Oxidative stress and altered endothelial cell function in preeclampsia. *Seminars in Reproductive Endocrinology*, 16, pp. 65-73.

Davison, J. M. *et al.* (2004) New Aspects in the Pathophysiology of Preeclampsia. *Journal of the American Society of Nephrology*, 15, pp. 2440-2448.

Dechend, R., *et al.* (2003) AT1 receptor agonistic antibodies from preeclamptic patients stimulate NADPH oxidase. *Circulation*, 107, pp. 1632-1639.

Diejomaoh, F. M. *et al.* (2004) Nitric oxide production is not altered in preeclampsia. *Archives of Gynecology and Obstetrics*, 269, pp. 237-243.

Ding, Z. Q. *et al.* (2002) Modulation of prostacyclin and thromboxane secretion by cytotrophoblasts from normal and pre-eclamptic human pregnancies. *Placenta*, 23, pp. 594-599.

Dotsch, J. *et al.* (2001) Increase of endothelial nitric oxide synthase and endothelin-1 mRNA expression in human placenta during gestation. *European Journal of Obstetrics, Gynecology and Reproductive Biology*, 97, pp. 163-167.

Duckitt, K. and Harrington, D. (2005) Risk factors for pre-eclampsia at antenatal booking: systematic review of controlled studies. *British Medical Journal*, 330, doi: 10.1136/bmj.38380.674340.E0.

Ellis, J. *et al.* (2001) Levels of dimethylarginines and cytokines in mild and severe preeclampsia. *Acta Obstetricia et Gynecologica Scandinavica*, 80, pp. 602-608.

Endemann, D. H. and Schiffrin, E.L. (2004) Endothelial dysfunction. *Journal of the American Society of Nephrology*, 15, pp. 1983-1992.

Facchinetti, F. *et al.* (1996) L-arginine infusion reduces preterm uterine contractions. *Journal of Perinatal Medicine*, 24, pp. 383-385.

Facchinetti, F. *et al.* (1999) L-Arginine infusion reduces blood pressure in preeclamptic women through nitric oxide release. *Journal of the Society for Gynecologic Investigation*, 6, pp. 202-207.

Fraser, R. (1998) Pre-eclampsia and diet. In: Strain, J. J. *et al.* (eds) *The Encyclopedia of Human Nutrition*. London: Academic Press, pp. 1620-1626.

Germain, A. M. *et al. (*2004) Evidence supporting a beneficial role for long-term L-arginine supplementation in high-risk pregnancies. *Hypertension*, 44, e1.

Gónzalez, R. R. *et al.* (2000) Leptin and leptin receptor are expressed in the human endometrium and endometrial leptin secretion is regulated by the human blastocyst. *Journal of Clinical Endocrinology and Metabolism*, 85, pp. 4883-4888.

Hassoun, P. M. *et al.* (1994) Regulation of endothelial cell xanthine dehydrogenase/xanthine oxidase gene expression by oxygen tension. *American Journal of Physiology*, 266, pp. 163-171.

Hishikawa, K. et al. (1992) Effects of systemic L-arginine administration on hemodynamics and nitric oxide release in man. *Japanese Heart Journal*, 33, pp. 41-48.

Holthe, M. R. et al. (2004) Leukocyte adhesion. Obstetrics and Gynecology, 103, pp. 913-922.

Hou, H. L. *et al.* (2008) Changes of clinical features in hydatidiform mole: analysis of 113 cases. *Journal of Reproductive Medicine*, 53, pp. 629-633.

Hubel, C. A. (1999) Oxidative stress in the pathogenesis of preeclampsia. *Proceedings of the Society for Experimental Biology and Medicine*, 222, pp. 222-235.

Hulstein, J. J. *et al.* (2006) Acute activation of the endothelium results in increased levels of active von Willebrand factor in hemolysis, elevated liver enzymes and low platelets (HELLP) syndrome. *Journal of Thrombosis and Haemostasis*, 4, pp. 2569-2575.

Hung, T. *et al.* (2001) In vitro ischemia-reperfusion injury in term human placenta as a model for oxidative stress in pathological pregnancies. *American Journal of Pathology*, 159, pp. 1031-1043.

Irving, J. A. and Lala, P. K. (1995) Functional role of cell surface integrins on human trophoblast cell migration regulation by TGF-beta, IGF-II and IGFBP-1. *Experimental Cell Research*, 217, pp. 419-427.

Jauniaix, E. et al. (2000) Onset of maternal arterial blood flow and placental oxidative stress. A possible factor in human early pregnancy failure. *American Journal of Pathology*, 157, pp. 2111-2122.

Jauniaux, E. *et al.* (2003) Trophoblastic oxidative stress in relation to temporal and regional differences in maternal placental blood flow in normal and abnormal early pregnancy. *American Journal of Pathology*, 162, pp. 115-125.

Karumanchi, S. A. and Bdolah, Y. (2004) Hypoxia and sFlt-1 in preeclampsia: The "Chicken-and-Egg" question. *Endocrinology,* 145, p. 4835-4837.

Kaur, G. et al. (2008) Alterations in lipid peroxidation and antioxidant status in pregnancy with preeclampsia. *Molecular and Cellular Biochemistry*, 313, pp. 37-44.

Khong, T. Y. *et al.* (1986) Inadequate maternal vascular response to placentation in pregnancies complicated by pre-eclampsia and by small-for-gestational age infants. *British Journal of Obstetrics and Gynaecology*, 93, pp. 1049-1059.

Kruithof, E. K. *et al.* (1995) Biological and clinical aspects of plasminogen activator inhibitor type 2. *Blood*, 86, pp. 4007-4024.

Kubes, P. *et al.* (1991) Nitric oxide: An endogenous modulator of leukocyte adhesion. *Proccedings of the National Academy of Sciences of the United States of America*, 88, pp. 4651-4655.

Labonté, J. *et al.* (2008) Distinct modulation of the endothelin-1 pathway in iNOS-/- and eNOS-/- mice. *Canadian Journal of Physiology and Pharmacology*, 86, pp. 516-525.

Lee, V. M. *et al.* (2003a) Neutrophil activation and reactive oxygen species production in pre-eclampsia. *Journal of Hypertension*, 21, pp. 395-402.

Lee, V. M. *et al.* (2003b) Neutrophil intracellular pH and Na+/H+ exchanger activity in pre-eclampsia. *Metabolism*, 52, pp. 87-93.

Lee, J. M. and Johnson, J. A. (2004) An important role of Nrf2-ARE pathway in the cellular defense mechanism. *Journal of Biochemistry and Molecular Biology*, 37, pp. 139-143.

Leitch, C. R. *et al.* (1997) The changing pattern of eclampsia over a 60 year period. *British Journal of Obstetrics and Gyneacology*, 104, pp. 917-922.

Levine, R. J. et al. (2004) Circulating angiogenic factors and the risk of preeclampsia. *The New England Journal of Medicine*, 350, pp. 672-683.

Liochev, S. I. and Fridovich, I. (1997) How does superoxide dismutase protect against tumor necrosis factor: a hypothesis informed by effect of superoxide on "free" iron. *Free Radical Biology and Medicin*e, 23, pp. 668-671.

Lowe, D. T. (2000) Nitric oxide dysfunction in the pathophysiology of preeclampsia. *Nitric Oxide*, 4, pp. 441-458.

Luscher, T. F. and Barton, M. (1997) Biology of the endothelium. *Clinical Cardiology*, 20, pp. 3-10.

Lyall, F. *et al.* (1997) Placental expression of vascular endothelial growth factors in placentae from pregnancies complicated by pre-eclampsia and intrauterine growth restriction does not support placental hypoxia at delivery. *Placenta*, 18, pp. 269-276.

Lyall, F. *et al.* (1995) Expression of cell adhesion molecules in placentae from pregnancies complicated by pre-eclampsia and intrauterine growth retardation. *Placenta*, 16, pp. 579-587.

Ma, Y. *et al.* (2002). Regulation of plasminogen activator inhibitor (PAI)-1 expression in a human trophoblast cell line by glucocorticoid (GC) and transforming growth factor (TGF)-beta. *Placenta*, 23, pp. 727-734.

Many, A. *et al.* (2000) Invasive cytotrophoblasts manifest evidence of oxidative stress in preeclampsia. *American Journal of Pathology*, 156, pp. 321-331.

Martin Jr, J. N., et al. (1999). The spectrum of severe preeclampsia: comparative analysis by HELLP (hemolysis, elevated liver enzyme levels, and low platelet count) syndrome classification. *American Journal of Obstetrics and Gynecology,* 180, pp. 1373-1384.

Martinez-Orgado, J. et al. (2004) Impairment of fetal endothelium-dependent relaxation in a rat model of pre-eclampsia by chronic NO synthase inhibition. *Journal of the Society for Gynecological Investigation*, 11, pp. 82-88.

Matsubara, S. et al. (2001a) Immuno-electron microscopic localization of endothelial nitric oxide synthase in human placental terminal villous trophoblasts-normal and pre-eclamptic pregnancy. *Placenta*, 22, p. 782.

Matsubara, S. *et al.* (2001b) Enzyme-cytochemically detectable glucose-6-phosphate dehydrogenase in human villous macrophages (Hofbauer cells). *Placenta,* 22, pp. 882-885.

Maynard, S.E. *et al.* (2003) Excess placental soluble fms-like tyrosine kinase 1 (sFlt1) may contribute to endothelial dysfunction, hypertension, and proteinuria in preeclampsia. *Journal of Clinical Investigation*, 111, pp. 649-658.

Maynard, S. E. and Karumanchi, S. A. (2011) Angiogenic factors and preeclampsia. *Seminars in Nephrology*, 31, pp. 33-46.

Meher, S. and Duley, L. (2005) Interventions for preventing pre-eclampsia and its consequences: generic protocol. *Cochrane Database of Systematic Reviews*, 2, doi: 10.1002/14651858.CD004659.pub2.

Merviel, P. *et al.* (2004) Pathophysiology of preeclampsia: links with implantation disorders. *Obstetrics and Gynecology*, 115, pp. 134-147.

Mignini, L. E. *et al.* (2006) Mapping the theories of preeclampsia: the need for systematic reviews of mechanisms of the disease. *American Journal of Obstetrics and Gynecology*, 194, pp. 317-321.

Moncada, S. and Higgs, E. A. (2006) The discovery of nitric oxide and its role in vascular biology. *British Journal of Pharmacology*, 147, pp. 193-201.

Moretti, M. *et al.* (2004) Increased breath markers of oxidative stress in normal pregnancy and in preeclampsia. *American Journal of Obstetrics and Gynecology*, 190, pp. 1184-1190.

Morris, N. H. *et al.* (1996) Nitric oxide, the endothelium, pregnancy and Preeclampsia. *British Journal of Obstetrics and Gynecology*, 103, pp. 4-15.

Myatt, L. and Webster, R.P. (2009) Vascular biology of preeclampsia. *Journal of Thrombosis and Haemostasis*, 7, pp. 375-384.

Myatt, L. and Cui, X. (2004) Oxidative stress in the placenta. *Histochemistry and Cell Biology*, 122, pp. 369-382.

Myatt, L. *et al.* (1993) Immunohistochemical localization of nitric oxide synthase in the human placenta. *Placenta*, 14, pp. 487-495.

Nadar, S. K. *et al.* (2004) Thrombomodulin, von Willebrand factor and E-selectin as plasma markers of endothelial damage/dysfunction and activation in pregnancy induced hypertension. *Thrombosis Research*, 113, pp. 123-128.

Napolitano, M. *et al.* (2000) Expression and relationship between endothelin-1 messenger ribonucleic acid *Journal of Clinical Endocrinology and Metabolism*, 85, pp. 2318-2323.

Neri, I. *et al.* (1996). Effects of L-arginine on utero-placental circulation in growth-retarded fetuses. *Acta Obstetricia et Gynecolica Scandinavica*, 75, pp. 208-212.

Neri, I. *et al.* (2010) L-arginine supplementation in women with chronic hypertension: impact on blood pressure and maternal and neonatal complications. *Journal of Maternal-Fetal and Neonatal Medicine*, 23, pp. 1456-1460.

Nobunaga, T. et al. (1996) Plasma nitric oxide levels in pregnant patients with preeclampsia and essential hypertension. *Gynecologic and Obstetric Investigation*, 41, pp. 189-193.

Noris, M. *et al.* (2004) L-arginine depletion in preeclampsia orients nitric oxide synthase toward oxidant species. *Hypertension*, 43, pp. 614-622.

Oh, M. J. *et al.* (2006) Vascular endothelial growth factor expression is unaltered in placentae and myometrial resistance arteries from pre-eclampsia patients. *Acta Obstetricia et Gynecologica Scandinavica*, 85, pp. 545-550.

Orange, S. J. *et al.* (2003) Placental endothelial nitric oxide synthase localization and expression in normal human pregnancy and pre-eclampsia. *Clinical and Experimental Pharmacology and Physiology*, 30, pp. 376-381.

Parra-Cordero, M. *et al.* (2011) Immunohistochemical expression of von Willebrand factor in the preeclamptic placenta. *Journal of Molecular Histology*, 42, pp. 459-465.

Peter-Stein, T. *et al.* (2008) Oxidative stress early in pregnancy and pregnancy outcome. Free Radical Research, 42, pp. 841-848.

Pijnenborg, R. *et al.* (1996) Evaluation of trophoblast invasion in placental bed biopsies of the baboon, with immunohistochemical localisation of cytokeratin, fibronectin, and laminin. *Journal of Medical Primatology*, 25, pp. 275-281.

Poston, L. and Raijmakers, M. T. (2004) Trophoblast oxidative stress, antioxidants and pregnancy outcome-a review. *Placenta*, 25, doi: 10.1016/j.placenta.2004.01.003.

Poston, L. et al. (2006) Vitamin C and vitamin E in pregnant women at risk for pre-eclampsia (VIP trial): randomised placebo-controlled trial. *Lancet,* 367, pp. 1145-1154.

Qanungo, S. and Mukherjea, M. (2000) Ontogenic profile of some antioxidants and lipid peroxidation in human placental and fetal tissues. *Molecular and Cellular Biochemistry*, 215, pp. 11-19.

Raijmakers, M. T. *et al.* (2004) Oxidative stress and preeclampsia: rationale for antioxidant clinical trials. *Hypertension*, 44, pp. 374-380.

Rector, T. S. *et al.* (1996) Randomized, double-blind placebo-controlled study of supplemental oral L-arginine in patients with heart failure. *Circulation*, 93, pp. 2135-2141.

Redman, C. W. (1991) Current topic: pre-eclampsia and the placenta. *Placenta*, 12, pp. 301-308.

Redman. C. W. and Sargent, I. L. (2005) Latest advances in understanding preeclampsia. *Science*, 308, pp. 1592-1594.

Rees, D.D. *et al.* (1989) Role of endothelium-derived nitric oxide in the regulation of blood pressure. *Proceedings of the National Academy of Sciences of the United States of America*, 86, pp. 3375-3378.

Reith, A. *et al.* (1993) Plasminogen activator inhibitors (PAI-1 and PAI-2) in normal pregnancies, pre-eclampsia and hydatidiform mole. *British Journal of Obstetrics and Gynaecology*, 100, pp. 370-374.

Roberts, J. M. *et al.* (1995) Endothelial dysfunction yes, cytotoxicity no!. *American Journal of Obstetrics and Gynecology*, 173, pp. 978-979.

Roberts, J. M. (1998) Endothelial dysfunction in preclampsia. *Seminars in Reproductive Endocrinology*, 16, pp. 5-15.

Roberts, J. M. and Hubel, C. A. (1999) Is oxidative stress the link in the two-stage model of pre-eclampsia? *Lancet*, 354, pp. 788-789.

Roberts, J. M. and Cooper, D. W. (2001) Pathogenesis and genetics of pre-eclampsia. *Lancet*, 357, pp. 53-56.

Rodgers, G. M. *et al.* (1998) PEE is associated with a serum factor cytotoxic to human endothelial cells. *American Journal of Obstetrics and Gynecology*, 159, pp. 908-914.

Rodrigo, R. *et al.* (2005) Pathophysiological basis for the prophylaxis of preeclampsia through early supplementation with antioxidant vitamins. *Pharmacology and Therapeutics*, 107, pp. 177-197.

Ronsmans, C. and Graham, W. J. (2006) Maternal Mortality: who, when, where, and why. *Lancet*, 368, pp. 1189-1200.

Rosano, G. M. C. *et al.* (1998) L-arginine improves endothelial function in newly diagnosed hypertensives. *Journal of the American College of Cardiology*, 31[Suppl], 262A (abstract).

Rumbold, A. R. *et al.* (2006) ACTS Study Group. Vitamins C and E and the risks of preeclampsia and perinatal complications. *The New England Journal of Medicine*, 354, pp. 1796-1806.

Rytlewski, *K.* et al. *(2005) Effects of prolonged oral supplementation with L-arginine on blood pressure and nitric oxide synthesis in pre-eclampsia. European Journal of Clinical Investigation,* 35, pp. 32-*37.*

Rytlewski, K. *et al.* (2006) Effects of oral L-Arginine on the foetal condition and neonatal outcome in preeclampsia: a preliminary report. *Basic and Clinical Pharmacology and Toxicology*, 99, pp. 146-152.

Sankaralingam, S. *et al.* (2009) Evidence for increased methylglyoxal in the vasculature of women with preeclampsia: role in upregulation of LOX-1 and arginase. *Hypertension*, 54, pp. 897-904.

Sankaralingam, S. *et al.* (2010). Arginase contributes to endothelial cell oxidative stress *Cardiovascular Research*, 85, pp. 194-203.

Saphier, C. J. and Repke, J. T. (1998). Hemolysis, elevated liver enzymes, and low platelets (HELLP) syndrome: a review of diagnosis and management. *Seminars in Perinatology*, 22, pp. 118-133.

Savvidou, M. D. *et al.* (2003) Endothelial dysfunction and raised plasma concentrations of asymmetric dimethylarginine in pregnant women who subsequently develop pre-eclampsia. *Lncet*, 361, pp. 1511-1517.

Scholz, H. et al. (2003) 8-isoprostane increases expression of interleukin-8**.** *Cardiovascular Research*, 59, pp. 945-954.

Scot, J. S. (1958) Pregnancy toxaemia associated with hydrops foetalis, hydatidiform mole and hydramnios. *Journal of Obstetrics and Gynaecology of the British Empire*, 65, pp. 689-701.

Sela, S. *et al.* (2008) A novel human-specific soluble vascular endothelial growth factor receptor 1: cell-type-specific splicing and implications to vascular endothelial growth factor homeostasis and preeclampsia. *Circulation Research,* 102, pp. 1566-1574.

Serdar, Z. *et al.* (2002) Placental and decidual lipid peroxidation and antioxidant defenses in preeclampsia. Lipid peroxidation in preeclampsia. *Pathophysiology*, 9, pp. 21-25.

Sgambati, E. *et al.* (2004) VEGF expression in the placenta from pregnancies complicated by hypertensive disorders. *British Journal of Obstetrics and Gynaecology*, 111, pp. 564-570.

Sibai, B. M. et al. (1991) Severe preeclampsia in the second trimester: recurrence risk and long-term prognosis. *American Journal of Obstetrics and Gynecology*, 165, pp. 1408-1412.

Sibai, B. *et al. (*2005) Pre-eclampsia. *Lancet*, 365, pp. 785-799.

Sies, H. (1991) Role of reactive oxygen species in biological processes. *Wien Klinike Wochenschrift*, 69, pp. 965-968.

Spinnato, J. A. *et al.* (2007) Antioxidant therapy *Obstetrics and Gynecology*, 110, pp. 1311-1318.

Staff, A. C. *et al.* (2004) Dietary supplementation with L-arginine or placebo in women with pre-eclampsia. *Acta Obstetricia et Gynecologica Scandinavica*, 83, pp. 103-107.

Subtil, D. *et al.* (2003) Randomised comparison of uterine artery Doppler and aspirin (100 mg) with placebo in nulliparous women: the Essai Régional Aspirine Mère-Enfant study (Part 2). *British Journal of Obstetrics and Gynaecology*, 110, pp. 485-491.

Szabo, I. *et al.* (2003) Fetal betamethasone treatment and neonatal outcome in preeclampsia and intrauterine growth restriction. *American Journal of Obstetrics and Gynecology*, 189, pp. 1812-1813.

Takagi, Y. *et al.* (2004) Levels of oxidative stress and redox-related molecules in the placenta in preeclampsia and fetal growth restriction. *Virchows Archives*, 444, pp. 49-55.

Tamura, T. *et al.* (2001) Plasma extracellular superoxide dismutase activity in healthy pregnant women is not influenced by zinc supplementation. *Biologic Trace Element Research*, 80, pp. 107-113.

Touyz, R. M. *et al.* (2005) p47phox associates with the cytoskeleton *Arteriosclerosis, Thrombosis, and Vascular Biology*, 25, pp. 512-518.

Tranquilli, A. L. *et al.* (2004) Amniotic vascular endothelial growth factor (VEGF) and nitric oxide (NO) in women with subsequent preeclampsia. *European Journal of Obstetrics, Gynecology and Reproductive Biology*, 113, pp. 7-20.

Trupin, L. S. *et al.* (1996) Change in paternity: a risk factor for preeclampsia in multiparas. *Epidemiology*, 7, pp. 240-244.

Tsukahara, H. *et al.* (2008) Determination of asymmetric dimethylarginine, an endogenous nitric oxide synthase inhibitor, in umbilical blood. *Metabolism*, 57, pp. 215-220.

Uzan, J. *et al.* (2011) Pre-eclampsia: pathophysiology, diagnosis, and management. *Vascular Health and Risk Management*, 7, pp. 467-474.

Vadillo-Ortega, F. *et al.* (2011) Effect of supplementation during pregnancy with L-arginine and antioxidant vitamins in medical food on pre-eclampsia in high risk population: randomised controlled trial. *British Medical Journal*, 342, doi: 10.1136/bmj.d2901.

van der Post, J. A. *et al.* (2011) The functions of microparticles in pre-eclampsia. *Seminars in Thrombosis and Hemostasis*, 37, pp. 146-152.

Vanderlelie, J. *et al.* (2008) Antioxidant gene expression in Preeclamptic Placentae – A preliminary Investigation. *Placenta*, 29, pp. 519-522.

Var, A. *et al.* (2003) Endothelial dysfunction in preeclampsia: increased homocysteine and decreased nitric oxide levels. *Gynecologic and Obstetrics Investigation*, 56, pp. 221-224.

Venkatesha, S. *et al.* (2006) Soluble endoglin contributes to the pathogenesis of preeclampsia. *Nature Medicine*, 12, pp. 642-629.

Visek, W. J. (1986) Arginine needs, physiological state and usual diets: a reevaluation. *Journal of Nutrition*, 116, pp. 36-46.

Walker, J. J. (2000) Preeclampsia. *Baillieres Best Practice and Research Clinical Obstetrics and Gynecology*, 14, pp. 57-71.

Wang, Y. *et al.* (2004) Evidence of endothelial dysfunction in preeclamps in endothelial cells from preeclampsia. *American Journal of Obstetrics and Gynecology*, 190, pp. 817-824.

Watson, A. L. *et al.* (1998) Changes in concentration, localization and activity of catalase within the human placenta during early gestation. *Placenta*, 19, pp. 27-34.

Woods, J. R. *et al.* (2001) Vitamins C and E: missing links in preventing preterm premature rupture of membranes?. *American Journal of Obstetrics and Gynecology*, 185, pp. 5-10.

Yu, C. K. *et al.* (2003) Medicine Foundation Second Trimester Screening Group. Randomized controlled trial using low-dose aspirin in the prevention of pre-eclampsia in women with abnormal uterine artery Doppler at 23 weeks' gestation. *Ultrasound in Obstetrics and Gynecology*, 22, pp. 233-239.

Zachary, I. (1998) Vascular endothelial growth factor. *International Journal of Biochemistry and Cell Biology*, 30, pp. 1169-1174.

Zachary, I. and Gliki, G. (2001) Signaling transduction mechanisms mediating biological actions of the vascular endothelial growth factor family. *Cardiovascular Research*, 49, pp. 568-581.

Zhou, Y. *et al.* (1997) Human cytotrophoblasts adopt a vascular phenotype as they differentiate. A strategy for successful endovascular invasion?. *Journal of Clinical Investigation*, 99, pp. 2139-2151.

Zou, M. H. *et al.* (1999) Selective nitration of prostacyclin synthase and defective vasorelaxation in atherosclerosic bovine coronary arteries. *American Journal of Pathology*, 54, pp. 1359-1365.

In: Hypotheses in Clinical Medicine
Editors: M.M. Shoja, P.S. Agutter et al.

ISBN: 978-1-62257-276-2

Chapter 23

A Unified Hypothesis for the Pathogenesis of Chronic Obstructive Pulmonary Disease and Atherosclerosis: The Role of Microvascular Flow Insufficiency and Functional Hypoxia

***Pentti Tuohimaa*[1,*] *and Matti Järvilehto*[2]**
[1]Fimlab Laboratories, Tampere, Finland
[2]Medical School University of Tampere, Finland
[2] Department of Bioloby, University of Oulu, Finland

Abstract

Atherosclerosis and chronic obstructive pulmonary disease (COPD) are among the leading causes of death and their incidences are increasing worldwide. There is a common risk factor for the two diseases as both are strongly associated with smoking. Several pathogenic mechanisms have been proposed, such as infection and inflammation for both diseases and dyslipidemia for atherosclerosis. However, the actual processes leading to the diseases are not very clear especially since none of the mechanisms suggested can explain the risk from smoking. We propose a simple logical hypothesis for these diseases, which includes all known risk factors as well as the previously proposed mechanisms: The diseases are caused by the anatomical and physiological weakness of the nutritive microvasculature, leading to hypoxia up to severe anoxia in the smooth muscle cells of the target organ. In the bronchi and arterial walls, smooth muscle cells contract rhythmically according to heart beat or breathing rhythm leading to high rates of oxygen consumption. Hypoxia induced by prolonged vasoconstriction (caused by nicotine or other vasoconstrictors) of the arterioles feeding the microvessels of the smooth muscles leads to inflammation of the capillary endothelium as well as the smooth muscle cells. The hypoxia and inflammation increase the permeability of the endo-

* E-mail: pentti.tuohimaa@uta.fi.

thelium, which then allows large particles such as cholesterol and bacteria to invade the tunica media of arteries and bronchiolar walls. Hypoxia also leads to prolonged contraction of the smooth muscles. Furthermore, it causes neoangiogenesis in the walls of both systems, which may improve nutrition and reduce cholesterol accumulation in atherosclerosis but also has harmful effects. In COPD, the increased vascular volume causes thickening of the wall, which increases bronchiolar resistance and results in air trapping in the alveoli, contributing to the pathogenesis of airway obstruction.

Introduction

The World Health Organization (WHO) reported this year that chronic obstructive pulmonary disease (COPD) ranked 4th among global causes of death (5.8% of deaths). This disease is common among smokers; it has been found in every third smoker over 50 years of age and in every second smoker over 70. The disease is progressive leading finally to incurable emphysema. Coronary heart disease (atherosclerosis of the coronary arteries) is the leading cause of death in western countries. The age-standardized death rate from coronary heart disease is 80.5 per 100,000 people. An important reason to evaluate the mechanisms of COPD and atherosclerosis together is their remarkable comorbid association (Bursi *et al.* 2010; Coulson *et al.* 2010; Couillard *et al.* 2010; Sinden and Stockley 2010).

There are two phenotypes of COPD (also known as chronic obstructive lung disease, COLD, chronic obstructive airway disease, COAD, chronic airway limitation, CAL or chronic obstructive respiratory disease, CORD). Bronchial COPD is characterized by chronic bronchitis, whereas the other type leads to emphysema. Long-term smoking is the major etiological factor in COPD, but the underlying pathogenic mechanisms have not been fully elucidated. Other risk factors include long-term exposure to industrial dust and chemicals as well as genetic factors (Eisner *et al.* 2010), which may determine the smokers who are more likely to get COPD. The chemical components of cigarette smoke that irritate the ciliary epithelium of the bronchial tree have been proposed to initiate an inflammatory reaction leading to COPD; however, less attention has been paid to the role of nicotine. In a recent study, both tobacco smoke and to a lesser degree nicotine caused relaxation of the bronchiolar smooth muscle (Streck *et al.* 2010), which, in fact, would facilitate air flow (in contrast to what is expected). The effect of smoking on blood circulation was not studied.

Cigarette smoking is also a risk factor for atherosclerosis, but there are several other risk factors for coronary disease such as hypertension, stress, dyslipidemia, low physical activity, male gender, obesity and diabetes mellitus. The dominant theory for the development of atherosclerosis is the cholesterol-dyslipidemia theory (Brown and Goldstein 1986). There is also evidence supporting the inflammatory (Ross 1999) and bacterial infection (Epstein *et al.* 1999) theories. In our recent study (Tuohimaa and Jarvilehto 2010), we concluded that the known risk or preventive factors of atherosclerosis do not completely support the cholesterol theory, but all are in agreement with functional hypoxia of the vasa vasorum (Jarvilehto and Tuohimaa 2009).

Microvasculature of the Bronchial Tree and the Coronary Arteries

Bronchial vessels originate from the aorta or intercostal arteries, entering the lung at the hilum and branching at the main stem bronchus to supply the lower trachea, extrapulmonary airways, and supporting structures; this fraction of the bronchial vasculature drains into the right heart via systemic veins. Bronchial vessels also supply the intrapulmonary airways as far as the level of the terminal bronchioles where they form extensive anastomoses with the pulmonary vasculature; this systemic-to-pulmonary blood drains via the pulmonary veins to the left heart (Baile 1996). The terminal bronchioles are the last part of the respiratory airway supplied by the vasa nutritia and therefore they are especially vulnerable to hypoxia, as shown in Figure 23.1. The bronchiolar vasa nutritia as well as the vasa vasorum are functionally end arteries. The bronchial vasculature consists of a continuous dense network of subepithelial capillaries that converge to form venules extending to a deeper plexus of larger venules on the adventitial side of the smooth muscle. The branches of small arteroli (vasa nutritia) form a plexus on the adventitial side of the smooth muscle layer. The two capillary plexuses supply oxygen and nutrients to the smooth muscle and epithelium, both of which are metabolically very active. The innervation is under the control of vasodilatory parasympathetic nerves that release acetylcholine and vasoactive intestinal polypeptide, vasoconstrictor sympathetic nerves that release norepinephrine and neuropeptide Y, and sensory nerves that release substance P, neurokinin A, and calcitonin gene-related peptide. Mechanical factors such as downstream pressure and alveolar pressure also influence the distribution of blood flow through the tracheal bronchial vasculature (Baile 1996). The critical areas of oxygen supply are the smooth muscle layer, which contracts rhythmically with breathing, and the epithelium because of its secretory activity.

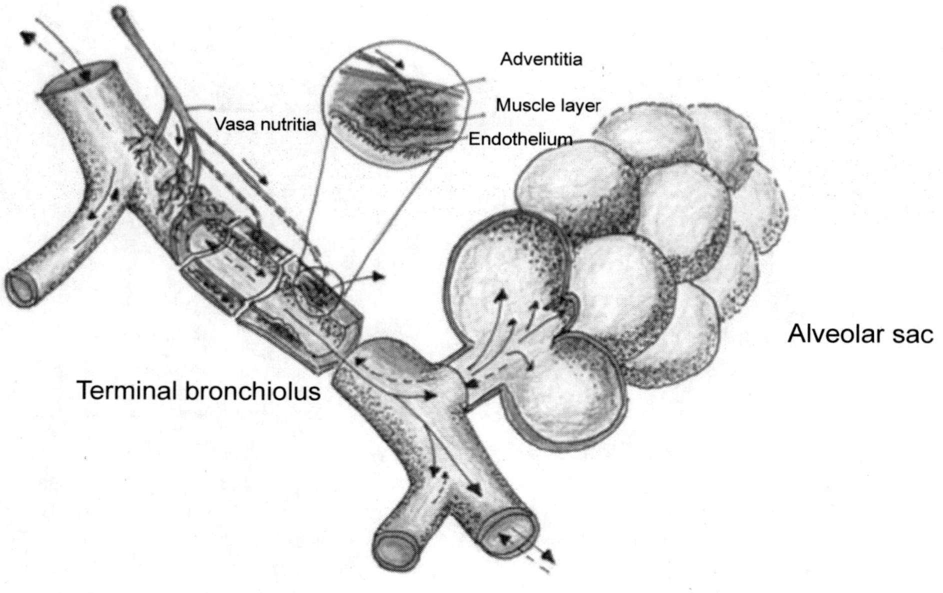

Figure 23.1. Anatomy of the vasa nutritia at the terminal bronchioli. The terminal branches are functionally end arteries forming the adventitial and intimal capillary plexuses, which are connected with alveolar capillaries and the vena pulmonalis. Hypoxia (blue color) develops in the terminal bronchioles owing to vasoconstriction of the vasa nutritia.

Microvessels (vasa vasorum) in the walls of coronary and other arteries originate from the concave side of the upstream arterial branch (external vasa vasorum) (Figure 23.2). The external branches form a tight plexus on the adventitial side of the smooth muscle layer (Galili *et al.* 2004). They supply oxygen and nutrients to the media (smooth muscle layer). The intima obtains its oxygen supply directly from the lumen of the main artery. Few direct arterial branches from the lumen of the main artery penetrate into the wall (internal vasa vasorum). The innervation of the vasa vasorum is similar to that of the vasa nutritia in the bronchioli. The systolic blood pressure wave and the systolic and diastolic blood pressures influence blood flow in the vasa vasorum. The critical area of oxygen supply seems to be the smooth muscle layer of the arterial branching area, as depicted in Figure 23.2, because the arteries are functionally end arteries and their blood flow is reversed (Jarvilehto and Tuohimaa 2009). Smooth muscle contracts rhythmically with the heartbeat and needs high oxygen supply, so even a small constriction of the vasa vasorum may lead to hypoxia.

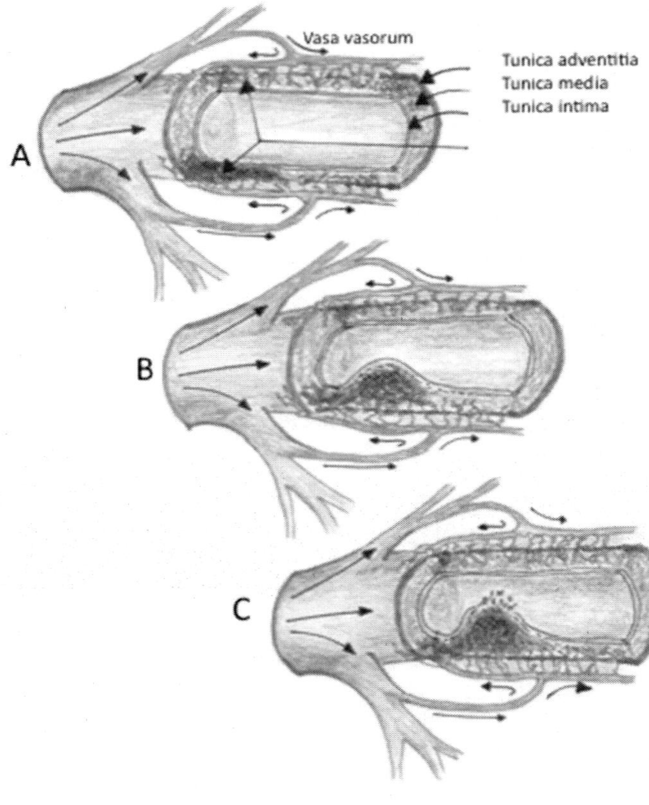

Figure 23.2. Anatomy of the external vasa vasorum and development of atherosclerosis. The most vulnerable site is the branching area, where atherosclerosis is initiated and the arterial supply has a reversed flow. Branches of the vasa vasorum are functionally end arteries, although they supply rich capillary plexuses on the smooth muscle. Hypoxia begins at the arterial branching site and causes inflammation. Different phases are shown: (A) hypoxia and inflammation characterized by contraction of the vasa vasorum, and damaged capillary endothelium; (B) development of atheroma characterized by the accumulation of large particles (LDL-cholesterol, HDL-cholesterol, lipids, cholesterol esters, and bacteria). This phase leads to an osmotic edema, reduced blood flow in the main artery and calcification; (C) atheroma rupture and thrombosis caused by increased pressure in the tunica media; damaged arterial endothelium.

Hypothesis

Functional Hypoxia in Microvessels May Initiate the Pathogenesis of COPD and Atherosclerosis

The pathogenesis of COPD is not clearly understood. It has been proposed that chemical compounds as well as the particles in cigarette smoke and dust inhibit ciliary movements and cause inflammation in the sub-epithelial intima (Cornwell *et al.* 2010; Criner and Celli 2010). The reduced ciliary activity causes an accumulation of mucus in the airway. The inflamemation is followed by neovascularization (Walters *et al.* 2008), which leads to a remodeling and narrowing of the lumen of the terminal bronchioli (Zanini *et al.* 2010). Here we propose an alternative sequence of events, beginning with a decrease in blood flow in the vasa nutritia and hypoxia of bronchiolar smooth muscle layer (media). We also extend this simple model to the pathogenesis of atherosclerosis.

According to this model, the initial stage of both diseases is mild or severe hypoxia of the smooth muscle cells of either the arteriolar or the bronchiolar wall. In both systems, the smooth muscle cell layer contracts rhythmically (with the heartbeat or breathing rhythm). Hypoxia can be induced by prolonged vasoconstriction in arterioles feeding the microvasculature of the smooth muscle layer, leading to injury and prolonged contraction of muscle cells. Hypoxia may also progress to a severe anoxia leading to regional inflammation. The hypoxically injured endothelia become more permeable, allowing large particles such as LDL- and HDL-cholesterol, bacteria etc. to invade the tunica media of the arteries as well as the walls of the bronchioles. In arteries, the cholesterol particles and bacteria accumulate (Renko *et al.* 2008), since the intact endothelium of the main artery does not allow secretion or exudation. The inflammatory reaction will lead to breakdown of the HDL and LDL particles, liberating cholesterol esters, which are water insoluble and accumulate in the media-intima. In bronchioli, cholesterol esters increase the osmotic pressure and thereby the volume of the interstitial tissue. Lipid/cholesterol metabolism seems to play an important role in inflammatory responses in the bronchi (Baldan *et al.* 2008), and the metabolites increase the osmotic pressure within the bronchial wall leading to edema (Wilson and Hii 2006). Cholesterol particles may also be transferred into the bronchial lumen via exudation (Hincman *et al.* 1990). The excreted/secreted cholesterol esters in the lumen may reduce the activity of the lung surfactant by binding to its lipophilic groups, thus promoting the development of emphysema. The hypoxia as well as inflammation may also cause angiogenesis in the walls of both systems, which may improve circulation and nutrition, but at the same time leads to the thickening of the wall, which further reduces the lumen of the artery or bronchiole. This consequently reduces blood flow in the vasa vasorum and vasa nutritia, creating a vicious circle with progressive injury. In the lung, progressive airflow obstruction ensues. Figure 23.3 illustrates schematically the similarities and differences between these two diseases.

Discussion

Chronic inflammatory pulmonary diseases such as COPD and asthma are highly prevalent and constitute a major health burden worldwide. Despite a wealth of biological and clinical information on normal and pathological airway structure and function, the primary causes and mechanisms of these diseases remain to a large extent unknown, preventing the development of more efficient diagnosis and treatment (Auffray *et al.* 2010). COPD is characterized by an abnormal, persistent inflammatory response to noxious environmental stimuli, most commonly cigarette smoke. Although cigarette smoking elicits airway inflammation in all of those who smoke, persistent inflammation and clinically significant COPD occur in only a minority.

The pathogenesis of COPD involves the recruitment and regulation of neutrophils, macrophages, and lymphocytes to the lung, as well as the induction of oxidative stress, all of which result in lung parenchymal destruction and airway remodeling (Cornwell *et al.* 2010). The epithelial inflammation hypothesis does not explain why COPD progresses even after smoking cessation, nor does it explain why the terminal bronchioli are the most vulnerable site; if epithelial inflammation were the origin of the disease, smoking would affect all parts of the respiratory tract equally.

Our hypothesis on the microvascular origin of COPD can better explain the initiation and progression of the disease. The most important factor in cigarette smoke is nicotine, which is a bronchodilator but is strongly vasoconstrictive in the peripheral arteries. Vasoconstriction of the vasa nutritia will lead to hypoxia especially within the smooth muscle layer, but also in the metabolically active ciliary epithelium.

Such hypoxia will cause prolonged smooth muscle contraction, increasing oxygen consumption and compressing the capillaries. This vicious circle continues even after cessation of smoking. Use of nicotine chewing gum instead of smoking would sustain the vicious circle.

Table 1. Risk and protective factors in atherosclerosis and their vascular effects

Risk factor (Vasoconstrictor)	Reference
Nicotine	Rahman and Laher 2007
Obesity	Reaven 1994
Stress	Rozanski *et al.* 1999
Hypertension	Touyz and Schiffrin 2003
Apnea	Drager *et al.* 2008
Protective factor (Vasodilatator)	**Reference**
Estrogen	Cruz *et al.* 2008
Vitamin D	Zittermann and Koerfer 2008
Phys. Exercise	Roberts *et al.* 2007
Alcohol	Deng and Deitrich 2007
Statins	Veillard and Mach 2002

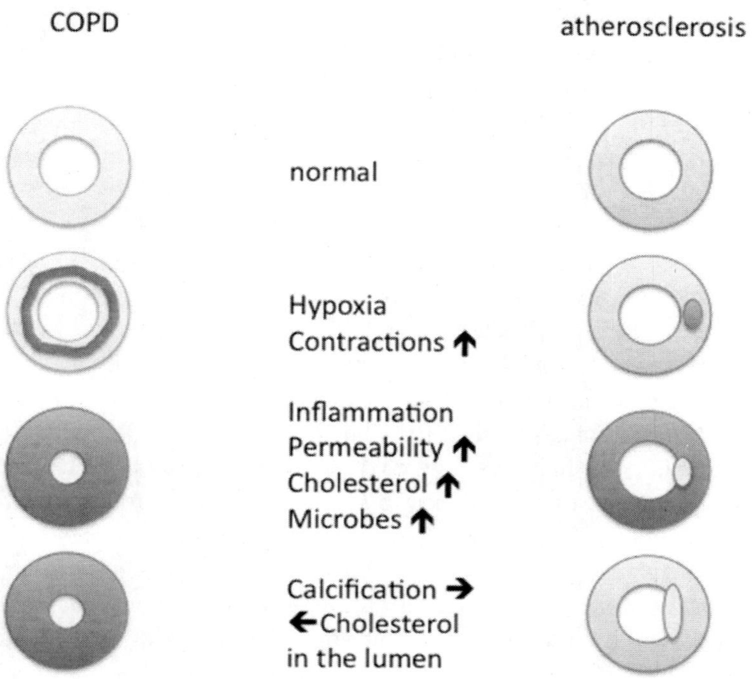

Figure 23.3. A schematic presentation of the three phases of pathogenesis of COPD and atherosclerosis. Both diseases begin with vasoconstriction of the vasa nutritia or vasa vasorum. This leads to hypoxia, which may develop to severe anoxia and tissue injury. Hypoxia will cause prolonged smooth muscle contraction, which will cause increased oxygen consumption leading to a vicious circle. Tissue damage will cause increased permeability of the capillaries and extravasation of HDL- and LDL-particles. Cholesterol is esterified. Intercellular edema will be a consequence of increased osmolarity. Cholesterol esters accumulate focally in atherosclerosis, whereas, in COPD, cholesterol esters are excreted/secreted into the lumen, where they can bind to the surfactant molecules, beginning the pathological process leading to emphysema.

The bronchial vasculature is the systemic arterial blood supply to the lung. Although small relative to the pulmonary vessels, it serves important functions and is modified in a variety of pulmonary and airway diseases. Congestion of the bronchial vasculature seems to narrow the airway lumen in inflammatory airway diseases, and formation of new bronchial vessels (angiogenesis) is implicated in the pathology of a variety of chronic inflammatory, infectious and ischemic pulmonary diseases. The remarkable ability of the bronchial vasculature to remodel has implications for the pathogenesis and especially for the progression of COPD (Charan *et al.* 1997). Although the role of microvessels in the progression of COPD has been recognized, it has been seen as secondary to inflammation. Our hypothesis proposes a new order of events beginning from a functional hypoxia, which is a strong stimulator of neovasculogenesis.

The bronchial circulation, like the pulmonary circulation, is subject to the mechanical effects of lung inflation with each breath. Lung inflation decreases bronchial blood flow in all species studied because of changes in both lung volume and intra-pulmonary pressure. With this reduction of flow there is a relative increase in the proportion of bronchial blood flow drained from the lung through the systemic veins. These changes are probably due to purely mechanical effects on the systemic-to-pulmonary anastomotic bronchial blood vessels, with both compression and stretching of the vessels (Deffebach 1990). Similarly, in coronary artery walls, the circulation is highly dependent on the heartbeat and the wave of systolic pressure, which compresses the microvessels especially in the arterial branching areas. Thus, the anatomical sites of both COPD and atherosclerosis strongly support the microvessel origin hypothesis.

Angiogenesis is a prominent feature of structural tissue remodeling that occurs in the chronic airway diseases of asthma, bronchiolitis obliterans syndrome (BOS, post-lung transplantation), and smoking-related chronic obstructive pulmonary disease (COPD). The hypervascular changes secondary to inflammation are regarded as a mechanism of pathogenesis of these diseases (Walters *et al.* 2008). In asthma, the microvasculature has been shown from early post-mortem series to contribute to airway-wall thickening and edema (Wilson and Hii, 2006). Inflammation seems to induce production of vascular endothelial growth factor (VEGF) (Zanini *et al.* 2010), but hypoxia is also known to enhance VEGF synthesis. According to our hypothesis, hypoxia or anoxia initiates VEGF production as well as inflammation. There is strong evidence to suggest that local production of VEGF and its receptor system is a major driver of angiogenesis in the airway component of COPD, though paradoxically emphysema seems to be due to lack of VEGF in the lung parenchyma (Walters *et al.* 2008). In terms of therapy, evidence for the effectiveness of anti-angiogenic treatment is strongest for inhaled corticosteroids (ICS) and long-acting beta-agonists (LABA) in asthma (Bergeron and Boulet 2006). According to our hypothesis, drugs that cause vasodilatation in the peripheral arteries would be most successful. They would prevent the earliest phase of COPD. Unfortunately, there are no useful direct peripheral vasodilators, because they cause a serious orthostatic hypotonia. Therefore development of new vasodilatory drugs is needed, which might be useful for preventing COPD and atherosclerosis. Statins and vitamin D have weak vasodilatatory properties and they are potential prophylactic drugs (Veillard and Mach 2002; Zittermann and Koerfer 2008).

Female gender is associated with reduction of lung function and more severe disease in subjects with COPD with early onset of disease or low smoking exposure (Sorheim *et al.* 2010). The reason for the gender difference is unknown, but there could be a sex difference in the microvessels, which are known being regulated by sex steroids (Verhave and Siegert 2010).

It is interesting that vitamin D may play a role in the development of both diseases. It is necessary for the calcification of atherosclerotic plaques (Verhave and Siegert 2010). Vitamin D deficiency is associated with increased carotid artery atherosclerosis (Carrelli *et al.* 2011). Genetic polymorphism of the vitamin-D-binding protein (VDBP-1F homozygosity) gene is considered a candidate for explaining the variation in susceptibility to COPD, whereas VDBP-2 has a protective effect in the Chinese Han population (Shen *et al.* 2010).

Finally, the known risk and protective factors strongly support our microvascular theory. Table 1 demonstrates that all risk factors for atherosclerosis (except hypercholesterolemia) cause vasoconstriction, but only obesity may influence serum cholesterol concentration (Tuohimaa and Järvilehto 2010). In contrast, all protective factors for atherosclerosis are associated with vasodilatation, but they are variably associated with serum cholesterol (Tuohimaa and Järvilehto 2010). There is only one clearly verified risk factor for COPD, cigarette smoking, which is known for its vasoconstrictive effect.

Conclusion

The pathogenesis of COPD is complex and not fully understood. The chemical components of cigarette smoke are known to depress ciliary activity so mucus clearance from the lower respiratory tract is impaired. There are several factors that affect expiration: edema of the terminal bronchioles, prolonged muscle contraction, neovascularization and poor mucus removal. Inflammation of the terminal bronchus degrades LDL and HDL particles to cholesterol esters, which are insoluble in water and increase the osmotic pressure in the intima and media layers leading to edema. In contrast to the arteries, where the endothelial barrier is tight, cholesterol esters do not accumulate in the intima of bronchioles but enter the lumen (Hincman *et al.* 1990). In the bronchiolar and alveolar lumen, cholesterol esters bind to surfactant molecules. The surfactant is a complex mixture of phospholipids, proteins, neutral lipids, carbohydrates and minor constituents including cholesterol and its esters (Frosolono *et al.* 1970). The surface tension of the surfactant varies with its content (Hills 1999; Ingenito *et al.* 2005). The putative inhibition of surfactant activity by increased levels of cholesterol esters may lead to emphysema. The role of the surfactant in the pathogenesis of emphysema is not well studied or has been entirely ignored (Ingenito *et al.* 2005), but our hypothesis recommends a closer look at this aspect.

References

Auffray, C. *et al.* (2010) An integrative systems biology approach to understanding pulmonary diseases. *Chest*, 137, pp. 1410-1416.

Baile, E. M. (1996) The anatomy and physiology of the bronchial circulation. *Journal of Aerosol Medicine*, 9, pp. 1-6.

Baldan, A. *et al.* (2008) Loss of ABCG1 results in chronic pulmonary inflammation. The *Journal of Immunology*, 180, pp. 3560-3568.

Bergeron, C. and Boulet, L. P. (2006) Structural changes in airway diseases: characteristics, mechanisms, consequences, and pharmacologic modulation. *Chest*, 129, pp. 1068-1087.

Brown, M. S. and Goldstein, J. L. (1986) A receptor-mediated pathway for cholesterol homeostasis. *Science*, 232, pp. 34-47.

Bursi, F. *et al.* (2010) Chronic obstructive pulmonary disease after myocardial infarction in the community. *American Heart Journal*, 160, pp. 95-101.

Carrelli, A. L. *et al.* (2011) Vitamin d deficiency is associated with subclinical carotid atherosclerosis: the northern Manhattan study. *Stroke*, 42, pp. 2240-2245.

Charan, N. B. *et al.* (1997) Bronchial vascular congestion and angiogenesis. *The European Respiratory Journal*, 10, pp. 1173-1180.

Cornwell, W. D. *et al.* (2010) Pathogenesis of inflammation and repair in advanced COPD. *Seminars in Respiratory and Critical Care Medicine*, 31, pp. 257-66.

Couillard, A. *et al.* (2010) COPD recent findings: impact on clinical practice. *Journal of Chronic Obstructive Pulmonary Disease*, 7, pp. 204-213.

Coulson, J. M. *et al.* (2010) Excessive aortic inflammation in chronic obstructive pulmonary disease: an 18F-FDG PET pilot study. *Journal of Nuclear Medicine*, 51, pp. 1357-1360.

Criner, G. J. and Celli, B. R. (2010) Advanced COPD: pathogenesis, evaluation, and treatment. *Seminars in Respiratory and Critical Care Medicine*, 31, p. 255.

Cruz, M. N. *et al.* (2008) Acute dilatation to phytoestrogens and estrogen receptor subtypes expression in small arteries from women with coronary heart disease. *Atherosclerosis*, 196, pp. 49-58.

Deffebach, M. E. (1990) Lung mechanical effects on the bronchial circulation. *The European Respiratory Journal - Supplement*, 12, pp. 586-590.

Deng, X. S. and Deitrich, R. A. (2007) Ethanol metabolism and effects: nitric oxide and its interaction. *Current Clinical Pharmacology*, 2, pp. 145-153.

Drager, L. F., *et al.* (2009) Additive Effects of Obstructive Sleep Apnea and Hypertension on Early Markers of Carotid Atherosclerosis. *Hypertension*, 53, pp. 64-69.

Eisner, M. D. *et al.* (2010) An official American Thoracic Society public policy statement: Novel risk factors and the global burden of chronic obstructive pulmonary disease. *American Journal of Respiratory and Critical Care Medicine*, 182, pp. 693-718.

Epstein, S. E. *et al.* (1999) Infection and atherosclerosis: emerging mechanistic paradigms. *Circulation*, 100, pp. 20-28.

Frosolono, M. F. *et al.* (1970) Isolation, characterization, and surface chemistry of a surface-active fraction from dog lung. *Journal of Lipid Research*, 11, pp. 439-457.

Galili, O. *et al.* (2004) Adventitial vasa vasorum heterogeneity among different vascular beds. *Journal of Vascular Surgery*, 40, pp. 529-535.

Hills, B. A. (1999) An alternative view of the role(s) of surfactant and the alveolar model. *Journal of Applied Physiology*, 87, pp. 1567-83.

Hincman, H. O. *et al.* (1990) Lipids in airway mucus of acute quadriplegic patients. *Experimental Lung Research*, 16, pp. 369-385.

Ingenito, E. P. *et al.* (2005) On the role of surface tension in the pathophysiology of emphysema. *American Journal of Respiratory and Critical Care Medicine*, 171, pp. 300-304.

Jarvilehto, M. and Tuohimaa, P. (2009) Vasa vasorum hypoxia: initiation of atherosclerosis. *Medical Hypotheses*, 73, pp. 40-41.

Rahman, M. M. and Laher, I. (2007) Structural and functional alteration of blood vessels caused by cigarette smoking: an overview of molecular mechanisms. *Current Vascular Pharmacology*, 5, pp. 276-292.

Reaven, G. M. (1994) Syndrome X: 6 years later. *Journal of Internal Medicine -Supplement*, 736, pp. 13-22.

Renko, J. *et al.* (2008) Bacterial signatures in atherosclerotic lesions represent human commensals and pathogens. *Atherosclerosis*, 201, pp. 192-197.

Roberts, C. K. *et al.* (2007) Effect of a short-term diet and exercise intervention in youth on atherosclerotic risk factors. *Atherosclerosis*, 191, pp. 98-106.

Ross, R. (1999) Atherosclerosis is an inflammatory disease. *American Heart Journal*, 138, pp. S419-20.

Rozanski, A. *et al.* (1999) Impact of psychological factors on the pathogenesis of cardiovascular disease and implications for therapy. *Circulation*, 99, pp. 2192-2217.

Shen, L. H. *et al.* (2010) Association of vitamin D binding protein variants with susceptibility to chronic obstructive pulmonary disease. *The Journal of International Medical Research*, 38, pp. 1093-1098.

Sinden, N. J. and Stockley, R. A. (2010) Systemic inflammation and comorbidity in COPD: a result of 'overspill' of inflammatory mediators from the lungs?: Review of the evidence. *Thorax*, 65, pp. 930-936.

Sorheim, I. C. *et al.* (2010) Gender differences in COPD: are women more susceptible to smoking effects than men? *Thorax*, 65, pp. 480-485.

Streck, E. *et al.* (2010) Effects of cigarette smoke extract and nicotine on bronchial tone and acetylcholine-induced airway contraction in mouse lung slices. *Journal of Investigational Allergology and Clinical Immunology*, 20, pp. 324-330.

Touyz, R. M. and Schiffrin, E. L. (2003) Role of endothelin in human hypertension. *Canadian Journal of Physiology and Pharmacology*, 81, pp. 533-541.

Tuohimaa, P. and Jarvilehto, M. (2010) Niacin in the prevention of atherosclerosis: Significance of vasodilatation. *Medical Hypotheses*, 75, pp. 397-400.

Walters, E. H. *et al.* (2008) Angiogenesis: a potentially critical part of remodelling in chronic airway diseases? *Pharmacology and Therapeutics*, 118, pp. 128-137.

Veillard, N. R. and Mach, F. (2002) Statins: the new aspirin?. *Cellular and Molecular Life Sciences*, 59, pp. 1771-1786.

Verhave, G. and Siegert, C. E. (2010) Role of vitamin D in cardiovascular disease. *The Netherlands Journal of Medicine*, 68, pp. 113-118.

Wilson, J. W. and Hii, S. (2006) The importance of the airway microvasculature in asthma. *Current Opinion in Allergy and Clinical Immunology*, 6, pp. 51-55.

Zanini, A. *et al.* (2010) The role of the bronchial microvasculature in the airway remodelling in asthma and COPD. *Respiratory Research*, 11, p. 132.

Zittermann, A. and Koerfer, R. (2008) Vitamin D in the prevention and treatment of coronary heart disease. *Current Opinion in Clinical Nutrition and Metabolic Care*, 11, pp. 752-757.

In: Hypotheses in Clinical Medicine
Editors: M.M. Shoja, P.S. Agutter et al.
ISBN: 978-1-62257-276-2

Chapter 24

Oral Foci in Systemic Diseases

***Shailesh M. Gondivkar*[1,*], *Amol R. Gadbail*[2] *and Rima V. Parikh*[3]**
[1]MGV's KBH Dental College and Hospital, Nashik, Maharashtra, India
[2]SPDC, Sawangi, Wardha, Maharashtra, India
[3]Nashik, Maharashtra, India

Abstract

A large number of publications have suggested that oral infections, especially periodontitis, are potential contributing factors to a variety of clinically important systemic diseases. Endocarditis has been studied most extensively. Several other systemic infections are caused by bacteria residing in the oral cavity. The final consequence of an occult odontogenic bacteremia is a protracted systemic inflammation. The heightened inflammatory reactions interfere with organ function and induce a variety of pathological conditions in susceptible (especially elderly) individuals. It is safe to assume that odontogenic bacteremias are likely to cause end-organ damage, but it is likely that most such infections remain occult and are dealt with swiftly by body defenses. In this chapter, a review of literature on this topic is presented with an emphasis on the hypothesis that the odontogenic bacteremias, which often remain clinically occult, can induce end-organ damage in susceptible patients.

Introduction

A current research controversy centers on a hypothesized connection between the presence of chronic oral infections and the development of adverse systemic health conditions. The recent findings have strongly suggested that oral health may be indicative of systemic health. Currently, the gap between general medicine and dental medicine is closing, owing to significant findings supporting associations between dental diseases and systemic conditions such as cardiovascular disease, type 2 diabetes mellitus, respiratory diseases,

* E-mail: shailesh_gondivkar@yahoo.com.

stroke, adverse pregnancy outcomes, osteoporosis, etc. Significant effort has brought numerous advances in revealing the etiopathological links between the chronic inflammatory dental disease and systemic conditions.

A focal infection can be generalized by the dissemination of microorganisms or toxic products from a focus of infection. The focus of infection refers to a circumscribed area of tissue that is infected with the exogenous pathogenic microorganisms and is usually located near a mucous or cutaneous surface (Sivapathasundharam 2006). The theory of focal infection, which was promulgated during the 19th and early 20th centuries, stated that "foci" of sepsis are responsible for the initiation and progression of a variety of inflammatory diseases such as arthritis, peptic ulcers and appendicitis (Scannapieco 1998). The therapeutic edentulation was then adopted as a result of the popularity of the focal infection theory. Since many teeth were extracted without evidence of infection, thereby providing no relief of symptoms, the theory was discredited and largely ignored for many years. Recent progress in classification and identification of oral microorganisms and the realization that certain microorganisms are normally found only in the oral cavity have opened the way for a more realistic assessment of the importance of oral focal infection. It has become increasingly clear that the oral cavity can act as the site of origin for dissemination of pathogenic organisms to the distant body sites, especially in immunocompromised hosts such as patients suffering from malignancies, diabetes mellitus, or rheumatoid arthritis or receiving corticosteroid or other immunosuppressive treatments.

Recent advances in bacterial identification methods have shown that oral niches are inhabited by more than six billion bacteria representing in excess of 700 species belonging to at least nine different phyla (de Lillo *et al.* 2006; Aas *et al.* 2005; Paster *et al.* 2001). The oral microbial flora, like most other resident floras of the human body such as those of the skin and the gut, exhibits commensalism, a survival mechanism that benefits the microbes without harming the host. Yet, these largely innocuous commensal residents of the human body have a propensity to become pathogenic in the event of translocation to a different niche (Henderson *et al.* 1998). Oral commensals, particularly those residing in periodontal niches, commonly exist in the form of biofilm communities on either non-shedding surfaces such as the teeth or prostheses, or shedding surfaces such as the epithelial linings of gingival crevices or periodontal pockets. A feature that is unique to the oral bacterial biofilm, particularly the subgingival plaque biofilm, is its close proximity to a highly vascularized milieu (Nanci *et al.* 2000). This environment is different from other sites where bacteria commonly reside in the human body. For example, the ingress of cutaneous flora into the circulation is prevented by the relatively thick and impermeable keratinized layers of the skin. Their covering epithelia are continuously shed at a quick rate, denying prolonged colonization by the bacterial flora. Although innate defense by polymorphonuclear neutrophils is highly developed at the dentogingival junction and backed up by a highly organized lymphatic system, the oral biofilms, if left undisturbed, can establish themselves permanently on non-shedding tooth surfaces subjacent to the dentogingival junction. Any disruption of the natural integrity between the biofilm and the subgingival epithelium, which is at most about 10 cell layers thick, could lead to a bacteremic state (Samaranayake 2006). The literature and guidelines on the prevention and management of bacteremia of odontogenic origin have been under constant review, particularly with regard to prophylactic antibiotics and dental procedures, with differing opinions (Gould *et al.* 2006; Richey *et al.* 2008). Yet, there are a number of other organs and body sites that may be affected by focal bacteremic spread from the oral cavity.

On the basis of current evidence, it is likely that bacteria gain entry into the bloodstream from oral niches through a number of mechanisms and a variety of portals:

1. When there is tissue trauma induced by procedures such as periodontal probing, scaling, instrumentation beyond the root apex, and tooth extractions, a breakage in capillaries and other small blood vessels that are located in the vicinity of the plaque biofilms may lead to spillage of bacteria into the systemic circulation. Obviously, a higher microbial load would facilitate such dissemination, as it is known that individuals with poor oral hygiene are at a higher risk of developing bacteremia during oral manipulative procedures (Forner *et al.* 2006).
2. Innate microbial factors may play a role in the latter phenomenon, as only a few species are detected in experimental bacteremia despite the multitude of diverse bacteria residing within the periodontal biofilm.

Triggering Factors in Odontogenic Bacteremia

The factors triggering the odontogenic bacteremia include:

1. Chewing
2. Personal oral hygiene measures
3. Periodontal procedures
4. Tooth extraction
5. Orthodontic procedures
6. Endodontic procedures
7. Miscellaneous oral procedures

Pathways Linking Oral Infection to Secondary Systemic Diseases

Three mechanisms or pathways linking oral infections to secondary systemic effects have been proposed (Thoden van Velzen *et al.* 1984):

- *Metastatic infection*: The microorganisms that gain entrance to the blood and circulate throughout the body are usually eliminated by the reticuloendothelial system within minutes (transient bacteremia) and as a rule lead to no other clinical symptoms than possibly a slight increase in body temperature (Thoden van Velzen *et al.* 1984; Kilian 1982). However, if the disseminated microorganisms find favorable conditions, they may settle at a given site and, after a certain time lag, start to multiply.
- *Metastatic injury*: Some Gram-positive and Gram-negative bacteria have the ability to produce diffusible proteins, or exotoxins, which include cytolytic enzymes and dimeric toxins with A and B subunits. The exotoxins have specific pharmacological actions and are considered the most powerful and lethal poisons known (Hammond

1992). In contrast, endotoxins are part of the outer membranes released after cell death. Endotoxin is compositionally a lipopolysaccharide that, when introduced into the host, gives rise to a large number of pathological manifestations.

- *Metastatic inflammation*: Soluble antigen may enter the bloodstream, react with circulating specific antibody, and form a macromolecular complex. These immuno-complexes may give rise to a variety of acute and chronic inflammatory reactions at the sites of deposition (Hunter 1911).

Systemic or End Organ Diseases with Oral Bacteria

Since 1911, when Hunter introduced the concept of the focal infection, interest has varied regarding the impact of an oral infection on distant sites in the body (Hunter 1911). Research has proliferated in recent years regarding the relationship of oral disease to systemic conditions. Although the science concerning all relationships between oral disease and systemic health is not conclusive (Michalowicz *et al.* 2006), it is imperative that oral health care providers stay abreast of the latest evidence about periodontal oral-systemic disease connections and potential risk factors, as they relate to patient assessment, diagnosis, treatment planning, and referral to dental specialists and medical providers.

Cardiovascular Disease

Cardiovascular disease (CVD) is a common cause of death, accounting for 29% of deaths worldwide (Amar and Hand 2003). CVDs such as atherosclerosis and myocardial infarction occur as a result of a complex set of genetic and environmental factors. Among other possible risk factors, evidence linking chronic infection and inflammation to CVD has been accumulating (Ridker *et al.* 1997). It is clear that periodontal disease is capable of predisposing individuals to CVD. This was proven by detecting the abundance of Gram-negative species involved, the readily detectable levels of proinflammatory cytokines, the heavy immune and inflammatory infiltrates involved, the association of high peripheral fibrinogen, and the white blood cell (WBC) counts. A number of reviews have been published that outline potential biological mechanisms linking oral infections and periodontal disease to CVD via both direct and indirect pathways.

Direct Pathways

Oral microbes and their by-products can gain systemic access via the circulatory system. Several triggering factors (described earlier) can induce bacteremia. By gaining systemic access, oral microbes have the potential directly to influence subclinical mediators of cardiovascular events such as hypercoagulability, atherosclerotic development or both. The evidence indicates that oral bacteria such as *Streptococcus sanguis* and *Porphyromonas gingivalis* induce platelet aggregation, which leads to thrombus formation (Herzberg *et al.* 1996). These organisms have a collagen-like molecule, the platelet aggregation-associated protein, on their surfaces (Herzberg *et al.* 1994). A mouse study demonstrated that intravenous inoculation with *P. gingivalis* accelerates atherosclerotic development (Li *et al.* 2002). Certain strains of *P. gingivalis* are capable of infecting macrophages and enhancing foam cell formation in the vascular wall, adding further credence to the ability of *P. gingivalis* to initiate or exacerbate the atherosclerotic process (Giacona *et al.* 2004). Thus, previous studies demonstrated the ability of these organisms to induce platelet aggregation and hypercoagulability, increasing the likelihood of thrombus formation, which can lead to ischemic cardiovascular events. Antibodies reactive to periodontal organisms could possibly localize in the heart and trigger complement activation, a series of events leading to sensitized T cells and heart disease (Herzberg *et al.* 1996).

Indirect Pathways

People with periodontal disease have elevated levels of systemic inflammatory markers such as C-reactive protein (CRP) (Slade *et al.* 2003), and treatment for periodontal disease has been reported to decrease systemic inflammation levels (D'Aiuto *et al.* 2004). There are many potential triggers for this enhanced systemic inflammatory response, including transient bacteremia and the local release of bacterial by-products such as lipopolysaccharides (LPS) (Elter *et al.* 2006; Mahanonda *et al.* 2004). Previous studies suggested that proteolytic enzymes referred to as gingipains R are released in large quantities from *P. gingivalis* (Potempa *et al.* 1997; Lourbakos *et al.* 2001). After entering the circulation, gingipains R can activate factor X, prothrombin, and protein C, promoting a thrombotic tendency through the ultimate release of thrombin, subsequent platelet aggregation, conversion of fibrinogen to fibrin, and intravascular thrombus formation. Another mechanism possibly involves the relationship between bacterial and inflammatory products of periodontitis and CVD. LPS from periodontal organisms being transferred to the serum as a result of bacteremia may have an effect on endothelia, so that atherosclerosis is promoted (Pesonen *et al.* 1981). LPS may also elicit recruitment of inflammatory cells into major blood vessels and stimulate proliferation of vascular smooth muscle, vascular fatty degeneration, intravascular coagulation, and blood platelet function.

Another plausible mechanism connecting oral infection and CVD is molecular mimicry, in which antibodies targeted toward bacterial (including periodontal) species inadvertently cross-react with host cells. For example, heat shock protein 60 (Hsp60) has been studied for its potential role in mediating infection-induced atherosclerosis, as human and bacterial Hsp60 are highly conserved. These instances of mistaken identity could lead to vascular inflammation and atherosclerosis (Ford *et al.* 2005). Another predictor of CVD, in particular coronary heart disease (CHD), may be serum levels of antibodies directed against periodontal pathogens such as *P. gingivalis* and *A. actinomyecetemcomitans,* suggesting that periodontal disease could play a role in the pathogenesis of CHD (Pussinen *et al.* 2003).

Subacute Bacterial Endocarditis (SABE)

Subacute bacterial endocarditis or infective endocarditis is a bacterial infection of the heart valves or the endothelium of the heart. It occurs when bacteria in the bloodstream lodge on abnormal heart valves or injured heart tissue. Infective endocarditis is a serious and often fatal systemic disease that has been associated with dental diseases and treatment. It appears that dental procedures, especially extractions and possibly scaling, are associated with bacterial endocarditis. Drangsholt (1998) reported the incidence of infective endocarditis between 0.70 and 6.8 per 100,000 person-years. Over 50% of all infective endocarditis cases are not associated with either an obvious procedural or infectious event three months prior to developing symptoms. Eight percent of all infective endocarditis cases are associated with periodontal or dental disease without a dental procedure. The risk of infective endocarditis after a dental procedure is probably in the range of 1 per 3,000 to 5,000 procedures; over 80% of all infective endocarditis cases are acquired in the community, and the associated bacteria are part of the host's endogenous flora.

A new causal model of dental disease and procedure-associated endocarditis has been proposed that involves early and late bacteremia. The early bacteremia may "prime" the endothelial surface of the heart valves over many years and promote early valve thickening. This renders the valves susceptible to late adherence and colonization with bacteria. The late bacteremia may work over days to weeks and allows bacteria to adhere to and colonize the valve, resulting in the characteristic fulminant infection (Drangsholt 1998).

Respiratory Infections

Pneumonia is an infection of pulmonary parenchyma caused by a wide variety of infectious agents, including bacteria, fungi, parasites, and viruses. Pneumonia can be a life-threatening infection, especially in the old and immunocompromised patient, and is a significant cause of morbidity and mortality in patients of all ages. Pneumonia includes community acquired and hospital acquired (nosocomial) pneumonia. Nosocomial pneumonia, occurring more than 48-72 h after admission to a hospital or nursing home, can be divided into two subtypes: ventilator-associated pneumonia (VAP) and non-VAP. Pulmonary infections consequent on odontogenic bacteremia have been described, although this is controversial because it can always be argued that bacteria could have translocated into the lung through direct anatomical routes. However, the involvement of more than one lung, the multiplicity of lesions, and the nature of the organisms favor an oral-hematogenous spread. It has therefore been argued that such episodes are a result of spread from an oral niche due to the presence of poor oral hygiene or recent orogingival manipulation.

Oral bacteria have been implicated in the pathogenesis of this disease and, in this regard, dental plaque that initiates periodontal disease and dental caries might be an important reservoir for the potential pathogens. Common potential respiratory pathogens (PRPs) such as *Streptococcus pneumoniae*, *Mycoplasma pneumoniae*, and *Haemophilus influenzae* can colonize the oropharynx. Pneumonia can result from infection by anaerobic bacteria. Dental plaque would seem to be a logical source of these bacteria, especially in patients with periodontal disease. Such patients harbor a large number of subgingival bacteria, particularly anaerobic species. Among the oral bacterial species implicated in pneumonia are *A. actinomycetemcomitans*, *Actinomyces israelii*, *Capnocytophaga* spp., *Eikenella corrodens*, *Prevotella intermedia*, and *Streptococcus constellatus*. These organisms also populate the oral cavity in certain settings, for example in institutionalized subjects and in people living in areas served by unsanitary water supplies, and can also be aspirated into the lower airways to cause pneumonia (Scannapieco, 1999; Lorenz and Weiss 1994; Morris *et al.* 1994).

Most commonly, bacterial pneumonia results from aspiration of oropharyngeal flora into the lower respiratory tract, failure of host defense mechanisms to eliminate them, multiplication of the microorganisms, and subsequent tissue destruction. It is likely that most pathogens first colonize the surfaces of the oral cavity or pharyngeal mucosa before aspiration

(Bonten *et al.* 1994). These pathogens can colonize from an exogenous source or emerge following overgrowth of the normal oral flora after antibiotic treatment. Cytokines and enzymes induced from the periodontally inflamed tissues by the oral biofilm may also be transferred into the lungs where they may stimulate local inflammatory processes preceding colonization of pathogens and the actual lung infection (Scannapieco *et al.* 2001). Other possible mechanisms of pulmonary infection are inhalation of airborne pathogens or translocation of bacteria from local infections via bacteremia.

There are several proposed mechanisms to explain the propensity for PRPs to colonize the oropharynx of susceptible patients. Compromised individuals such as diabetics and alcoholics may be prone to oropharyngeal colonization by PRPs (Scannapieco *et al.* 1996). Thus, the extensive dental plaque of these subjects could provide surfaces to which PRPs might adhere to provide a reservoir for infection to distal portions of the respiratory tract. Mechanically ventilated patients in ICUs, with no ability to clear oral secretions by swallowing or by coughing, are at risk for VAP especially if the ventilation lasts for more than 48 h (Estes *et al.* 1995). Oral bacterial load increases during intubation and higher dental plaque scores predict risk of pneumonia.

Diabetes Mellitus

Diabetes mellitus (DM) is a condition in which the body either fails to respond properly to its own insulin, does not make enough insulin, or both. This causes glucose to accumulate in the blood, often leading to various complications such as acute/chronic infection, vascular diseases, neuropathy, nephropathy, and retinopathy (The Diabetes Control and Complications Trial Research Group 1993; Wild *et al.* 2007). DM is commonly categorized as type 1 or insulin dependent, type 2 or non-insulin dependent and gestational. Severe periodontal disease often coexists with severe DM. Diabetes is a risk factor for severe periodontal disease. The converse possibility that periodontal disease either predisposes or exacerbates the diabetic condition has been receiving increasing attention.

A recent hypothesis links chronic subclinical inflammation with insulin resistance, initiating the development of type 2 diabetes. The triggers of inflammation are many and potentially include oral infection, which may lead to a cascade of events including increased cytokine production, activation of acute-phase protein synthesis, and consequent insulin resistance that ultimately leads type 2 diabetes (Amar *et al.* 2003). Once periodontal pathogens are established in the diabetic host, periodontal infection may aggravate micro-vascular complications (retinopathy, nephropathy, and neuropathy), that can progress to macrovascular complications (coronary artery disease, cerebrovascular disease, and peripheral vascular disease) (Amar *et al.* 2003). In patients with periodontal disease, chronic low-level systemic exposure to periodontal microorganisms may exist, leading to significant changes in plasma levels of cytokines and hormones. Owing to the dynamic nature of the inflamed periodontium, the tissue may serve as an endocrine-like source of inflammatory mediators. In type II diabetes mellitus, serum inflammatory cytokines, especially tumor necrosis factor (TNF)-α , have effects on insulin sensitivity, while those cytokines induced by periodontitis are considered to be related to metabolic abnormalities associated with DM (Grossi 2001). *P. gingivalis* and its components, including fimbriae and LPS, reportedly activate various host cells resulting in the release of cytokines such as interleukin (IL)-1, IL-6,

IL-8, and TNF-α (Amano *et al.* 2004). Successful periodontal treatment has been suggested to improve diabetes metabolic control, possibly through reduced TNF-α and improved insulin resistance.

Grossi and Genco (1998) suggested that severe periodontal disease increases the severity of DM and complicates metabolic control. They proposed infection-mediated up-regulation of cycle of cytokine synthesis and secretion by chronic stimulus from LPS and products of periodontopathic organisms. This may amplify the magnitude of the advanced glycation end product (AGE)-mediated cytokine response that is operative in DM. The combination of these two pathways, infection and AGE-mediated cytokine up-regulation, helps to explain the increase in tissue destruction seen in diabetic periodontitis and how periodontal infection may complicate the severity of diabetes and the degree of metabolic control. This results in a two-way relationship between DM and periodontal disease or infection. Shlossman *et al.* (1990) noticed that severe periodontitis at baseline is associated with increased risk of poor glycemic control. These findings suggest that severe periodontitis may be an important risk factor in the progression of diabetes, and control of periodontal infection is essential for achieving long-term control of diabetes mellitus. Interestingly, *P. gingivalis* was detected more frequently in subjects with increased HbA1c levels after periodontal treatment than in those with decreased levels. Furthermore, *P. gingivalis* organisms with type II fimbriae were detected only in subjects with elevated HbA1c, while improvements in HbA1c levels were observed only in subjects without type II clones. These results suggest that glycemic level in DM is affected by the persistence of *P. gingivalis* in periodontal pockets, especially clones with type II fimbriae (Makiura *et al.* 2008).

Adverse Pregnancy Outcomes

Preterm low-birth weight (PLBW) constitutes a set of leading perinatal problems worldwide that have evident public health implications, because their incidence has not decreased despite the many attempts at their prevention. PLBW as defined by the 29th World Health assembly in 1976 is a birth weight of less than 2500 g with a gestational age of less than 37 weeks. This obstetric complication is usually a direct result of preterm labor, in which case it is referred to as preterm delivery of low-birth-weight infants (McGaw 2002). It is known that various risk factors, such as older (greater than 34 years) and younger (less than 17 years) maternal age, inadequate prenatal care, smoking, drug and alcohol abuse, hypertension, genitourinary tract infection, diabetes mellitus, and multiple pregnancies contribute to adverse pregnancy outcomes (McGaw 2002; Garcia *et al.* 2001). Other than local infection of the genitourinary tract, potential infections distant from the placental complex or the genitourinary tract, due to an indirect action of translocated bacterial products such as LPS and/or the action of maternally induced inflammatory mediators, can adversely affect pregnancy outcomes (McGaw 2002; Offenbacher *et al.* 1996a). Therefore, periodontal disease might be a newly considered risk factor of adverse pregnancy outcomes. Initially, the relationship between periodontal disease and PLBW was not so evident in case control studies (Wang *et al.* 2003). Despite these studies, which actually showed a negative correlation between periodontal disease and PLBW, a growing number of studies have shown a positive association (Offenbacher *et al.* 2001; Moreu *et al.* 2005).

Periodontal disease is associated with chronic Gram-negative infections, which result in local and systemic elevations of proinflammatory prostaglandins and cytokines. Hence, maternal periodontal disease may be connected with preterm delivery through mechanisms involving inflammatory mediators or a direct bacterial assault on the amnion. During the second trimester of pregnancy, the proportion of Gram-negative anaerobic bacteria in dental plaque increases with respect to aerobic bacteria (Li *et al.* 2000). *Fusobacterium nucleatum* and other subspecies from the oral flora have been found in the amniotic fluid of women with preterm births (Offenbacher *et al.* 1998a). The Gram-negative bacteria associated with progressive disease can produce a variety of bioactive molecules that may directly affect the host (Li *et al.* 2000). A microbial component, LPS, can activate macrophages and other cells to synthesize and secrete a wide spectrum of molecules, including cytokines IL-1ß, TNF-α, IL-6 and PGE2 and matrix metalloproteinases (MMPs) (Offenbacher *et al.* 1998b). If these components travel to the blood stream and cross over the placental barrier, the physiological levels of PGE2 and TNF-α in the amniotic fluid may increase and induce a preterm birth (Li *et al.* 2000).

Periodontal pathogens including *P. gingivalis* were detected using a PCR assay in the amniotic fluid of pregnant women with a diagnosis of threatened premature labor as well as in placentas of women with preeclampsia (Leon *et al.* 2007; Barak *et al.* 2007). In an immunocytochemical examination, localization of *P. gingivalis* was also shown in placental tissues, including syncytiotrophoblasts, chorionic trophoblasts, decidual cells, and amniotic epithelial cells, as well as vascular cells, which were obtained from women with chorio-amnionitis at fewer than 37 weeks of gestation (Katz *et al.* 2009). In 2005, Bogges *et al.* suggested that prematurity risk may increase when the fetus is exposed to periodontal bacteria and an inflammatory response is generated (Boggess *et al.* 2005). Immunological studies have also revealed higher levels of periodontopathogen-specific immunoglobulin M in umbilical cord blood from babies born preterm (Boggess 2005). However, it should be noted that periodontal disease pathogens are necessary but not sufficient for periodontal disease expression. The role of the host's inflammatory response appears to be the critical determinant of susceptibility and severity (Offenbacher 1996b). The association between periodontal disease and low birth weight may reflect an altered immune-inflammatory trait that places the patient at risk for both conditions. Thus, periodontitis may be a marker for preterm delivery susceptibility as well as a potential risk factor.

Osteoporosis

Osteoporosis, an age-related condition, is defined as a systemic skeletal disease characterized by low bone mass and micro-architectural deterioration, with a consequent increase in bone fragility and susceptibility to fracture. Osteopenia is a reduction in bone mass due to an imbalance between bone resorption and bone formation favoring resorption, resulting in demineralization and leading to osteoporosis. Periodontal disease, tooth loss, and osteoporosis are major public health problems that affect large numbers of elders. From the viewpoint of public health, prevention and early detection of both periodontal disease and osteoporosis have been recognized to be of great importance.

In inflammatory processes, activated T lymphocytes expresses receptor activator of nuclear factor-κB ligand (RANKL), and it is therefore possible that cell-to-cell contact between T lymphocytes and monocyte/osteoclast precursor cells is involved in osteoclast formation. The activation of mature osteoclasts is inhibited by osteoprotegerin (OPG). In periodontal infection, dense infiltrates of mononuclear leukocytes are found in the gingiva, including T lymphocytes and monocyte/osteoclast progenitor cells, and these results in osteoclast formation. Interestingly, RANKL mRNA is up-regulated in the gingiva of patients with advanced periodontitis. In contrast, OPG mRNA is down-regulated (Taubman *et al.* 2001; Liu *et al.* 2003). The hypothesis linking OPG and periodontal disease is strengthened by studies involving Gram-negative bacteria (Jiang *et al.* 2002). Owing to the transient nature of infection by these pathogens, exposure to periodontal infection may trigger RANKL activation and subsequent osteoclast activation and activity, inducing osteoporosis in patients with periodontal infection. Estrogen deficiency is another dominant pathogenic factor for osteoporosis in women (Jacobs *et al.* 1996). Estrogen deficiency modulates the cytokines that initiate an increase in the number of osteoclasts. Periodontitis also activates the host proinflammatory response, recruiting cytokines such as IL-1 beta, TNF-α, IL-6, and IL-8 and prostanoids, leading to the activation of osteoclasts, and thus inducing bone resorption. Hence, many investigations have found a statistically significant positive correlation between periodontal disease and estrogen deficiency (Tezal *et al.* 2000).

Stroke

Stroke is a cerebrovascular disease that affects blood vessels supplying blood to the brain. It occurs when a blood vessel bringing oxygen and nutrients to the brain bursts or is clogged by local thrombus formation or by aggregates of bacteria and fibrin from other sources such as the heart. An inflamed periodontium or other intraoral pathologies such as caries or periapical osteitis will release inflammatory cytokines, LPS, and bacteria into the systemic circulation. Bacteria circulating in the bloodstream could ingress into the CNS through the blood-brain barrier. In addition, because of anatomical proximity, organisms could directly ascend to the brain or the upper part of the spinal cord from oral niches. For these reasons, it is apparent that the CNS could be a vulnerable relocation site for oral bacteria. All these pathogenic bacteria, cytokines and LPS in the systemic circulation may promote atherosclerosis and affect blood coagulation, the function of platelets (Herzberg and Meyer 1996), and PG synthesis, thereby contributing to the onset of stroke. In most of the studies, a correlation between CNS infections and the organisms that are the members of resident oral flora has been found. The commonly noticed bacteria include *S. intermedius*, *S. oralis*, *S. constellatus*, *Fusobacterium* spp., *F. nucleatum*, *Aggregatibacter actinomycetemcomitans*, and *P. gingivalis* (Heckmann *et al.* 2003; Iida *et al.* 2004; Kazanci *et al.* 2005; Khouzam *et al.* 2006). In most reports, there is concomitant circumstantial evidence of poor oral hygiene, periodontitis, dental abscesses, mucositis with oral ulcerations, and the CNS lesions.

Gastrointestinal Diseases

Gastrointestinal (GI) diseases have been periodically related to oral foci of infection. Gastric and duodenal ulcers have reportedly been produced experimentally by the injection of streptococci. Some workers have proposed that the constant swallowing of microorganisms might lead to a variety of GI diseases. In most instances, however, the low pH of the gastric secretions is an adequate defense against such infection.

Helicobacter pylori infection is considered as one of the most prevalent infectious diseases throughout the world; the carriage rate of *H. pylori* is reported to be 20-80% for adults in the developed world, and more than 90% in the developing world (Taylor and Blaser 1991). This infection has a central role in the development and progress of active and chronic gastritis, peptic ulcers and duodenal diseases (Lee *et al.* 1993; Dixon 1991), which afflict more than 10% of individuals during their lifetime. Moreover, *H. pylori* has been designated a type I, or definite, carcinogen by the World Health Organization (International Agency for Research on Cancer 1994) through its association with the development of gastric adenocarcinoma, the second most commonly diagnosed fatal cancer worldwide. While the evidence is less convincing, *H. pylori* has also been shown to be associated with non-Hodgkin's lymphomas of gastric mucosa-associated lymphoid tissue (MALT) (Wotherspoon *et al.* 1991). The reservoir of *H. pylori* and its mode of transmission are unclear. A fecal-oral, oral-oral, and in developing countries a waterborne route of infection have been suggested (Kelein *et al.* 1991; Mai *et al.* 1989). *H. pylori* has been detected by various methods in dental plaque (Khandaker *et al.* 1991), which has led to the suggestion that dental plaque may be responsible for the transmission of the bacteria and possibly serve as a source of reinfection after eradication treatment. *H. pylori* has also been isolated from saliva (Mapstone *et al.* 1993), gastric juice (Tompkin *et al.* 1989), and feces (Thomas *et al.* 1992). Dentures, in common with most other restorations, provide hard surfaces that become colonized by oral bacteria. It is not known, however, whether their presence increases the risk of infection with *H. pylori*. However, the exact role of the oral cavity in this transmission remains under discussion and is the subject of controversy.

Results of several studies have suggested a positive association between oral and gastric *H. pylori* detection (Oshowo *et al.* 1998), whereas others have not (Olsson *et al.* 1993; Song *et al.* 2000); the latter correlate the temporary residence of the bacterium in the oral cavity with gastroesophagal reflux (Savoldi *et al.* 1998; Mattana *et al.* 1998). Interestingly, within these studies, different methods were used for the diagnosis of gastric infection and for the detection of oral *H. pylori*; hence, with differences in sensitivity and specificity between methods being likely, conclusions should be treated cautiously. Not only is the oral cavity a potential reservoir for *H. pylori* infection of the stomach, but it is also a potential reservoir for re-infection, so that even if oral *H. pylori* is initially acquired from the stomach *via* a gastro-oral route, it could still be detrimental to gastric health. Relapse following treatment of gastric infection is common, with re-isolation of the initial infecting strain. It has been proposed that this is due to re-colonization of the gastric mucosa by *H. pylori* originating from dental plaque, an environment that may be inaccessible to systemic antibiotics. In support of this premise, it has been demonstrated that cure of gastric infection does not consistently promote disappearance of *H. pylori* from the oral cavity (Dore-Davin *et al.* 1999), and the success of gastric eradication is significantly lower in oral *H. pylori*-positive than -negative cases (Miyabayashi *et al.* 2000). A few studies have hypothesized that those working close to the oral cavity may be at increased risk of *H. pylori* infection. Japanese dentists have been reported to be at higher risk for *H. pylori* infection than age-matched controls, although, for indiscernible reasons, the risk appears to be greater in younger dentists (Honda *et al.* 2001). In contrast, Banatvala *et al.* in 1995 suggested that dentists do not appear to have a higher carriage rate than pre-clinical dental students (Banatvala *et al.* 1995).

In summary: The presence of *H. pylori* in the oral cavity seems to be transient, but there is increasing evidence for a role of the oral cavity in transmission of this organism. It appears that oral cavity *H. pylori* in hosts with balanced immunological status may not be sufficient to be a source of infection and reinfection of the stomach. However, in changing environmental conditions that would promote the growth of bacteria, such as immunodeficiency or disturbed oral biofilm balance, as in patients with dentures, the number of bacteria can increase and could possibly be sufficient for gastric infection. However, this subject requires considerably more investigation before definite involvement of the oral cavity can be confirmed and preventive measures can be tailored toward the prevention of oral spread.

Rheumatoid Arthritis

Rheumatoid arthritis (RA) is a systemic autoimmune disease characterized by progressive joint destruction and a variety of systemic manifestations resulting from chronic inflammation. RA occurs worldwide and affects approximately 1% of the world population in a female/male ratio of 3:1 and has a peak incidence of onset in women in the fourth and fifth decades of life (Arnett *et al.* 1988). Periodontitis and RA share similar clinical and pathogenic characteristics (Mercado *et al.* 2003). Clinically, both diseases are characterized by local destruction of hard and soft tissues as a consequence of inflammation, and the pathogenesis includes the release of cytokines and MMPs from inflammatory cells (Birkedal-Hansen *et al.* 1993; Bendtzen 1994). The expression of proinflammatory cytokines such as TNF-α leads to the propagation of inflammation and the extensive release of inflammatory mediators that result in bone destruction (Lerner 2006).

Recent studies suggest a significant relationship between RA and periodontitis (Ramamurthy *et al.* 2005; Mercado *et al.* 2001); RA may have a negative impact on periodontal condition and vice versa. Previous studies reported a higher prevalence of RA in patients with periodontitis than in the general population (Mercado *et al.* 2001). Oral bacterial DNAs are detected in serum and synovial fluid of RA patients (Ramamurthy *et al.* 2005). RA patients were also found to have a significantly higher level of IgG antibody against *P. gingivalis, P. intermedia, and B. forsythus* (Moen *et al.* 2006). Furthermore, two recent clinical trials have suggested that treatment of periodontal disease might have a significant impact on RA severity (Riberio *et al.* 2005; Al-Katma *et al.* 2007). A relationship between the reduction of rheumatoid factor (RF) and periodontal treatment complemented by tooth extractions has been reported in the literature (Takahashi *et al.* 1995). In vivo and in vitro studies have shown that LPS from bacteria associated with periodontal disease can stimulate the production of RF, antierythrocyte, anti-DNA and antithymocyte antibodies (Dresser 1978; Hara *et al.* 1996). Human studies have also indicated a relationship between periodontal bacteria and local or systemic production of RF in periodontal disease patients (Gargiulo *et al.* 1982). It is thus reasonable to suggest that treatment of periodontal disease could induce a reduction in LPS production and consequently reduce the levels of RF.

With the realization that an imbalance between pro-inflammatory and anti-inflammatory cytokines exists in the pathogenesis of RA in periodontitis, emerging therapies are focusing on the inhibition of pro-inflammatory cytokines and destructive proteases. The development of chemically engineered bio-active molecules, gene therapy and MMP inhibitors is being aimed at restoring the dysregulation in the pathogenesis of chronic inflammatory diseases. These new therapies hold great promise for patients in altering the course of progressive forms of RA and periodontitis.

Renal Diseases

Renal diseases of certain types are sometimes attributed to foci of infection. The type of microorganism most commonly involved in urinary infections is *Escherichia coli*, although other *Staphylococci* and *Streptococci* may also be cultured. Of the *Streptococci*, *Streptococcus hemolyticus* seems to be the most common. This is an uncommon inhabitant of dental root canals or periapical and gingival areas. Since the microorganisms commonly involved in oral infection are only infrequently involved in renal infections, it appears that oral foci of infection play a minor role even when the possibility of superimposition on a damaged urinary tract exists.

In 2007, Shultis and associates reported that periodontitis predicts the development of overt nephropathy and end-stage renal disease (ESRD) in a dose-dependent manner in individuals with little or no pre-existing kidney disease after adjustment for age, sex, duration of diabetes, BMI, and current smoking. These findings confirm the emerging evidence for an independent association between periodontitis and the development of diabetic kidney disease (Saremi *et al.* 2005; Shultis *et al.* 2007). Hyperglycemia is a known risk factor for kidney disease (104) and previous studies have proved that the level of glycemia rises as a consequence of periodontitis (Shlossman *et al.* 1990; Nelson *et al.* 1990; Taylor 2001; Taylor *et al.* 1996). HbA1C may therefore be both a confounder and an intermediate variable in the causal pathway between periodontitis and kidney disease. A proposed mechanism for the effect of periodontitis on the development of kidney disease is systemic inflammation. Both periodontitis and kidney disease are associated with inflammatory markers such as CRP (Fried *et al.* 2004), and chronic low-level inflammation associated with periodontitis may lead to endothelial dysfunction, which plays a role in the pathogenesis of kidney disease (Seinost *et al.* 2005). Recently, Ardalan *et al.* (2011) supported that the causative link between peritoneal disease and glomerulonephritis might be plausible through both invasion of the glomeruli by periodontal pathogens directly, and systemic inflammatory burden of chronic periodontitis indirectly. In edentulous individuals, potentially deleterious effects of systemic inflammation on kidney function could occur during the period of active periodontal infection and accumulate during the lifetime of the individual. This hypothesis is supported by the observation that the strongest predictive effect of periodontal status on kidney disease was found in edentulous individuals (Shultis *et al.* 2007). Limited studies on the general population suggest that effective periodontal therapy may decrease CRP levels. Therefore, periodontitis in ESRD populations may be a covert source of systemic inflammation that can be managed through effective periodontal therapy.

Conclusion

In the era of evidence-based medicine, a large number of publications have suggested that oral infections, especially periodontitis, are a potential contributing factor to a variety of clinically important systemic diseases. Endocarditis has been studied most extensively. It appears that dental procedures and oral infection meet currently accepted epidemiological criteria for the causation of endocarditis. Apart from bacterial endocarditis, there are a number of other systemic infections caused by bacteria residing in the oral cavity. However, most records of such infections are presented in the literature in the form of case reports or as a summary of a few cases. It is safe to assume that odontogenic bacteremias are likely to cause systemic infections and end-organ damage, but it is likely that most such infections remain occult and are dealt with swiftly by body defenses. The available data provide us only a glimpse of the reality, and much more work on the genetic relatedness of organisms, rather than their phenotypes, sophisticated sampling, detection, and analytical techniques, needs to be done to establish the associations noted above.

References

Aas, J. A. *et al.* (2005) Defining the normal bacterial flora of the oral cavity. *Journal of Clinical Microbiology*, 43, pp. 5721-5732.

Al-Katma, M. K. *et al.* (2007): Control of periodontal infection reduces the severity of active rheumatoid arthritis. *Journal of Clinical Rheumatology*, 13, pp. 134-147.

Amano, A. *et al.* (2004): Variations of Porphyromonas gingivalis fimbriae in relation to microbial pathogenesis. *Journal of Periodontal Research*, 39, pp. 136-142.

Amar, S. *et al.* (2003) Periodontal disease is associated with brachial artery endothelial dysfunction and systemic inflammation. *Arteriosclerosis, Thrombosis and Vascular Biology*, 23, pp. 1245-1249.

Amar, S. and Han, X. (2003) The impact of periodontal infection on systemic diseases. *Medical Science Monitor*, 9, pp. RA291-299.

Ardalan, M. R. *et al.* (2011) A causative link between periodontal disease and glomerulonephritis: a preliminary study. *Therapeutics and Clinical Risk Management*, 7, pp. 93-98.

Arnett, F. et al. (1988) The American Rheumatism Association 1987 revised criteria for the classification of rheumatoid arthritis. Arthritis and Rheumatism, 31, pp. 315-324.

Banatvala, N. et al. (1995) Helicobacter pylori infection in dentists: a case-control study. Scandinavian Journal of Infectious Diseases, 27, pp. 149-151.

Barak, S. *et al.* (2007) Evidence of periopathogenic microorganisms in placentas of women with preeclampsia. *Journal of Periodontology*, 78, pp. 670-676.

Bendtzen, K. (1994) Cytokines and natural regulators of cytokines. *Immunology Letters*, 43, pp. 111-123.

Birkedal-Hansen, H. *et al.* (1993) Matrix metalloproteinases: A review. Critical *Reviews in Oral Biology and Medicine*, 4, pp. 197-250.

Boggess, K. A. *et al.* (2005) Fetal immune response to oral pathogens and risk of preterm birth. *American Journal of Obstetrics and Gynecology*, 193, pp. 1121-1126.

Boggess, K. A. (2005) Pathophysiology of preterm birth: emerging concepts of maternal infection. *Clinics in Perinatology*, 32, pp. 561-569.

Bonten, M. J. *et al.* (1994) The stomach is not a source for colonization of the upper respiratory tract and pneumonia in ICU patients. *Chest*, 105, pp. 878-884.

D'Aiuto, F. *et al.* (2004) Periodontitis and systemic inflammation: control of the local infection is associated with a reduction in serum inflammatory markers. *Journal of Dental Research*, 83, pp. 156-160.

De Lillo, A. *et al.* (2006) Novel subgingival bacterial phylotypes detected using multiple universal polymerase chain reaction primer sets. *Oral Microbiology and Immunology*, 21, pp. 61-68.

Dixon, M. F. (1991) Helicobacter Pylori and peptic ulceration: Histopathological aspects. *Journal of Gastroenetrology and Hepatology*, 6, pp. 125-130.

Dore-Davin, C. *et al.* (1999) Helicobacter pylori in the oral cavity reflects handling of contaminants but not gastric infection. *Digestion*, 60, pp. 196-202.

Drangsholt, M. T. (1998) A new causal model of dental diseases associated with endocarditis. *Annals of Periodontology*, 3, pp. 184-196.

Dresser, D. W. (1978) Most IgM-producing cells in the mouse secrete auto-antibodies (rheumatoid factor). *Nature*, 74, pp. 480-448.

Elter, J. R. *et al.* (2006) The effects of periodontal therapy on vascular endothelial function: a pilot trial. *American Heart Journal*, 151, doi: 10.1016/j.ahj.2005.10.002.

Estes, R. J. and Meduri, G. U. (1995) The pathogenesis of ventilator-associated pneumonia: I. Mechanisms of bacterial transcolonization and airway inoculation. *Intensive Care Medicine*, 21, pp. 365-383.

Ford, P. *et al.* (2005) Characterization of heat shock protein-specific T cells in atherosclerosis. *Clinical and Diagnostic Laboratory Immunology*, 12, pp. 259-267.

Forner, L. T. *et al.* (2006) Incidence of bacteremia after chewing, tooth brushing and scaling in individuals with periodontal inflammation. *Journal of Clinical Periodontology*, 33, pp. 401-407.

Fried, L. *et al.* (2004) Inflammatory and prothrombotic markers and the progression of renal disease in elderly individuals. *Journal of American Society of Nephrology*, 15, pp. 3184-3191.

Garcia, R. I. *et al.* (2000) Relationship between periodontal disease and systemic health. *Periodontology*, 25, pp. 21-36.

Gargiulo, A. V. *et al.* (1982) Identification of rheumatoid factor in periodontal diseases. *Journal of Periodontology*, 53, pp. 568-577.

Giacona, M. B. *et al.* (2004) Porphyromonas gingivalis induces its uptake by human macrophages and promotes foam cell formation in vitro. *FEMS Microbiology Letter*, 241, pp. 95-101.

Gould, F. K. *et al.* (2006) Guidelines for the prevention of endocarditis: report of the Working Party of the British Society for Antimicrobial Chemotherapy. *Journal of Antimicrobial Chemotherapy*, 57, pp. 1035-1042.

Grossi, S. G. and Genco, R. J. (1998) Periodontal disease and diabetes mellitus: a two-way relationship. *Annals of Periodontology*, 3, pp. 51-61.

Grossi, S. G. (2001) Treatment of periodontal disease and control of diabetes: an assessment of the evidence and need for future research. *Annals of Periodontology*, 6, pp. 138-145.

Hammond, B. F. (1992) Major bacterial diseases. In: Slots, J. and Taubman, M. A. (eds) *Contemporary Oral Microbiology and Immunology*. St. Louis: Mosby, pp. 165-190.

Hara, Y. *et al.* (1996) Serum rheumatoid factor induced by intraperitoneal administration of periodontopathic bacterial lipopolysaccharide in mice. *Journal of Periodontal Research*, 31, pp. 502-507.

Heckmann, J. G. *et al.* (2003) Multiple brain abscesses caused by Fusobacterium nucleatum treated conservatively. *Canadian Journal of Neurological Sciences*, 30, pp. 266-268.

Henderson, B. and Wilson, M. (1998) Commensal communism and the oral cavity. *Journal of Dental Research*, 77, pp. 1674-1683.

Herzberg, M. C. *et al.* (1994) The platelet as an inflammatory cell in periodontal disease: interactions with Porphyromonas gingivalis. In: Genco, R. *et al.* (eds) *Molecular Pathogenesis of Periodontal Disease*. Washington: American Society for Microbiology, pp. 247-255.

Herzberg, M. C. and Meyer, M. W. (1996) Effects of oral flora on platelets: possible consequences in cardiovascular disease. *Journal of Periodontology*, 67, pp. 1138-1142.

Honda, K. *et al.* (2001) High risk of Helicobacter pylori infection in young Japanese dentists. *Journal of Gastroenterology and Hepatology*, 16, pp. 862-865.

Hunter, W. (1911) An address on the role of sepsis and antisepsis in medicine. *Lancet*, 1, pp. 79-86.

Iida, Y. K. *et al.* (2004) Brain abscess in which Porphyromonas gingivalis was detected in cerebrospinal fluid. *British Journal of Oral and Maxillofacial Surgery*, 42, p. 180.

Jacobs, R. *et al.* (1996) Long-term bone mass evaluation of mandible and lumbar spine in a group of women receiving hormone replacement therapy. *Europian Journal of Oral Sciences*, 104, pp. 10-16.

Jiang, Y. *et al.* (2002) Bacteria induce osteoclastogenesis via an osteoblastindependent pathway. *Infection and Immunity*, 70, pp. 3143-3148.

Katz, J. *et al.* (2009) Localization of P.gingivalis in preterm delivery placenta. *Journal of Dental Research*, 88, pp. 575-578.

Kazanci, E. *et al.* (2005) Streptococcus oralis as a risk factor for middle cerebral artery thrombosis. *Journal of Child Neurology*, 20, pp. 611-613.

Kelein, D. K. *et al.* (1991) Water source as risk factor for Helicobacter pylori infection in Peruvian children. *Lancet*, 337, pp. 1503-1506.

Khandaker, M. A. *et al.* (1991) Do teeth predispose to duodenal ulcer relapse?. *Gut*, 32, p. A1207.

Khouzam, R. N. *et al.* (2006) Undiagnosed patent foramen ovale presenting as a cryptogenic brain abscess: case report and review of the literature. *Heart Lung*, 35, pp. 108-111.

Kilian, M. (1982) Systemic disease: manifestations of oral bacteria. In: Mcghee, J. R. *et al.* (eds) *Dental Microbiology*. Philadelphia: Harpers and Row, pp. 832-838.

Lee, A. *et al.* (1993) Pathogenecity of Helicobacter pylori: a perspec-tive. *Infection and Immunity*, 61, pp. 1601-1610.

Leon, R. *et al.* (2007) Detection of Porphyromonas gingivalis in the amniotic fluid in pregnant women with a diagnosis of threatened premature labor. *Journal of Periodontology*, 78, pp. 1249-1255.

Lerner, U. H. (2006) Inflammation-induced bone remodeling in periodontal disease and the influence of postmenopausal osteoporosis. *Journal of Dental Research*, 85, pp. 596-607.

Li, L. *et al.* (2002) Porphyromonas gingivalis infection accelerates the progression of atherosclerosis in a heterozygous apolipoprotein E-deficient murine model. *Circulation*, 105, pp. 861-867.

Li, X. *et al.* (2000) Systemic diseases caused by oral infection. *Clinical Microbiology Reviews*, 13, 547-558.

Liu, D. *et al.* (2003) Expression of RANKL and OPG mRnNA in periodontal disease. Possible involvement in bone destruction. *International Journal of Molecular Medicine*, 11, pp. 17-21.

Lorenz, K. A. and Weiss, P. J. (1994) Capnocytophagal pneumonia in a healthy man. *The Western Journal of Medicine*, 160, pp. 79-80.

Lourbakos, A. *et al.* (2001) Activation of protease-activated receptors by gingipains from Porphyromonas gingivalis leads to platelet aggregation: a new trait in microbial athogenicity. *Blood*, 12, pp. 3790-3797.

Mahanonda, R. *et al.* (2004) Monocyte activation by Porphyromonas gingivalis LPS in aggressive periodontitis with the use of whole-blood cultures. *Journal of Dental Research*, 83, 540-545.

Mai, U. *et al.* (1989) Route of infection in Campylobacter pylori (CP) disease. *Gastroenterology*, 96, p. 315.

Makiura, N. *et al.* (2008) Relationship of Porphyromonas gingivalis with glycemic level in patients with type 2 diabetes following periodontal treatment. *Oral Microbiology and Immunology*, 23, pp. 348-351.

Mapstone, N. P. *et al.* (1993) Identification of Helicobacter infection DNA in the mouths and stomach of patients with gastritis using PCR. *Journal of Clinical Pathology*, 46, pp. 540-543.

Mattana, C. M. *et al.* (1998) Isolation of Helicobacter pylori from dental plaque. *Revista Argentina de Microbiologica*, 30, pp. 93-95.

McGaw, T. (2002) Periodontal disease and preterm delivery of low birth-weight infants. *Journal of Canadian Dental Association*, 68, pp. 165-169.

Mercado, F. B. *et al.* (2003) Inter-relationships between rheumatoid arthritis and periodontal disease: A review. *Journal of Clinical Periodontology*, 30, pp. 761-772.

Mercado, F. B. *et al.* (2001) Relationship between rheumatoid arthritis and periodontitis. *Journal of Periodontology*, 72, pp. 779-787.

Michalowicz, B. S. *et al.* (2006) Treatment of periodontal disease and the risk of preterm birth. *The New England Journal of Medicine*, 355, pp. 1885-1894.

Miyabayashi, H. *et al.* (2000) Influence of oral Helicobacter pylori on the success of eradication therapy against gastric Helicobacter pylori. *Helicobacter*, 5, pp. 30-37.

Moen, K. *et al.* (2006) Synovial inflammation in active rheumatoid arthritis and psoriatic arthritis facilitates trapping of a variety of oral bacterial DNAs. *Clinical and Experimental Rheumatology*, 24, pp. 656-663.

Moreu, G. *et al.* (2005) Relationship between maternal periodontal disease and low-birth-weight pre-term infants. *Journal of Clinical Periodontology*, 32, pp. 622-627.

Morris, J. F. and Sewell, D. L. (1994) Necrotizing pneumonia caused by mixed infection with Actinobacillus actinomycetemcomitans and Actinomyces israelii: case report and review. *Clinical Infectious Diseases*, 18, pp. 450-452.

Nanci, A. and Bosshardt, D. D. (2000) Structure of periodontal tissues in health and disease. *Periodontology*, 40, pp. 11-28.

Nelson, R. G. *et al.* (1990) Periodontal disease and NIDDM in Pima Indians. *Diabetes Care*, 13, pp. 836-840.

Offenbacher, S. *et al.* (1996a) Periodontal infection as a possible risk factor for preterm low birth weight. *Journal of Periodontology*, 67[10 Suupl], pp. 1103-1113. Offenbacher, S. (1996b) Periodontal diseases: pathogenesis. *Annals of Periodontology*, 1, pp. 821-878.

Offenbacher, S. *et al.* (1998a) Potential pathogenic mechanisms of periodontitis associated pregnancy complications. *Annals of Periodontology*, 3, pp. 233-250. Offenbacher, S. *et al.* (1998b) Role of periodontitis in systemic health: spontaneous preterm birth. *Journal of Dental Education*, 62, pp. 852-858.

Offenbacher, S. *et al.* (2001) Maternal periodontitis and prematurity. Part I: obstetric outcome of prematurity and growth restriction. *Annals of Periodontology*, 6, pp. 164-174.

Olsson, K. *et al.* (1993) H. pylori in dental plaques (letter). *Lancet*, 341, pp. 956-957.

Oshowo, A. *et al.* (1998) Oral colonization is unlikely to play an important role in Helicobacter pylori infection. *British Journal of Surgery*, 85, pp. 850-852.

Paster, B. J. *et al.* (2001) Bacterial diversity in human subgingival plaque. *Journal of Bacteriology*, 183, pp. 3770-3783.

Pesonen, E. E. *et al.* (1981) Endothelial cell damage in piglet coronary artery after intravenous administration of E. coli endotoxin: a scanning and transmission electron-microscopic study. *Atherosclerosis*, 40, pp. 65-73.

Potempa, J. *et al.* (1997) Titration and mapping of the active site of cysteine proteinases from Porphyromonas gingivalis (gingipains) using peptidyl chloromethanes. *Biological Chemistry*, 378, pp. 223-230.

Pussinen, P. J. *et al.* (2003) Antibodies to periodontal pathogens are associated with coronary heart disease. *Arteriosclerosis, Thrombosis and Vascular Biology*, 23, pp. 1250-1254.

Ramamurthy, N. S. *et al.* (2005) Experimental arthritis in rats induces biomarkers of periodontitis which are ameliorated by gene therapy with tissue inhibitor of matrix metalloproteinases. *Journal of Periodontology*, 76, pp. 229-233.

Riberio, J. *et al.* (2005) Periodontal infection as a possible severity factor for rheumatoid arthritis. *Journal of Clinical Periodontology*, 32, pp. 412-416.

Richey, R. D. *et al.* (2008) Prophylaxis against infective endocarditis: summary of NICE guidance. *British Medical Journal*, 336, pp. 770-771.

Ridker, P. M. *et al.* (1997) Inflammation, aspirin, and the risk of cardiovascular disease in apparently healthy men. *The New England Journal of Medicine*, 336, pp. 973-979.

Samaranayake, L. P. (2006) *Essential Microbiology for Dentistry, 3rd Edition*. Philadelphia: Elsevier, pp. 275-285.

Saremi, A. *et al.* (2005) Periodontal disease and mortality in type 2 diabetes. *Diabetes Care*, 28, pp. 27-32.

Savoldi, E. *et al.* (1998) Absence of Helicobacter pylori in dental plaque determined by im-munoperoxidase. *Helicobacter*, 3, pp. 283-287.

Scannapieco, F. A. and Mylotte, J. M. (1996) Relationships between periodontal disease and bacterial pneumonia. *Journal of Periodontology*, 67, pp. 1114-1122.

Scannapieco, F. A. (1998) Position paper: periodontal disease as a potential risk factor for systemic diseases. *Journal of Periodontology*, 69, pp. 841-850.

Scannapieco, F. A. (1999) Role of oral bacteria in respiratory infection. *Journal of Periodontology*; 70, pp. 793-802.

Scannapieco, F. A. *et al.* (2001) Oral bacteria and respiratory infection: effects on respiratory pathogen adhesion and epithelial cell proinflammatory cytokine production. *Annals of Periodontology*, 6, pp. 78-86.

Seinost, G. *et al.* (2005) Periodontal treatment improves endothelial dysfunction in patients with severe periodontitis. *American Heart Journal*, 149, pp. 1050-1054.

Shlossman, M. *et al.* (1990) Type 2 diabetes mellitus and periodontal disease. *Journal of American Dental Association*, 121, pp. 532-536.

Shultis, W. A. *et al.* (2007) Effect of periodontitis on overt nephropathy and end-stage renal disease in type 2 diabetes. *Diabetes Care*, 30, pp. 306-311.

Sivapathasundharam, B. (2006) Spread of oral infection. In: Rajendran, R. and Sivapathasundharam, B. (eds) *Textbook of Oral Pathology, 5th Edition*. Elsevier, p. 709.

Slade, G. D. *et al.* (2003) Relationship between periodontal disease and C-reactive protein among adults in the Atherosclerosis Risk in Communities study. *Archives of Internal Medicine*, 163, pp. 1172-1179.

Song, Q. *et al.* (2000) Characteristic distribution pattern of Helicobacter pylori in dental plaque and saliva detected with nested PCR. *Journal of Medical Microbiology*, 49, pp. 349-353.

Takahashi, K. *et al.* (1995) Clinical and laboratory studies on a patient with early onset periodontitis and her family members: a case report. *Journal of Periodontology*, 66, pp. 403-412.

Taubman, M. A. and Kawai, T. (2001) Involvement of T-lymphocytes in periodontal disease and in direct and indirect induction of bone resoprtion. *Critical Reviews in Oral Biology and Medicine*, 12, pp. 125-35.

Taylor, D. N. and Blaser, M. J. (1991) The epidemiology of Helicobacter pylori infection. *Epidemiological Reviews*, 13, pp. 42-59.

Taylor, G. W. *et al.* (1996) Severe periodontitis and risk for poor glycemic control in patients with non-insulin- dependent diabetes mellitus. *Journal of Periodontology*, 67, pp. 1085-1093.

Taylor, G. W. (2001) Bidirectional interrelationships between diabetes and periodontal diseases: an epidemiologic perspective. *Annals of Periodontology*, 6, pp. 99-112.

Tezal, M. *et al.* (2000) The relationship between bone mineral density and periodontitis in postmenopausal women. *Journal of Periodontology*, 71, pp. 1492-1498.

The Diabetes Control and Complications Trial Research Group (1993) The effect of intensive treatment of diabetes on the development and progression of long term complications in insulin-dependent diabetes mellitus. *The New England Journal of Medicine*, 329, pp. 977-986.

Thoden van Velzen, S.K. *et al.*(1984) Plaque and systemic disease: a reappraisal of the focal infection concept. *Journal of Clinical Periodontology*, 11, pp. 209-220.

Thomas, J. E. *et al.* (1992) Isolation of Helicobacter pylori from human faeces. *Lancet*, 340, pp. 1194-1195.

Tompkin, D. S. *et al.* (1989) Campylobacter pylori in gastric juice. In: Megaraud, F. and Lamouliatte, H. (eds) *Gastroduodenal pathology and Campylobacter Pylori*. Amsterdam: Elsevier Science, pp. 24-28.

Wang, C. H. *et al.* (2003) C-reactive protein upregulates angiotensin type 1 receptors in vascular smooth muscle. *Circulation*, 107, pp. 1783-1790.

Wild, S. *et al.* (2007) Global prevalence of diabetes. Estimates for the year 2000 and projections for 2030. *Diabetes Care*, 27, pp. 1047-1053.

Wotherspoon, A. C. *et al.* (1991) Helicobacter pylori-associated gastritis and primary B-cell gastric lymphoma. *Lancet*, 338, pp. 1175-1176.

In: Hypotheses in Clinical Medicine
Editors: M.M. Shoja, P.S. Agutter et al.

ISBN: 978-1-62257-276-2

Chapter 25

Stress and the Flaws of the Stress Response: The Good, the Bad and the Ugly in the Evolution of the Stress Response

Deepak Kumar Singh[1,*] and Lekha Tuli[2]
[1]Department of General Surgery, Institute of Medical Sciences, Banaras Hindu University, Varanasi, Uttar Pradesh, India
[2]Department of Microbiology, Mahamaya Rajkiya Allopathic Medical College, Ambedkarnagar (Akbarpur), Uttar Pradesh, India

Abstract

In this chapter, the general aspects of stress and its effect on the body are discussed. A hypothesis is then discussed emphasizing that the physiological response to stress has been a subject of neglect in the evolutionary path, and is restricted by several flaws including the lack of specificity to the stressor, and the lack of an internal system to estimate stress levels, which would be a prerequisite for proper adaptation.

Introduction

Stress is a very commonly used term, both in scientific and vernacular language. It ranges from stress at a cellular level due to an adverse external environment, to a psychological level where it can be the cause of anxiety or depression. In biology, stress is any stimulus that causes an alteration in the peace of body, mind and psyche. Stress is a subjective phenomenon, at times confusing and too wide-ranging to be explained by a single definition. Hans Selye coined the term 'stress' in 1936. He observed that when rats are subjected to

* E-mail: deepakbhu@gmail.com.

stress they show some pathological changes similar to those found in humans, such as stomach ulcerations and adrenal enlargement. He can be proclaimed as the 'father of stress' for his serendipitous but keen observations. He also demonstrated the development of various diseases (similar to heart disease, stroke, kidney disease and rheumatoid arthritis in humans) in animals under persistent stress. He later described the '*General Adaptation Syndrome (GAS)*'. In 1975, he extended his model of stress and divided it into *Eustress* and *Distress* (Selye 1975). He coined a new word, *stressor*, for the stimulus or the cause of stress. However, the term 'stress' was later synonymously used with 'distress', and the word 'eustress' sank into obscurity (in this chapter the word stress is synonymously used for distress). Selye struggled to find a definition for stress, and the term became too common, too diverse, and too frequently used, to be restrained into a phrase or to apprehend through a single definition, and it remains so even today. One author even asserted: "stress, in addition to being itself, was also the cause of itself and the result of itself" (Roberts 1950).

The neurologist Walter Cannon described stressors as either physical or emotional. He demonstrated the "fight or flight" response and deciphered the role of the adrenal medulla in the release of the neurotransmitters (epinephrine and norepinephrine), which cause this response. The brief history of stress portrays it as a controversial subject. This can be attributed to the vastness of the subject and the deep ramifications in the etiology of various diseases, so much so that it can be linked to majority of diseases.

"General Adaptation Syndrome" Model

Selye introduced the GAS model to predict the stress response of an organism. It has three stages. The first stage is the '*alarm*', which is triggered after a stressor is recognized and the recognition is followed by an imminent response. It is the stage of hypothalamic-pituitary-adrenal (HPA) axis activation and the 'fight or flight' response. This is followed by the '*resistance*' stage in cases where the stressor persists. Here, the body tries to resist the damage from the stressor, but it is unable to continue this indefinitely. Finally, in the last stage of '*exhaustion*', the body is unable to carry on its normal functions and there is depletion of its resources. Extended '*exhaustion*' may result in decompensation and lasting damage to the body.

The 'Physical' Origin of the Stress Response

If the origin of the stress response is due to exposure to a predator, protection from the predator requires a prompt response to flee away to a safe shelter. This process includes early recognition of danger and an adequate 'fight or flight' response. In our ancestors, this need led to the evolution of the stress response in the form of the HPA axis, epinephrine secretion and activation of the sympathetic nervous system, which manifested as the 'fight or flight' response. Numerous changes take place during the 'fight or flight' response. The pupils are dilated to facilitate distance vision for early recognition of an approaching predator. Glucose levels in the body are increased, gluconeogenesis begins, and the vascular supply is concentrated to heart, brain and muscles as opposed to low perfusion in the gastroenteric and reproductive systems (concomitant with the inhibition of feeding and reproductive behaviors).

The rise in heart rate and blood pressure increases tissue perfusion and glucose delivery. Piloerection due to sympathetic activation is used to intimidate predators or competitors as it causes a virtual increase in body size. This is accompanied by a behavioral response leading to a state of alertness, heightened awareness and reduced pain perception.

Dynamics of the Stress Response

The hormonal axis associated with stress is well-understood. However, the neural circuitry and interaction between the different components of this circuit remain elusive. Monitoring of individual neurons in the prefrontal region showed the firing of neurons within 0.12 seconds of seeing an aversive image (Rossi *et al.* 2001). This clearly delineates the spontaneity of the stress response and the minimal time lag between the stressor and the stress response. All the biological components of the stress response are enumerated below.

Global Alarm System (Locus Ceruleus-Norepinephrine (LC/NE) System)

The locus ceruleus (LC) and certain noradrenergic cell groups are together known as the LC/NE system, which serves as a global alarm system (Tsigos and Chrousos 2002). Epinephrine secretion from the brain after activation of the LC/NE system initiates the various neuroendocrine and autonomic responses. A multitude of inputs are received by the LC from the prefrontal cortex, amygdala, medulla and paraventricular nucleus, and outputs are forwarded to the cortex, brainstem, limbic system (which performs memory review and emotional analysis of the situation) and spinal cord. Activation of the LC increases alertness or vigilance, and modulates the action of the autonomic nervous system.

The Hypothalamic-pituitary-adrenal Axis

The hypothalamic-pituitary-adrenal axis is responsible for the maintenance of metabolic homeostasis and the mediation of the neuroendocrine response to stress. It consists primarily of the corticotropin releasing hormone (CRH), adrenocorticotropic hormone (ACTH) and the adrenocortical steroids; CRH is released from the paraventricular nucleus (PVN) of the hypothalamus and stimulates the synthesis and secretion of ACTH. The paraventricular nucleus is activated by the amygdala and lateral thalamus. The hippocampus (source of painful memories), locus ceruleus, prefrontal cortex and brain stem are other sources of inputs to the PVN. ACTH, in turn, stimulates steroidogenesis in the adrenal cortex and results in the production and release of cortisol (a glucocorticoid).

Release of ACTH has a circadian rhythm, with a peak early in the morning and a nadir at midnight. As a result, cortisol secretion also peaks in the morning and falls at midnight, simulating the circadian rhythm of ACTH. Normally, this axis is under negative feedback control by cortisol through suppression of CRH secretion and direct inhibition of ACTH release. It also decreases the expression of the gene responsible for the synthesis of ACTH. Such a negative feedback loop keeps a check on the blood levels of cortisol. However, this axis is activated in cases of stress, through external (toxins) or internal (cytokines or neural) signals. Finally, it leads to untoward secretion of cortisol. The peculiarity of cortisol release in a stressful situation is that it is unable to result in a negative feedback on the HPA axis. The reason behind this phenomenon is, in some cases, the release of cytokines inducing a state of central glucocorticoid receptor resistance. In cases of severe depression, there is an elevation of plasma cortisol with deranged diurnal variation in its secretion.

Cortisol: A Multi-systemic Hormone

Cortisol release is immediate, and it produces responses within minutes of stress. The stress can be physiological (fever and hypoglycemia), psychological (anxiety, panic attack or depression), physical (exercise, trauma) or psychosocial (performance anxiety). Cortisol is responsible for the majority of changes occurring in the body, both in acute and chronic stress, to the extent that it can be referred to as the stress hormone. It not only mediates changes directly, but also brings into play other hormones. Its effects include regulation of carbohydrate, lipid, protein and even nucleic acid metabolism.

The primary action of cortisol, the principal glucocorticoid, is the regulation of glucose metabolism. It raises the blood glucose level by inhibiting peripheral glucose uptake and promoting gluconeogenesis (hepatic glucose synthesis from amino acids, etc.). This helps the body to cope with the acute crisis (especially hypoglycemia). Fat metabolism is also affected by cortisol, resulting in a peculiar fat distribution pattern. The central areas of the body accumulate fat while the extremities and peripheral tissues are drained of it. This may lead to weight gain and central obesity, which could be the harbinger of diabetes mellitus in predisposed individuals, and other health problems (Park 2009). Cortisol is mostly a catabolic hormone. It enhances protein breakdown and excretion of nitrogen. It reduces amino acid uptake and inhibits protein synthesis. The protein breakdown is facilitated in areas such as bone, muscle, skin and other connective tissues. The amino acids (glycogenic amino acids) released are used in the process of gluconeogenesis. In layman's terms, the body is fed upon by cortisol to generate glucose for the vital organs of the body during a stressful situation. The metabolic changes may lead to muscle weakness and easy fatigability, accompanied by osteoporosis (predisposing to fractures), and these changes are profound in the case of Cushing's syndrome or following prolonged use of exogenous glucocorticoids.

Several hormonal systems are altered by the action of cortisol. Cortisol decreases the secretion, and even antagonizes the action, of insulin, leading to impaired glucose tolerance and increased insulin resistance. Glucagon secretion is also stimulated by rising blood amino acid levels. Secretion of ACTH, β-lipotropin and β-endorphin from the pituitary gland, and CRH from the hypothalamus, are also decreased by cortisol, and it suppresses the secretion of vasopressin (which in turn promotes increased loss of water from the kidneys) and has a weak mineralocorticoid-like action of its own. Cortisol makes the retrieval of long-term memories difficult, dampens the thinking process, and impairs temporary retrieval of memory (Dominique *et al.* 1998). Psychological changes such as irritability, personality changes, confusion, depression, emotional lability and psychosis may also be seen. Skin is adversely affected by cortisol, with atrophy, friability and bruisability due to the loss of collagen fibers in the dermis. These adverse effects are seen only after a chronic rise in blood cortisol levels.

The immuno-modulatory properties of cortisol are well known, and have many therapeutic applications. Glucocorticoids are used as an immunosuppressant and in chemotherapeutic regimens. Cortisol has anti-inflammatory properties, decreases capillary permeability during inflammation, and facilitates vasoconstriction by circulating vaso-constrictors. It causes leukocytosis (an increase in the number of leukocytes in the blood) by releasing more leukocytes from the bone marrow and preventing their exit through the vessel wall. However, it decreases the number of circulating T cells by redistributing them and even decreasing their production (causing impairment of cell-mediated immunity). Its anti-inflammatory properties are also attributed to the inhibition of prostaglandin, leukotriene and interferon synthesis (inhibition of the latter is responsible for the antipyretic action) and a reduction in antibody production.

Most of the above mentioned effects are not found in an acute condition, and are evident only after continuous secretion (due to stress or any other pathological state) or chronic corticosteroid intake. After expounding all the effects of raised cortisol levels, we can conclude that not all its effects are necessary or useful, and are beneficial only in the short term, during the stage of acute stress. If high cortisol levels remain chronic and persistent, they have adverse health outcomes, not only of a physical but also of a psychological nature. Therefore, avoidance of chronic stress is the only way to prevent the complications brought about by this vital but dangerous hormone. Nonetheless, the principal role of this hormone in human metabolism is obvious from the very fact that, in cases of multi-hormone deficiencies, glucocorticoids are the first hormone to be administered to the patient.

Extrahypothalamic CRH Systems

Many regions in the brain apart from the hypothalamic PVN contain CRH-producing cells and influence the LC. For example, the CRH terminals from the brain activate the LC and increase its firing. There is a co nstant overlap between the different parts of the CRH system in the brain.

Autonomic Nervous System and 'Fight or Flight' Response

As discussed earlier, activation of the sympathetic nervous system and release of neurotransmitters (epinephrine and norepinephrine) constitute the immediate response to stress, or the basis of the 'fight or flight' response. The activation of the sympathetic nervous system is initiated primarily through LC firing, and is associated with the withdrawal of the parasympathetic nervous system. Ultimately, these alterations bring about various cardiovascular, respiratory, renal, gastrointestinal and hormonal changes in the body.

We Create Our Own Stress

"Stress is actually a shift in the homeostasis of the body and a trigger or change (real or imaginary) that forces the organism to respond in a manner different from its routine". As a result, both marriage and divorce will be categorized as stressful events. The categorization of stress is based on different parameters, on duration, origin, or even the type of stressor. We will not delve much into the etiology of stress, as it is not the topic of interest here. Generally, stress may present as an acute, episodic incidence such as marriage, entry into a new college, first sexual encounter, loss of a loved one, dealing with a project at work, getting stuck in a traffic jam, having an asthma attack, or any acute inflammatory disease. In the most deleterious and protracted cases, chronic stress ensues. Presumably, chronic stress sensitizes the stress response system, making it more responsive to the subsequent stresses.

Adverse Effects of Stress on Health

Stress upsets the dynamic equilibrium, or homeostasis, of the body. The effects of stress are innumerable. Some surveys show that stress-related complaints account for the majority (70-90%) of patient visits to primary care physicians. Given the varied symptoms, signs, manifestations and diseases caused by stress, the list is endless and ever expanding. However, a recollection of all the symptoms is necessary to prove its impact on clinical medicine. These symptoms have been segregated into different groups showing the permeating impact of stress on all the specialties of clinical medicine and every aspect of human life.

General or non-specific manifestations of stress include an array of symptoms: frequent headaches, jaw clenching, pain, blushing, sweating, cold or sweaty hands and feet, rashes, itching, hives, piloerection, fever, increased or decreased appetite, weight gain or loss, improper dietary intake, and obesity. Frequent and unexplained 'allergy' symptoms exaggerate under stress. Faintness, light headedness, dizziness, ringing, buzzing sounds, confusion, constant tiredness, weakness and fatigue are other symptoms which not only trouble us, but pose difficulty in diagnosing an underlying pathology. Chest pain and palpitations are symptoms indicating involvement of the cardiovascular system (American Psychological Association 2010, n.d.). Direct biochemical injury to heart muscle has been implicated in "cardiac muscle necroses", experimentally reproduced by Selye (Selye 1958). Stress can also lead to coronary occlusion and accelerated atherosclerosis, and stress-induced coronary vasospasm has a role in the presentation of clinical symptoms (Gersch *et al.* 1981). Accruing evidence for the causes of hypertension, heart attack, or even sudden death, following acute and severe emotional stress is very conspicuous (Rosch 1994a, 1994b). Increased secretion of neuropeptide Y in stressed mice led to proliferation and angiogenesis in fat cells, resulting in abdominal obesity and a metabolic syndrome-like condition (Kuo *et al.* 2007). A direct relationship between job stress and cardiovascular diseases has been well-demonstrated (Karasek and Theorell 1990). Many trials provide compelling evidence in favor of an increased sympathetic drive and catecholamine secretion related to stress. Reduction in mortality after administration of propanolol led to premature cessation of the trial to avoid delay in extending the benefits to other patients (Beta-Blocker Heart Attack Study Group 1981, 1982). The same scenario was encountered with the stress reduction techniques employed for Type A behavior (Thoresen *et al.* 1982; Friedman *et al.* 1982).

Stress As a Cause of Cancer?

Stress as a cause of neoplastic growth can be an indigestible assumption for many. Paul Rosch (1997) has elaborated numerous ideas and facts on the matter. We will shed light only on some favorite arguments:

- *Overreaction to a trigger or stimulus*: Development of keloid causing disfigurement is due to the overreaction of the normal process of wound healing. Secondly, development of lip cancer occurs in response to constant irritation and healing attempts in a smoker. Rosch (1997) refers to this as the theory of opportunism, which explains that an organism responds to fill a need in whatever way it can, even if the response is detrimental or worthless.
- *A dying response*: The neoplastic growth can be a remnant of the regenerative potential found in lower animals like starfish, earthworms or salamanders. During experiments certain carcinogens, when injected into the limb of a salamander, caused the growth of an accessory limb (Tsonis and Eguchi 1982). This further strengthens this hypothesis.
- *Deranged immunity*: Trial of a 6-week stress management intervention carried out on a group of early stage melanoma patients reduced the rate of recurrence and deaths by 50% (Fawzy *et al.* 1990). It enhanced the immunity status of the study group as compared to the controls. Stress can influence cancers with an immunological component, and may even play an etiological role.
- *Infective carcinogens*: Infections caused by the human papilloma virus (HPV), Epstein-Bar virus (EBV), *Helicobacter pylori*, human immunodeficiency virus (HIV), and hepatitis B and hepatitis C viruses may complicate and cause cancer. Stress may expedite this process through vulnerability to some of these infections and decreased immunity.

A rising incidence of breast cancer in middle-aged females in cities, as compared to homemakers from native places, may be attributed to increased stress levels. The possibility of hormonal derangements caused by stress cannot be ruled out in the causation of breast cancer. It is worth assuming that there are certain forms of cancer that may be aggravated or complicated due to stress.

Dual Damage by Stressor and Stress Response

In the above sections we have learned about the diseases caused by stress and the problems we encounter when the body mounts a stress response. As a result, both stress and the stress response can be detrimental to human health. Stress causes direct injury to the body and overzealous stress responses can cause physiological and metabolic derangements.

Assessment of Stress

Several tests have been introduced to measure stress levels. The Holmes and Rahe stress test was one of the initial attempts at measuring stress (Holmes and Rahe 1967). It only gives a rough estimate. The Trier social stress test, on the other hand, involves the induction of stress under laboratory conditions (Kirschbaum *et al.* 1993). While the stress tests determine the number of stressors and the level of stress an individual has, the burnout tests, in contrast, determine his or her ability to cope with the stress (Truby 2009). Certain tests, such as the measurement of salivary cortisol or alpha amylase, could help in assessing the burden of stress as well. Human salivary alpha amylase has been shown to have a positive correlation with the sympathetic activity during stress, and thus can be useful as a tool for measuring stress levels (Nater *et al.* 2006). The Corocometer is a recently introduced handheld device for measuring salivary amylase (Shankar and Dandekar 2009).

Evolution

Evolution is a mystical process if its understanding is merely based on the results we see and observe objectively. In spite of being an invisible phenomenon, it is at the helm of development and improvisation for all life forms. Life forms evolve for good reasons; to survive, to reproduce and to flourish. The intent of evolution is the improvement of existing life forms. Taking animals as an example, warm-blooded animals have evolved from cold-blooded animals. The former are better suited for survival than the latter because they can maintain their body temperature invariably and independently of the external environment. This is an ideal representation of 'intent to improve', the underlying principle of evolution.

In the path of evolution, individual preferences are often selected at the expense of whole species. Compromises and tradeoffs are occasionally made for a greater good. For example, the immune response protects us from pathogens, but an over-responsive immune response is responsible for causing tissue and organ injury. However, it is a price the body pays to prevent invasion by dreadful infectious agents. A similar impact of evolution on the development of the stress response will be discussed in the following sections.

The lack of retrospection and foresight represents flaws in evolution. Evolution is a one-way path and there is no possibility of retracing the steps and altering what has already been selected. The most important impact of this property is that any variation, once selected, cannot be suddenly dropped in the future. That would also require a long-duration evolutionary process. Evolution only affects life forms and has no means to predict the future of the external environment. It cannot predict that an ice age will arrive or a meteor will strike. As a result, it cannot equip or evolve organisms against any unforeseen future disasters. These incidences are the turning points in evolutionary biology as the evolutionary process inadvertently continues with what is left of 'life'.

Evolution has a very slow pace and even if it is due to genetic drift or shift, it takes time before a change is actually observed. The most serious consequence is that once a change is accepted, it requires a long period to root it out of the system or modify it after it becomes redundant or futile. An example is piloerection in humans due to activation of the sympathetic system in response to stress. This manifestation is seemingly redundant in humans, but might have helped earlier species.

In a nutshell, evolution is a very slow and steady phenomenon, which fathoms all aspects of life. It has played a very important role in carving and shaping life as we know it today. It permeates all characteristics of any population and involves every attribute/quality/property to enhance the survival and propagation of a given population. Every species has the prime goal of survival in the face of changing external and internal influences. As a result, every improvement through evolution depends solely on the vitality of the attribute for maintenance of the species, which funnels down to the enhancement of reproductive efficiency, and is observed in the form of increased numbers of offspring or longer life spans.

To sum up bluntly, every species in due course acquires the genetic variations that enable it to outnumber other species.

The Hypothesis

Evolutionary Neglect of Stress Response

It is postulated that, in the process of evolution, stress coping abilities fail to achieve a higher preference, probably because of the minimal role they play in the propagation of a given population. Neglecting this property may have minimal effects on a population, but it is of great significance when an individual organism's health and survival is at stake. To conclude, stress coping abilities or the stress response have not had a significant effect on the direction of human evolution. The inadequateness of the stress response can be judged by the fact that it comprises few physiological components; the stimulation of the HPA axis and sympathetic system is the predominant response to stress, be it physical or psychological. It is supplemented by local mediators, which add minor improvements to stress-coping abilities.

We have already hypothesized that the stress response is, in fact, a subject of neglect during the process of evolution. Now, we turn our focus to the pace of its evolutionary development. It has been so slow that humans have inevitably stuck to a common pathway (e.g., the HPA axis) to ward off every type of stress they encounter. There are no varied metabolic changes specific for different variants of stress, and it clearly unveils the infantile status of the stress responses as compared to other evolutionary developments. 'The response that was once a coveted need fails to serve much purpose presently.'

Internal Flaws of Stress Response

The rise in cortisol level in response to stress, is not a graded response that matchs the level of stress inflicted upon an individual, but instead manifests more like an "on and off" switch. There is no demarcation as to when, and to what degree, this switch is turned on or off. The response itself is nonspecific. For example, in a hypoglycemic state, the body needs to increase its blood glucose level and glucose utilization. Hormones such as adrenaline, growth hormone, thyroxin and cortisol not only help to increase blood glucose levels, heart rate and tissue perfusion, but also induce a myriad range of changes in the metabolic state that are seldom necessary. Likewise, we can state innumerable examples delineating the non-specific and wasteful processes in a stress response. This phenomenon could be described as a "blunderbuss response". This display of priming the whole body against both a real threat and a trivial and innocuous stressor is not cost-effective. Furthermore, the actual demarcation between the acute and chronic stress responses is obscure, hardly being distinguished by the predominant cortisol release in the chronic stage as opposed to a concomitant adrenaline upsurge in the acute stage.

Biological systems use two types of feedback mechanism to achieve homeostasis, i.e. positive and negative feedbacks. A perfect example of positive feedback is the luteinizing hormone (LH) upsurge at the time of ovulation; this triggers further LH secretion that finally culminates in ovulation. On the other hand, negative feedback is exemplified by the interplay of thyroxin and thyroxin-stimulating hormone (TSH); TSH stimulates the release of thyroxin, and in turn a rise in thyroxin level decreases the release of TSH. Reduced TSH release decreases any further increase in thyroxin secretion. Thus, thyroxin self-controls its blood levels through a negative feedback. The HPA axis is under negative feedback control by cortisol under normal, physiological conditions. In certain stressful situations, the feedback control of glucocorticoids is lost (as mentioned earlier). Cortisol injures the hippocampus, hindering its inhibition of the hypothalamus and cortisol secretion (Khalsa and Stauth 1999). The resulting uninhibited rise in cortisol levels causes further damage to the hippocampus and a vicious cycle is established.

Inadequateness of the Stress Response and the Concept of a 'Stress Meter'

The stress in our daily lives has increased tremendously, and every new generation is bound to face more complexities in life. Although the physical stress has minimized, the psychological and environmental stresses show an upward trend over time. However, the pace of development of stress-coping abilities has been slow. A core issue presented as a real problem here is that the human body cannot measure the amount of stress. It can only have a subjective assessment and vague idea about the level of stress it is facing, and it lacks any mechanism or 'stress meter' to quantify it. Thus, further adaptation of the system for varying and elevating degrees of stress is subject to the bias of individualized perception because of the lack of an internal 'stress meter'.

Does Avoiding Stress Benefit Health? The Concept of Eustress

The next topic of interest would be whether avoiding stress could increase life spans. This assumption may seem reasonable, but is not promising as indicated by the report of the Longevity project and the concept of Eustress. The longevity report is the result of a study that spanned approximately 90 years. The late psychologist Louis Terman and subsequent researchers studied 1,500 children who were just 10 years old when they were first studied in 1921. Friedman and Martin (2011), who led the study for 20 years from 1991, prepared the final report. Surprisingly, the results showed that those who did not work hard or stress themselves were not the ones who lived the longest. On the contrary, the individuals committed to their jobs, who worked hard, lived the longest. Pessimistic people survived longer than optimistic individuals. Ignorance of real threat and stressors could thus have adverse effects on health and survival. Therefore, optimism may not be good medicine after all.

At the end, the beneficial effects of stress should be mentioned. The concept of eustress is as old as the concept of stress. Its existence is very plausible. Eustress is that level of stress which optimizes the functioning of one's body and mind, and even helps to improve performance. An example to illustrate this is the performance anxiety before a presentation, which makes one more aware of the surroundings and potentially improves the performance (Bosch *et al.* 2001). Instead, the performance anxiety may worsen and turn into a stressful condition if it runs out of the control; generalized anxiety and panic attacks are some of its consequences.

We conclude from the longevity report that a certain amount of stress is indeed required for a long and healthy life. It provides a concrete background for the existence of eustress. Of the several underlying metabolic and hormonal changes proposed to substantiate the biological basis of eustress, only a few of them are promising. A transient increase in the levels of hormones such as oxytocin and norepinephrine may be relevant. Oxytocin makes people less anxious and more social. Norepinephrine is an excitatory neurotransmitter and is responsible for the elevation of mood and the formation of new memories. It encourages creative thinking and helps to form new connections in the brain. Exercise can be considered an ideal example of eustress; an exercising body is subjected to physical and mental stress, which proves rewarding both temporarily and permanently. The release of endorphins during exercise mediates a variety of actions in the body such as analgesia, euphoria, etc.

Conclusion

One may conclude the relevance of a certain amount of stress as a necessity for a healthy long life. However, the human is unable to calibrate that amount, and very often overstressing ensues. The core hypothesis discussed in this chapter suggests that the stress response has been a subject of neglect in the evolutionary path, and is restricted by several flaws including the lack of an internal "stress meter" for proper adaptation and the lack of specificity and graded response to stress.

References

American Psychological Association (2010) *Stress in America Findings*. [www] Official Website of the American Psychological Association. Available from: http://www.apa.org/news/press/releases/stress [Accessed 14/1/2012].

American Psychological Association (n.d.) *Stress* [www] Official Website of the American Psychological Association. Available from: http://www. apa.org/topics/stress/index.aspx [Accessed 28/6/2011].

Beta-Blocker Heart Attack Study Group (1981) Beta-blocker heart attack trial. *Journal of American Medical Association*, 246, pp. 2073-2074.

Beta-Blocker Heart Attack Study Group (1982) Beta-blocker heart attack trial, *Journal of American Medical Association*, 247, pp. 1701-1714.

Bosch, J. A. *et al.* (2001) Differential effects of active versus passive coping on secretory immunity. *Nieuw Amerongen*, 38, pp. 836-846.

Dominique, J. *et al.* (1998) Stress and glucocorticoids impair retrieval of long-term spatial memory. *Nature*, 394, pp. 787-790.

Fawzy, F. I. *et al.* (1990) A structured psychiatric intervention for cancer patients. I. Changes over time in methods of coping and affective disturbance. *Archives of General Psychiatry*, 47, pp. 720-725.

Friedman, H. S. and Martin, L. R. (2011) *The Longevity Project: Surprising Discoveries for Health and Long Life from the Landmark Eight-Decade Study*. New York: Hudson Street Press.

Friedman, M. *et al.* (1982) Feasibility of altering type A behavior pattern after myocardial infarction. Recurrent Coronary Prevention Project Study: methods, baseline results and preliminary findings. *Circulation*, 66, pp. 83-92.

Holmes, T. H. and Rahe, R. H. (1967) The Social Readjustment Rating Scale. *Journal of Psychosomatic Response*, 11, pp. 213-218.

Karasek, R. A. and Theorell, T. (1990) *Healthy Work: Stress, Productivity, and the Reconstruction of Working Life*. New York: Basic Books.

Khalsa, D. S. and Stauth, C. (1999) *Brain Longevity: The Breakthrough Medical Program that Improves Your Mind and Memory*. New York: Warner Books.

Kirschbaum, C. *et al.* (1993) The Trier Social Stress Test-a tool for investigating psychobiological stress responses in a laboratory setting. *Neuropsychobiology*, 28, pp. 76-81.

Kuo, L. E. *et al.* (2007) Neuropeptide Y acts directly in the periphery on fat tissue and mediates stress-induced obesity and metabolic syndrome. *Nature Medicine*, 13, pp. 803-811.

Nater, U. M. *et al.* (2006) Stress-induced changes in human salivary alpha-amylase activity-associations with adrenergic activity. *Psychoneuroendo-crinology*, 31, pp. 49-58.

Park, A. (2009) *Fat-bellied monkeys suggest why stress sucks* [www] Time Magazine Website. Available from: http://www.time.com/time/health/ article/0,8599,1915237,00 .html [Accessed on 9/8/2010].

Roberts, F. F. (1950) Stress and general adaptation syndrome. *British Medical Journal*, 2, pp. 104.

Rosch, P. J. (1994b) Can Stress Cause Coronary Heart Disease?. *Stress Medicine*, 10, pp. 207-210.

Rosch, P. J. (1994a) Does Stress Cause Hypertension?. *Stress Medicine*, 10, pp.141-143.

Rosch, P. J. (1997) Stress and cancer. *Journal of Royal Society of Medicine*, 90, p. 238.

Rossi, S. *et al.* (2001) Prefrontal cortex in long-term memory: an "interference" approach using magnetic stimulation. *Nature Neuroscience*, 4, pp. 948-952.

Selye, H. (1958) *The Chemical Prevention of Cardiac Necrosis*. New York: Ronald Press.

Selye, H. (1975) Confusion and controversy in the stress field. *Journal of Human Stress*, 1, p. 37.

Shankar, A. A. and Dandekar, R. C. (2009) *Assessment of stress in patients with Recurrent Aphthous Stomatitis, by salivary alpha amylase using a Corocometer*. Unpublished thesis, Maharashtra University of Health Sciences-India.

Thoresen, C. E. *et al.* (1982) The recurrent coronary prevention project: Some preliminary findings. *Acta medica Scandinavica*, 660, pp. 172-192.

Truby, B. (2009) *What is stress?* [Film] Truby Achievements Website. Available from: http://www.trubyachievements.com/Business/Stress _Management/Stress_Test.html [Accessed 15/1/12].

Tsigos, C. and Chrousos, G. P. (2002) Hypothalamic-pituitary-adrenal axis, neuroendocrine factors, and stress. *Journal of Psychosomatic Research*, 53, pp. 865-871.

Tsonis, P. A. and Eguchi, G. (1982) Abnormal limb regeneration without tumor production in adult newts directed by carcinogens, 20-methylcholanthrene and benzo (α) pyrene. *Development, Growth and Differentiation*, 24, pp. 183-190.

In: Hypotheses in Clinical Medicine
Editors: M.M. Shoja, P.S. Agutter et al.
ISBN: 978-1-62257-276-2

Chapter 26

Outbreaks of Red Mite (*Dermanyssus Gallinae*) Dermatitis in City-dwellers: An Emerging Urban Epizoonosis

Maria Assunta Cafiero[1,*], *Antonio Camarda*[2], *Domenico Galante*[1], *Giuseppe Mancini*[1], *Elena Circella*[2], *Nicola Cavaliere*[1], *Gianfranco Santagada*[1], *Mauro Caiazzo*[3] *and Michele Lomuto*[1]

[1]Istituto Zooprofilattico Sperimentale della Puglia e della Basilicata, Foggia, Italy
[2]Dipartimento di Sanità Pubblica e Zootecnia,
Università degli Studi di Bari, Bari, Italy
[3]Azienda Sanitaria Locale, Foggia, Italy

Abstract

The poultry red mite, *Dermanyssus gallinae, De Geer 1778,* is a blood-sucking mite of birds worldwide, including feral pigeons. The mite only visits its host for blood meals, having to do so repeatedly every 2-3 days. The rest of the time, it lives in crevices and cracks in roosting and nesting sites. When the avian host is not available, it can move to and bite humans, causing a non-specific dermatitis with intense itching. From 2001 to 2009, we observed 11 outbreaks of Red Mite Dermatitis (RMD) in city-dwellers in Southern Italy, where all cases were initially misdiagnosed and medical care failed to solve the dermatitis. Mites infested the patients in their dwellings/workplaces, and the source of the infestation was found in abandoned pigeons' nests in close proximity to the habitations. Cutaneous reactions resulting from contact with *D. gallinae* are uncharacteristic, and usually remain unrecognized when they arise in atypical contexts such as urban areas. This has led to scarce information being available on this subject. However, feral pigeons are very abundant in cities worldwide, and are well-known source of zoonotic ectoparasites, including red mites. This poses a considerable risk of

* E-mail: ma.cafiero@izsfg.it. Istituto Zooprofilattico Sperimentale della Puglia e della Basilicata, Dipartimento di Virologia, Via Manfredonia, 20, 71121 Foggia; tel +039 0881786326.

RMD in city-dwellers due to their contact with this nidicolous arthropod. Physicians and dermatologists should be made more aware of the occurrence of this urban epizoonosis. The management of this skin disorder requires correct identification of the mite and its eradication in the environment with removal of nests and appropriate disinfestation of infested areas.

Introduction

The increasing populations of feral pigeons (*Columba livia*) in modern cities are a serious cause for concern due to the repercussions on human health. These birds are well known as reservoirs of zoonotic pathogens and ectoparasites, including the red mite *Dermanyssus gallinae* (Haag-Wackernagel and Moch 2004; Haag-Wackernagel 2005). This arthropod can migrate to humans for a brief blood meal (Kirkwood 1963), even in the absence of direct human contact with birds, and causes a scabies-like dermatitis which is frequently misdiagnosed by physicians. By providing information on the parasite, its urban source, and the main aspects of the infestations, this chapter proposes that red mite dermatitis (RMD) may be an under-diagnosed entity in metropolitan areas. The information provided here could help physicians and dermatologists to identify and manage red mite dermatitis (RMD) in humans, especially in urban settings.

Dermanyssus gallinae: Life Cycle and Biology

The chicken mite or poultry red mite, *Dermanyssus gallinae* (De Geer 1778) (Figure 26.1) belongs to the phylum Arthropoda, class Arachnida (adults with four pairs of legs, as opposed to three in insects), order Parasitiformes, suborder Mesostigmata (= Gamasida), family Dermanyssidae (Krantz 1978). It presents an unsegmented body (idiosoma) and a tiny gnathosoma with its mouthparts, and is an obligate blood-feeder that generally parasitizes chickens and turkeys, but can also be found on a wide variety of other wild/synanthropic birds, including feral pigeons (Varma 1993).

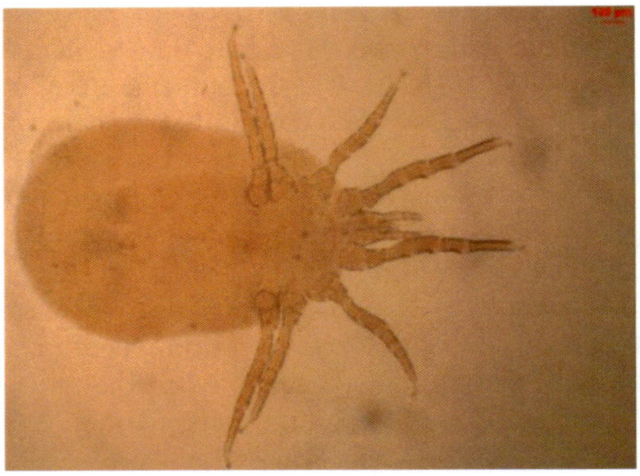

Figure 26.1. Red mite *Dermanyssus gallinae*: female.

When the avian hosts are not available, these mites can also feed on mammals, including humans in their close proximity (Neveu-Lemaire 1938; Varma 1993). Unfed *D. gallinae* females are approximately 0.70 mm long and 0.40 mm wide, but after a blood meal the female's body can increase to more than 1 mm (Varma 1993). The male is somewhat smaller. Reproduction occurs through copulation, and is possible only if the female has fed on its proper host. Twelve to 24 hours after feeding the fertilized female mite lays tiny (400 x 270∝), pearly-white, oval eggs, and 2-3 days later the six-legged *larvae* emerge (Kettle 1984) (Figures 26.2 and 26.3). Within her reproductive life-span the highly fertile female mite can lay hundreds of eggs, but each deposition must be preceded by a blood meal. The feeding-oviposition cycle of *D. gallinae* repeats approximately every third day (Kirkwood 1963; Desch 1984 as cited in Nordenfors and Chirico 2001). The larvae do not feed, and within 24-48 hours they are transformed into eight-legged *protonymphs*. After their first blood meal the *protonymphs* become *deuteronymphs* which, in turn, become adult mites after an interval of about two days (Baker 1999). The *egg-to-egg* cycle is completed within about one week when an avian host is present and optimum environmental conditions are met (Kettle 1984; Robinson 2005). *D. gallinae* remain on the host's body only long enough to complete the blood meal (1-2 hours) (Kirkwood 1963), withdrawing thereafter to the nearest hiding place (cracks and fissures in the walls and floors, birds' nests, cages, etc.) (Kettle 1984). Feeding occurs mainly during the night (Kirkwood 1963), although under certain conditions (high temperatures in particular) daytime feeding can also be observed (Haag-Wackernagel 2005). Adults are able to survive for 4-5 months without feeding (Kettle 1984), but under laboratory conditions some specimens have survived fasts as long as 34 weeks (Kirkwood 1963). *D. gallinae* are very rapid crawlers and, when a host is available, the mites can move very quickly over open spaces to reach the areas they inhabit. It is essential to note the possibility that *D. gallinae* can be a potential vector/reservoir of such zoonotic agents as *Pasteurella multocida, Salmonella spp, Erysipelothrix rhusiopathiae* and encephalopathic viruses (Chirico *et al.* 2003; Valiente-Moro *et al.* 2007).

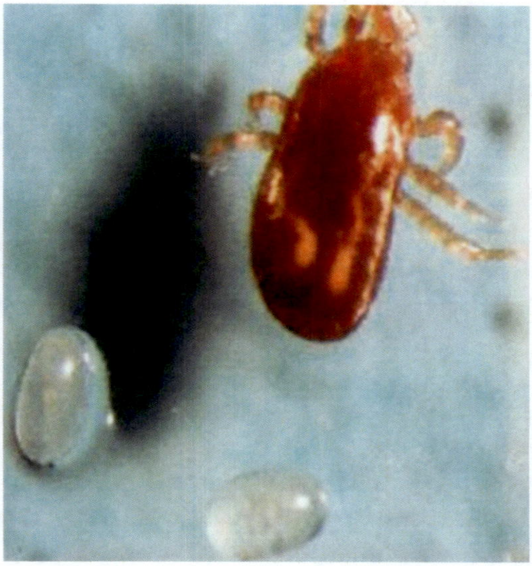

Figure 26.2. Red mite *Dermanyssus gallinae*: female and eggs.

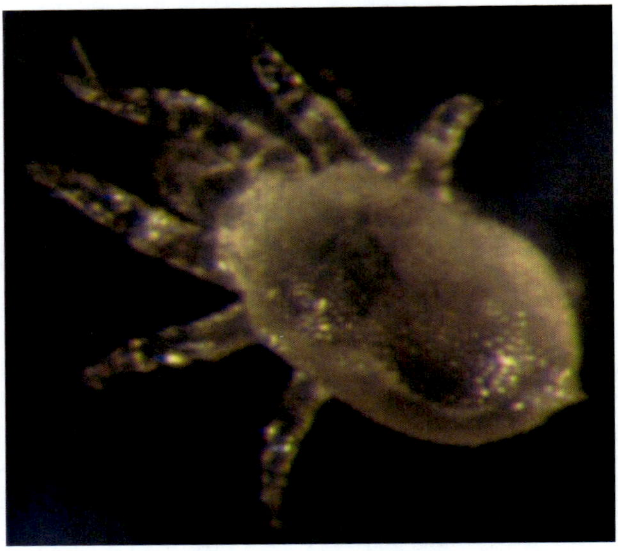

Figure 26.3. Red mite *Dermanyssus gallinae*: six-legged larva.

The Feral Pigeon (*Columba livia*): The Main Urban Reservoir of the Poultry Red Mite

Feral pigeons (*Columba livia* Gmelin, 1789) are the descendants of domesticated forms of the wild-living rock pigeon, and are among the most successful avian settlers in our cities, where they live close to the human population (Haag-Wackernagel 2005). The average feral pigeon population is around 1 pigeon per 10–20 city inhabitants (Johnston 1984; Vater 1998 as cited in Haag-Wackernagel and Birtcher 2010). In modern cities, the abundance of food supplies and the absence of the predators that normally prey on them, their eggs and hatchlings, allow increased urban pigeon populations to develop. As a result, the birds are increasingly choosing city buildings as nesting sites, and this brings them into close contact with the human population. The nests are often constructed under eaves, on balconies, or near heating/air-conditioning units, which the pigeons abandon after their eggs have hatched and the young birds have left the nest, or sometimes earlier if adult birds are threatened. Abandoned pigeons' nests can be a source of zoonotic ectoparasites, including red mites. Masses of these mites attack young chicks, and may cause death due to blood loss. When the avian host is not available, they can move very rapidly and migrate in search of new hosts, including humans, which can supply them with blood.

Red Mite Dermatitis in City-dwellers: Clinical Manifestations and Therapy

The parasitosis presents as a scabies-like dermatitis that is indistinguishable from other forms of pseudoscabies, even on histology (Yassien *et al.* 1966; Kowalska and Kupis 1976). Laboratory tests are within normal limits and blood eosinophilia is lacking (Kowalska and Kupis 1976). There are tiny erythematous papules, and occasionally vesicles, that cause intense pruritus and are often excoriated as a result of scratching; in some cases, there may be urticarioid manifestations (Rockwell 1953; De Oreo 1958; Sexton and Barton 1975). The intensity of the pruritus varies depending on the sensitivity of the host, but it is always referred to as "severe". The bites may be painful and can be located anywhere on the body of the patient. However, stings are not found in interdigital spaces, genitals or skin folds (Haag-Wackernagel and Bircher 2010). In the case of bedroom infestation, the skin lesions are more intense on the backs of the hands, forearms, ankles and feet (Regan *et al.* 1987). Our experience has also shown that the symptoms start on these body areas, spreading rapidly to the remaining parts of the body. In red mite dermatitis occurring in workplaces, lesions are almost always limited to arms and legs. Patients with dermatitis related to the red mite should temporarily leave the infested environment and take either a shower or a full bath so as to remove any mites from the body. This aids rapid healing of the dermatitis and pruritus, because the red mite is only a temporary visitor to human skin.

If treatment is needed, it is purely symptomatic. Topical anti-inflammatory agents can accelerate healing of the skin lesions, and antihistamines may be prescribed to reduce itching and prevent the development of impetigo. In cases of diffuse lesions and of allergic subjects, local and/or systemic steroid therapy may be necessary. However, there have been reports of persistent infestations in farmers close to poultry that involved unexpected sites such as the ear (auditory meatus) (Rossiter 1997) and the scalp (Pampiglione *et al.* 2001; Dogramaci *et al.* 2010). These cases have been treated with permethrin.

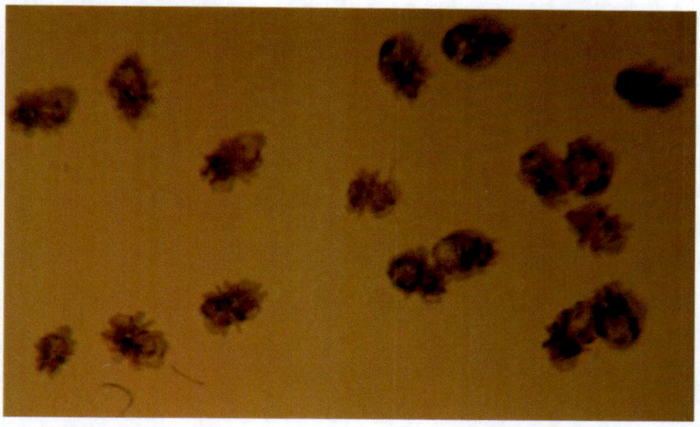

Figure 26.4. Red mites found in a bedroom in one of the eleven cases.

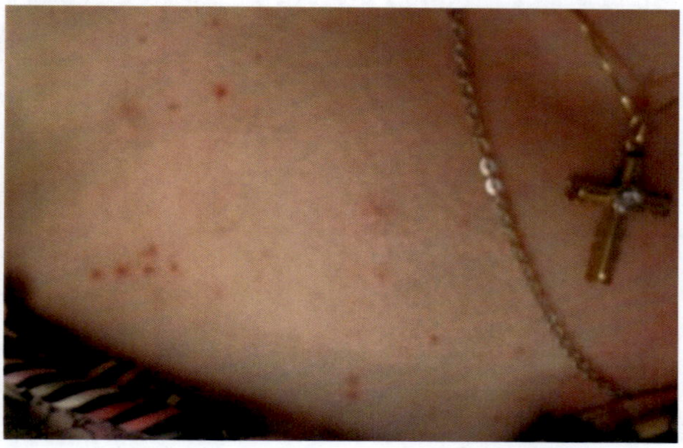

Figure 26.5. A 69-year-old woman with red-mite bites on her chest.

Table 1. Summary of history, clinical manifestations and treatment of the patients

Case	Date[1] and Location	Ambience	Duration of symptoms (weeks)	Number of people affected	Lesion sites	Mite collection site	Initial treatment
1	5/2001 Basilicata	Private Apartment	4	2 (1M, 1F)	Generalized	Bedroom (Furnitures, Walls, Bed Linen); Patient	Antiparasitic Shampoo, Steroids, Antihistamines
2	7/2003 Apulia	Office	5	10 (4M, 6F)	Arms, Legs	Office Room (Desktop, Floor)	Steroids, Antihistamines
3	1/2005 Apulia	Private Apartment (Holiday House)	36 (Recurrent)	2 (1M, 1F)	Generalized	Bedroom (Furnitures, Walls)	Steroids, antihistamines
4	5/2005 Apulia	Private Apartment	2	1 (1M)	Arms, Legs, Chest	Bedroom (Walls Behind the Bed)	NR
5	6/2005 Apulia	Office	4	7 (3M, 4F)	Arms, Legs	Conference Room (Wall Near the Balcony)	Steroids, Antihistamines
6	5/2007 Apulia	Private Apartment	8	4 (1M, 2F, 1C)	Generalized	Bedroom (Furnitures, Walls, Bed Linen, Cordless, Clock)	Steroids, Antibiotic, Tranquilizer
7	3/2007 Campania	Private Apartment	5	1 (1M)	Generalized	Bedroom (Furnitures, Computer, Desk); Patient	Steroids, Antihistamines
8	5/2008 Apulia	Private Apartment	24	3 (1M, 1F, 1C)	Generalized	Bedroom (Furnitures, Bed Linen)	Steroids, Antihistamines
9	6/2008 Apulia	Private Apartment	7	3 (1M, 2F)	Generalized	Bedroom (Furnitures, Bed); Bathroom	Steroids, Antihistamines
10	5/2008 Basilicata	Private Apartment	1	3 (1M, 2F)	Arms, Legs, Chest	Bedroom Furnitures	NR
11	6/2009 Apulia	Private Apartment	5	1 (1F)	Generalized	Bedroom (Furnitures, Walls, Bed Linen)	Steroids, Antihistamines

[1] Date when red mite detected; NR, not required; M, male; F, female; C, children.

Sanitation of Infested Areas and Actions to Prevent Red Mite Infestations

Regarding the disinfestation of urban environments, there is no specific literature about the used molecules or the number of the needed treatments. The mites present in human living spaces should be removed with a vacuum cleaner. We used pyrethroid sprays in two-three cycles of fumigation, and the treatment was very effective. However, the identification and complete elimination of the source of infestation is crucial. Usually, it is an abandoned pigeons' nest. Sometimes, its removal from within or near working and living areas is challenging, especially if located in hard-to-reach spots. The infested loci should subsequently be disinfested by specialized pest control companies.

To prevent further nesting, pigeon access to buildings should be deterred. Breeding sites (window-sills, ventilation and air-conditioning intakes) should be protected with an appropriate pigeon deterrent system (Haag-Wackernagel 2005). Crevices and holes in the outer walls of the building can be filled with cement to prevent their use as nesting sites by pigeons and other synanthropic birds. These operations are very important during the nesting season and in proximity to public buildings such as schools and hospitals, in order to prevent mass outbreaks.

Cases Series

From 2001 to 2009, the *Istituto Zooprofilattico Sperimentale della Puglia e della Basilicata*, Italy (IZSPB) received arthropod specimens for analysis (Figure 26.4). The arthropods were related to 11 dermatitis outbreaks and were collected by the patients in the bedrooms of private apartments (9/11) or in offices (2/11) (Table 1). Nine cases occurred in 2001, 2005 and 2007-2009 involving twenty individuals (18 adults and 2 children) living in six different Italian towns in the Apulia, Campania and Basilicata regions. The affected individuals presented itching and bites and had no pets or any contact with other animals. In all cases, the patients had from two weeks to six months history of pruritic dermatitis and the lesions started on the lower extremities and spread rapidly to the rest of the body (Figure 26.5). The remaining two outbreaks (2/11) came from Veterinary Services, and occurred in 2003 and 2005. They involved office employees in different cities in the Apulia Region (Italy). All the patients (total of 17) suffered from dermatitis on the arms and legs for several weeks. The itching and sensation of "bites or stings" were more severe during working hours.

Owing to the intense pruritic symptoms, almost all the patients had consulted general practitioners and dermatologists, and in one case a pediatrician. The presumptive diagnoses ranged from *prurigo, atopy, pseudoscabies of unknown origin, insect bites and stings, acariasis caused by parasites other than those responsible for scabies,* and *psychogenic pruritus.* The patients were treated with antihistamines and cortisone, and one woman was even given a tranquilizer, but the symptoms returned when symptomatic treatment stopped. The mites were later identified by IZSPB staff as *Dermanyssus gallinae,* De Geer 1778, using *Baker's* (Baker 1999) and *Varma's* (Varma 1993) morphological keys. Inspection by IZS staff at all the reported sites revealed the presence of abandoned pigeons' nests near the infested rooms (Figure 26.6). Removal of the nests coupled with disinfestation using pyrethroids in two cycles of fumigation at the subjects' homes/workplaces was associated with complete regression of the symptoms. There was no evidence of mites or dermatitis during the subsequent follow-up.

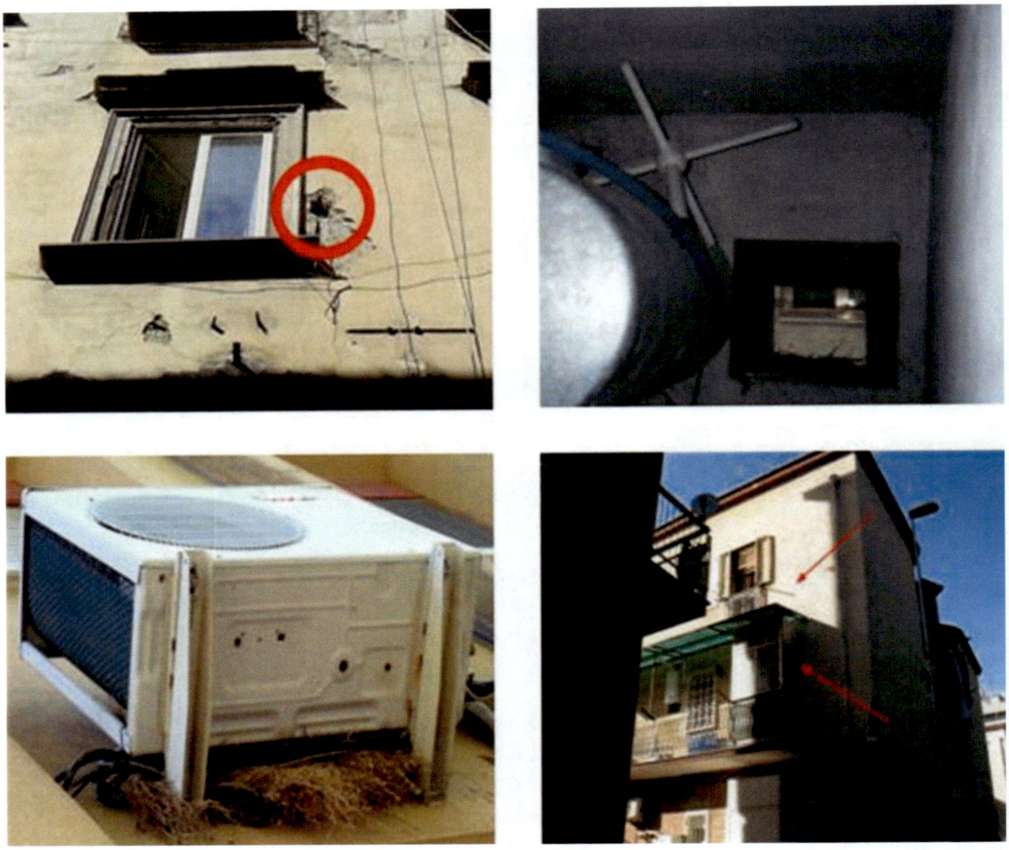

Figure 26.6. Pigeon nesting sites in four of the 11 cases observed (from Cafiero et al. 2007 – reproduced with permission from Obiettivi e Documenti Veterinari).

Discussion

Parasitology and medical entomology textbooks classically cite *D. gallinae* infestations as a normal occurrence in personnel working in the poultry industry (farmers, technicians, veterinarians). In these environments, cutaneous disorders related to the red mite are relatively easy to diagnose. In contrast, when patients have no apparent contact with rural environments , the dermatitis is frequently misdiagnosed. Most physicians, in fact, are keenly aware of dermatoses associated with burrowing mites (e.g. *Sarcoptes scabiei*). If the cutaneous manifestation is caused by epizoonotic parasites such as red mite, it is often misdiagnosed because there is little information available on this topic in medical textbooks. In addition, its detection in the infested environment can be difficult because of the characteristics of the parasitic life cycle, and its accurate identification can also be problematic. These factors all contribute to the current tendency to underestimate the frequency of this parasitosis in city-dwellers. The cases reported here suggest that the true incidence of this dermatitis in urban areas is much greater than that reported by the relatively sparse literature.

In fact, in modern cities there are all the epidemiological conditions needed to promote contact between men and red mites. It is a nidicolous species, and is the most common parasite of feral pigeons. These birds are very abundant in our cities, where they have few enemies and food is always copious. Food is either given deliberately by human "pigeon lovers", or accidentally by incorrect disposal, resulting in an ever-increasing population of pigeons, which build their nests close to human dwellings. At times when these pigeons are not on their nests, mites may migrate into nearby houses and bite humans. Among the parasites affecting feral pigeons, *D. gallinae* represents the main ectoparasite that humans may acquire, together with *Argas reflexus* (Haag-Wackernagel 2005). Both human infestations have recently been described (Haag-Wackernagel and Bircher 2010).

The medical literature reports the majority of RMD cases arising in the spring to early summer. We have also observed this seasonality and we maintain that it is probably related to the peak of the red mite population in this period. Although the reproductive behavior of pigeons is subject to variation, it is well known that, in temperate zones like Southern Italy, this activity peaks between April and June. Therefore, more nests are probably built and abandoned during the spring months, and red mites are more likely to be found in buildings inhabited by humans, searching for new hosts. The occurrence of feral pigeon ectoparasites has been proven to occur with increasing host density (i.e. feral pigeon) (Haag-Wackernagel 1991). Furthermore, the hot temperatures during this season also favor reproduction and movement (crawling) of the mites. The climate in these months explains the increasing risk of man-red mite contact.

The cases of RMD reported here confirm observations by other investigators regarding the increased frequency of these forms of dermatitis in humans living in apartments located on the top floors of buildings (Varma 1993), and reflect the birds' tendency to build their nests under the eaves of a building, on balconies, outside attics, or near terraces. The very high survival ability of the mite, even during prolonged fasting, may be epidemiologically relevant and of practical importance. It can result in recurrent episodes of RMD, as previously observed in an occasionally-used building (i.e. holiday homes). In these cases, pruritic skin lesions can occur each time people return to the infested places, even when the apartments are completely uninhabited for months (Cafiero *et al.* 2007; Cafiero *et al.* 2009).

It is interesting to note that in two of the described urban RM outbreaks, the mites were repeatedly found on electrical appliances located in infested rooms (e.g. cordless phone, television, alarm clock, personal computer). The electrical devices frequently run in stand-by mode, thus generating heat, and this may well be a factor attracting the mites, as it could simulate a pigeon's body temperature (about 42°C). The attracting force of the heat generated by these appliances might have practical applications (e.g. for detecting mites), and be interesting for diagnostic purposes since physicians, in cases of suspected infestation, could advise their patients to check these particular places.

In the episodes observed from 2001 to 2009, patients consulted physicians, most of whom were dermatologists, though they were requesting medical care just for the severe pruritus. They often described feeling as if they had been "bitten or stung by insects", especially during sleep. The medical diagnoses were consistently generic, and even when the eruption was attributed to acariasis, the possibility of zoonosis was never suspected, and none of the consulted physicians advised patients to inspect their living quarters for parasites. At this stage, they had usually not yet found any arthropods. In fact, mites feed preferentially at night, when the availability and immobility of their hosts and the darkness favor their ectoparasitic activity and enable them to return undisturbed to their hiding places. However, after the identification of the mites by IZS staff, a thorough epidemiological investigation revealed that, at the time of their medical examinations, some patients had already noticed these mites in the infested premises, mainly on electrical appliances. They were described as ''tiny, light-colored, rapidly crawling insects'' or as "dust" and the description strongly suggests that they could have been unengorged red mites. Despite being intrigued by their presence, the patients did not associate the symptoms with these mites, and so made no mention of them to the dermatologist. The behavior of patients is entirely different when they find engorged mites. Capturing fed mites is generally alarming enough to prompt the patient to seek help in identifying these arthropods (Cafiero *et al.* 2009). In all of the reported episodes, they went to the Veterinary Services to identify them. Once the source of the pruritus is found, most patients do not go back to the dermatologist, who is not sufficiently well-informed about the true cause of this skin disorder.

Dermatologists should be aware of the biology of this mite and of its morphological variations that depend upon its nutritional state. In the presence of the above symptoms, the dermatologist should provide the patient with complete instructions on how to inspect their living quarters and identify the mite (i.e. shape, different color and size of the mite, nocturnal feeding habits, typical hiding places). Our experience has shown that the use of white bed linen could favor the detection of red mites.

Conclusion

In conclusion, the differential diagnosis of nonspecific dermatitis in persons living in urban settings should always include pseudoscabies caused by *D. gallinae*, particularly when the lesions develop in the spring/summer and the patients live or work on the upper floors of a building. When the clinical presentation is nonspecific and the arthropod cannot be found, the only hope for a correct diagnosis lies in a thorough environmental anamnesis. Merely focusing on the symptoms can be misleading, as it is important to carry out an accurate anamnesis for every case. If arthropods are found in living/workspaces, a careful consideration of the exact position, size, and morphology of the several structures of the body of the collected specimens is essential for a correct identification. This task should be entrusted to entomologists. Recently, molecular analysis has been also proposed for the genetic study and the identification of *D. gallinae* (Marangi *et al.* 2009; Potenza *et al.* 2009).

Infestations may occur in schools, hospitals, offices, etc., and can easily lead to mass outbreaks. Dermatologists may play a fundamental role in underlining the zoonotic role of this mite in urban environments. Co-operation and dialogue between physicians and patients, as well as the interaction between human and veterinary medicine, is a crucial factor in preventing and managing these dermatites and other epizoonotic parasitoses.

References

Baker, A. S. (1999) *Mites and ticks of domestic animals*. An identification guide and information source. London: HM Stationery Office.

Cafiero, M. A. *et al.* (2007) Infestazione da *Dermanyssus gallinae* nell'uomo. *Obiettivi e Documenti Veterinari,* 6, pp. 41-45.

Cafiero, M. A. *et al.* (2009) An urban *International Journal of Dermatology*. 48, pp. 1119-1121.

Chirico, J. *et al.* (2003) The poultry red mite, *Dermanyssus gallinae,* a potential vector of *Erysipelothrix rhusiopathiae* causing erysipelas in hens. *Medical and Veterinary Entomology*, 17, pp. 232-234.

Deoreo, G. A. (1958) Pigeons acting as vector in acariasis caused by *Dermanyssus gallinae* (de Geer, 1778). *Archives of Dermatology,* 77, pp. 422-429.

Desch, C. E. (1984) Biology of biting mites (*Mesostigmata*). In: Nutting, W. B. (ed) *Mammalian diseases and Arachnids,* Volume 1. Boca Raton, FL: CRC, pp. 83-109.

Dogramaci, A. C. *et al.* (2010) D. gallinae infestation: an unusual cause of scalp pruritus *The Journal of Dermatological Treatment,* 21, pp. 319-321.

Haag-Wackernagel, D. (1991) Population density as a regulator of mortality among eggs and nestlings of feral pigeons (*Columbia livia domestica*) in Basel, Switzerland. In: Pinowski, J. *et al.* (eds) *Nestling Mortality of Granivorous Birds due to Microorganisms and Toxic Substances*. Warsaw: Polish Scientific Publishers, pp. 21-31.

Haag-Wackernagel, D. (2005) Parasites from feral pigeons as a health hazard for humans. *The Annals of Applied Biology*, 147, pp. 203-210.

Haag-Wackernagel, D. and Bircher, A. J. (2010) Ectoparasites from feral pigeons affecting humans. *Dermatology,* 220, pp. 82-92.

Haag-Wackernagel, D. and Moch, H. (2004) Health hazards posed by feral pigeons. *Journal of Infection*, 48: pp. 307-313.

Johnston, R. F. (1984) Reproductive ecology of the feral pigeon *(Columba livia). Occasional papers of the University of Kansas Museum of Natural History*, 114: pp. 1-8.

Kettle, D. S. (1984) *Medical and Veterinary Entomology*. London: Croom Helm Press, pp. 380-405.

Kirkwood, A. C. (1963) Longevity of the mites *Dermanyssus gallinae* and *Lyponyssus sylviarum. Experimental Parasitology,* 14, pp. 358-366.

Kowalska, M. and Kupis, B. (1976) Gamasoidosis (gamasidiosis)-not infrequent skin *Polish Medical Science and History Bulletin*, 15-16, pp. 391-394.

Krantz, G. W. (1978) *A Manual of Acarology*. Second edition. Corvallis, OR: Oregon State University.

Marangi, M. *et al.* (2009) Phylogenetic relationship between *Dermanyssus gallinae* populations in European countries based on mitochondrial COI gene sequences. *Experimental and Applied Acarology*, 48, pp. 143-155.

Neveu-Lemaire, M. (1938) *Traité d'Entomologie Médicale et Vétérinaire*. Paris: Vigot Frères Ed, pp. 458-462.

Nordenfors, H. and Chirico, J. (2001) Evaluation of sampling trap for *Dermanyssus gallinae* (Acari: Dermanyssidae). *Journal of Economic Entomology*, 94, pp. 1617-1621.

Pampiglione, S. *et al.* (2001) Infestazione persistente del cuoio capelluto da *D. gallinae* in una contadina emiliana. *Parassitologia*, 43, pp. 113-115.

Potenza, L. *et al.* (2009) Characterization of *Dermanyssus gallinae* (Acarina: Dermanissydae) by sequence analysis of the ribosomal internal transcribed spacer regions. *Veterinary Research Communications*, 33, pp. 611-618.

Regan, A. M. *et al.* (1987) Nosocomial dermatitis and pruritus caused by pigeon mite infestation. *Archives of Internal Medicine*, 147, pp. 2185-2187.

Robinson, H. W. (2005) *Artrhopoda in Urban Insects and Arachnids: A Handbook of Urban Entomology*. Cambridge: Cambridge University Press, pp. 389- 440.

Rockwell, E. M. (1953) *Dermatitis due to Dermanyssus gallinae of pigeons*. Archives of Dermatology and Siphilogy, 68, pp. 82.

Rossiter, A. (1997) Occupational otitis externa in Chicken catchers. *The Journal of Laryngology and Otology,* 111, pp. 366-367.

Sexton D. J. and Barton H. (1975) Bird-mite infestation in a university hospital. *The Lancet*, 7904, p. 445.

Valiente-Moro C., *et al.* (2007) Experimental infection of *Salmonella Enteritidis* by the poultry red mite, *D. gallinae. Veterinary Parasitology*, 146, pp. 329-336.

Varma, M. G. (1993) Ticks and Mites (Acari). In: Lane, R. P. and Crosskey, R. W. (eds) *Medical Insects and Arachnids*. Cambrige: Cambrige University Press, pp. 597-658.

Vater, G. (1998) Wie viele Tauben gibt es in mitteleuropäischen Städten? *Der Praktische Schädlingsbekämpfung*, 50, pp. 12-17.

Yassien, N. A. *et al.* (1966) Immunohistopathological status of the skin in cases infested with 3 species of mites. *Journal of the Egyptian Society of Parasitology*, 26, pp. 567-573.

In: Hypotheses in Clinical Medicine
Editors: M.M. Shoja, P.S. Agutter et al.

ISBN: 978-1-62257-276-2

Chapter 27

House Dust Mites Do not Live in House Dust: Evidence and Implications for the Current Understanding of House Dust Mite Allergy

Thorkil E. Hallas*
Allergy Clinic, Dermato-Allergological Department
Copenhagen University Hospital Gentofte, Hellerup, Denmark

Abstract

Since the discovery fifty years ago that house dust allergy was caused by house dust mites *(Dermatophagoides spp.),* it has been implicitly understood that these mites live in our dwellings. Consequently, efforts to minimize exposure have focused on reducing the concentrations of these mites indoor. In the meantime, evidence has appeared that points to another explanation for their presence in house dust samples. A new hypothesis suggests that house dust mites found indoor represent contamination from the outside. They do not live indoors. Instead, findings of house dust mites in house dust samples are consequent on their life cycles in the open. There are several major reasons for believing this hypothesis to be correct. The mites appear discontinuously (sometimes present, sometimes not) in house dust samples - a pattern that could be explained by the assumption that only the migrant stages, not the resting stages, are transferred from the outside. In addition, it seem impossible to remove them permanently from indoors. This can be explained if the mites are already dead or moribund when they sediment in our dwellings and are readily replaced by new specimens arriving as contamination from the outside. House dust mites are not the only kind of mites that appear this way in house dust samples: the house mite (*Glycyphagus domesticus*) and the small mite *Tarsonemus sp.* behave similarly. Adoption of the hypothesis implies that most of the advice on how to avoid house dust mite exposure in homes will lose its value. Indeed, the recognition that exposure to house dust mites may also take place outdoors will give a more accurate picture of the causes of house dust mite allergy.

* E-mail: thallas@hotmail.com.

Introduction

In 1964, the Dutch physician Reindert Voorhorst and his colleagues at the University Hospital of Leiden, Netherlands, published a paper claiming that mites of the species *Dermatophagoides pteronyssinus* and *D. farinae* (and others) were the cause of what had formerly been known as "house-dust allergy" (Voorhorst *et al.* 1964). From then on, these mites came to be known as "house dust mites". Today, house dust mite allergy remains a widespread and troublesome disease and there is an overwhelming amount of literature about house dust mites (for references, see the monograph by Colloff 2009). There is no doubt that house dust mites are the cause of the disease.

Mites of the genus *Dermatophagoides* are known to science as outdoor-living mites from birds' nests and - on very rare occasions - also from stored products. They were not reported in dwellings before the use of vacuuming as a method for collecting house dust samples. In order to explain their presence in such samples (and because no other explanation was offered), it was assumed that they must live where they were found (Bronsjwijk *et al.* 1971). Therefore, today's guidelines for avoidance of house-dust mites in patients' homes are still based upon the idea of mites living in the indoor environment.

I have worked as an entomologist for about forty years. A considerable part of my career has involved research into the biology of mites, including house dust mites. During my work in the laboratory, I gradually became aware that house dust mites probably do not live where they have been found. Rather, their presence in samples from the homes might be due to a natural phenomenon not hitherto considered as an explanation. This understanding is summarized in a new hypothesis about house dust mite allergy (Hallas 2010). The hypothesis suggests that house dust mites found in houses represent contamination from the outside. They do not live indoors. Findings of house dust mites in house dust samples are a consequence of their life cycles in the open. In this chapter, some of the main arguments for the hypothesis and some new perspectives on our understanding of house dust mite allergy are presented. Many details, however, wait to be further explored. That is why it still is a hypothesis.

Lack of Evidence for Indoor Life of House Dust Mites

Let me start by explaining why it is very likely that the mites we encounter in house dust samples do not come from a living, breeding indoor mite population. Surprisingly, some common beliefs - even among scientists - about the mites have not been scientifically verified. Moreover, standard research methods for mite exposure studies preclude those beliefs. A closer look at our knowledge will reveal that signs of normal house dust mite life are missing indoors, and mites in our homes do not react as we expect live mites to do.

Popular Beliefs about House Dust Mites Have not Been Verified by Science

Despite the beliefs of many, there seem to be no published scientific records demonstrating that house-dust mites actually *live* in our homes (i.e. are alive and breed in our homes). The correct and objective statement is that mite specimens *are found in our homes.* Unfortunately, patients are routinely told that house dust mites *live* in our dwellings, particularly in mattresses and bedding; the mites supposedly ingest skin scales in beds and leave allergenic excrement that makes people sick. We also tell patients that the mites are associated with house dust and benefit from the indoor temperature and humidity and from lack of hygiene. Patients and their advisers seem convinced that all this is true, but from a biologist's point of view, none of these statements have been satisfactorily verified. Impressive pictures and films of living mites often appear alongside the information to illustrate the idea of a living, indoor population of house dust mites. But when details of such images are given, it is invariably revealed that the photographers have used mites from a mite culture (i.e. mites that have been bred in a laboratory) and not living specimens from a sample of indoor house dust.

Standard Monitoring Methods May Perhaps Only Count Dead Mites from Dust Samples

To explain why most people to date have agreed that mites found indoors come from a living and breeding population, it is important to understand how mites are found in dust samples. Only in very rare cases can live house dust mites be seen moving around in these samples. I have not observed them myself but I do not exclude the possibility that others may occasionally have seen such mites. On looking into freshly collected dust samples, one may recognize the mites as shrunken bodies, looking dry and dead, often missing some limbs. Such mite bodies are very hard to find, count and identify. Therefore, the samples are treated directly by adding concentrated lactic acid solution with a few grains of Lignin Pink, which colors the mites. It also makes them swell so they appear puffy and life-like. When prepared in this manner it is easy to recognize and count the mites in a Petri dish under a magnification of 25x and identify selected specimens by picking them up on a needle for transfer to slides to be examined under higher magnification and normal phase-contrast microscopy.

Because we cannot know whether the specimens were actually alive when collected it has become standard practice in the literature to report the number of mites simply as "number of *Dermatophagoides* spp". This number does not imply that the mites were alive when collected. There is no way to tell. And because both dead and live mites have an allergenic load, whether the mites were dead or alive when the sample was taken has not been considered important for exposure. Furthermore, it has been considered implicit that the dead specimens seen under the microscope must have lived in the very place where they were found. This is a tempting but incorrect assumption, which may have led to wrong inferences.

Signs of Normal Mite Life Are Missing Indoors

If house dust mites really lived indoors, we would expect to see signs of the full spectrum of their life cycles including mites moving about, mites feeding, and the presence of all developmental stages. Active developmental stages should walk restlessly around on all surfaces, so even if the mites are small we should be able to see them moving where light conditions are adequate. They should also aggregate in places where they are easy to recognize either visually or by their smell. (House dust mites held in cultures have a sweetish, rotten smell from the decay of many dead bodies. In addition, when they go from one developmental stage to the next, a sticky, unpleasant smell is emitted.) If caught by vacuuming, live active mites should react to the disturbance by walking away from the dust sample collected. None of the signs of life mentioned seem to have been described for house dust mites collected indoors. From my observations it can be added that food pellets are generally absent from the stomachs of mites collected indoors, which means that those mites have not eaten recently. Perhaps house dust mites neither ingest human skin scales nor (consequently) produce fecal pellets in our dwellings. They do not possess the enzyme keratinase to digest keratin, a major structural protein of shed skin scales, and nobody seems to have reported observations of mites eating such (raw) scales. Active, live mites, however, do eat all the time, so probably the mites were already dead when collected. An important criterion for establishing that the mites live indoors with us is that all developmental stages of their life cycles must be found in house dust samples; not necessarily in the same samples or in representative amounts (because there may be collection bias, and if a developmental morph is of short duration it might be under-represented), but all developmental stages should at least be present to some extent.

Table 1. Distribution of developmental stages of house dust mites in indoor samples. From examination of house dust samples, it has been noted that developmental stages of house dust mites representing about half of a mite's developmental time was generally absent

Development morphs in order*	Resting stages	Migrant stages
Prelarva (inside the eggshell)	absent	
Larva		present
Moulting larva to protonymph	absent	
Protonymph		present
Moulting protonymph to tritonymph	absent	
Tritonymph		present
Moulting Tritonymph to Adult	absent	
Adult		present

* Undifferentiated eggs may be found, too, but usually in very small numbers.

As Table 1 shows, quite a few of the developmental stages are missing or under-represented in house dust samples. This indicates that house dust mites do not carry out their life cycles in our dwellings. Rather, it suggests that their development takes place elsewhere, and what we find in our houses are the migrant stages only. Consequently, they must complete their full life cycles only in the outdoor environment. If researchers fifty years ago had been curious enough, they might have been able to draw the same inference. In conclusion, key signs of active, living mites are missing indoors because: there are no signs of mites moving about, there are no signs of feeding activity, and essential developmental stages are missing.

House Dust Mites Found Indoors Cannot Be Eradicated...

Living house dust mites will respond to control methods, e. g. heat, drought, pesticides. We know this from observing how mites *in situ* or in laboratory cultures react. So it is tempting to try to control house dust mites in the same way we manage other common indoor pests. A multitude of methods have been tested, but in clinical testing none has led to a substantial reduction in exposure to allergens as experienced by patients (Gøtzsche and Johansen 2008). Similarly, much effort has been devoted to identifying environmental parameters or variations in patients' behavior that can explain why mites seem to be found in substantial numbers in their homes. But so far, no such factors have been consistently identified. Because we have been fixated on the idea of indoor living house dust mites we have focused on the collection of mites on surfaces, rooms, furniture etc. where we thought that allergens were produced and emitted. In this context we have to recall that in reality vacuuming is merely a method for collecting particles suspended in air. Higher concentrations of mites have been reported in mattresses than on floors, and higher concentrations on carpeted than hard floors. However, these findings do not indicate preferred living places, as mites become suspended in the air because of the vacuuming process. Therefore, these concentrations should rather be explained as being proportional to the volume of air filtered during vacuuming and not interpreted as if the mites were situated on the surfaces being vacuumed. Since the mites in our homes do not react as we expect live mites to do, it is likely that they are not affected by the treatment (are resistant or not present where we think they are) or alternatively that they are not alive. Thorough cleaning with the purpose of wiping out house dust mites seems to work; however, after a short time they are found there again. This could be explained by the arrival of new mites, either from other places in the house or from the outside. Other places in the house could potentially be inside mattresses, in upholstered furniture, inside pillows etc., but almost five decades of research have failed to document the presence of such "reservoirs" of house dust mites inside our homes. Consequently, we are left with the implication that new house dust mites arrive from the outside. They may be dead on arrival, or they may be alive but die shortly thereafter.

House Dust Mites in House Dust Samples Area Consequence of the Life Cycle of Mites from Outdoors

If house dust mites do not live in house dust, then why do we find them in such numbers in dust samples? The hypothesis suggests that their presence is a by-product of house dust mite biology in the open, where synchronal bursts of migrating mites move into new places.

They may be distributed into our houses in the same manner as other components of dust (e.g. pollen). In other words, mites accumulate inside our houses because of sedimentation in an environment with relatively little movement of air. The same phenomenon is actually seen with other mite species. In the following I will explore these aspects further.

Dead Mites and Absolute Humidity

House dust mites produce their own water from the metabolism of food and they are actually net producers of water. Surplus water is a waste product they have to excrete. So they do not need free water in their environment to survive. Therefore, it is strange that the number of mites in house dust samples (often but not always) increases with increasing absolute humidity, AH (g H_2O per m^3 or kg of dry air) (Korsgaard and Hallas 1979; Gunnarsen *et al.* 2002).

The phenomenon is interesting in the context of the new hypothesis that house dust mites result from contamination from the outside: What we measure is AH. Because the outdoor relative humidity does not vary much and the indoor temperature is fairly constant, variations in indoor AH are merely an expression of variations in outdoor temperature (Hallas *et al.* 2004). Therefore, the phenomenon of mite concentration and humidity can be reformulated as: Higher outdoor temperature results in more mites in the indoor dust. This could be due to higher migration activity in the mites or could simply be ascribed to a greater air exchange ratio between the indoor and outdoor environments in warmer weather, and thus the introduction of larger volumes of outdoor air into our homes.

Airing in warm weather may thus bring more particles into a house whereas the production of particles of indoor origin does not increase correspondingly. In consequence, dust of outdoor origin may make up a larger proportion of the indoor dust and we will experience higher concentrations of mites in the house dust samples and probably also of other particles from the open. A positive correlation between the number of mites in house dust samples and the absolute humidity is also known for the mites *Tarsonemus* spp. (Korsgaard and Hallas 1979) and it might be a common feature for all kind of particles of outdoor origin distributed by air.

Mites Might Be Distributed in a Similar Way to Pollen

Particles from the outside air frequently occur in house dust samples, e.g. pollens of various kinds. They appear at the same time as in the outside air and disappear when the concentration of outside pollens decreases. So from studying indoor dust samples we could actually obtain reliable knowledge of the kind of pollen that is present outside, and when there are many or few of pollen grains in the outside air. Mite bodies suspended in the outdoor air may act in the same way.

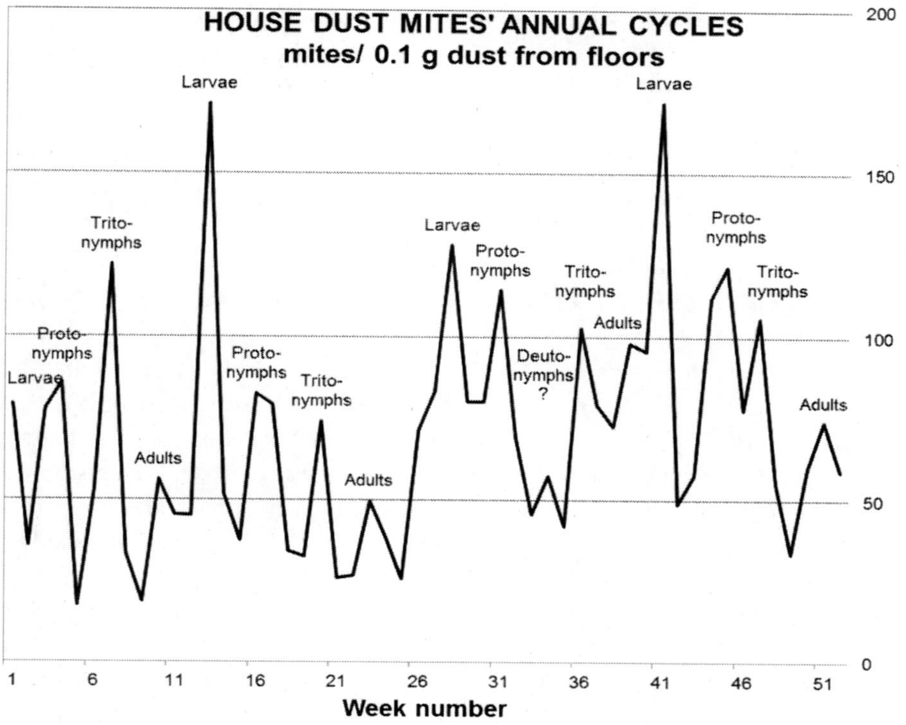

Figure 27.1. The exposure levels vary with time and reflect the biology of the mites (Redrawn from Hallas and Korsgaard 1997). That only migrant development stages are found in the indoor samples tells us that that the mites do not live indoor but may arrive from outdoor sources.

This assumption was confirmed 15 years ago in a large array of house dust samples (Hallas and Korsgaard 1997). In this study, peak concentrations of mites alternated between spikes of high concentration and periods of time where only a small background concentration was found. The material was provided over 11 years from c. 2000 individual patients with newly-diagnosed house dust mite allergies; each of them sent in 1-3 samples of their house dust for mite examination. This association with time had not been noted before because researchers normally do not collect samples simultaneously, and because they had tried to relate mite levels to factors that might explain why they "lived" in some houses and not others. As can be seen from Figure 27.1, time is a major determinant of the observed variation in mite occurrences among indoor-collected dust samples.

There were 16 peaks per year and they were repeated every year in a nationwide synchrony. Thus, there are peak periods when both mites and their allergens are present, alternating with periods when both allergens and mites are almost absent. This contradicts the assumption that house dust mites carry out their life cycles in our homes. It also shows that they do not accumulate. The number of patients having had a bad experience of exposure to house dust mites appeared in corresponding peaks every year (Hallas and Korsgaard 1997). A positive correlation was later found between FEV-reduction in a small number of patients and the weeks of the year when the annual high concentrations of mites in the samples were expected (Hallas and Korsgaard 1998).

According to the new hypothesis, we are exposed to aerosols of migrant stages of the mites from the outside. They could come as a flux through our dwellings possibly with the ventilation air, although there might be other explanations. Thus, house dust mites are not connected with human dwellings as such. We may be exposed there or elsewhere.

From Figure 27.1 we can localize the allergen liberation to the emergence of newly molted, migrating specimens of the stages in question. This indicates that the allergens may originate from the molting fluid between old and new cuticle, which is released as an aerosol when molting takes place.

A Similar Phenomenon in Other Mite Species

House dust mites found inside our homes are a by-product of house dust mite biology in the open where synchronal bursts of migrating developmental stages are on the move and some of them end up, dead or alive, in our houses. Normally nothing further happens. We now have the outline of which stages and when during the year we will encounter them (Figure 27.1) and thus also an idea of what may cause allergy attacks and when these may take place. The studies I refer to (Hallas and Korsgaard 1997, 1998) took place in Denmark; the schedule may differ in other geographical areas.

According to my experience, synchrony of progressing developmental stages also seems to be a common feature in other free-living mites: the initial phases of *Lepidoglyphus destructor* in stored grain in Denmark and *Acarus siro* s.l. in Icelandic hay (Hallas and Iversen 1996), *Glycyphagus domesticus* and *Tarsonemus* spp. in house dust samples (Hallas and Korsgaard 1997) and *Tyrophagus similis* in old fields in Northern Iceland (Hallas and Gudleifsson 2008). Among these, the house mite *G. domesticus* is particularly interesting because in many ways it is a behavioral analog of house dust mites.

Glycyphagus domesticus is a long-haired mite. The long hairs and a slightly larger size than house dust mites make this species more readily seen even without a microscope. House mites are sometime reported indoors because people observe them crawling on surfaces or they appear as a layer of fine whitish dust. They are microbial grazers from the outdoor environment and may sometimes benefit from the growth of microfungi on surfaces in unheated rooms. The name does not indicate that they live in houses, just the custom of naming pest mites according to their interface with us.

In the decade 1900-1910, there was a series of reports of very large indoor populations of house mites appearing as living dust (Ludwig 1904). According to Ludwig they were mainly *Glycyphagus domesticus*, but *Glycyphagus spinipes* was also found. The latter is today known as *Lepidoglyphus destructor*, and is a very common mite in decaying plant materials. They were then thought to have developed from vegetable stuffing material for furniture. It was frequently reported that mites were suddenly absent but then appeared in masses weeks later. They were also impossible to control either by harsh chemical means or cleaning. The list of means that failed to work is impressive: insect powder, camphor, naphthalene, kerosene, lysol, white spirit, borax, corrosive sublimate, diethyl ether, ethyl acetate, sulfur dioxide, sodium hypochlorite, hydrochloric acid, hydrogen cyanide, heat treatment, disinfection of furniture and mattresses in an autoclave at 110 degree Celsius. Surprisingly, no one at that time came up with the idea that the mites might have continued to come from the outside.

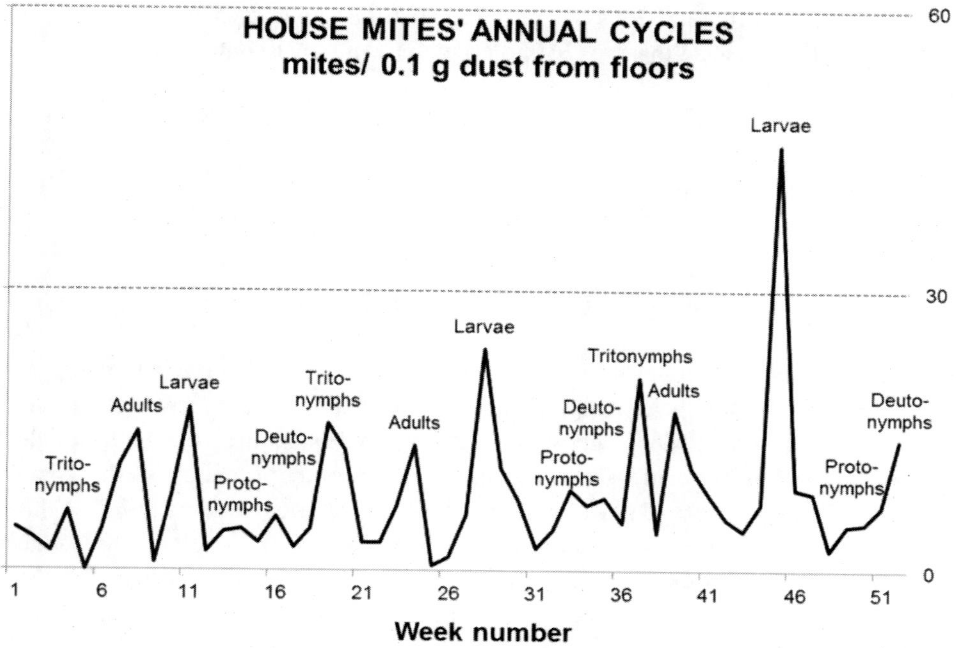

Figure 27.2. The concentration of the house mite *Glycyphagus domesticus* in house dust samples does vary with time in a characteristic way (Redrawn from Hallas and Korsgaard 1997). House mites - in this example from Denmark - have three generations each year. Only migrant developmental stages are found, as in house dust mites.

Recently, it was discovered that moderate outbreaks of house mites in dwellings might be due to nationwide-synchronized developmental stages, and as in house dust mites the pauses indicate that molting (immobile) stages were absent. It was demonstrated first for the autumn generation from public inquiries to the Danish Pest Infestation Laboratory (Hallas and Iversen 1996), and later from examination of house dust samples from new patients for the entire calendar year (Hallas and Korsgaard 1997).

Such bursts of specimens of house mites may be a common phenomenon. Many inquiries mention sudden, unexplained appearances of whitish dust on floors and furniture. This was assumed at the time to be woodworm (*Anobium punctatum*) dust. Woodworm biology, however, shows no such periodic activities (Hallas 1996).

Researchers 100 years ago were unaware of the synchronous behavior of house mites. They believed that moldy stuffing material used in furniture was infested with house mites and that this was the cause of the massive indoor occurrences. Now we realize that infestation of moldy materials was probably not the cause, but rather the consequence of the invasion of large numbers of starving house mites from outdoor sources.

In house mites there are three synchronized generations per annum. In house dust mites there are four. The winter generation in the house mite seems the smallest while the autumn generation is the largest. The annual generations of house dust mites appear to be almost the same size. Apart from this difference the phenomenon is similar in both house dust mites and in house mites: Sudden bursts of active (migrating) specimens of the same developmental stage, followed by a pause where no specimens are found, and then the next stage, etc. Cleaning or use of chemical treatments has no durable effect. The characteristics that there are a whole number of generations per year and that the annual synchrony is nationwide in both species indicate instead that we have to do with a window to outdoor populations of both kind of mites.

Many other species of mites are occasionally found in house dust samples, but none of them have yet been analyzed for possible synchrony of developmental stages in house dust, as in house dust mites, house mites and *Tarsonemus* spp.

Outside Exposure

Traditionally, sensitization to house dust mites has been explained by exposure in bedrooms because we all spend a significant amount of time there. Even pet cats and dogs were thought to be sensitized in bedrooms. But a consequence of the understanding that findings of house dust mites in indoor dust only mirrors outdoor activity is that exposure to house dust mites may also take place outdoors. Indeed, allergic reactions to house dust mites have been verified in horses with atopic dermatitis (Baxter and Vogelnest 2008) where the connection with human dwellings is dubious.

In addition, there are situations where neither the house dust mites nor their allergens are found in dwellings in an area (e. g. Reykjavik; Hallas *et al.* 2004), but the average sensitization to the allergens appeared to be the same as in rural areas where house dust mites are found in some homes (Hallas *et al.* 2011). These observations support the new understanding that sensitization to house dust mites can be due to outdoor exposure, and weakens the argument that indoor exposure makes a difference.

At present we do not know whether there are sufficient concentrations of mites or allergens in the outdoor air to cause sensitization or asthma attacks in humans or in animals. Such exposure should logically take place near foci where migrating synchronized stages of house dust mites are emitted. Possible locations for large numbers of mites might be birds' nests where house dust mites have been reported, but more investigations are required to clarify the outdoor biology of house dust mites.

Conclusion

Consequences of the Hypothesis

The present hypothesis should probably be considered a working hypothesis that can be refined and modified in light of additional research. If the hypothesis can be confirmed it will have several important consequences. First of all, patients should not need to feel embarrassed because they develop house dust mite allergy: the mites are not associated with them because of poor hygiene standards or lack of compliance with doctors' advice, or because they did not buy e.g. a mattress cover or other marketed device.

The hypothesis could represent a paradigm in allergy research. Realizing that house dust exposure takes place outside will allow us to focus on more effective ways of managing house dust mite exposure and allergic reactions. It may also enable us to recognize cases of house dust mite allergy where exposure takes place in the outside environment, i.e. cases that might have been neglected under the current understanding of the phenomenon. If the hypothesis is basically correct and the mites accumulate inside our houses because of sedimentation there might be a simple way to maintain low indoor exposure: Do the vacuuming while windows are open.

How Can the Hypothesis Be Confirmed?

Experimental evidence documenting the transmission of mites and their allergens from outdoor sources to the indoor dust would be the best way to confirm the hypothesis. Alternatively, if it can be properly documented that live, progressive populations of house dust mites are a common phenomenon in our dwellings, the entire hypothesis should be rejected.

It is part of the hypothesis that there is some regularity in the timing of exposure for house dust mites or their allergens (as shown in Figure 27.1). This aspect has been overlooked to date because of the idea that more or less permanent house dust mite populations live in dwellings. But the existence of synchronized bursts of migration stages from the outside might be verified from records of when and where asthma attacks or drastic FEV-reductions take place. Here, any patient or doctor having such diaries may be able to contribute.

Furthermore, we should seek to identify conditions that allow house dust mites (and other relatively harmless species of mites) to behave synchronously and thus temporarily cause high risk for allergic reactions in humans. In laboratory cultures, synchrony is met less often because the optimization to produce many new specimens includes selection of environmental factors that allow females to live long and lay many eggs that subsequently hatch over many weeks. Perhaps synchrony is possible only because of certain environmental factors that we have not previously considered relevant and therefore remain unrecognized.

References

Baxter, C. G. and Vogelnest, L. J. (2008) Determination of threshold concentrations of multiple allergenic extracts for equine intradermal testing using normal horses in three seasons. *Veterinary Dermatology*, 19, pp. 305-313.

Bronsjwijk, J. E. *et al.* (1971) On the abundance of *Dermatophagoides pteronyssinus* (Trouessart, 1897) in house dust. *Researches on Population Ecology*, 13, pp. 67-79.

Colloff, M. J. (2009) *Dust Mites*. Dordrecht: Springer.

Gøtzsche, P. C. and Johansen, H. K. (2008) House dust mite control measures for asthma. *Cochrane Database of Systematic Reviews*, 2, doi: 10. 1002/ 14651858.CD001187.pub3.

Gunnarsen, L. *et al.* (2002) House dust mites, humidity of room air and flooring materials. *Proceedings of Indoor Air*, 4, pp. 725-731.

Hallas, T. E. (1996) Dust from woodworm holes may also be the result of house mite activity. *International Pest Control*, 40, p. 157.

Hallas, T. E. and Iversen, M. (1996) Sources of exposure for storage mites in the farming environment. *Annals of Agricultural and Environmental Medicine*, 3, pp. 9-12.

Hallas, T. E. and Korsgaard, J. (1997) Systematic variations in the appearance of house-dust mites, house mites and of *Tarsonemus sp.* in dust from dwellings. *Revista Española de Alergología e Inmunología Clínica*, 12, pp. 173-177.

Hallas, T. E. and Korsgaard, J. (1998) Peak expiration flow variations may reflect house-dust mite exposure and patient reactivity. *Allergy*, 53[Suppl 48], pp. 101-103.

Hallas, T. E. *et al.* (2004) Sensitization to house dust mites in Reykjavik, Iceland, in the absence of domestic exposure to mites. *Allergy*, 59, pp. 515-519.

Hallas, T. E. and Gudleifsson, B. E. (2008) Summer occurrence of Tyrophagus similis Volgin (Acari, Acaridae) in hayfields in Northern Iceland may include a facultative deutonymph. *Journal of the Acarological Society of Japan*, 17, pp. 101-106.

Hallas, T. E. (2010) House-dust mites in our homes are a contamination from outdoor sources. *Medical Hypotheses*, 74, pp. 777-779.

Hallas, T. E. *et al.* (2011) Mite allergy and mite exposure in Iceland. *Annals of Agricultural and Environmental Medicine*, 18, pp. 31-35.

Korsgaard, J. and Hallas, T. E. (1979) Tarsonemid mites in Danish house-dust. *Allergy*, 34, pp. 225-232.

Ludwig, F. (1904) Die Milbenplage der Wohnungen, Ihre Entstehung und Bekämpfung. *Sammlung naturwissenschaftlich-pädagogischer Abhandlungen, Leipzig und Berlin*, 8, pp. 9-12.

Voorhorst, R. *et al.* (1964) Is a mite (Dermatophagoides sp.) the producer of the house-dust allergen? *Allergie und Asthma*, 10, pp. 329-334.

In: Hypotheses in Clinical Medicine
Editors: M.M. Shoja, P.S. Agutter et al.

ISBN: 978-1-62257-276-2

Chapter 28

The Role of UV Irradiation in the Progression of Diabetic Retinopathy

Liat Avdian[1], *Alon Harris*[2], *R. Shane Tubbs*[3], *Marios Loukas*[4], *Ghaffar Shokouhi*[5], *Kamyar Ghabili*[6], *Paul S. Agutter*[7], *Brent A. Siesky*[8], *Yochai Shoshani*[9] *and Mohammadali M. Shoja*[10]

[1] Department of Ophthalmology, Indiana University School of Medicine, Indianapolis, Indiana, US
[2] Department of Ophthalmology, Indiana University School of Medicine, Indianapolis, Indiana, US
[3] Pediatric Neurosurgery, Children's Hospital, Birmingham, Alabama, US
[4] Department of Anatomical Sciences, St. George's University, Grenada, West Indies
[5] Neuroscience Research Center, Tabriz University of Medical Sciences, Tabriz, Iran
[6] Medical Philosophy and History Research Center, Tabriz University of Medical Sciences, Tabriz, Iran
[7] Theoretical Medicine and Biology Group, Glossop, Derbyshire, UK
[8] Department of Ophthalmology, Indiana University School of Medicine, Indianapolis, Indiana, US
[9] Department of Ophthalmology, Indiana University School of Medicine, Indianapolis, Indiana, US
[10] Pediatric Neurosurgery, Children's Hospital, Birmingham, Alabama, US Division of Neurological Surgery, Department of Surgery, University of Alabama at Birmingham, Birmingham, Alabama, US Tuberculosis and Lung Disease Research Center, Tabriz University of Medical Sciences, Tabriz, Iran

Abstract

Diabetic retinopathy is a major cause of blindness. Underlying pathogenic mechanisms that have been suggested include the non-enzymatic glycosylation pathway and production of advanced glycation end-products (AGEs), retinal neurodegeneration and inflammation, and enhanced reactive oxygen species (ROS) generation. Here, the authors discuss how the UV component of solar radiation may potentially enhance the progression of diabetic retinopathy. The mechanisms we suggest are: (1) In high-temperature environments with intense solar radiation, the amount of UV reaching the retina is sufficient to increase *de novo* ROS generation. (2) Under UV-A irradiation, AGEs generate ROS. (3) Enhanced oxidative stress promotes generation of AGEs. (4) UV-B may enhance intraocular inflammation (production of endothelin and IL-6) in DR patients, and this in turn may accelerate AGE generation. (5) UV-B and ROS independently up-regulate VEGF expression, inducing fibrovascular proliferation and inflammation. (6) ROS induce apoptosis of the retinal neurons and pericytes. (7) Oxidation of the glycated proteins and lipids produces potentially toxic substances within the retina. Thus, UV irradiation could enhance the progression of diabetic retinopathy, so strategies to limit UV exposure such as wearing protective sunglasses or using photochromic lenses that could attenuate this progression will become increasingly important as humans are exposed to greater levels of solar radiation.

Introduction

Energies that move at the speed of light are collectively referred to as electromagnetic radiation. This radiation conveys stellar energy efficiently to planets and its wavelength or frequency is used to differentiate among the varying ranges in the electromagnetic spectrum (Vazquez and Haslmeier 2006). The visible light wavelength range is between 400 nm and 700 nm. Ultraviolet (UV) radiation is in the range of the spectrum where the wavelength is shorter than blue light. It is divided into three categories. UV-A (400-320 nm) does not interact with ozone. Thus, organisms are exposed to it at all times. UV-B (320-280 nm) breaks the bonds between the oxygen atoms in molecules of ozone. UV-C (280-250 nm) is effectively absorbed by the ozone layer. Depletion of the ozone layer leads to increased exposure to UV-B radiation at ground level (Lumsden 1997). Recent measurements show that stratospheric ozone is at a very low level and the level of UV-B radiation is very high (Madronich *et al.* 1998). Naturally, levels of UV absorption vary according to location and conditions (latitude and elevation, cloud cover, proximity to an industrial area). It is important to study these different factors and their effects in order to understand better how to take protective measures in the future. Ultraviolet radiation constitutes only ~5% of the solar energy reaching the earth's surface (Hilgenkamp 2006; Koleske 1995) but it has major effects on biological systems, accelerating tissue aging.

UV Irradiation and the Eye

It injures ocular structures (cornea, lens and retina) more readily than the skin (Sliney 2001); in particular, it has a causal role in cataract (Vinson 2006). UV-A induces photoxidation of histidine, tryptophan and cysteine residues in the insoluble protein fraction of the lens. Cysteine oxidation, involving hydrogen peroxide production, leads to protein cross-linking by disulfide bridge formation and this appears to be a significant contributor to cataract (Linetsky and Ortwerth 1995). The formation of advanced glycation end-products (AGEs) in the lens is potentiated by oxidation of ascorbic acid (Linetsky and Ortwerth 1996);

glucose oxidation is also an important contributor (Fuentealba *et al.* 2007), though it appears not to lead to cross-linking of lens proteins (Linetsky *et al.* 2008).

These mechanisms are well established, but the possibility that UV radiation also injures the retina in humans has not been explored in detail. Such injury is possible unless the UV is filtered out by the lens (Sliney 2001), though epidemiological findings are inconsistent (Sliney 2002). Blue light is injurious to the retina (Augustin *et al.* 2002), suggesting that at least UV-A irradiation may also be retinopathic, and the anterior segment structures are at particular risk of UV exposure. About one week of light exposure reduced the thickness of the outer nuclear layer of the retina to less than one fifth of normal in a rat model (Joly *et al.* 2006). Despite these data, a comprehensive account of the ocular effects of UV irradiation in healthy and disease conditions remains to be provided.

Can Diabetic Retinopathy (DR) Be Exacerbated by Continuous Exposure to UV Light?

Diabetic retinopathy (DR) is a major cause of blindness worldwide. Pathologically, DR is characterized by (a) apoptosis of retinal neurons, (b) the loss of retinal arteriolar pericytes and microaneurysm formation, (c) increased vascular permeability, (d) hypertrophy of basement membranes, (e) capillary occlusions, and (f) neovascularization and fibrovascular proliferation (Kastelan *et al.* 2007). Several mechanisms have been proposed to explain these pathological events. Non-enzymatic glycosylation pathways and AGEs have a role (Stitt 2003), and there are speculations concerning early retinal dysfunction and neurodegeneration due to insulin deficiency, retinal inflammation (Antonetti *et al.* 2006), enhanced autoimmune reactions and generation of free radicals (Stitt 2003; Suzuma *et al.* 2007). In this chapter, we discuss how UV irradiation could, directly or indirectly, accelerate retinal injury in diabetic patients.

Generation of Reactive Oxygen Species (ROS) and AGEs in the Eye

UV irradiation enhances the generation of reactive oxygen species (ROS) in different cell types (Brauchle *et al.* 1996). For example, UV-A irradiation increases H_2O_2 production in the human lens (Linetsky *et al.* 1996). Activation of the ROS-mediated caspase cascades induces apoptosis in porcine retinal pericytes and this mechanism could contribute to the hypertension-related exacerbation of DR (Suzuma *et al.* 2007). ROS, largely generated from the mitochondrial apoptosis pathway, play a significant role in the development of DR and are closely linked to the activation pathways of AGEs (Gillery 2006). Increased oxidative stress associated with uremia promotes AGE production (Miyata *et al.* 1997). Also, oxidative products such as malondialdehyde may bind to proteins and amplify glycoxidation-generated lesions (Gillery 2006). *In vitro*, UV-A irradiation of glycated lens proteins produced considerably more singlet oxygen than irradiation of unmodified proteins and reduced lens epithelial cell-mediated protection against UV-A-induced cytotoxicity (Argirova and Breipohl 2002).

Conversely, UV-A-irradiated AGEs generate ROS, enhancing their cytotoxicity (Masaki *et al.* 1999). AGEs can potentiate UV-mediated oxidation of glycosylated proteins; they photosensitize tissues (Fuentealba *et al.* 2007). The irreversible oxidative cleavage of the carbohydrate moieties of glycosylated proteins yields N-carboxymethyllysine and erythronic acid; this reaction involves superoxide radicals and hydrogen peroxide and proceeds through a free radical-mediated pathway. Increases in N-carboxymethyllysine have been correlated with the severity of retinopathy in diabetic and elderly patients, and there are high levels in the elastic membrane of the arterial wall in diabetic patients (Schleicher *et al.* 1997).

This positive feedback effect between AGE production and ROS production suggests that even the small amount of solar UV that reaches the retina could be pathogenic, particularly in cases of DR. The cornea is largely opaque to radiation of wavelengths below 295 nm and the lens to wavelengths below 400 nm, so only about one part in 100 of the incident UV on the eye surface reaches the retina. Nevertheless, that may be sufficient to exert significant toxic effects (Sliney 2002). In high-temperature environments where the horizon is visible and the ground surface is reflective, there is evidence that the superior retina receives significant UV doses (Sliney 2001).

UV, Inflammation and AGEs

UV-B exposure increases cutaneous endothelin-1 concentration (Metz *et al.* 2006). Endothelin-1 induces interleukin-6 (IL-6) production and secretion from endothelial cells (Xin *et al.* 1995). Reciprocally, IL-6 enhances endothelin-1 secretion from endothelial cells (Kahaleh and Fan 1997). UV irradiation may similarly increase intraocular and retinal endothelin-1 and IL-6. Indeed, IL-6 levels are elevated in patients with proliferative DR (Mocan *et al.* 2006), and this is likely to increase vascular permeability leading to macular edema (Funatsu *et al.* 2001). Moreover, aqueous humor levels of VEGF and IL-6 are positively correlated in patients with DR (Funatsu *et al.* 2003). Such inflammatory processes may accelerate the formation of AGEs (Hein *et al.* 2005).

Regulation of Vascular Endothelial Growth Factor (VEGF) Levels

The level of vascular endothelial growth factor (VEGF) is elevated in the intraocular fluid of patients with diabetic macular edema, and this elevation is associated with the breakdown of the blood-retinal barrier in animal models of diabetes (Starita *et al.* 2007). Isoforms of VEGF may induce fibrovascular proliferation, as well as expression of retinal intercellular adhesion molecule-1, which favors leukostasis and inflammation (Ishida *et al.* 2003). Interestingly, UV-B and H_2O_2 may up-regulate VEGF expression independently (Li *et al.* 2006; Suzuma *et al.* 2007). UV-B radiation also increases hypoxia-inducible factor-1α expression in a dose- and time-dependent manner in human keratinocytes *in vitro*, and this correlates with the degree of angiogenesis (Li *et al.* 2006). ROS increase VEGF release from skeletal myotubes via a PI3K/Akt-dependent pathway (Kosmidou *et al.* 2001).

The Hypothesis

The foregoing lines of evidence suggest that the UV component of solar radiation may enhance the progression of DR by the following mechanisms. (1) In high-temperature environments with intense solar radiation, the amount of UV reaching the retina is sufficient to increase *de novo* ROS generation. (2) Under UV-A irradiation, AGEs generate ROS. (3) Enhanced oxidative stress promotes generation of AGEs. (4) UV-B may enhance intraocular inflammation (production of endothelin-1 and IL-6) in DR patients, and this in turn may accelerate AGE generation. (5) UV-B and ROS independently up-regulate VEGF expression, inducing fibrovascular proliferation and inflammation. (6) ROS induce apoptosis of the retinal neurons and pericytes. (7) Oxidation of the glycated proteins and lipids produces potentially toxic substances within the retina.

This hypothesis could be tested by longitudinal studies on cohorts of diabetic patients and age/sex-matched non-diabetic control subjects. Also, established methods (Adamiec-Mroczek *et al.* 2010; Sasaki *et al.* 2010; Sun *et al.* 2010; Yoshimura *et al.* 2009) could be used to compare the levels of VEGF, IL-6, endothelin-1 and ROS in the retinas of diabetic and non-diabetic rats or mice of the same strain exposed to UV-A and UV-B irradiation, or in cultured human retinal endothelial cells exposed to the same insults; the hypothesis predicts significantly greater levels in the diabetic cases.

Conclusion

Taking the available evidence together, we suggest that exposure to intense sunlight might potentially contribute to accelerated retinopathy in diabetic patients. Hence, strategies to limit UV exposure such as wearing protective sunglasses or using photochromic lenses may potentially attenuate the progression of DR (Sliney 2001). Such strategies are warranted since worldwide depletion of the ozone layer exposes humans to greater amounts of UV radiation (Williams and Langley 2001; Murray and Zentner 2001; Maser *et al.* 1999). Pharmaceutical measures may also prove effective, such as the use of p38 MAPK inhibitors (Du *et al.* 2010) or VEGF inhibitors (Zheng *et al.* 2009); however, less expensive and invasive alternatives such as proposed here may be preferred by both clinicians and patients (cf. Maser *et al.* 1999).

References

Adamiec-mroczek, J. *et al.* (2010) Roles of endothelin-1 and selected proinflammatory cytokines in the pathogenesis of proliferative diabetic retinopathy: Analysis of vitreous samples. *Cytokine*, 49, pp. 269-274.

Antonetti, D.A. *et al.* (2006) Diabetic retinopathy: seeing beyond glucose-induced microvascular disease. *Diabetes*, 55, pp. 2401-2411.

Argirova, M.D. and breipohl, W. (2002) Glycated proteins can enhance photooxidative stress in aged and diabetic lenses. *Free Radical Research*, 36, pp. 1251-1259.

Augustin, A.J. *et al.* (2002) The significance of oxidative mechanisms in diseases of the retina. *Klinische Monatsblätter für Augenheilkunde*, 219, pp. 631-643.

Brauchle, M. *et al.* (1996) Ultraviolet B and H2O2 are potent inducers of vascular endothelial growth factor expression in cultured keratinocytes. *The Journal of Biological Chemistry*, 271, pp. 21793-21797.

Fuentealba, D. *et al.* (2007) Photosensitizing activity of advanced glycation endproducts on tryptophan, glucose 6-phosphate dehydrogenase, human serum albumin and ascorbic acid evaluated at low oxygen pressure. *Photochemistry and Photobiology*, 83, pp. 563-569.

Funatsu, H. *et al.* (2001) Relationship between vascular endothelial growth factor and interleukin-6 in diabetic retinopathy. *Retina*, 21, pp. 469-477.

Funatsu, H. *et al.* (2003) Vitreous levels of interleukin-6 and vascular endothelial growth factor are related to diabetic macular edema. *Ophthalmology*, 110, pp. 1690-1696.

Gillery, P. (2006) Oxidative stress and protein glycation in diabetes mellitus. *Annales de Biologie Clinique (Paris)*, 64, pp. 309-314.

Hein, G.E. *et al.* (2005) The advanced glycation end product pentosidine correlates to IL-6 and other relevant inflammatory markers in rheumatoid arthritis. *Rheumatology International*, 26, pp. 137-141.

Hilgenkamp, K. (2006) *Environmental Health: Ecological Perspectives*. Ontario: Jones & Bartlett Publishers, Inc., p. 223.

Ishida, S. *et al.* (2003) VEGF164 is proinflammatory in the diabetic retina. *Investigative Ophthalmology and Visual Science*, 44, pp. 2155-2162.

Joly, S. *et al.* (2006) Light-induced retinopathy: comparing adult and juvenile rats. *Investigative Ophthalmology and Visual Science*, 47, pp. 3202-3212.

Kahaleh, M.B. and FAN, P.S. (1997) Effect of cytokines on the production of endothelin by endothelial cells. *Clinical and Experimental Rheumatology*, 15, pp. 163-167.

Kastelan, S. *et al.* (2007) Could diabetic retinopathy be an autoimmune disease?. *Medical Hypotheses*, 68, pp. 1016-1018.

Koleske, J.V. (1995) *Paint and Coating Testing Manual: Fourteenth Edition of the Gardner-Sward Handbook*. Ann Arbor: ASTM International.

Kosmidou, I. *et al.* (2001) Reactive oxygen species stimulate VEGF production from C(2)C(12) skeletal myotubes through a PI3K/Akt pathway. *American Journal Of Physiology - Lung Cellular and Molecular Physiology*, 280, pp. L585-L592.

Li, Y. *et al.* (2006) UVB radiation induces expression of HIF-1alpha and VEGF through the EGFR/PI3K/DEC1 pathway. *International Journal of Molecular Medicine*, 18, pp. 713-719.

Linetsky, M. and ortwerth, B.J. (1995) The generation of hydrogen peroxide by the UVA irradiation of human lens proteins. *Photochemistry and Photobiology*, 62, pp. 87-93.

Linetsky, M. *et al.* (1996) The generation of superoxide anion by the UVA irradiation of human lens proteins. *Experimental Eye Research*, 63, pp. 67-74.

Linetsky, M. and ortwerth, B.J. (1996) Quantitation of the reactive oxygen species generated by the UVA irradiation of ascorbic acid-glycated lens proteins. *Photochemistry and Photobiology*, 63, pp. 649-655.

Linetsky, M. *et al.* (2008) Glycation by ascorbic acid oxidation products leads to the aggregation of lens proteins. *Biochimica et Biophysica Acta*, 1782, pp. 22-34.

Lumsden, P. (ed) (1997) *Plants and UV-B Responses to Environmental Change*. Cambridge: Cambridge University Press.

Madronich, S. *et al.* (1998) Changes in biologically active ultraviolet radiation reaching the earth's surface. In: *Environmental Effects Of Ozone Depletion*. Nairobi: United National Environment Program.

Masaki, H. *et al.* (1999) Generation of active oxygen species from advanced glycation end-products (AGEs) during ultraviolet light A (UVA) irradiation and a possible mechanism for cell damaging. *Biochimica et Biophysica Acta*, 1428, pp. 45-56.

Maser, R.E. *et al.* (1999) Over-the-counter yellow ultraviolet light protective lenses: any benefit for individuals with diabetes mellitus? *Delaware Medical Journal*, 71, pp. 287-290.

Metz, M. *et al.* (2006) Inflammatory murine skin responses to UV-B light are partially dependent on endothelin-1 and mast cells. *American Journal of Pathology*, 169, pp. 815-822.

Miyata, T. *et al.* (1997) Oxidation conspires with glycation to generate noxious advanced glycation end products in renal failure. *Nephrology, Dialysis and Transplantation*, 12, pp. 255-258.

Mocan, M.C. *et al.* (2006) Elevated intravitreal interleukin-6 levels in patients with proliferative diabetic retinopathy. *Canadian Journal of Ophthalmology*, 41, pp. 747-752.

Murray, R.B. and zentner, J.P. (2001) *Health Promotion Strategies through the Life Span*. 7th ed. Englewood Cliffs: Prentice-Hall.

Sasaki, M. *et al.* (2010) Neurodegenerative influence of oxidative stress in the retina of a murine model of diabetes. *Diabetologia*, 53, pp. 971-979.

Schleicher, E.D. *et al.* (1997) Increased accumulation of the glycoxidation product N(epsilon)-(carboxymethyl)lysine in human tissues in diabetes and aging. *Journal of Clinical Investigation*, 99, pp. 457-468.

Sliney, D.H. (2001) Photoprotection of the eye - UV radiation and sunglasses. *Journal of Photochemistry and Photobiology. B: Biology*, 64, pp. 166-175.

Sliney, D.H. (2002) How light reaches the eye and its components. *International Journal of Toxicology*. 21, pp. 501-509.

Sliney, D.H. (2002) Geometrical gradients in the distribution of temperature and absorbed ultraviolet radiation in ocular tissues. *Developmental Ophthalmology*, 35, pp. 40-59.

Starita, C. *et al.* (2007) Vascular endothelial growth factor and the potential therapeutic use of pegaptanib (macugen) in diabetic retinopathy. *Developments in Ophthalmology*, 39, pp. 122-148.

Stitt, A.W. (2003) The role of advanced glycation in the pathogenesis of diabetic retinopathy. *Experimental and Molecular Pathology*, 75, pp. 95-108.

Sun J, *et al.* (2010) Intermittent high glucose enhances cell proliferation and VEGF expression in retinal endothelial cells: the role of mitochondrial reactive oxygen species. *Molecular and Cellular Biochemistry*, 343, pp. 27-35.

Suzuma, I. *et al.* (2007) Cyclic stretch-induced reactive oxygen species generation enhances apoptosis in retinal pericytes through c-jun NH2-terminal kinase activation. *Hypertension*, 49, pp. 347-354.

Vazquez, M. and haslmeier, A. (2006) *Ultraviolet Radiation in the Solar System*. Dordrecht: Springer.

Vinson, J.A. (2006) Oxidative stress in cataracts. *Pathophysiology*, 13, pp. 151-162.

Williams, L.K. and langley, R.L. (2001) *Environmental Health Secrets*. Philadelphia: Hanley & Belfus, Inc.

Xin, X. *et al.* (1995) Endothelin-induced interleukin-6 production by rat aortic endothelial cells. *Endocrinology*, 136, pp. 132-137.

Yoshimura, T. *et al.* (2009) Comprehensive analysis of inflammatory immune mediators in vitreoretinal diseases. *PLoS One*, 4, doi: 10.1371/journal.pone.0008158.

Zheng, Z. *et al.* (2009) Protective effect of perindopril on diabetic retinopathy is associated with decreased vascular endothelial growth factor-to-pigment epithelium-derived factor ratio: involvement of a mitochondria-reactive oxygen species pathway. *Diabetes*, 58, pp. 954-964.

In: Hypotheses in Clinical Medicine
Editors: M.M. Shoja, P.S. Agutter et al.

ISBN: 978-1-62257-276-2

Chapter 29

Nonalcoholic Steatohepatitis (NASH) Revisited by Crossing the Boundaries between Physical Chemistry and Histomorphology

***Sven Gunia*[*,1] *and Andreas Erbersdobler*[2]**

[1]Institute of Pathology, HELIOS Klinikum Bad Saarow,
Charité-University Medicine Teaching Hospital, Bad Saarow, Germany
[2]Institute of Pathology, University of Rostock, Rostock, Germany

Abstract

Nonalcoholic steatohepatits (NASH) shares substantial histomorphological overlap with alcoholic steatohepatitis but, by definition, occurs in subjects with "insignificant" alcohol consumption. Histologically, NASH is characterized by hepatocellular ballooning, steatosis, necroinflammation, and fibrosis as well as the formation of Mallory's hyaline (MH) as a response to hepatocellular injury. MH comprises poorly formed "wispy" structures containing keratin 8/18, ubiquitin, and p62 that are frequently encountered in ballooned hepatocytes. Concerning the histological distribution patterns of steatosis and MH in NASH, it is intriguing to observe that hepatocytes featuring substantial steatosis are commonly devoid of MH. According to the prevailing pathogenetic concept of NASH, steatosis precedes the formation of MH; so by applying the laws of statistical thermodynamics, the present hypothesis suggests a possible interplay between liver triglyceride accumulation (cytoplasmic fat droplets) and the major constituents of MH, preventing the latter from aggregating to form MH.

[*] E-mail: sven.gunia@helios-kliniken.de.

Introduction

Nonalcoholic steatohepatits (NASH) by definition occurs in subjects with "insignificant" alcohol consumption. According to the prevailing concept, its pathogenesis follows a sequential process starting with nonalcoholic fatty liver disease (NAFLD) characterized by steatosis, which may be purely macrovesicular or a combination of large and small fat droplets. Subsequently, NASH supervenes; it might either resolve or enter a final cirrhotic pathway (Lewis and Mohanty 2010). In addition to steatosis, NASH features hepatocellular ballooning, varying degrees of mixed lobular inflammation (portal inflammation is commonly mild or absent and is predominantly chronic), fibrosis, and the formation Mallory's hyaline (MH) morphologically characterized by poorly formed "wispy" structures frequently encountered in the cytoplasm of ballooned hepatocytes (Figure 29.1) (Brunt 2005). The aim of the present chapter is to explain the rarity of MH in hepatocytes featuring steatosis.

Possible Interactions between the Major Constituents of MH and Cytoplasmic Fat Droplets from the Thermodynamic Point of View

Basically, MH contains ubiquitin (Ub), p62, and keratin 8/18 (Brunt 2005; Stumptner *et al.* 2007). Ub is a centrally important component of the ubiquitin-proteasome system (UPS) that is covalently attached to various cellular proteins through a highly regulated process (Shabek and Ciechanover 2010). Briefly, UPS and autophagy are the two major mechanisms responsible for protein degradation in eukaryotic cells (Gao *et al.* 2010). The 26S proteasome is a non-lysosomal protease mediating Ub-mediated proteolysis, and the attached Ub binds to other proteins to target them for proteolysis (Banner *et al.* 2000; Matias *et al.* 2010). P62 is a stress-inducible adapter protein that links ubiquitinated species to other proteins and mediates autophagic degradation of polyubiquitin aggregates in the cell (Gao *et al.* 2010; Stumptner *et al.* 1999; Stumptner *et al.* 2007). Considering the remaining structural component of MH, keratin 8/18, it merits emphasis that hepatocellular ballooning is associated with a disturbance of the keratin-intermediate filament cytoskeleton (Denk *et al.* 2001). In particular, in its early stage, this imbalance is characterized by over-expression and hyperphosphorylation of soluble keratin 8 (Denk *et al.* 2001). Owing to the resulting perturbation of the physiological 1:1 ratio of keratins 8 and 18, the increased levels of soluble keratin 8 monomers become sensitive to misfolding and inevitably experience degradation or aggregation leading to the formation of MH (Denk *et al.* 2001). Given that these mechanisms might occur in a hepatocyte harboring large cytoplasmic fat droplets, the space-occupying surface of the latter will force the cytoplasmic keratins (including the increased soluble keratin 8) together into the remaining rim of cytoplasm, bringing these molecules much closer together (Figure 29.2). As a consequence, hydrogen bonds and also dispersion forces and van der Waals attraction forces will lead to stabilization of the preexisting structural organization of the keratin polpypetide chains (that is, either helical structures or beta pleated sheets) (Denk *et al.* 2001; Marzec 2001; Parry *et al.* 2006; Atkins 2006). This increase in stabilization (abbreviated by the symbol s) might counteract protein misfolding. The structural change from a helical polypeptide chain to a statistical tangle represents a so-called *cooperative conversion* (Atkins

2006). Considering a polypeptide chain encompassing a total of n amino acids, its rate of conversion (RC) to a statistical tangle is given by the equation:

$$RC = 1/n \times d(\ln q)/d(\ln s) \times \ln q$$

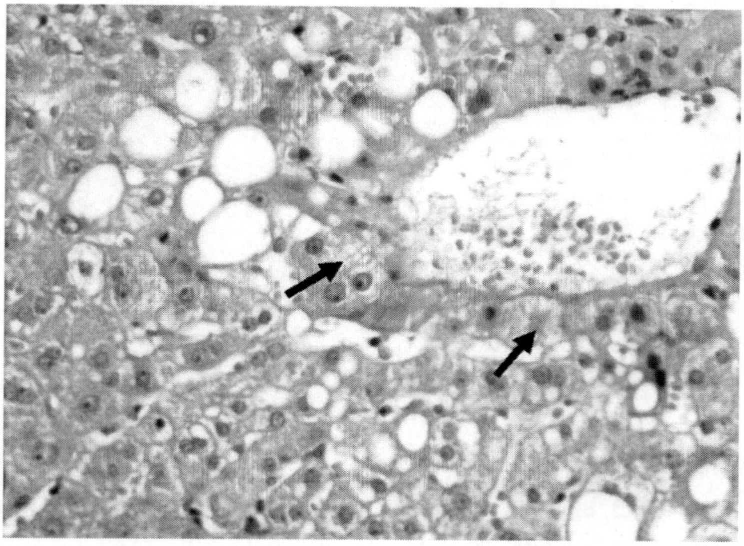

Figure 29.1. Nonalcoholic steatohepatitis (NASH). There is centrilobular steatosis along with Mallory's hyaline (arrows) encountered in ballooned hepatocytes devoid of cytoplasmic fat droplets. Hematoxylin-eosin stain, original magnification 20×.

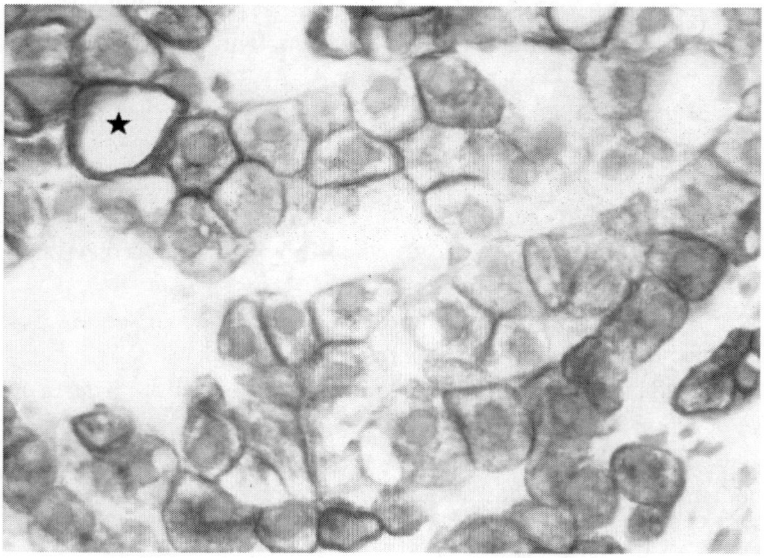

Figure 29.2. The space-occupying fat droplet (asterisk) forces the cytoplasmic keratins together into the remaining rim of cytoplasm, hence giving rise to apparently intense dark cytoplasmic immunostaining around the fat vacuole. Although cytoplasmic staining intensity encountered in the surrounding hepatocytes might also be moderate to strong from cell to cell, the staining quality observed in the fat-containing hepatocyte (asterisk) stands out and fails to fade towards the cell nucleus, in contrast to the adjacent hepatocytes. Anti-CK8/18 immunostaining, original magnification 40×.

in which q represents the sum of all possible states of the polypeptide chain (Atkins 2006). From this equation, it becomes readily apparent that the increase in stability (*s*) of the preexisting structure (helix or beta pleated sheet) of keratin 8 brought about by space-occupying cytoplasmic fat droplets inevitably decreases its rate of conversion to a statistical tangle which, together with Ub and p62, forms the structural basis for what is histologically designated as MH.

Conclusion

In conclusion, the present theoretical consideration suggests that space-occupying cytoplasmic fat droplets might counteract the aggregation of the diverse major structural constituents of MH, which might explain the histologically observed rarity of MH in hepatocytes containing large cytoplasmic fat droplets.

References

Atkins, P.W. (2006) *Physical Chemistry*. 4th ed. Weinheim: Wiley-VCH.

Banner, B.F. *et al.* (2000) Ubiquitin as a marker of cell injury in nonalcoholic steatohepatitis. *American Journal of Clinical Pathology*, 114, pp. 860-866.

Brunt, E.M. (2005) Nonalcoholic steatohepatitis: pathologic features and differential diagnosis. *Seminars in Diagnostic Pathology*, 22, pp. 330-338.

Denk, H. *et al.* (2001) Alcoholic and nonalcoholic steatohepatitis. Histopathologic and pathogenetic considerations [German]. *Der Pathologe*, 22, pp. 388-398.

Gao, Z. *et al.* (2010) Processing of autophagic protein LC3 by the 20S proteasome. *Autophagy*, 6, pp. 126-137.

Lewis, J.R. and MOHANTY, S.R. (2010) Nonalcoholic fatty liver disease: a review and update. *Digestive Diseases and Sciences*, 55, pp. 560-578.

Marzec, E. (2001) Analysis of the dielectric properties of keratin in the alpha-dispersion electric field region. Medical and biological engineering and computing, 39, pp. 558-561.

Matias, R.C. *et al.* (2010) Chaperone-assisted assembly of the proteasome core particle. *Biochemical Society Transactions*, 38, pp. 29-33.

Parry, D.A. et al. (2006) Human hair keratin-associated proteins: sequence regularities and structural implications. *Journal of Structural Biology,* 155, 361-369.

Shabek, N. and Ciechanovera, A. (2010) Degradation of ubiquitin: The fate of the cellular reaper. *Cell Cycle*, 9, 523-530.

Stumptner, C. *et al.* (1999) Analysis of intracytoplasmic hyaline bodies in a hepatocellular carcinoma. Demonstration of p62 as a major constituent. *American Journal of Pathology*, 154, pp. 1701-1710.

Stumptner, C. *et al.* (2007) In vitro production of Mallory bodies and intracellular hyaline bodies: the central role of sequestome 1/p62. *Hepatology*, 46, pp. 851-860.

In: Hypotheses in Clinical Medicine
Editors: M.M. Shoja, P.S. Agutter et al.
ISBN: 978-1-62257-276-2

Chapter 30

Is the Iliotibial Band Syndrome Really a Friction Syndrome?

Frederick Michels*[*,1], Jan Van Der Bauwhede[1] and Stéphane Jambou[2]
[1]Department of Orthopaedic Surgery, AZ Groeninge, Kortrijk, Belgium
[2]Department of Orthopaedic Surgery, Sports Clinic Mérignac, Bordeaux, France

Abstract

In this chapter, evidence is presented to support the idea that iliotibial band (ITB) syndrome is a form of enthesopathy of the insertion of the ITB to the lower end of the femur. The ITB is firmly attached to the distal femur by strong fibrous strands. This femoral anchorage prevents the ITB from rolling over the epicondyle. Thus, friction of the ITB over the bony prominence of the femoral epicondyle seems to be an illusion. From a practical point of view, if the inflammation is limited to the fibrous attachments to the femur (i.e., enthesitis) and the surrounding fat, there is no need to manipulate the ITB surgically.

Introduction

Iliotibial band syndrome (ITBS) is an overuse syndrome mainly affecting runners but also found in cyclists. The syndrome is relatively common among athletes and distant runners with an incidence up to 12% (Lavine 2010). The diagnosis is primarily based on history and physical examination. ITBS causes pain in the region of the lateral femoral epicondyle. Symptoms increase with running. Physical examination reveals a local tenderness of the lateral femoral epicondyle. Initial treatment of ITBS may consist of activity modification, correction of training errors, a trial of nonsteroidal anti-inflammatory drugs, local modalities, stretching, physical therapy, shoe modification, and possibly a cortisone injection. Only in recalcitrant cases is surgery needed. Several surgical procedures have been described. Most

[*] E-mail: frederick_michels@hotmail.com.

techniques resect a part of the ITB to lower the tension. Some authors recommend performing an associated arthroscopy to address any associated intra-articular pathology (Hariri *et al.* 2009; Richards *et al.* 2003).

Mainstream Hypothesis

The ITB Syndrome is a Friction Syndrome

Initially, ITBS was considered a friction syndrome. The concept of a friction syndrome was developed because of several observations. History of the ITBS reveals a correlation between the symptoms and repetitive flexion and extension of the knee. Symptoms typically increase with running. The longer the distance, the worse the pain until the runner is forced to stop. The pain is more severe when running downhill. The pain may be prevented by walking with a stiff knee. Physical examination reveals a typical correlation between pain and position of the knee. Noble's test is a well-known diagnostic test for ITB syndrome. The examiner applies pressure on the lateral side of the knee directly over the femoral epicondyle. The knee is straightened from a 90° position. In a positive test, the patient feels pain when the knee reaches about 30° flexion (Noble 1979). Magnetic resonance imaging (MRI) might be indicated. Ekman showed a thickened ITB on MRI in patients with ITBS (Ekman *et al.* 1994). An underlying bursa was found. Some biomechanical factors are linked to ITBS. Excessive tightness of the ITB may increase the pressure abnormally (Noble 1979). Hip abductor weakness or increased hip adduction during the stance phase of gait is associated with ITBS (Fredericson *et al.* 2000). Those findings lead to the following hypothesis for the pathogenesis of ITB syndrome. If the ITB is too tight, it repetitively shifts forward and backward over the prominent lateral femoral epicondyle and causes friction. This friction results in inflammation of the underlying bursa.

Practical Implication

Stretching of the ITB and strengthening of the hip abductors are frequently recommended in treatment of ITBS. Most published surgical procedures involve debridement or lengthening of the ITB. In 1979, Noble described a 2-cm incision across the fibers of the posterior ITB (Noble 1979). Martens *et al.* (1989) resected a triangular piece of the ITB with a posterior base (base 2 cm, height 1.5 cm). Holmes *et al.* (1993) did not succeed with a percutaneous release and alternatively performed an elliptical resection. Drogset *et al.* (1999) performed a more extensive resection. Others reported a mesh technique or Z-lengthening (Richards *et al.* 2003; Sangkaew 2007).

New Hypothesis

The ITB Syndrome is a form of Enthesopathy

In 1996, Nemeth and Sanders performed a cadaver study to characterize the tissue deep to the ITB and its relationship to the lateral knee joint capsule. They found in each specimen a lateral extension of the joint capsule, which they referred to as the lateral recess (Figure 30.1). A specific effort was made to find a separate bursa deep to the ITB, but no bursa was found in any specimen. In another cadaver study, Fairclough *et al.* (2006) found that the ITB was firmly anchored to the distal femur by fibrous strands, closely associated with a richly innervated layer and vascularised fatty tissue. The ITB was not a separate structure but rather a thickening in the lateral part of the fascia lata. No bursa was identified in any of the examined specimens. Fairclough *et al.* found dense, regular, fibrous connective tissue with some fibroblasts in the strands that linked the ITB to the femur. Biopsies of this lateral recess in patients with ITBS showed histopathological changes consistent with chronic inflammation, fibrosis and mucoid degeneration (Nemeth and Sanders 1996). Because of the mesodermal synovial structure, the lateral recess can histopathologically be mistaken for a bursa.

In 1999, Muhle and colleagues performed a study on 16 patients with ITBS. They found a correlation between the ITBS and alterations in MRI signal intensity in the fatty tissue deep to the ITB (Muhle *et al.* 1999). Similar MRI signal changes were found in other studies (Fairclough *et al.* 2006; Isusi *et al.*, 2007; Murphy *et al.* 1992). No thickening of the ITB was found. In a minority of the patients, a circumscribed fluid collection was observed. Magnetic resonance imaging of the knee at 30° flexion and full extension showed that the ITB is compressed against the lateral epicondyle at 30° flexion. The area beneath the ITB was occupied by fatty tissue (Fairclough *et al.* 2006).

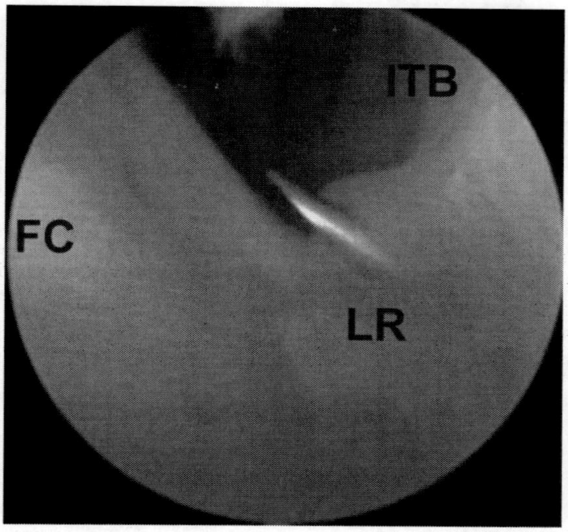

Figure 30.1. The arthroscopic view of the lateral gutter with femoral condyle (FC), needle in lateral recess (LR) and iliotibial band (ITB).

Nemeth and Sanders (1996) studied the lateral synovial recess in patients undergoing knee surgery for other problems. During open surgery for total knee reconstruction or lateral joint reconstruction, the anatomical relationship between the ITB and the underlying synovial recess was observed in all 35 patients. In knee arthroscopy, this lateral synovial recess was found in the lateral gutter. Michels *et al.* (2009) described 36 patients with ITBS treated with an arthroscopic technique. They reported very good results after resection of the lateral synovial recess leaving the ITB intact. In two patients a meniscal lesion was found. Hariri *et al.* treated 12 patients with an open technique resecting the tissue underlying the ITB (Hariri *et al.* 2009). At the end of the procedure, they repaired the surgical split of the ITB. The underlying tissue was seen as a pathological bursa, though no pathological or MRI examination was performed to confirm this identification. The good result of this procedure supports the view that the underlying tissue, and not the ITB itself, is the pain generator in ITBS. ITBS presents as a diagnostic challenge. Given that an intra-articular lesion could possibly cause the knee pain, a diagnostic arthroscopy maximizes the chance of finding and treating such lesions.

Anatomical and imaging studies have shown that the ITB is firmly attached to the distal femur by strong, obliquely oriented, fibrous strands that can be regarded as tendon entheses (Fairclough *et al.* 2006). This femoral anchorage prevents the ITB from rolling over the epicondyle. The impression of a rolling mechanics is probably an illusion created by the sequential shifting of the tension in the ITB. The presence of fat beneath the ITB can be compared with the fat present at many tendon and ligament entheses (Benjamin *et al.* 2004). If there is no shear movement, referring to ITBS as a 'friction' syndrome should be avoided. As no pathological findings have been observed in the ITB itself, ITBS should be considered a form of enthesopathy of the insertion of the ITB to the lower end of the femur.

Conclusion: The Practical Implications of the New Hypothesis

The practical consequence of this new hypothesis is interesting because successful surgical treatment of ITBS must address the underlying pathological causes. If the inflammation is limited to the fibrous attachments to the femur and the surrounding fat, there is no need to manipulate the ITB in the event of surgery. An open technique preserving the structure and length of the ITB can result in good outcome. The arthroscopic approach seems very promising because it allows the synovial recess to be resected in a minimally invasive manner leaving the ITB intact. Several studies report meniscal tears in patients (mis)-diagnosed as ITBS. Therefore, an associated arthroscopy is recommended by some authors. The arthroscopic management of ITBS allows any concomitant intra-articular pathology to be assessed and treated properly.

References

Benjamin, M. *et al.* (2004) Adipose tissue at entheses: the rheumatological implications of its distribution. A potential site of pain and stress dissipation? *Annals of the Rheumatic Diseases, 63, pp. 1549-1555.*

Drogset, J. *et al.* (1999) Surgical treatment of iliotibial band friction syndrome. A retrospective study of 45 patients. *Scandinavian Journal of Medicine and Science in Sports*, 9, pp. 296-298.

Ekman, E.F. *et al.* (1994) Magnetic resonance imaging of iliotibial band syndrome. *The American Journal of Sports Medicine,* 22, pp. 851-854.

Fairclough, J. *et al.* (2006) The functional anatomy of the iliotibial band during flexion and extension of the knee: implications for understanding iliotibial band syndrome. *Journal of Anatomy*, 208, pp. 309-316.

Fredericson, M. *et al.* (2000) Hip abductor weakness in distance runners with iliotibial band syndrome. *Clinical Journal of Sport Medicine*, 10, pp. 169-175.

Hariri, S. *et al.* (2009) Treatment of recalcitrant iliotibial band syndrome with open iliotibial band bursectomy: indications, technique, and clinical outcomes. *The American Journal of Sports Medicine*, 37, pp. 1417-1424.

Holmes, J.C. *et al.* (1993) Iliotibial band syndrome in cyclists. *The American Journal of Sports Medicine,* 21, pp. 419-424.

Isusi, M. *et al.* (2007) MRI findings in iliotibial band friction syndrome: a report of two cases. *Radiologia*, 6, pp. 433-435.

Lavine, R. (2010) Iliotibial band friction syndrome. *Current Reviews in Musculoskeletal Medicine*, 3, pp. 18-22.

Martens, M. *et al.* (1989) Surgical treatment of the iliotibial band syndrome. *The American Journal of Sports Medicine*, 17, pp. 651-654.

Michels, F. *et al.* (2009) An arthroscopic technique to treat the iliotibial band syndrome. *Knee Surgery, Sports Traumatology and Arthroscopy*, 17, pp. 233-236.

Muhle, C. *et al.* (1999) Iliotibial band friction syndrome: MRI imaging findings in 16 patients and MR arthrographic study of six cadaveric knees. *Radiology*, 212, pp. 103-110.

Murphy, B.J. *et al.* (1992) Iliotibial friction syndrome: MR imaging findings. *Radiology*, 185, 569-571.

Nemeth, W.C. and Sanders, B.L. (1996) The lateral synovial recess of the knee: Anatomy and role in chronic iliotibial band friction syndrome. *Arthroscopy*, 12, pp. 574-580.

Noble C. (1979) The treatment of iliotibial band friction syndrome. *British Journal of Sports Medicine*, 13, pp. 51-54.

Richards D, *et al.* (2003) Iliotibial band Z-lengthening. *Arthroscopy*, 19, pp. 326-329.

Sangkaew, C. (2007) Surgical treatment of iliotibial friction syndrome with mesh technique. *Archives of Orthopaedic and Trauma Surgery*, 127, pp. 303-306.

In: Hypotheses in Clinical Medicine
Editors: M.M. Shoja, P.S. Agutter et al.

ISBN: 978-1-62257-276-2

Chapter 31

Thirty Years Lost in Medical Theory: Hans Selye's Unified Theory of Medicine and the Stress Repair Mechanism

Lewis S. Coleman*
Barnes Dental Surgery Center, California, US

Abstract

In 1951, Hans Selye hypothesized that a single mechanism continuously repairs and maintains the vertebrate body. The discovery of this mechanism would enable a "Unified Theory of Medicine" by explaining the nature of physiology, pathology, stress, and their relationships. Such a theory would vastly enhance pharmaceutical development and medical treatment. Soon after Selye published his theory, the discovery of DNA inspired great excitement in medicine and biology. Many believed that the secret of life was at hand. It was widely anticipated that the stress mechanism works closely with DNA to enable embryological developments. DNA would then resume quiescence, but the stress mechanism would remain active to maintain and repair mature structures. These powerfully simple ideas inspired an intense international search for the stress mechanism that lasted 30 years and consumed hundreds of research careers, thousands of test animals, and millions of dollars. Stress researchers proposed two important theories to facilitate their research. Capillary gate theory postulates a submicroscopic mechanism that governs capillary blood flow and provides a superior explanation of hemodynamic physiology. Tissue repair theory postulates a single mechanism that governs tissue repair. Unfortunately, the two theories seemed incompatible. The era of stress research produced numerous important scientific advances, but no clue could be found to the existence of testable mechanisms that could confirm either capillary gate theory or tissue repair theory, let alone a single mechanism that explains both. Stress research was mostly abandoned after 30 years of fruitless effort. Since then, the DNA paradigm has dominated biological research, but it has failed to explain either embryological development or adult

* E-mail: lewis_coleman@yahoo.com.

biology in complex life forms. Now, 60 years after Selye's original prediction, fresh evidence from unrelated research has enabled the first crude description of the long-sought "stress repair mechanism" (SRM) that maintains and repairs the vertebrate body. It closely resembles the "coagulation cascade" that appeared during the heyday of stress research, but fresh information enables the SRM to provide detailed explanations for hemodynamic physiology, hemostasis, and tissue repair, while the coagulation cascade provides only a crude description of clot formation. The SRM incorporates both the capillary gate and tissue repair theories in the form of semi-independent sub-components, each of whose activity exaggerates that of the other. The extrinsic pathway of the coagulation cascade is analogous to the tissue repair component of the SRM, and the intrinsic pathway of the coagulation cascade is analogous to the capillary gate component of the SRM. Their combined activities enable the SRM to focus its powerful effects to maintain and repair tissues, and explain how it generates a bewildering variety of dynamic effects. The appearance of the SRM explains the Cambrian Explosion, and it provides fresh insights to embryology and evolution. It enables Selye's Unified Theory of Medicine that encompasses cohesive new theories of pathophysiology. The SRM thus fulfills all the predictions and expectations of the previous generation of stress researchers. It is now poised to complement and rejuvenate the DNA paradigm, and introduce a new era of medical research and progress.

Introduction

The ultimate objective of medical science is a theory that explains physiology, pathology, stress, and their relationships. Such a theory would vastly enhance the effectiveness and reliability of medical treatments, and enable efficient and profitable pharmaceutical development. Unfortunately, vertebrate biology remains stubbornly mysterious and confusing. Vertebrates obviously possess the means to maintain and repair their body structure, but the means remains unknown. Despite the discovery of DNA, embryological development remains a mystery. The physiological differences among reptiles, amphibians, birds, and mammals remain obscure. The nature of blood pressure, the palpable pulse, atherosclerosis, cancer, eclampsia, apoptosis, amyloidosis, sepsis, eclampsia, rheumatoid diseases, hemoglobin encapsulation, and the regulation of blood flow and cardiac output remain obscure. Lacking such understanding, medicine remains an art based on experiment, where physicians must judge their treatments in terms of symptoms, so that they are at risk of being inefficient, unpredictable, or counterproductive.

In 1951, Hans Selye postulated the presence of a "stress mechanism" that continuously repairs and maintains vertebrate tissues. Selye's theory provided the simplest explanation of physiology, pathology, stress, and their relationships, and it promised a revolutionary "Unified Theory of Medicine" (Selye 1954; Selye 1976; Wolak *et al.* 2004). Only three years later, Watson and Crick discovered DNA. Their unprecedented achievement caused enormous excitement that is difficult to appreciate from our distant perspective. Many believed that the secret of life was at hand. It was widely expected that the stress mechanism converts DNA genetic information into embryological development, and then remains active throughout life to maintain mature structures, while the DNA mechanism resumes quiescence once embryological development is complete.

Selye's pioneering ideas established a science; introduced the concepts of *stress, stressor, eustress, distress, fight or flight,* and the *general adaptation syndrome*. They inspired an international search for the putative stress mechanism that lasted 30 years and consumed a generation of researchers, thousands of test animals, and millions of dollars. These efforts produced *capillary gate theory*, which postulates a sub-microscopic mechanism that regulates capillary flow, and *tissue repair theory*, which postulates a single mechanism that regulates the orderly sequence of tissue repair. The intense scientific research during this era clarified photosynthesis, identified the coagulation cascade and the Krebs cycle, and established the relationship of hypothalamic-pituitary-adrenal (HPA) hormones and immune system activity to stress. It accumulated a solid body of evidence that stress induces HPA hormone release, elevates immune activity, and otherwise induces harmful effects in the vertebrate body that are inhibited by anesthesia and analgesia. More recently, the terms *allostasis* and *allostatic load* have supplanted Selye's classical terms to acknowledge the ability of animals to adjust their behavior and physiology to maintain homeostasis in the presence of stress, but explanations of these phenomena have never been satisfactory for lack of an explanation of tissue repair.

The DNA paradigm has dominated medical science and research for the past 30 years since stress theory was abandoned. The DNA mechanism by itself does not explain how genetic information is converted into embryological development. In theory, continuous DNA/RNA signaling might explain adult biology, but despite more than 60 years of intense research, there is no convincing evidence that supports this idea. On the contrary, available evidence indicates that environmental factors are the most significant influence in adult biology, and this is difficult to explain purely in terms of DNA/RNA signaling. There is growing frustration with the lack of progress in biological research, most of which is inspired by the DNA/RNA paradigm, and attempts to rationalize adult biology in terms of DNA/RNA signaling are ever more strained, complex, and tenuous. This suggests that the DNA/RNA paradigm has reached the limits of its utility. Meanwhile, Selye's idea was never disproved, and its theoretical potency remains undiminished, even though the search for the stress mechanism was almost completely abandoned after no clue to its existence could be found. Since then, prominent experts have pronounced that no single mechanism could possibly explain the seemingly incompatible capillary gate and tissue repair theories, as well as the bewildering multitude of stress manifestations (Fink 2005; Yehuda and McEwen 2005). However, this turns out not to be the case.

Powerful scientific theories often appear long before their time, and must await the death of critics and the accumulation of supporting evidence before they are embraced. That seems to be the fate of Selye's ideas. Sixty years after its origin and 30 years after its demise, fresh evidence has finally enabled the first testable description of the long sought "*stress repair mechanism*" (SRM) that explains stress theory (Coleman 2010) (Figure 1). The SRM was identified after fresh information about coagulation factor VIII (Petrovitch 2003) inspired an extensive review of scientific literature. The distinctive physical and enzymatic properties of factor VIII served as a "Rosetta Stone" that deciphered SRM characteristics and first yielded a fresh explanation for coagulation (Coleman 2005), soon followed by explanations of atherosclerosis (Coleman 2005; Coleman 2006), capillary gate theory (Coleman 2005; Coleman 2005; Coleman 2007), and tissue repair theory (Coleman 2006, 2007). Finally, all of these seemingly disparate mechanisms were comprehended as elements of a single cohesive mechanism, and it became possible to describe the SRM (Coleman 2010).

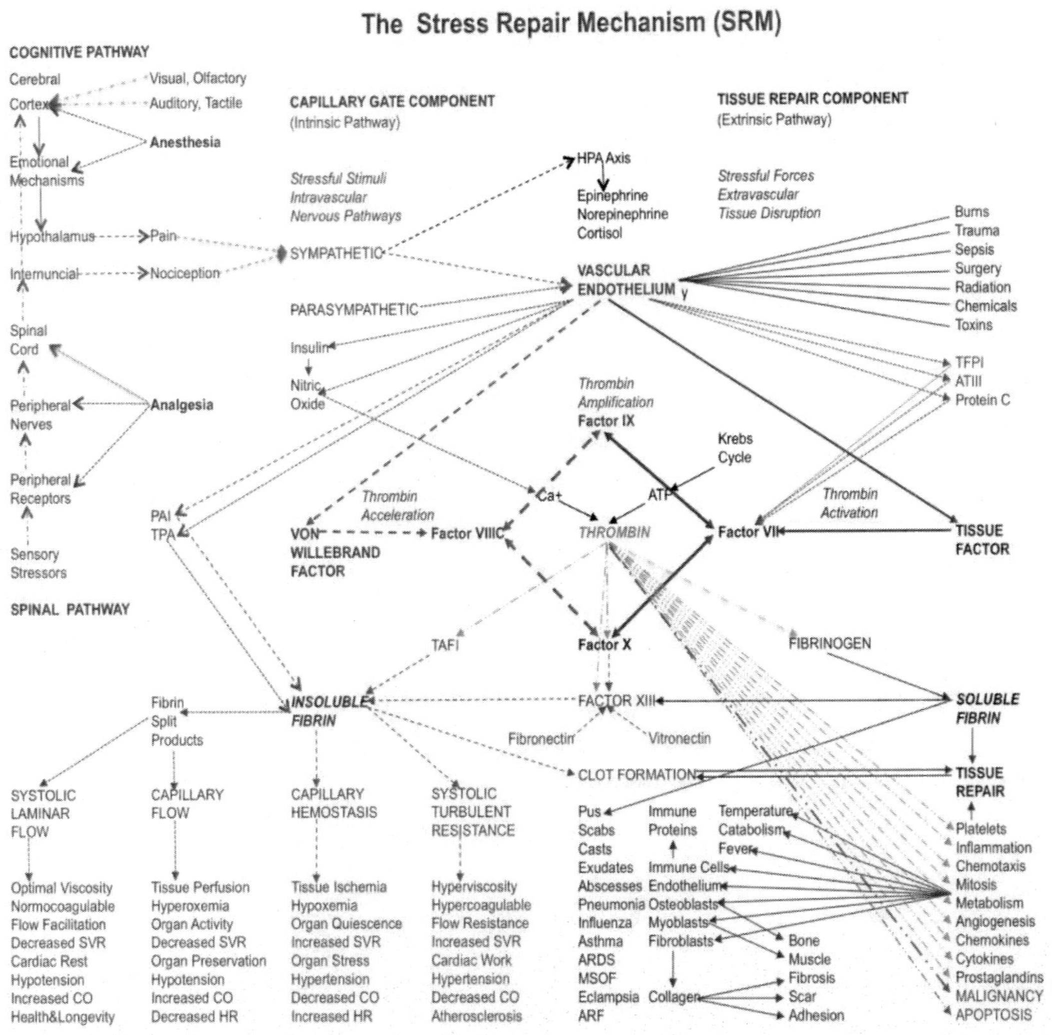

Figure 1. The Stress Repair Mechanism. The SRM appears complex, but its underlying structure is simple and symmetrical. Arrows represent the influence (direct and indirect) that one biological function or reaction brings to bear on another. The SRM is analogous to the older coagulation cascade concept, but it combines more recent research information with capillary gate theory and tissue repair theory to explain tissue repair, physiology and pathology as well as coagulation. The capillary gate component (red) corresponds to the intrinsic pathway of the coagulation cascade. The tissue repair component (blue) corresponds to the extrinsic pathway of the coagulation cascade. Both the SRM and the coagulation cascade generate thrombin (orange) plus soluble and insoluble fibrins. Inhibitory pathways appear in green. ARDS, adult respiratory distress syndrome; ARF, acute renal failure; ATIII, stoichiometric antithrombin III; ATP, adenosine triphosphate; CO, cardiac output; DIC, disseminated intravascular coagulation; HAPE, high-altitude pulmonary edema; HR, heart rate; MSOF, multi-system organ failure; SVR, systemic vascular resistance; TFPI, tissue factor pathway inhibitor.

Perhaps it is unsurprising that the SRM has remained elusive, because it is complex, counterintuitive, and at odds with most prevailing medical beliefs, practices, and assumptions. Daunting evidence of the relationships between coagulation, tissue repair, and nervous activity has long existed, but missing pieces of the puzzle have made it impossible to explain until very recently. Without an effective explanation, medical science has treated coagulation as an independent process that is unrelated to nervous system activity, hemodynamic physiology, and tissue repair, and whose sole purpose is to stem blood loss. Practitioners and researchers may therefore be startled to learn that coagulation enzymes are key elements of a cohesive mechanism that regulates tissue repair, hemodynamic physiology, and hemostasis in accord with combinations of neural activity and tissue disruption.

The previous generation of stress researchers was closer to success than they could have known. As they suspected, the vascular endothelium and blood-borne "coagulation" enzymes are the focus of SRM activity. They would be gratified that their capillary gate and tissue repair theories paved the path to SRM discovery, but surprised that these seemingly incompatible concepts represent sub-components of a cohesive mechanism. They might also be startled to see that the coagulation cascade that appeared during the heyday of stress research is strikingly similar to the SRM. Its "intrinsic pathway" is analogous to the "tissue repair component" of the SRM. Its "extrinsic pathway" is analogous to the "capillary gate component" of the SRM. Its "final common pathway" is clarified and extended by the previously unappreciated roles of thrombin, soluble fibrin, and insoluble fibrin. The two SRM components operate independently, but they share the dynamic interaction of coagulation factors VII, VIII, IX, and X that generates thrombin, soluble fibrin, and insoluble fibrin, whose combined effects account for all SRM manifestations. The extravascular tissue repair component regulates factor VII to generate thrombin and soluble fibrin for tissue repair. The intravascular capillary gate component regulates factor VIII, which accelerates thrombin generation to convert soluble fibrin into insoluble fibrin to enable hemostasis and regulate tissue perfusion, organ function, and tissue repair. Because they share the same enzymes, the activity of each component exaggerates that of the other to induce positive feedback that produces rapid, powerful, and focused responses to stressors, and their independent fluctuations explain the bewildering multitude of SRM manifestations that belie the presence of a single mechanism. If stressors subside, the subsequent tissue repair process invokes negative feedback in the form of tissue repair that restores SRM activity to maintenance levels. However, prolonged and exaggerated stressor activity causes positive feedback to overwhelm negative feedback with pathological consequences. Therefore, control of the SRM confers the ability to improve outcome in numerous pathological conditions. The SRM thus enables Selye's Unified Theory of Medicine. This chapter will describe the SRM and discuss its operation and its implications in detail.

Stress Theory and the SRM

SRM activity explains tissue repair and other manifestations of stress, homeostasis, allostasis, allostatic load and their relationships that cannot be explained by HPA hormones and immune activity alone. Without an effective explanation of tissue repair, the effects of stress have often been attributed to immune activity or stress hormones (epinephrine, norepinephrine, cortisol, glucagon, chemokines, cytokines, and so forth), both of which are routinely elevated in accord with SRM hyperactivity. For example, diabetes and rheumatoid diseases are imputed to be "autoimmune" phenomena. These and other mysterious pathologies are better explained by dysfunctional SRM hyperactivity that elevates immune activity and releases chemokines, cytokines, and other substances that are normally generated by the SRM during tissue repair. Surgical stress illustrates these differences because it stimulates sympathetic nervous system (SNS) activity that increases both SRM activity and HPA hormone release. The HPA hormones typically normalize within 24 hours, and therefore cannot explain the distant manifestations of surgical stress. Meanwhile, SRM hyperactivity peaks around 48 hours and persists for months. SRM hyperactivity explains all known manifestations of the surgical stress syndrome, including increases in heart disease and malignancy in the distant aftermath of surgery (see "surgical stress syndrome" below) (Hampton *et al.* 1991; Adembri *et al.* 2004; Monk *et al.* 2005; Exadaktylos *et al.* 2006; Modesti *et al.* 2009).

The SRM clarifies stress theory terms, as follows:

Allostasis is the process that enables an organism to maintain homeostasis in the presence of environmental stress via physiological and behavioral adaptation (Korte *et al.* 2005; Ganzel *et al.* 2010). Allostasis is known to involve the autonomic nervous system, the HPA axis, and cardiovascular, metabolic, and immune effects that are assumed to protect the body by responding to internal and external stimuli. SRM operation provides a fresh explanation. Emotional mechanisms continually adapt to environmental circumstances by altering autonomic balance to regulate hemodynamic physiology and facilitate "fight or flight" (see "allostasis" below) (Ahmed *et al.* 2001; Adamiec *et al.* 2003).

Allostatic Load is physiological "wear and tear" on the body that results from ongoing adaptive efforts to maintain stability (homeostasis) in response to environmental factors (von Kanel *et al.* 2003; von Kanel *et al.* 2006; Juster *et al.* 2010). Such "wear and tear" is explained by SRM hyperactivity that produces harmful excesses of SRM products and depletes reserves of their precursors and components, which sometimes causes abnormal SRM function.

The SRM similarly explains classical stress theory terms. *Eustress* is SRM activity that restores or enhances function. The SRM restores body structure following injury. Strength training causes the SRM to induce muscle cell proliferation and hypertrophy that increases muscle capacity (Chinni *et al.* 1999; Brostrom *et al.* 2003). Endurance conditioning causes the SRM to induce angiogenesis (capillary proliferation) that reduces vascular resistance, increases ejection fraction (which lowers resting heart rate), and increases exercise capacity (Wijnen *et al.* 1994; Ades *et al.* 1996; Prior *et al.* 2003; Franzoni *et al.* 2004; Sandercock *et al.* 2005; Rao *et al.* 2007; Zanesco and Antunes 2007). *Distress* is synonymous with disease. Harmful SRM hyperactivity produces excessive or defective quantities of thrombin, soluble fibrin, and insoluble fibrin. This can exhaust their precursors and cause abnormal SRM activity (see "DIC" below) (Genovese *et al.* 1980; Genovese *et al.* 1980; Genovese *et al.* 1982; Genovese *et al.* 1983; Genovese *et al.* 1983; Goudemand 1983; Chohan *et al.* 1984; Stevens *et al.* 1986; Ciavarella *et al.* 1987).

The SRM is consistent with the *general adaption syndrome* and extends it. *Alarm* is cognitive pathway activity (see "cognitive pathway" below) that detects and assesses danger, chooses between fight and flight, and activates the capillary gate component via hypothalamic pathways (see "capillary gate component" below). *Resistance* is persistent positive feedback caused by unrelenting stressors that perturb hemodynamic physiology, disrupt organ function, and deplete SRM reserves of ATP, fibrinogen, vitronectin, fibronectin, and enzymes. *Exhaustion* is stressor-induced organ failure and critical depletion of SRM resources.

The Three SRM Products: Thrombin, Soluble Fibrin and Insoluble Fibrin

Thrombin is the "universal enzyme of extracellular energy transduction." Though it is conventionally regarded as a "coagulation enzyme," it also energizes tissue repair. It transforms ATP energy into both cell and enzyme activities (Sutherland and Schurman 1987; Murakami *et al.* 1995; Goldsack *et al.* 1998; Warkentin *et al.* 1999; Armstrong *et al.* 2000; Mahajan *et al.* 2000; Sambrano *et al.* 2001; Haas 2002; Hedner 2002; Mann *et al.* 2003b; Moser and Patterson 2003; Archiniegas *et al.* 2004; Luo *et al.* 2005). Thrombin affects all cell types thus far tested via their protease activated receptors (PAR). These vary in type and number according to individual cell types (Brass and Molino 1997; Bretschneider *et al.* 1999; Chinni *et al.* 1999; Mahajan *et al.* 2000; Wang *et al.* 2000; Naldini *et al.* 2002; Chalmers *et al.* 2003; Pagel *et al.* 2003; Wang and Reiser 2003; Gorbacheva *et al.* 2005; Day *et al.* 2006). Thrombin activity requires ionized calcium (Ca^{2+}). Parathyroid glands regulate extracellular Ca^{2+} to optimize thrombin activity (Brass *et al.* 1978; Sakata and Aoki 1980; Sakariassen *et al.* 1984; von Brecht *et al.* 1986; Gurrieri 1990; Murdoch *et al.* 1994; Shapiro and Mistry 1996; Davies *et al.* 1997; Zuccala *et al.* 1997; Zuccala *et al.* 2000; Bobe *et al.* 2003; Brostrom *et al.* 2003; Butenas *et al.* 2003; James and Roche 2004; Jeng *et al.* 2004). Mg^+ competitively inhibits Ca^+ and mitigates thrombin activity (Erodi 1973; Sakariassen *et al.* 1984; Menzel *et al.* 1985; Fehlinger *et al.* 1986; Elin 1988; Seelig 1990; Galland 1991; Dedhia and Banks 1994; Fuentes *et al.* 1995; Scheibe *et al.* 2000; Mussoni *et al.* 2001; Baker and Worthley 2002a,b; Kondo *et al.* 2002; Rukshin *et al.* 2002; James and Cronje 2004; James and Roche 2004; Elsharnouby and Elsharnouby 2006; Barbagallo *et al.* 2007). Thrombin increases intracellular calcium levels and mitochondrial activity via PAR-1 receptors (Fuentes *et al.* 1995; Garcia *et al.* 1995; Bretschneider *et al.* 1999; Mahajan *et al.* 2000; Archiniegas *et al.* 2004; Jeng *et al.* 2004; Kaushal *et al.* 2004; Song *et al.* 2005; Zania *et al.* 2006). All cells thus far tested possess PAR (thrombin) receptors that are present in various combinations that are characteristic of specific cell types, and these determine cellular reactions to thrombin (Sabri *et al.* 2000; Karp *et al.* 2005). PAR (thrombin) receptors can be over-expressed during both malignancy and normal wound healing (Luo *et al.* 2005; Tantivejkul *et al.* 2005).

The SRM continuously generates thrombin in all tissues to energize tissue maintenance (Fenton *et al.* 1998; Stewart *et al.* 1999). It accelerates thrombin generation to energize hemostasis immediately after injury (Brummel *et al.* 2002). It then maintains lesser thrombin elevations to energize tissue repair (Karp *et al.* 2005). As healing nears completion, it reduces thrombin to maintenance levels, causing clot disintegration and apoptosis of repair cells that facilitates wound closure (Chinni *et al.* 1999; Chalmers *et al.* 2003). Thrombin energizes and orchestrates all elements of tissue maintenance and repair including the following:

- Chemotaxis of platelets, osteocytes, white blood cells, and other tissue repair cells (Hong and Levine 1976; Sabri *et al.* 2000; Brostrom *et al.* 2003; Karp *et al.* 2005)
- Mitosis (Pohl *et al.* 1979; Fenton *et al.* 1998; Brostrom *et al.* 2003; Wang and Reiser 2003, 2003)
- Metabolism (Brostrom *et al.* 2003)
- Hypertrophy (Glembotski *et al.* 1993; Rothman *et al.* 1994; Sabri *et al.* 2000; Brostrom *et al.* 2003; Imamura 2004; Okada *et al.* 2006)

- Angiogenesis (Tsopanoglou and Maragoudakis 1998; Archiniegas *et al.* 2004; Zania *et al.* 2006)
- Platelet activation, chemotaxis, and thromboxane release (Hornstra and Hemker 1979; Hornstra 1981; Tate and Rittenhouse 1993; Henriksen *et al.* 1997; Sambrano *et al.* 2001)
- Proliferation, spreading and gap formation in the vascular endothelium (Garcia *et al.* 1995; Asero *et al.* 2006)
- Release of chemokines, cytokines, interleukins, bradykinins, caspases, and prostaglandins (Hong and Levine 1976; Ueno *et al.* 1996; Naldini *et al.* 1998; Naldini *et al.* 2000; Naldini *et al.* 2002; Naldini *et al.* 2002; Naldini *et al.* 2003; Naldini *et al.* 2004; Ben Amor *et al.* 2005; Naldini *et al.* 2005; Okada *et al.* 2006; Naldini *et al.* 2006)
- Production of bone, muscle, collagen and immune activity by osteocytes, myocytes, fibroblasts, and immune cells (Pohl *et al.* 1979; Kuznik *et al.* 1985; Glembotski *et al.* 1993; Howells *et al.* 1993; Naldini *et al.* 1993; Tordai *et al.* 1993 ; Rothman *et al.* 1994; Naldini and Carney 1996; Goldsack *et al.* 1998; Chinni *et al.* 1999; Huang *et al.* 2000; Sabri *et al.* 2000; Howell *et al.* 2001; Laudes *et al.* 2002; Bobe *et al.* 2003; Hua *et al.* 2003; Tran and Stewart 2003; Vlahos *et al.* 2003; Song *et al.* 2005; Asero *et al.* 2006)
- Conversion of fibrinogen to soluble fibrin (Gurrieri 1990) that facilitates tissue repair
- Conversion of fibrillar soluble fibrin to three-dimensional insoluble fibrin (Brass *et al.* 1976; Holm *et al.* 1985; Malik 1987; Davies *et al.* 1997; Brummel *et al.* 1999; Brummel *et al.* 2002; Butenas and Mann 2002; Juhan-Vague and Hans 2003; Mosesson 2005; Weisel 2005; Bouma and Mosnier 2006) that enables hemostasis and regulates tissue repair and hemodynamic physiology
- Inflammation, which dissolves the "basement membrane" that binds cells in tight formation with one another and with the Vascular Endothelium to facilitate chemotaxis (Bretschneider *et al.* 1999; Bobe *et al.* 2003).
- Proliferation of astrocytes and glial cells in brain tissue (Wang and Reiser 2003, 2003).
- Activation of gelsolin that neutralizes actin (Smith *et al.* 1987)
- Complement activation that attacks foreign antigens (Gong *et al.* 2005)
- T-cell activation independent of an immune response (Howells *et al.* 1993; Day *et al.* 2006)
- Blast transformation in lymphocytes
- Increased macrophage phagocytic activity (Kuznik *et al.* 1985; Howells *et al.* 1993; Augustin *et al.* 1995; Tsopanoglou and Maragoudakis 1998; Jeng *et al.* 2004; Day *et al.* 2006; Zania *et al.* 2006)
- Activation of plasma (immune) cells and neutrophils (Kuznik *et al.* 1985; Malik 1987; Birkenbach *et al.* 1993)
- Release of "tumor necrosis factor" from microglial cells (Suo *et al.* 2003)
- Tumor growth, malignancy, and fibrosis (Chinni *et al.* 1999; Huang *et al.* 2000; Zain *et al.* 2000; Howell *et al.* 2001; Haas 2002; Chalmers *et al.* 2003; Hua *et al.* 2003; Pagel *et al.* 2003; Tsopanoglou and Maragoudakis 2004)

- Inhibits apoptosis (Turgeon *et al.* 1998; Mahajan *et al.* 2000; Wang *et al.* 2000; Choi *et al.* 2003; Pagel *et al.* 2003; Gorbacheva *et al.* 2005)
- Intracellular gap formation in the vascular endothelium that increases permeability (Garcia *et al.* 1995)
- Embryological development, tissue maintenance, wound healing (Fenton *et al.* 1998; Stewart *et al.* 1999; Schiller *et al.* 2002; Moser and Patterson 2003; Kaushal *et al.* 2004). Defects in factors VII, X and tissue factor that disrupt thrombin generation necessary for embryological development and tissue repair are generally lethal (Uprichard and Perry 2002)

Older studies have confused fibrinogen, soluble fibrin and insoluble fibrin, because they are nearly identical chemically (Bredbacka *et al.* 1994; Bredbacka and Edner 1994; Lip *et al.* 1995; Idell 2002; Weisel 2005). Their fluctuating equilibrium determines blood viscosity and coagulability (see "The capillary gate component" below).

Fibrinogen is a structurally complex protein molecule that exists in more than one form. It is the precursor of both soluble and insoluble fibrin. The liver produces and releases fibrinogen into the blood at steady rates. It cannot escape the intact vasculature. It is not directly involved in either tissue repair or hemostasis, but defective forms of insoluble fibrin are produced when fibrinogen is depleted (Holm *et al.* 1985; Plendl *et al.* 2002). It consists of alpha, beta and gamma subunits that are connected by disulfide bonds (Weisel 2005). Thrombin disrupts the disulfide bonds and enables the alpha, beta, and gamma fibrinogen subunits to polymerize into fibrillar (two-dimensional) strands of "soluble fibrin" (Gurrieri 1990; Garcia *et al.* 1995; Mosesson 2005).

Soluble fibrin is the universal protein of tissue repair. It is the precursor of insoluble fibrin, but it has no direct effect on blood viscosity and coagulability. It is the substance of pus, scabs, mucus, exudates, renal casts, and hyaline deposits (Gartner 1994; Idell 2002). Thrombin-generated soluble fibrin escapes from the vascular system through thrombin-induced inflammatory gaps in the vascular endothelium into thrombin-inflamed extravascular tissues to form a structural matrix that facilitates the formation of granulation tissue that fills wound cavities (Pohl *et al.* 1979; Malik 1987; Gurrieri 1990; Garcia *et al.* 1995; Goldsack *et al.* 1998; Idell 2002; Juhan-Vague and Hans 2003). Excessive soluble fibrin generation causes tissue edema and disrupts organ function. For example, soluble fibrin causes proteinuria and hyaline casts. It disrupts pulmonary function by flooding alveoli in pneumonia and influenza, and narrowing airway passages in asthma (Widdicombe 1992; Idell 2002, 2002; Kawada *et al.* 2003). Soluble fibrin deposits promote collagen production, fibrosis, sclerosis, adhesions, and scar formation (Fairley *et al.* 1983; Bredbacka *et al.* 1986; Tighe *et al.* 1989; Bredbacka *et al.* 1994; Bredbacka and Edner 1994; Ventura *et al.* 1997; Akassoglou *et al.* 2000; Fan *et al.* 2000; Rath *et al.* 2000; Rodriguez-Inigo *et al.* 2001; Akassoglou and Strickland 2002; Akassoglou *et al.* 2002; Laudes *et al.* 2002; Akassoglou *et al.* 2003; Fiorucci *et al.* 2004). For example, peritoneal soluble fibrin deposits produce peritoneal adhesions after surgery and infection, and alveolar soluble fibrin evolves into pulmonary fibrosis in the aftermath of acute respiratory distress syndrome (ARDS), chronic asthma, and prolonged pulmonary infection. Thrombin inhibition mitigates soluble fibrin generation and collagen production (Howell *et al.* 2001), but most anticoagulants have minimal effect on soluble fibrin deposits and collagen scars once they have formed (Schoots *et al.* 2004).

Insoluble fibrin is the universal polymer of hemostasis. It cannot escape the intact vascular system. It binds red cells and platelets together, and this produces several seemingly unrelated effects. It increases blood viscosity and coagulability, accelerates atherosclerosis, activates capillary hemostasis, and forms viscoelastic clots that stem blood loss and then regulate tissue repair (Vehar and Davie 1977; Goudemand 1983; Dufner and Marbet 2002; Wilmer *et al.* 2002; He *et al.* 2003; McIntosh *et al.* 2003; Kawasaki *et al.* 2004; Nielsen *et al.* 2004; Wettstein *et al.* 2004; Dargaud *et al.* 2005; Mosesson 2005). The generation and disintegration of insoluble fibrin explains viscoelastic clot formation, capillary hemostasis, hemodynamic physiology, organ regulation, tissue repair regulation, atherosclerosis acceleration, infarction, and the effects of anticoagulants and "vasoactive" drugs (Holemans 1965).

The conversion of soluble fibrin to insoluble fibrin occurs in a series of complex enzymatic interactions. Factor VIII accelerates thrombin generation to energize its enzymatic conversion of factor X to factor XIII (Vehar and Davie 1977; Dufner and Marbet 2002; Wettstein *et al.* 2004). Factor XIII adds plasminogen and fibronectin cross-links to fibrillar soluble fibrin to generate three-dimensional insoluble fibrin that spontaneously polymerizes into strands that bind red cells and platelets together (Tamaki and Aoki 1981; Goudemand 1983; Wilmer *et al.* 2002). The plasminogen cross-links spontaneously deteriorate into plasmin that disintegrates insoluble fibrin into inert fibrin split products (FSP, or d-Dimer), unless plasminogen is continuously stabilized by thrombin via thrombin activated fibrinolysis inhibitor (TAFI) (Castellino 1981; Walsh and Ahmad 2002; Juhan-Vague and Hans 2003; Castoldi and Rosing 2004; Stasko *et al.* 2004). Parasympathetic nervous system (PNS) activity stimulates the release of nitric oxide, which binds avidly to Ca^{2+}, inactivates thrombin, and accelerates the disintegration of insoluble fibrin (James and Roche 2004). The effects of insoluble fibrin are thus readily reversible, and this could explain the fluctuations of blood viscosity, tissue perfusion, and organ regulation in accord with autonomic balance.

Hemophilia and von Willebrand disease coagulopathies illustrate the difference between soluble fibrin and insoluble fibrin. Both conditions paralyze factor VIII activity, which impairs the ability to convert soluble fibrin to insoluble fibrin for hemostasis. Afflicted patients retain the normal ability to generate soluble fibrin to repair tissues and produce pus, scabs, exudates, soluble fibrin deposits, fibrosis, scars, and adhesions (Willert *et al.* 1983; Markakis *et al.* 1984). Like normal individuals, they produce excessive quantities of soluble fibrin in accord with pneumonia, influenza, ARDS, multi-organ failure syndrome (MOFS), asthma, and eclampsia (Roberts *et al.* 1989; Tighe *et al.* 1989; Widdicombe 1992; Ventura *et al.* 1997; Rath *et al.* 2000; Kawada *et al.* 2003). However, their inability to produce factor VIII in normal quality and/or quantity inhibits their ability to accelerate thrombin generation to activate platelets, energize the enzymatic conversion of soluble fibrin to insoluble fibrin, and stabilize the insoluble fibrin molecule via "thrombin-activated fibrinolysis inhibitor" (TAFI) (Hornstra and Hemker 1979; Antovic *et al.* 2002; Grunewald *et al.* 2002; Grunewald *et al.* 2002; Malyszko *et al.* 2002; Setian *et al.* 2002; Wilmer *et al.* 2002; Lisman *et al.* 2003; Stasko *et al.* 2004; Malyszko *et al.* 2006). This explains why they exhibit abnormally low blood viscosity and coagulability, retarded atherosclerosis, and reduced incidence of heart disease, as well as defective coagulation and capillary hemostasis (Rosendaal *et al.* 1990; Koumbarelis *et al.* 1994; Cheras *et al.* 1997). Defects or deficiencies in factor XIII also disrupt the conversion of soluble fibrin to insoluble fibrin by inhibiting the installation of plasminogen and fibronectin cross-links in the insoluble fibrin structure, but these coagulopathies do not impair thrombin generation and platelet activation and are usually less severe (Tamaki and Aoki 1982; Zlokovic *et al.* 1995; Zhang *et al.* 1999).

Insoluble fibrin elevations cause increased viscosity and coagulability that pre-disposes to disseminated intravascular coagulation (DIC), thrombophlebitis, pulmonary embolus, and accelerated atherosclerosis (Tran *et al.* 1984; Gutstein 1988; O'Donnell *et al.* 2000; O'Donnell *et al.* 2001; Lip *et al.* 2002; Toh and Dennis 2003). Insoluble fibrin generation also closes the capillary gate and disrupts perfusion and oxygenation in organs and tissues (see "Capillary Gate Component" below). This predisposes to stroke (Wu *et al.* 1998; Jaeger and Labarrere 2003), mental disturbances (Zerbino and Lukasevich 1982, 1983), myocardial infarction (Kent and Epstein 1976; Taylor *et al.* 1987; Wu *et al.* 1998; Gerber *et al.* 2000; Osterud and Bjorklid 2001), renal dysfunction (Gartner 1994), bowel infarction, bowel ileus, and increased vascular resistance.

The Central Role of the Vascular Endothelium

The vascular endothelium is the focus of SRM activity. It is a ubiquitous, diaphanous, selectively permeable layer of cells, one cell thick, that lines all blood vessels and is the sole constituent of capillary walls. It controls the dynamic interaction of enzymatic factors VII, VIII, IX, and X. The vascular endothelium secretes tissue factor hormone into extravascular tissues and then insulates it from the factor VII flowing freely in blood, so that tissue damage exposes tissue factor to blood-borne factor VII and activates the tissue repair component (see "Tissue Repair Component" below) (Weiss *et al.* 1989; Fleck *et al.* 1990; Stvrtinova *et al.* 1998; Siegbahn 2000; Siegbahn *et al.* 2000; Bajaj *et al.* 2001; Sajadi *et al.* 2003).

The vascular endothelium also functions as a neuroendocrine organ that releases nitric oxide hormone and von Willebrand factor into blood in accord with autonomic balance to regulate the capillary gate component (see "Capillary Gate Component" below) (Itakura *et al.* 1977; Lau *et al.* 1991; Burnstock and Ralevic 1994; van Zwieten and Doods 1995; Muller *et al.* 2002; Kvasnicka 2003). Endothelial cells respond to their immediate surroundings and communicate with one another via electrical signals. Endothelial cells also produce fibronectin, vitronectin (Goudemand 1983), tissue factor pathway inhibitor (TFPI) (Bajaj *et al.* 2001), protein C (Esmon 2004), and tissue plasminogen activator (TPA) to enable and regulate SRM function (Zlokovic 1997; Idell 2002).

The Dynamic Interaction of Factors VII, VIII, IX, and X

The interaction of hepatic enzyme factors VII, VIII, IX, and X generates thrombin, soluble fibrin, and insoluble fibrin. Tissue factor activates factor VII to *initiate* the interaction (Weiss *et al.* 1989; Fleck *et al.* 1990; McVey 1999; Butenas *et al.* 2000; Siegbahn 2000; Rodriguez-Inigo *et al.* 2001; Welty-Wolf *et al.* 2001; Butenas *et al.* 2002; Butenas and Mann 2002; Butenas *et al.* 2003; Butenas *et al.* 2003; Himber *et al.* 2003; Cirillo *et al.* 2004; Hjortoe *et al.* 2004). Factor VII slowly and continuously penetrates the intact vascular endothelium and enters extravascular tissues, where tissue factor activates it. This continuously generates small amounts of thrombin in all tissues to energize tissue maintenance (Stewart *et al.* 1999; Mullins *et al.* 2009), but thrombin generated by factor VII alone is insufficient for hemostasis or tissue repair (Butenas and Mann 2002). Tissue injury disrupts the vascular endothelium and exposes tissue factor to factors VII, VIII, IX and X simultaneously. The resulting interaction accelerates thrombin generation to energize platelet activation and clot formation. The viscoelastic clot then substitutes for the damaged vascular endothelium and regulates contact between blood enzymes and tissue factor in injured tissues. Factor VIII cannot penetrate the clot due to its large molecular size. Factors VII, IX, and X penetrate the clot to interact with tissue factor and generate thrombin in levels that energize tissue repair (see "Tissue Repair Component" below) (Vehar and Davie 1977; Goudemand 1983; Butenas and Mann 2002; Dufner and Marbet 2002; Wilmer *et al.* 2002; He *et al.* 2003; McIntosh *et al.* 2003; Nielsen *et al.* 2004; Wettstein *et al.* 2004; Dargaud *et al.* 2005; Mosesson 2005; Audu *et al.* 2006).

The priority of tissue development, maintenance, and repair is illustrated by anti-coagulants and defects that affect factors VII and X and tissue factor, and disrupt embryological development, tissue maintenance, and tissue repair (Brass *et al.* 1978; Vinckier and Vermylen 1984; Fenton *et al.* 1998; Dalen *et al.* 1999; Stewart *et al.* 1999; Warkentin *et al.* 1999; Howell *et al.* 2001). In contrast, defects in hemostasis factors VIII, IX and XIII are non-teratogenic and survivable (Willert *et al.* 1983). Heparin is non-teratogenic because it affects only factor VIII.

The SRM Components

The SRM consists of a *tissue repair component* that governs factor VII activity in extravascular tissues, and a *capillary gate component* that governs factor VIII activity in flowing blood. Factors IX and X are produced continuously, so they do not fluctuate. Both components share the enzymatic interaction of factors VII, VIII, IX, and X, so that the activity of each synergistically exaggerates that of the other. This explains how the SRM generates and focuses positive feedback, and produces complex manifestations.

The Tissue Repair Component

The *tissue repair component* continuously maintains and repairs tissues by elevating thrombin levels in injured tissues. It consists of the vascular endothelium, tissue factor hormone, and the enzymatic interaction of factors VII, VIII, IX, and X. The selectively permeable vascular endothelium allows the slow, continuous penetration of factor VII from blood into healthy extravascular tissues, where tissue factor activates it to generate small amounts of thrombin that energize fibroblast mitosis and collagen production to maintain tissues (Stewart *et al.* 1999; Howell *et al.* 2001; Fiorucci *et al.* 2004).

Trauma disrupts the fragile vascular endothelium and directly exposes tissue factor to blood enzymes (Weiss *et al.* 1989; Fleck *et al.* 1990; Imamura 2004). Factor VII activation by tissue factor *initiates* the enzymatic interaction and determines its magnitude and location (Weiss *et al.* 1989; Himber *et al.* 2003; Cirillo *et al.* 2004). Factors IX and X *amplify* thrombin production to moderate levels that energize tissue repair (Sutherland and Schurman 1987; Butenas and Mann 2002; Audu *et al.* 2006). Factor VIII *accelerates* thrombin production to high levels to energize its conversion of factor X to factor XIII to generate insoluble fibrin for hemostasis (Barnhart 1978; Hornstra and Hemker 1979; Hornstra 1981; Chesebro *et al.* 1995; Butenas and Mann 2002; Grunewald *et al.* 2002; Hedner 2002). Pulsatile blood flow thrusts platelets into damaged tissues (Tangelder *et al.* 1985), where thrombin chemotaxis attracts them and insoluble fibrin binds them into a short-lived "white clot" (Hornstra 1981). Thrombin-activated platelets release thromboxane that induces local vasoconstriction to temporarily reduce flow and turbulence, which increases coagulability. Rising levels of insoluble fibrin increase local blood viscosity to reduce pulsatile turbulent mixing below a threshold (see "turbulence mechanism" below), whereupon insoluble fibrin binds red cells into a durable, viscoelastic, selectively permeable "red clot" that substitutes for the damaged vascular endothelium by isolating damaged tissues from flowing blood (Brummel *et al.* 2002; Puckett *et al.* 2003; Alexandrov *et al.* 2004; Kawasaki *et al.* 2004; Wettstein *et al.* 2004). The enormous molecular size of factor VIII prevents it from penetrating the clot and interacting with the other enzymes, so that clot formation is self-limiting.

The red clot regulates thrombin in damaged tissues (Schramm *et al.* 1977; van Gelder *et al.* 1994). Factors VII, IX, and X penetrate the clot and interact with tissue factor to generate thrombin, which enhances insoluble fibrin generation and preservation, reduces clot permeability, and constrains thrombin production in the manner of negative feedback. This maintains thrombin at levels optimal for tissue repair (Schramm *et al.* 1977; Weiss *et al.* 1989; van Gelder *et al.* 1994; Scott 1998; Haas 2002; Stasko *et al.* 2004). Tissue repair then proceeds in predictable stages (Choi *et al.* 2003). Bradykinins, caspases, prostaglandins, chemokines, cytokines, and interleukins induce inflammation and enable cell-to-cell communications that coordinate cell repair activities and determine the stages of wound healing (Hu and Xie 1994; Kenny *et al.* 2002; Nakase *et al.* 2003; Chanson *et al.* 2005; Xia *et al.* 2010). Inflammation loosens cell connections to facilitate the entry and movement of soluble fibrin and repair cells (Garcia *et al.* 1995). Soluble fibrin creates a structural matrix that facilitates the formation of granulation tissue that fills empty wound spaces (Akassoglou *et al.* 2003). Chemotaxis attracts fibroblasts, myoblasts, osteocytes, and immune cells into inflamed tissues, where they proliferate and produce collagen, muscle, bone, and immune activity to replace damaged tissues, inhibit infection, and remove debris and foreign substances (Howells *et al.* 1993; Howell *et al.* 2001; Fiorucci *et al.* 2004). Angiogenesis perfuses proliferating repair tissues. Increases in cell metabolism cause temperature elevation in healing tissues (Zain *et al.* 2000). As tissue repair nears completion, proliferation and spreading of the vascular endothelium restores the normal barrier between blood and extravascular tissues, which reduces thrombin generation to maintenance levels. This undermines clot integrity and repair cell viability, so that the clot disintegrates, apoptosis facilitates wound closure by actomyosin, and structural integrity is restored (Henson *et al.* 2002; Chalmers *et al.* 2003; Pagel *et al.* 2003; Sersa *et al.* 2007).

The tissue repair component automatically forms abscesses, furuncles, and fistulas that isolate and expel bacteria and foreign substances. Trauma, burns, toxic chemicals, sepsis, and radiation disrupt the vascular endothelium, activate the tissue repair component (Welty-Wolf *et al.* 2001), and release inflammatory substances that activate the capillary gate component by stimulating its nervous sensors.

The Capillary Gate Component

The *capillary gate component* consists of factors VII, VIIIC, IX and X, the autonomic nervous system, the vascular endothelium, von Willebrand factor, and nitric oxide. It generates and disintegrates insoluble fibrin in accord with autonomic balance to simultaneously govern a *capillary gate mechanism* (see below) that regulates tissue perfusion, capillary hemostasis, and organ function, and a *turbulence mechanism* (see below) that regulates blood viscosity (flow resistance), blood coagulability, and atherosclerosis (Schneider 1949; Burnstock and Ralevic 1994; Groebe 1996; Park 2002). The capillary gate component explains why von Willebrand factor, factor VIII, insoluble fibrin, d-dimer (fibrin split products), blood viscosity, blood coagulability, blood pressure, cardiac output, heart rate, capillary hemostasis, tissue perfusion, tissue oxygenation, atherosclerosis, and organ function all fluctuate in accord with autonomic balance (Schneider 1949; Chohan *et al.* 1977; Itakura *et al.* 1977; von Kries *et al.* 1981; Cahalan *et al.* 1987; Nees 1989, 1989; Penny *et al.* 1991; Burnstock and Ralevic 1994; Akca *et al.* 1999; Beyak *et al.* 2000; Kocsis *et al.* 2000; Sielenkamper *et al.* 2000; Klingel *et al.* 2002; Beyak *et al.* 2003; Toda *et al.* 2005, 2007; Kang *et al.* 2008). Its *acute* hyperactivation causes infarction, pulmonary embolus, thrombophlebitis, and high altitude pulmonary edema (HAPE) (Chohan *et al.* 1974; Kloner *et al.* 1974; Kent and Epstein 1976; Genovese *et al.* 1980; Chiariello *et al.* 1983; O'Brodovich *et al.* 1984; Bartsch *et al.* 1987; Barinov *et al.* 1989; Bartsch *et al.* 1989; Gasser *et al.* 1995; Ito *et al.* 1996; Wu *et al.* 1998; Gibson *et al.* 1999; Ito *et al.* 1999; O'Donnell *et al.* 2000; O'Donnell *et al.* 2001; Roe *et al.* 2001; Segler 2001; Rezkalla and Kloner 2002; Kario *et al.* 2003; Mann *et al.* 2003a; Das *et al.* 2004; Wittstein *et al.* 2005; Fagenholz *et al.* 2007). Its *chronic* hyperactivation accelerates atherosclerosis and capillary senescence, and causes diabetes, hypertension, and organ failure (Schneider 1949; Penny *et al.* 1991; Friedman *et al.* 1997; Lip *et al.* 1997; Cicco *et al.* 1999; Vicaut 1999; Veyradier *et al.* 2000; Esler *et al.* 2001; Naeije and Vachiery 2001; Bogar 2002; Hlubocka *et al.* 2002; Muller *et al.* 2002; Das *et al.* 2004; Choi 2005; Farkas *et al.* 2005; Danson and Paterson 2006; Savoia and Schiffrin 2006).

The chimeric factor VIII complex links the sympathetic nervous system (SNS) to the enzymatic interaction of factors VII, VIIIC, IX and X. Factor VIII consists of von Willebrand factor (VWF) produced by the vascular endothelium and factor VIIIC produced by the liver. These bind together to form factor VIII in blood circulation and exert their effects in concert. Factor VIIIC is a hepatic enzyme that is released into blood at constant rates, but it is so labile that it cannot exert its enzymatic effects unless it is continuously stabilized by VWF. SNS activity releases VWF into blood, so that VWF blood levels constantly fluctuate in accord with stressful stimuli. SNS activity thus regulates the activity and half-life of factor VIII. Factor VIII interacts with factors VII, IX, and X to accelerate thrombin generation to energize its conversion of factor X to factor XIII. Factor XIII installs "cross-links" of fibronectin and plasminogen to convert soluble fibrin to insoluble fibrin in capillaries and flowing blood to "close" the capillary gate (Mannucci *et al.* 1971; Grant 1990; Lau *et al.* 1991; Sadler 1991; van Mourik *et al.* 1999; Federici 2003; Sadler *et al.* 2006; Hovinga *et al.* 2007). Continued factor VIII activity inhibits the spontaneous disintegration of insoluble fibrin into inert fibrin split products via thrombin activated fibrinolysis inhibitor (TAFI) (von Kries *et al.* 1981; Wilmer *et al.* 2002; Stasko *et al.* 2004; Bouma and Mosnier 2006; Malyszko *et al.* 2006).

Parasympathetic nervous system activity disintegrates insoluble fibrin by releasing nitric oxide from the vascular endothelium to "open" the capillary gate. Nitric oxide is a ubiquitous gaseous signaling molecule that binds avidly to Ca^{2+}, which inactivates thrombin, and thereby accelerates the spontaneous disintegration of insoluble fibrin (Epstein *et al.* 1976; Brugger *et al.* 1985; Amano *et al.* 1994; van Zwieten and Doods 1995; Fricchione *et al.* 1996; Hudetz 1997; Webb *et al.* 2000; Si and Lee 2002; Hudetz 2003; Baskurt *et al.* 2004; Dijkstra *et al.* 2004; Toda *et al.* 2005; Anderson *et al.* 2006). Nitric oxide is also bactericidal, so that PNS activity inhibits infection as well as promotes tissue perfusion and oxygenation (Saraiva *et al.* 2011).

Capillary gate component operation requires the continuous "leakage" of tissue factor from extravascular tissues into blood circulation to activate factor VII, without which factors VIII, IX, and X remain inert. The vascular endothelium releases stoichiometric antithrombin III (ATIII), tissue factor pathway inhibitor (TFPI), and protein C hormones into blood to quench excessive factor VII activity. Otherwise, factors VIII, IX, and X could interact with activated factor VII to exaggerate thrombin generation harmfully in flowing blood (Taylor *et al.* 1987; Weiss *et al.* 1989; Butenas *et al.* 2000; Bajaj *et al.* 2001; Hoppensteadt *et al.* 2001; Butenas and Mann 2002; Walsh and Ahmad 2002; Esmon 2004; van der Poll *et al.* 2005; Audu *et al.* 2006; Robriquet *et al.* 2006; Griffin *et al.* 2007; Mosnier *et al.* 2007).

The Capillary Gate Mechanism

Capillary perfusion is the essence of hemodynamic physiology. Athletic conditioning induces angiogenesis that enhances tissue perfusion and oxygenation, mitigates flow resistance, reduces blood pressure, and enhances ejection fraction, which slows heart rate via the Starling mechanism (Eichner 1983; Baron 1994; Wijnen *et al.* 1994; Ades *et al.* 1996; Yi *et al.* 1999; Lee *et al.* 2000; van den Burg *et al.* 2000; Carr 2001; Long *et al.* 2001; Moser and Patterson 2003; Prior *et al.* 2003; Franzoni *et al.* 2004; Schmermund 2004; Choi 2005; Lloyd *et al.* 2005; Sandercock *et al.* 2005; Rao *et al.* 2007; Zanesco and Antunes 2007). Allostatic load accelerates capillary senescence (Rakusan and Nagai 1994; Phillip *et al.* 2003; Chen and Goligorsky 2006), which increases vascular resistance, impairs tissue and organ perfusion, inhibits glucose uptake, and causes diabetes and essential hypertension (Schneider 1949; Ventura *et al.* 1984; Penny *et al.* 1991; Lip *et al.* 1995; Lip *et al.* 1997; Boudier 1999; Vicaut 1999; Esler *et al.* 2001; Lip *et al.* 2001; Naeije and Vachiery 2001; Lip *et al.* 2002; Lip *et al.* 2002; Lip *et al.* 2002; Kawut *et al.* 2005; Kawut *et al.* 2005; Savoia and Schiffrin 2006).

The capillary gate is a sub-microscopic, molecular mechanism that governs capillary flow, tissue perfusion, organ function, and capillary hemostasis despite the absence of contractile musculature in capillaries (Itakura *et al.* 1977; Huang *et al.* 1990; Hudetz 1997; Ito and Iwakura 1998; Ito *et al.* 1999; Hudetz 2003). It operates efficiently, because capillary flow, pressure, and turbulence are minimal, and capillary surface area is greater than that of all other vessels combined. The capillary gate explains hemodynamic physiology and "vasoactive" drug effects in terms of fibrinogenesis and fibrinolysis (the generation and disintegration of insoluble fibrin) as opposed to "vasoconstriction," "vasodilation," and "stiffness" of muscular arterioles that become rapidly exhausted (Holemans 1965; Chohan *et al.* 1977; Barinov *et al.* 1989; Nees 1989, 1989; Grant 1990; Groebe 1996; Ito *et al.* 1999;

Ciardella 2004; James and Cronje 2004; Trachte *et al.* 2005; Korom *et al.* 2006; Behr-Roussel *et al.* 2007; Lewis *et al.* 2007).

SNS activity "closes" the capillary gate by causing the vascular endothelium cells of the capillary walls to release von Willebrand factor (Mannucci *et al.* 1971; Sadler 1991; Veyradier *et al.* 2000; Federici 2003; Sadler *et al.* 2006). This release activates factor VIIIC, which converts fibrinogen and fibronectin at adjacent binding sites into polymerizing strands of insoluble fibrin that bind to passing red cells and halt capillary flow (Goudemand 1983; Witte 1984; Zhang *et al.* 1999; Esler *et al.* 2001; Casonato *et al.* 2003; Kawasaki *et al.* 2004).

PNS activity "opens" the capillary gate by releasing nitric oxide from the vascular endothelium in visceral organs, including eye, brain, lung, gastrointestinal tract, urinary tract, and pancreas via direct parasympathetic innervation (van Zwieten and Doods 1995; Hudetz 1997; Si and Lee 2002; Hudetz 2003; Wojtarowicz *et al.* 2003; Dijkstra *et al.* 2004; Toda *et al.* 2005; Anderson *et al.* 2006). PNS activity also releases insulin, which releases nitric oxide from the capillaries of skeletal muscle and other peripheral tissues where direct PNS innervation is absent (Wamhoff *et al.* 1976; Belcaro *et al.* 1992; Morita-Tsuzuki *et al.* 1993; Watkins *et al.* 2000; Martin *et al.* 2001; Kvist-Reimer *et al.* 2002; Vincent *et al.* 2003; Colantuoni *et al.* 2005; Ahmed 2006; Ali and Rakkah 2007; Ayala *et al.* 2007; Behr-Roussel *et al.* 2007). This explains why insulin prolongs bleeding time, reduces systemic vascular resistance, increases cardiac index, aggravates angina, and counteracts "vasopressor" (fibrinogenic) drugs (Wamhoff *et al.* 1976; Figueras *et al.* 1979; Rich *et al.* 1992; Singh *et al.* 1993; Baron 1994; Lee *et al.* 2000; Carr 2001; Ciardella 2004; Parker *et al.* 2007); why allostatic load inhibits insulin effects(Brandi *et al.* 1990); and why diabetes and hypertension are closely related (Schneider 1949; Hassoun *et al.* 1989; He 1990; Penny *et al.* 1991; Boudier 1999; Cicco *et al.* 1999; Vicaut 1999; Yi *et al.* 1999; Lee *et al.* 2000; McDonagh and Hokama 2000; Veyradier *et al.* 2000; Esler *et al.* 2001; Long *et al.* 2001; Naeije and Vachiery 2001; Bogar 2002; Hlubocka *et al.* 2002; Muller *et al.* 2002; Adamiec *et al.* 2003; Choi 2005; Colantuoni *et al.* 2005; Kawut *et al.* 2005; Kawut *et al.* 2005; Khan *et al.* 2005; Wallis *et al.* 2005; Caruso *et al.* 2006; Caruso *et al.* 2006; Savoia and Schiffrin 2006; Messerli *et al.* 2007; Schafer *et al.* 2008). Nitric oxide is also bactericidal, so that PNS activity inhibits infection as well as enhances tissue perfusion and oxygenation (Saraiva *et al.* 2011).

The vascular endothelium additionally regulates capillary flow via TPA (tissue plasminogen activator) that disintegrates insoluble fibrin, and its rapid inhibitor, plasminogen activator inhibitor (PAI-1) (Zlokovic *et al.* 1995; Zlokovic 1997; Kranenburg *et al.* 2002; Kim *et al.* 2003). Astrocytes proliferate when exposed to thrombin and release TPA to ensure brain perfusion (Zlokovic 1997; Wang and Reiser 2003). Their anticoagulant effects necessitate abundant tissue factor, which explains the exaggerated morbidity of brain injury (Fleck *et al.* 1990; Bredbacka and Edner 1994; Hua *et al.* 2003).

Angiodysplasia, Angioneurotic Edema, Coagulopathy, and the Capillary Gate Mechanism

Coagulopathies reveal capillary gate characteristics. Capillary structural integrity requires VWF, so that chronic VWF damage and/or deficiency cause flow-related capillary damage called *angiodysplasia* as well as von Willebrand coagulopathy (Rosborough and Swaim 1978;

O'Brien 1996; Fujita *et al.* 2000; Koscielny *et al.* 2000; Veyradier *et al.* 2001; Rodeghiero 2002; Warkentin *et al.* 2003; Basso and Keeling 2004; Leibovitz *et al.* 2004). Sudden VWF destruction by complement (usually triggered by bee sting and other antigens) disrupts capillary gate structure, causing angioneurotic edema (anaphylaxis) wherein vascular resistance and blood pressure drop sharply as blood shifts from larger vessels into capillaries, causing lethal airway edema, while coagulation enzymes and cardiac output remain unaffected (Ferrell *et al.* 1983; Bergamaschini *et al.* 1995; Bergamaschini *et al.* 1996). VWF is released from the vascular endothelium in accord with SNS activity, and this may explain the fluctuating severity of the coagulopathy in individual patients. Defective VIIIC (true hemophilia) paralyzes capillary gate regulation, causing exercise intolerance, but capillary gate structure is not affected and patients remain susceptible to anaphylaxis (Koch *et al.* 1984; Jadhav and Warrier 2000; Kadar *et al.* 2007).

A sex-linked gene controls VIIIC production. Defects in this gene that affect the quality or quantity of VIIIC production cause true hemophilia, which is transmitted by female "carriers" and primarily afflicts their male offspring. This infamous genetic defect plagued the royal families of Europe in the previous century. The condition causes a severe bleeding diathesis in most victims, but the severity varies in individual cases, depending on the ability of the individual patient to generate functional insoluble fibrin. This is reflected by 20-fold individual differences in blood viscosity (Rodeghiero 2002) and variable individual response to factor VII therapy in hemophilia patients (Casonato *et al.* 2003; Federici 2003).

A somatic gene controls the production of VWF (Lindenfeld *et al.* 1985, 2005). Defects in the quality or quantity of its production cause von Willebrand's disease, which afflicts males and females equally (Kurth *et al.* 1999). Its severe forms cause a bleeding diathesis that cannot be clinically distinguished from true hemophilia. Von Willebrand disease is more common and usually much less severe than true hemophilia. Fluctuating levels of SNS activity that affect VWF levels and therefore affect factor VIII activity and half-life explain the fluctuating severity of the bleeding disorder observed in individual von Willebrand's disease patients (Gleick 1988; Rodeghiero 2002).

The Turbulence Mechanism

Hemoglobin encapsulation does not enhance oxygen delivery. Instead, red cell morphology alters blood turbulence, and thereby beneficially alters blood viscosity, coagulability, atherosclerosis, and hemodynamic efficiency (Lindenfeld *et al.* 1985; Cinar *et al.* 1999; Suttner *et al.* 2004; Tous *et al.* 2004; Lindenfeld et al. 2005). This explains why red cells are present in far greater quantities than needed for effective oxygen delivery.

In "Newtonian" fluids such as water and oil, pipe flow turbulence causes viscosity (flow resistance) to increase exponentially with velocity (Hof et al. 2004; see Figure 2). Mammalian blood, however, is a "non-Newtonian" fluid that exhibits exponential *declines* in viscosity with increasing velocity. This is because bi-concave mammalian red cells spontaneously form highly efficient, self-organizing "aggregate" flow patterns that suppress systolic turbulence to optimize blood acceleration, cardiac output, and peak end-systolic velocity (Seo *et al.* 1991; Baskurt and Meiselman 2003; Baskurt *et al.* 2004; Rampling *et al.* 2004; Yalcin *et al.* 2004; Baskurt and Meiselman 2007; Meiselman *et al.* 2007; Baskurt and Meiselman 2008). The resulting hemodynamic efficiency explains why the hearts of both elephant and mouse weigh only 0.6% of their body weight (Holt *et al.* 1968). Diastolic deceleration disrupts the aggregates, and suddenly converts their kinetic energy into Newtonian turbulence that dissipates in a traveling pulse wave (see Figure 3). The pulse wave periodically increases viscosity, halts flow, generates *turbulent mixing* that inhibits coagulation and atherosclerosis, and induces *turbulent lateral forces* that explain blood pressure and the palpable pulse (Parker 1977; Laurent *et al.* 2003). Diastolic turbulence is inversely related to red cell mass. Polycythemia decreases turbulence, increases coagulability, and accelerates atherosclerosis. Anemia progressively increases turbulence, paralyses coagulation, and retards atherosclerosis (Fernandez *et al.* 1985; Couch and Stumpf 1990; Quaknine-Orlando *et al.* 1999; Casonato *et al.* 2001; Malyszko *et al.* 2002; Kwaan and Wang 2003; Bogar *et al.* 2005; Hardy *et al.* 2006).

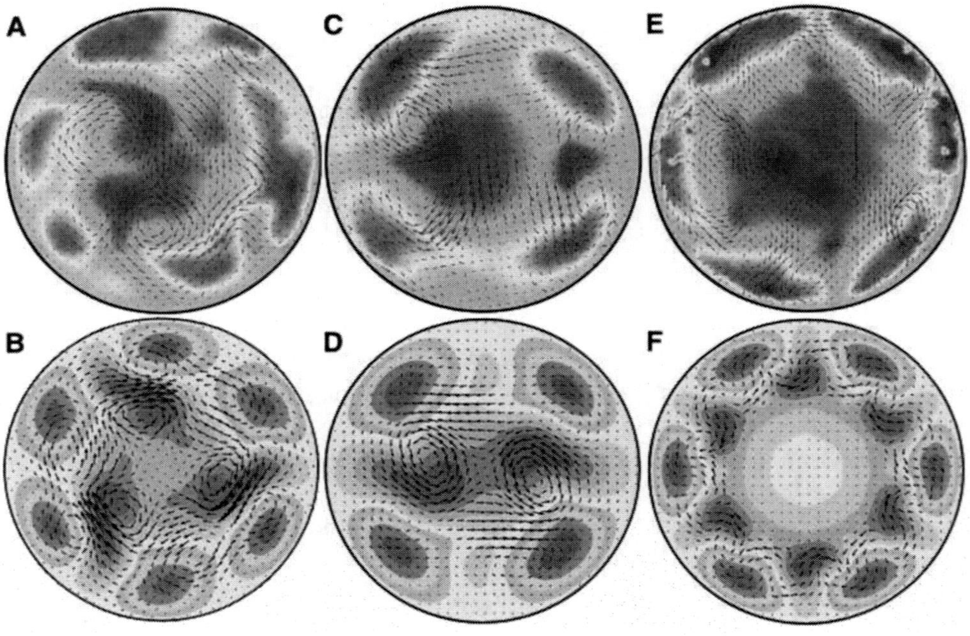

Figure 2. Newtonian pipe flow turbulence (from Hof *et al.* 2004 – reproduced with permission from the American Association for the Advancement of Science). Turbulent forward flow appears as fast-moving "jet streams" (shown in red) that form along the inner walls of pipes and force slow-moving fluid to the center, where it moves *backward* (shown in blue), causing increased viscosity (flow resistance). A, C and E are laser photographs that show "fast (A), faster (C) and fastest (E)" flow acceleration that produce "small (A), medium (C) and large (E)" increases in turbulent intensity. B, D and F are computer simulations that predicted the experimental results shown by A, C and E. Similar arterial turbulence during diastole mobilizes particulate deposits from arterial walls to prevent atherosclerosis. It also generates lateral forces that press on the inner walls of the vessel, which explains blood pressure and the palpable pulse.

Oil must flow through a pipeline at high rates to generate enough turbulence to prevent corrosive sludge deposits (Woodyard *et al.* 2006). Similarly, pulsatile arterial flow operates at the threshold of peak diastolic turbulence to prevent atherosclerosis. The vascular endothelium adjusts arterial diameter via neuromuscular control of vascular smooth muscle to optimize diastolic turbulent mixing, which mobilizes particulate deposits from arterial walls

(Glagov *et al.* 1988; Nees 1989; Giddens *et al.* 1993; Glagov *et al.* 1995). Without adequate turbulence, deposits form on the inner walls of arteries. This activates the tissue repair component, causing thrombin and soluble fibrin generation, inflammation, tissue factor accumulation, fibrosis, and cholesterol trapping that forms atherosclerotic plaque (Kaunitz 1977; Ventura *et al.* 1984; Gordon *et al.* 1989; Bassiouny *et al.* 1994; Burnstock and Ralevic 1994; Chesebro *et al.* 1995; Davies 1995; Malek *et al.* 1999; Ross 1999; Silber *et al.* 2001; Jaeger and Labarrere 2003; Kensey 2003; Sajadi *et al.* 2003).

Increased blood viscosity enhances turbulent lateral forces at the expense of turbulent mixing effects, and vice-versa. This explains how stress increases blood pressure and accelerates atherosclerosis, while stress control reduces blood pressure and retards atherosclerosis. The washing machine provides a convenient analogy. The rotor mechanism of the washing machine corresponds to the heart. The clothing load corresponds to blood viscosity. With reasonable clothing loads, the rotor mechanism induces turbulent mixing that increases contact between soap and dirt, and cleaning proceeds efficiently. If the machine is overloaded, the rotor energy is shifted in favor of turbulent lateral forces at the expense of turbulent mixing, and the clothes are not cleaned properly.

Atherosclerosis begins on the greater curvatures of arteries, where shear stress and systolic velocity decline and turbulence decreases exponentially (Nerem and Seed 1972; Ku *et al.* 1985; Glagov *et al.* 1988; Giddens *et al.* 1993; Glagov *et al.* 1995; Zhao *et al.* 2000; Zhao *et al.* 2002; Katritsis *et al.* 2007). Diastolic turbulence increases exponentially with end-systolic velocity. Exercise increases cardiac contractility, elevates peak end-systolic velocity, exaggerates diastolic pulsatile turbulence, and inhibits atherosclerosis. Myxedema, congestive heart failure, and sedentary life style reduce cardiac contractility, retard peak end-systolic velocity, decrease diastolic cleansing turbulence, and accelerate atherosclerosis (Roguski *et al.* 1964; Eichner 1983; Powell *et al.* 1987; Donders *et al.* 1993; Rosenson *et al.* 2001; Biondi *et al.* 2002; Chambless *et al.* 2003; Mehta and Singhal 2003; Biondi and Klein 2004; Fazio *et al.* 2004; Schmermund 2004; Wolak *et al.* 2004).

Diastolic turbulence inhibits coagulation (Alexandrov *et al.* 2004). Thrombosis is rare in arteries, where turbulence is intense, but thrombophlebitis is common in veins, where turbulence is sluggish (Britton *et al.* 1974). Insoluble fibrin fluctuates in blood in accord with SNS activity, which is increased by allostatic load. Insoluble fibrin entangles red cells and disrupts aggregate patterns, which induces systolic turbulence that increases viscosity, decreases ejection fraction, and increases heart rate via the Starling mechanism (Stuart *et al.* 1981; Seo *et al.* 1991; Bogar 2002; Kawasaki *et al.* 2004; Rao *et al.* 2007). Insoluble fibrin elevations disrupt red cell aggregates and induce turbulence during systolic acceleration that strains and collapses structurally defective red cells, causing sickle-cell anemia crisis in susceptible individuals (Salvaggio *et al.* 1963; Devine *et al.* 1986; Famodu 1988; Francis 1989; Aluoch 1998; Solomon 2008). Systolic turbulence also retards peak end-systolic blood velocity, which exaggerates diastolic turbulent lateral forces at the expense of turbulent mixing, elevates blood pressure, increases blood coagulability, and accelerates atherosclerosis (Mori *et al.* 1989; Rosendaal *et al.* 1990; Koumbarelis *et al.* 1994; Kim *et al.* 1997; Cinar *et al.* 1999; Meiselman 1999; Kullo *et al.* 2000; Koenig *et al.* 2001; Bogar 2002; Chang *et al.* 2002; Reich *et al.* 2002; Chambless *et al.* 2003; Jaeger and Labarrere 2003; Koenig 2003; Laurent *et al.* 2003; Prandoni *et al.* 2003; Alexandrov *et al.* 2004; London *et al.* 2004; Bouma and Mosnier 2006; Rudnicka *et al.* 2006).

Insoluble fibrin binds red cells into a clot after it reduces turbulent mixing below a threshold (Puckett *et al.* 2003; Alexandrov *et al.* 2004; Kawasaki *et al.* 2004).

Blood turbulence normally occurs below the threshold of hearing. Blood pressure cuff inflation constricts arterial diameter, increases flow velocity, alters the turbulent pulse wave and elevates turbulent frequencies above audible levels at the distal edge of the cuff to produce *Korotkoff sounds* that are analogous to bruit sounds (Tavel *et al.* 1969). The blood pressure cuff measures the diastolic turbulent lateral force in arteries, as opposed to the forward force imparted by cardiac contraction that induces laminar systolic blood flow, so that blood pressure is not directly related to perfusion.

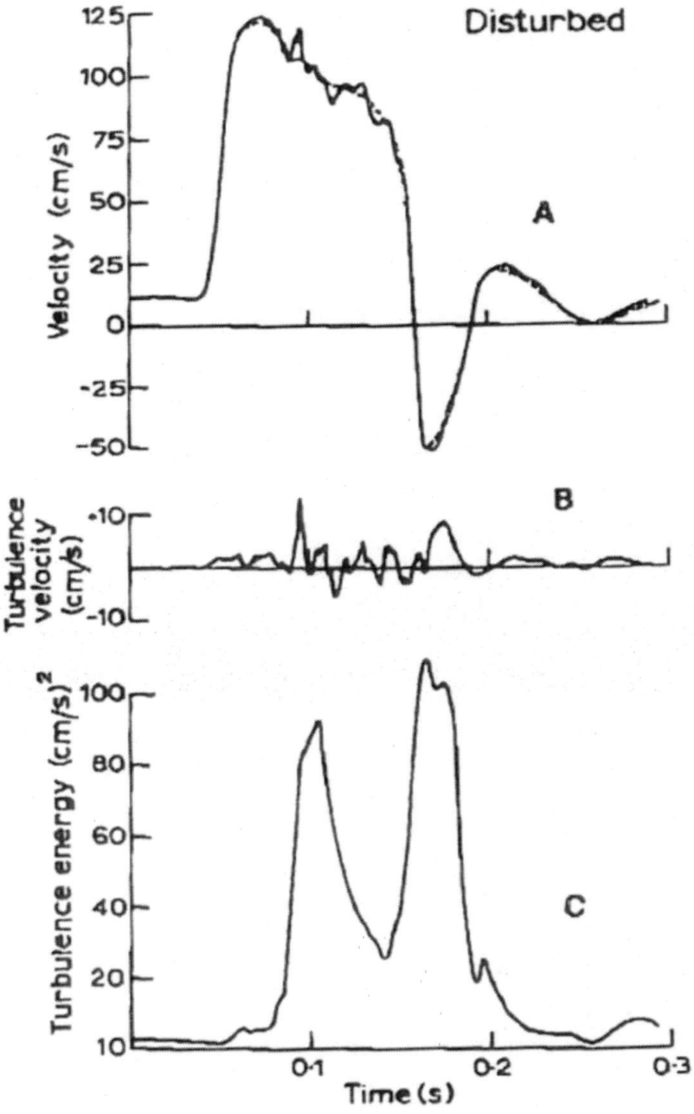

Figure 3. Turbulence and velocity in pulsatile blood flow in a dog (reproduced with permission from Parker 1977).

Blood viscosity that fluctuates in accord with autonomic balance is the main variable that affects blood pressure. Stressful stimuli activate the SNS, which causes the release of VWF from the vascular endothelium into flowing blood. This generates insoluble fibrin that elevates blood viscosity, reduces stroke volume, elevates heart rate via the Starling mechanism, decreases cardiac output and tissue perfusion, increases blood pressure, and accelerates atherosclerosis. Stress reduction and parasympathetic activity decreases blood viscosity, increases stroke volume, retards atherosclerosis, reduces heart rate and blood pressure, and enhances tissue perfusion and organ function. Sleep is a state of minimal stress that is characterized by hypotension, bradycardia, enhanced tissue perfusion, and increased cardiac efficiency.

Hemodynamic relationships usually appear linear because turbulent variables are maintained within narrow ranges by mammalian physiology. Blood pressure is strikingly similar among most mammalian species because cardiac power generation is proportional to body size (Holt *et al.* 1968). However, turbulent relationships are exponential in nature, so that small changes can produce large differences (Gleick 1988). Multiple factors affect blood turbulence, including cardiac inotropy and chronotropy, arterial diameter and length, body temperature and lipoprotein solidification, red cell mass and morphology, and blood viscosity. Hemodynamic parameters are affected by complex fluctuating exponential interactions of inotropy, chronotropy, temperature, and viscosity that can produce non-linear perturbations. This explains why blood pressure and cardiac output are not linearly related (Gleick 1988; Biais *et al.* 2008).

Reptilian red cells enhance systolic turbulence at the expense of exercise tolerance to prevent atherosclerosis caused by lipoprotein solidification at low temperatures that sharply increases blood viscosity (Dintenfass 1965). Reptiles thrive in warm environments, but their activity is sluggish at low temperatures. Mammals achieve superior exercise tolerance and dominate cold environments by maintaining their body temperature above the level of lipoprotein liquefaction, which enables their bi-concave red cells to simultaneously optimize hemodynamic efficiency and atherosclerosis resistance, but this necessitates substantially greater caloric intake (Dintenfass 1965; Rim *et al.* 2001; Hardy *et al.* 2004; Dirkmann *et al.* 2008). Mammalian red blood cells spontaneously form aggregates that suppress turbulence during systole to enable rapid and efficient blood acceleration. Diastolic deceleration disrupts the aggregates and converts laminar systolic flow into diastolic turbulence that halts net forward flow (Parker 1977). In humans, the brief flow reversal in the distal aorta inhibits turbulent cleansing and accelerates atherosclerosis relative to the proximal aorta (Bassiouny *et al.* 1994).

Anesthesia, Analgesia, and the Three Pathways of SRM Activation

Three independent pathways activate the SRM and focus its powerful effects: the *spinal pathway*, the *cognitive pathway*, and the *tissue pathway*. Individual stressors and combinations of stressors activate these synergistic pathways in various magnitudes, locations, intervals, and combinations, so that the manifestations of SRM activity appear chaotic and confusing. Analgesia inhibits the spinal pathway, and anesthesia inhibits the cognitive pathway. There are no clinically available means to inhibit the tissue pathway.

The Spinal Pathway

The spinal pathway consists of peripheral nociceptors in the skin and internal organs that detect noxious stimuli and activate the SNS via peripheral nerves and spinal cord internuncial pathways. Nociceptors detect vibration, temperature, inflammation and tissue disruption, but are insensitive to radiation, sepsis, and many toxic chemicals (Hahnenkamp *et al.* 2002). Spinal pathway activity is called *nociception*. Descending cortical pathways inhibit nociception, so that their absence exaggerates nociception (Melzack and Wall 1965). Analgesic agents inhibit nociception by disrupting spinal pathway activity. Cyclo-oxygenase (COX) inhibitors prevent inflammation that activates nociceptors. Opioids inhibit spinal cord nociception pathways. Lidocaine, marcaine, and other local analgesics block the function of peripheral nerves, spinal cord pathways, and autonomic nerve endings that conduct nociception signals.

The following examples illustrate spinal pathway function:

1. *Spinal pathway nociception resists anesthesia* in safe and practical doses (Bredbacka *et al.* 1986; Breslow *et al.* 1993; Kuitunen *et al.* 1993; Groeben *et al.* 1994; Bromage 1996; Groudine *et al.* 1998; Groban *et al.* 2004). This explains the release of stress hormones (VWF, cortisol, epinephrine, glucagon, etc.) during surgery despite dangerously deep levels of anesthesia. It also explains spinal cord "windup" syndrome that causes problematic muscle tension and unexpected muscular movements during surgery despite deep levels of anesthesia.
2. Spinal cord damage at/or above the level of T5 causes autonomic dysreflexia. The cognitive pathway no longer responds to nociception, so that pain is eliminated, but spinal pathway nociception, freed from descending cortical inhibition, causes harmful SNS hyperactivity that is little affected by anesthesia (Melzack and Wall 1965).
3. Cortical inhibition remains intact in spinal cord damage below the level of T5, and it inhibits spinal cord nociception pathways and synergizes the effects of general anesthetic agents in a manner analogous to analgesia (Yeager *et al.* 1987; Yoo *et al.* 2006; Zhang *et al.* 2007).
4. Analgesia prevents both nociception and pain and thereby reduces surgical morbidity and mortality more effectively than anesthesia, which prevents only pain, fear, and apprehension (see "Cognitive Pathway" below) (Pflug and Halter 1981; Sebel and Bovil 1982; Modig *et al.* 1983; Modig *et al.* 1983; Woolf 1983; Modig 1985; Tverskoy *et al.* 1985; Bredbacka *et al.* 1986; Davis *et al.* 1986; Woolf and Wall 1986; Yeager *et al.* 1987; Giesecke *et al.* 1988; Roizen 1988; Tverskoy *et al.* 1990; Christopherson *et al.* 1993; Kuitunen *et al.* 1993; Rosenfeld *et al.* 1993; Woolf and Chong 1993; Moore *et al.* 1995; Christopherson *et al.* 1996; Rodgers *et al.* 2000; Treschan *et al.* 2003; Filimonovic *et al.* 2005; Exadaktylos *et al.* 2006).

5. Pediatric anesthetic methods such as the once popular "Liverpool technique" that rely on inhalation agent supplemented by muscle relaxants do not adequately control stress. Fetuses and newborn babies cannot understand language and perceive danger, but their nociception pathways are fully functional so that they require analgesia as well as anesthesia for surgical safety (Edde 1981; von Kries *et al.* 1981; Anand *et al.* 1987; Anand *et al.* 1990; Hickey and Hansen 1991; Anand and Hickey 1992; Fisk *et al.* 2001).
6. I hypothesize that cortical damage sometimes impairs descending inhibition of spinal cord activity, so that spinal cord nociception pathway activity is exaggerated in the manner of autonomic dysreflexia (see item 2 above). I further hypothesize that general anesthesia without supplemental analgesia exaggerates nociception by inhibiting cortical activity that is essential for descending pathway inhibition.
7. Nociceptors are not directly sensitive to radiation and some toxic chemicals, but they are indirectly and belatedly activated by inflammation that is induced by these forms of stress. For example, sunburn is initially painless, but becomes painful the day after sun exposure due to the inflammatory effects of radiation damage.

The Cognitive Pathway

The cognitive pathway consists of conscious awareness generated by corticofugal mechanisms that assesses environmental hazards via sensory input including sight, smell, sound, vibration, and nociception. It activates the SNS and the HPA axis via hypothalamic pathways that are independent of the spinal pathway (Khomulo *et al.* 1976; Gutstein *et al.* 1978; Gutstein and Parl 1978; Khomulo *et al.* 1980; Gutstein 1988; Kario *et al.* 2003). The cognitive pathway also inhibits spinal pathway nociception via descending pathways from the brain to the spinal cord (Melzack and Wall 1965). Conscious awareness interprets nociception as *pain* (Parker *et al.* 2006; Price 2008). Inhalation anesthetics are hypnotic agents that obtund consciousness. Even moderate inhibition of conscious awareness by hypnotic agents can eliminate pain, but hypnotic agents have little effect on nociception. The benefits of hypnotic inhalation anesthetic agents such as ether, halothane, chloroform, ethrane, isoforane, desflurane and sevoflurane are equivalent to those of intravenous hypnotic agents such as benzodiazepines, barbiturates, propofol, ketamine, etomidate, althesin, viadril, and alcohol.

Emotional mechanisms modulate cognitive pathway activity. This explains *allostasis*, which is the subconscious alteration of behavior and physiology in accord with prior experience. Hyperthymestic syndrome demonstrates that the brain automatically records permanent audiovisual memories of all waking moments throughout life, and that these normally suppressed memories activate emotions and SNS activity (Hobson 1997). Sleep halts the recording process while the emotional mechanism engages in the process of dreaming, wherein it automatically compares and contrasts previously stored memories to identify threatening circumstances (Khomulo *et al.* 1976; Khomulo *et al.* 1980; Wittstein *et al.* 2005; Chapman *et al.* 2008). This enables the pre-emptive perception of danger, whereupon emotional mechanisms automatically generate anxiety, rage, fear and apprehension, and activate the SNS and the HPA axis to facilitate "fight or flight" (Feigl *et al.* 1987; Jern *et al.* 1989). This activates capillary hemostasis, and, increases blood viscosity

(Freeman *et al.* 1987), which limits blood loss in the event of subsequent injury. It also concentrates blood flow in critical organs such as heart, lung, and brain, whose tissues resist capillary hemostasis. The HPA axis simultaneously releases epinephrine, glucagon, cortisol, and other stress hormones. These combined effects explain the tachycardia, hypertension, and hyperglycemia, other reactions associated with acute and chronic allostasis, and how these reactions are progressively altered by accumulating memories and their ongoing manipulation by emotional mechanisms (Sano and Itoh 1998).

The emotional mechanism plays an important survival role in animals, which often face life or death confrontations and lack the reasoning ability of humans. Idiopathic insomnia demonstrates that sleep and dreaming are not essential in humans (Bovill *et al.* 1983; Wong 1983; Bovill *et al.* 1984; Freeman *et al.* 1987; Park 2002). However, occult allostasis explains neurosis in humans. It also explains how emotions alter the perception of pain and danger, which suggests new treatments for chronic pain and neurosis (Behar 2007).

The following examples illustrate cognitive pathway activity:

1. The cognitive pathway activates the SNS despite the absence of nociception. One may not sense the pain of a dentist's drill, but one can still perceive vibration, pressure, the noise of the drill, and the comments of the dentist and his staff. One anticipates pain and danger consciously, even if none is present, and this activates the SNS (Bovill *et al.* 1983; Wong 1983; Bovill *et al.* 1984; Dorges *et al.* 2002; Park 2002; Hoffmeister *et al.* 2003; Wannamethee *et al.* 2003; Mukamal *et al.* 2004).
2. The cognitive pathway resists analgesia in clinically practical doses, because sight, smell, vibration, and sound perception remain intact. Spinal and epidural analgesia, analgesic block techniques, and high-dose opioid analgesia for cardiac surgery often require supplementation with hypnotic agents to prevent sharp increases in blood pressure, pulse rate and muscle activity caused by frightening sounds and sensations, even though nociception and pain are absent (Bredbacka *et al.* 1986; Mangano *et al.* 1992; Breslow *et al.* 1993; Groeben *et al.* 1994; Bromage 1996; Groudine *et al.* 1998; Myles *et al.* 2002; Groban *et al.* 2004).
3. Anesthesia increases surgical safety by abolishing consciousness, fear, apprehension, and pain, but it cannot prevent harmful spinal pathway nociception in clinically practical doses (Freeman *et al.* 1987; Kario and Matsuo 1995; Kario *et al.* 1996; Kario *et al.* 1997; Matsuo *et al.* 1997; Kario *et al.* 1998; Matsuo *et al.* 1998; Matsuo *et al.* 1998; Dorges *et al.* 2002; Pignalberi *et al.* 2002; Kario *et al.* 2003; Wittstein *et al.* 2005; von Kanel *et al.* 2006).
4. Acute allostatic load, such as occurs in uninjured earthquake victims, activates the cognitive pathway and causes acute and residual elevations of VWF, factor VIII activity, blood viscosity, blood coagulability, myocardial infarction, stroke, heart rate and blood pressure in accord with the severity of fear. This explains how people are sometimes frightened to death (Chang *et al.* 2002).
5. Chronic emotional allostatic load, such as job difficulties, elevates VWF and factor VIII activity, accelerates atherosclerosis, and shortens life span (Gutstein *et al.* 1978; Gutstein 1988; Jern *et al.* 1989; Park 2002; Hoffmeister *et al.* 2003; Wannamethee *et al.* 2003; Mukamal *et al.* 2004; Hao *et al.* 2005; Ranjbar *et al.* 2007).

6. Moderate alcohol consumption inhibits consciousness and mitigates emotional distress, which reduces SNS activity, thus explaining its ability to prevent heart disease and enhance longevity (Mangano *et al.* 1991; Mangano *et al.* 1992; Landesberg *et al.* 2001).
7. Analgesia prevents infarction during anesthetic emergence, when the sudden restoration of cognitive pathway function and the ability to perceive pain and danger synergizes with spinal pathway nociception to harmfully exaggerate capillary gate component activity (Fleck *et al.* 1990).

The Tissue Pathway

The tissue pathway consists of the vascular endothelium, tissue factor, and factor VII. The vascular endothelium manufactures tissue factor, excretes it into extravascular tissues, and insulates it from flowing blood. Tissue damage disrupts the vascular endothelium and exposes tissue factor to factor VII in flowing blood, which activates factor VII and initiates tissue repair. The tissue pathway activates the tissue repair component in accord with the magnitude and location of injurious forces that disrupt the vascular endothelium, expose tissue factor to factor VII in blood, and release tissue factor into blood circulation with systemic consequences.

Brain, lung, nerves, autonomic ganglia, cervix, adventitia of blood vessels, epithelium of skin, mucosa, glomeruli, and placenta are rich in tissue factor (Fleck *et al.* 1990; Welty-Wolf *et al.* 2001; Idell 2002, 2002; Kipnis *et al.* 2004; van der Poll *et al.* 2005; Fornek *et al.* 2007). This explains why these tissues are "targets" for positive feedback in stress-related conditions. For example, severe brain and burn injuries release tissue factor into systemic circulation and exaggerate morbidity and mortality. Lung tissue reacts violently to microbes, antigens, and chemicals, causing lethal overproduction of soluble fibrin that floods alveolar spaces and airway passages and disrupts gas exchange in asthma, pneumonia, influenza, and poison gas exposure. Brain, lung, kidney, nerves, cervix, and peri-arterial tissues are more likely to develop malignancies or be the site of metastasis than other tissues. Placenta, brain, kidney and lung function are primary targets in eclampsia. Adult respiratory distress syndrome (ARDS) is usually the first manifestation of multi-organ failure syndrome (MOFS) that primarily affects lung, brain, and kidney.

The following examples illustrate tissue pathway activity:

1. Pneumonia and influenza insensibly disrupt the vascular endothelium in lung tissues that are rich in tissue factor, causing profuse soluble fibrin exudates that flood alveolar spaces, disrupt gas exchange, and promote collagen generation (fibrosis) (Widdicombe 1992; Bonacci *et al.* 2003; Kawada *et al.* 2003).
2. Inhaled antigens imperceptibly deposit on airway passages and induce soluble fibrin generation on their inner walls. This has minor effect during inhalation, when airway diameters are increased, but inhibits airflow during exhalation, when airway diameters are reduced, causing asthma (Hesselvik *et al.* 1989; Bredbacka *et al.* 1994; Garcia *et al.* 1995; Welty-Wolf *et al.* 2001; Healy 2002; Akassoglou *et al.* 2003; Hovinga *et al.* 2007).

3. Bacterial products that enter the bloodstream cause sepsis by insensibly increasing the permeability of the vascular endothelium and releasing tissue factor into the blood, causing positive feedback that exaggerates thrombin and soluble fibrin generation. Thrombin energizes inflammatory changes that enable soluble fibrin to enter extravascular tissues, causing tissue edema and organ dysfunction (Warr *et al.* 1990; Bredbacka and Edner 1994).
4. Brain and burn injuries release large amounts of tissue factor into blood circulation, causing abnormal systemic factor VII activation that overwhelms inhibitory mechanisms and induces SRM hyperactivity and positive feedback that exaggerates morbidity and mortality (Welty-Wolf *et al.* 2001).
5. Radiation does not directly activate peripheral nociceptors, but it damages the vascular endothelium, causing thrombin generation and positive feedback that energizes the release of inflammatory substances that activate nociceptors, causing belated pain. For example, skin damage due to sun exposure is initially painless and invisible, but the gradual onset of inflammatory effects caused by radiation damage produces a delayed painful reaction.
6. Site-inactivated tissue factor neutralizes the tissue pathway and inhibits the effects of sepsis (Angelov 1989; Lockwood *et al.* 1991; Lau and Chui 1994).
7. Amniotic fluid is rich in tissue factor. Amniotic fluid embolus suddenly introduces large amounts of tissue factor into circulation, which activates factor VII and induces capillary gate component hyperactivity that triggers spontaneous systemic coagulation activity that depletes coagulation precursors such as fibrinogen and fibronectin, causing defective coagulation activity known as disseminated intravascular coagulation (DIC; see below) (Cheras *et al.* 1997).

Positive and Negative Feedback

The *tissue repair pathway* activates the *tissue repair component* in accord with the magnitude and location of injurious forces that affect the vascular endothelium. For example, invasive surgery releases greater amounts of tissue factor into circulation than minor surgery, thereby exaggerating morbidity and mortality (Gleick 1988). The semi-independent and synergistic *spinal* and *cognitive pathways* both activate the capillary gate component, in accord with combinations of sight, sound, smell, vibration, and nociception. Combinations of anesthesia and analgesia synergistically inhibit sympathetic nervous system activity and control capillary gate component activity.

The tissue repair component activates factor VII, amplifies thrombin production, and generates soluble fibrin (Antovic *et al.* 2002; Basso and Keeling 2004). The capillary gate component activates factor VIII, accelerates thrombin production, and generates insoluble fibrin (Bredbacka *et al.* 1994; Bredbacka and Edner 1994; Fenton *et al.* 1998; Adembri *et al.* 2004; Garvin *et al.* 2010; Modesti *et al.* 2009). The activity of each component exaggerates that of the other in a "chaotic" manner (Gleick 1988), because both share the enzymatic interaction of factors VII, VIII, IX and X (Griffin *et al.* 2007). The simultaneous, synergistic activation of both components induces "positive feedback", so that peak SRM activity occurs several hours after injury (Walsh and Ahmad 2002). The constantly fluctuating activities of the three synergistic pathways enable the SRM to focus its powerful effects and generate an infinite variety of manifestations (Woolf 1983; Wall and Woolf 1986; Woolf and Wall 1986; Coderre and Melzack 1987; Cousins 1989; Woolf and Chong 1993; Kario *et al.* 1998; van Mourik *et al.* 1999; Herrero *et al.* 2000; Hovinga *et al.* 2007; Ofek and Defrin 2007).

As stressors subside, "negative feedback" restores homeostasis via clot formation and tissue repair that progressively reduces thrombin production to maintenance levels. Likewise, parasympathetic activity, stoichiometric ATIII, TFPI, TPA and protein C mobilization (Berglund *et al.* 1988; Bredbacka *et al.* 1994; Fan *et al.* 2000; Inoue *et al.* 2004; Baum *et al.* 2005; Hovinga *et al.* 2007) restores homeostasis by inhibiting factor VII and factor VIII activity and accelerating the spontaneous disintegration of insoluble fibrin (Avikainen 1977; Hesselvik *et al.* 1989; Wei 1990; Abraham 1991; Bredbacka *et al.* 1994; Garrison *et al.* 1998; Sielenkamper *et al.* 2001; Laudes *et al.* 2002; Weijer *et al.* 2004; Hovinga *et al.* 2007; Chapman *et al.* 2008). However, prolonged factor VIII half-life and spinal cord "wind up" can cause residual capillary gate component hyperactivity to linger long after stressors subside (Modig *et al.* 1983; Moalli *et al.* 1989; Tighe *et al.* 1989; Fleck *et al.* 1990; Rubin *et al.* 1990; Fan *et al.* 2000; Idell 2002, 2002).

Eclampsia, ARDS, MSOF and DIC

Positive feedback that induces SRM hyperactivity explains the similarities of MSOF, ARDS, eclampsia, malignancy, DIC, and the surgical stress syndrome (Thornton and Bonnar 1977; Inglis *et al.* 1982; Weiner and Brandt 1982; Ogawa *et al.* 1983; Scholtes *et al.* 1983; Roberts *et al.* 1989; Gartner 1994; Ventura *et al.* 1997; Rath *et al.* 2000; Carr 2001; Roy *et al.* 2001; Anim-Nyame *et al.* 2003; Bryson *et al.* 2003; Kabon *et al.* 2004; Harskamp and Zeeman 2007). Placenta, lung, cervix, brain, and peri-arterial tissues are especially vulnerable to SRM hyperactivity because they possess abundant tissue factor. MSOF commonly occurs after extensive injuries or sepsis, especially when both are present (Newman *et al.* 2001). ARDS is typically the first manifestation of MSOF, because lung tissue possesses abundant tissue and is therefore affected sooner than other organs (Fitzgerald 1979; Poste and Greig 1982; Bruhn *et al.* 1983; Kuznik *et al.* 1985; Dvorak 1986; Sporn 1991; Farber 1995; Klementsen and Jorgensen 1997; Huang *et al.* 2000; Zain *et al.* 2000; De Vos *et al.* 2001; Schiller *et al.* 2002; Bobe *et al.* 2003; Darmoul *et al.* 2003; Versteeg *et al.* 2004; Cao *et al.* 2005; Tantivejkul *et al.* 2005). Eclampsia is a form of MSOF that is unique to pregnancy, which is a stressful condition. Additional forms of stress are invariably present in eclampsia, such as obesity, diabetes, rheumatoid disease, and urinary tract infection (Augustin *et al.* 1995; Jin *et al.* 2003; Archiniegas *et al.* 2004; Versteeg *et al.* 2004; Tantivejkul *et al.* 2005). Smoking mitigates the severity of eclampsia by tranquilizing cognitive pathway activity (Fidler and Kripke 1977; Warr *et al.* 1990; Schiller *et al.* 2002; Hua *et al.* 2003; Tsopanoglou and Maragoudakis 2004; Versteeg *et al.* 2004). SRM hyperactivity induced by eclampsia predisposes to DIC, especially in the event of amniotic fluid embolus that introduces tissue factor into blood circulation (see "DIC" below). Magnesium sulfate (MgSO4) therapy mitigates the symptoms of eclampsia by competing with Ca^{2+} and inhibiting thrombin activity (see "Pharmacology and the SRM" below).

Malignancy

Devra Davis discusses the origin of the currently prevailing belief that defective DNA is the cause of cancer in her book "*The Secret History of the War on Cancer*" (Davis 2007). Goodman and Gilman of pharmacology textbook fame conducted government-funded war gas research during WWII, shortly before Watson and Crick discovered DNA. They demonstrated that toxic war gases reduce white blood cell counts in leukemia, which they believed was beneficial. They subsequently tested their gas treatment on a mouse with a solid tumor, whereupon the tumor shrank dramatically. Though subsequent experiments produced far less impressive results, they believed that they had discovered an effective means to treat cancer. The coincidental discovery of DNA around this same time synergized with the toxic gas research and led to the seemingly reasonable assumption that defective DNA causes cancer, and that cells thus infested must be killed to effect a cure. This belief provides the basis for currently prevailing forms of cancer treatment, including surgical tumor excision, chemotherapy, and radiation therapy. The limited success of these treatments can be explained by the fact that malignant cells are more vulnerable to these destructive treatments than normal cells. However, the belief that defective DNA is the cause of cancer remains scientifically unfounded. Some evidence is at odds with this idea and indicates that cancer is caused by environmental stress. This explains why the incidence of cancer is rising in recent years despite these "modern" forms of treatment, and why conventional cancer treatments that produce "cures" are often bedeviled by the subsequent appearance of other, seemingly unrelated, forms of cancer, not to mention increased morbidity and mortality from heart disease, stroke, and pulmonary embolus (Bradlow *et al.* 1997).

The SRM provides an improved explanation of cancer. Malignancy is aberrant repair-cell hyperactivity caused by SRM positive feedback that induces persistent abnormal thrombin elevations (Fleck *et al.* 1990; Hjortoe *et al.* 2004; Levi *et al.* 2006). It may involve re-activated embryological thrombin receptor configurations (see "Evolution, Embryology and the SRM" below) (Fitzgerald 1979; McCoy and Wynder 1979; Bhatia *et al.* 1996; Sala-Serra *et al.* 1996; 1997; von Tempelhoff *et al.* 2000; Coussens and Werb 2002; von Tempelhoff *et al.* 2002; Hjortoe *et al.* 2004; Pankhurst *et al.* 2004; Jee *et al.* 2005; Wang *et al.* 2005; Elikowski *et al.* 2006; Smedby *et al.* 2006; Davis 2007). Malignant cells invade normal tissues, release tissue factor, and activate nervous sensors, causing a "vicious cycle" of positive feedback that sustains abnormal thrombin elevations, promotes angiogenesis, and inhibits apoptosis and resolution that normally occurs at the conclusion of the tissue repair process (Vinckier and Vermylen 1984; Fenton *et al.* 1998; Dalen *et al.* 1999; Haas 2002; Asanuma *et al.* 2004; Bobek and Kovarik 2004; Holzheimer 2004; Cao *et al.* 2005). Brain, nerve, ovary, placenta, lung, artery, and cervix tissues that are rich in tissue factor are especially vulnerable to both malignancy and metastasis (Fleck *et al.* 1990; Warr *et al.* 1990; Weissman 1990; Hampton *et al.* 1991; Samama *et al.* 2001; Adembri *et al.* 2004; Modesti *et al.* 2009). This explains the close association of malignancy with allostatic load including chronic disease and environmental stressors, inflammatory symptoms, elevated factor VII and factor VIII activity, increased blood viscosity and coagulability, accelerated atherosclerosis, and seemingly unrelated forms of malignancy (McDaniel *et al.* 1984; Chernow *et al.* 1987; Kavarana *et al.* 2003; Adembri *et al.* 2004; Inoue *et al.* 2004; Monk *et al.* 2005; Liberzon *et al.* 2006; Garvin *et al.* 2010; Modesti *et al.* 2009). Surgical excision of malignant tumors, radiation therapy and chemotherapy all activate the SRM and elevate thrombin generation, which explains why these treatments produce unreliable results and increase the risk of subsequent heart disease, stroke, pulmonary embolus, and seemingly unrelated forms of cancer. Combinations of analgesia that inhibits the spinal pathway, anesthesia that inhibits the cognitive pathway, and anticoagulants that inhibit the tissue pathway can potentially induce apoptosis and cure cancer quickly, safely, comfortably and reliably (Anand *et al.* 1987; Anand *et al.* 1990; Anand and Hickey 1992; Abram and Yaksh 1993, 1994).

Anesthesia, Analgesia, and the Surgical Stress Syndrome

The SRM provides a long-sought theory of anesthesia, analgesia, and allostasis that enables the alteration of anesthesia technique to optimize surgical outcome. Invasive surgery was avoided until anesthesia provided a practical means to ablate consciousness. This reduced stress, improved survival, and revolutionized surgery. However, anesthesia alone cannot prevent the "surgical stress syndrome", which consists of pathological symptoms that appear distant from the time and location of surgery. Even deep levels of anesthesia must be supplemented with muscle relaxants to prevent unexpected movements and troublesome muscle tension. An effective theory must explain these problems.

Attempts to establish anesthesia theory began with Meyer and Overton around 1896, but their lipid solubility theory proved invalid, and no subsequent effort has succeeded. The challenge became more daunting after 1914, when George Washington Crile, founder of the Cleveland Clinic, demonstrated that adding analgesia to anesthesia improves surgical safety (Crile and Lower 1914). This means that an effective theory must explain the confusing and overlapping effects of both anesthesia and analgesia. However, most efforts have focused on anesthesia and neglected analgesia (Orser *et al.* 2002; Campagna *et al.* 2003; John and Prichep 2005). The need for an effective theory has recently become more urgent after clinical research produced unexpected evidence that anesthesia technique affects cancer and heart disease in the distant aftermath of surgery (Monk *et al.* 2005).

Impediments to Anesthesia Theory

Pre-existing beliefs, entrenched habits, and defective standards have obstructed anesthesia research, patient safety, and theory development. Most of these originated during the "Golden Era of Ether" that lasted from approximately 1860 to 1960, when anesthesia practitioners routinely observed that ether progressively reduces blood pressure and abolishes pain before it eliminates conscious awareness. This conveyed the conviction that anesthesia has dose-related analgesic properties that prevent Sympathetic Nervous System (SNS) stimulation by surgical stress. This lingering assumption has caused most theorists to neglect nociception pathways that bypass the brain and remain active despite anesthesia (John and Prichep 2005).

Also problematic is the counterintuitive mystery of hemodynamic physiology. The nature of blood pressure and the palpable pulse has never been understood. They became basic monitoring standards for lack of alternatives. Decreased cardiac output and tissue perfusion usually accompanies tachycardia and hypertension, while bradycardia and hypotension characterize enhanced cardiac efficiency and tissue perfusion, as in normal sleep and resting athletes. Nevertheless, researchers and practitioners usually equate hypertension with effective cardiac function and tissue perfusion, and regard hypotension as a harbinger of disaster.

Hemodynamic physiology is customarily explained by autonomic innervation that regulates cardiac inotropy and arteriolar diameter, but this explanation is weak. Were this true, the blood pressure force would appear simultaneously and equally throughout the arterial tree, for blood, like water, is incompressible. Instead, it appears as a traveling wave that generates lateral forces that vary in accord with arterial length and diameter, blood viscosity, red cell mass, and temperature. Furthermore, chronic hypertension causes sustained increases in cardiac work that induces congestive heart failure, and vascular smooth muscle contraction is energy-intensive, limited in duration, and soon followed by obligatory relaxation. Thus, neither cardiac inotropy nor vasoconstriction can readily explain sustained hypertension. In addition, exercise causes little change in the heart, but instead causes capillary proliferation that reduces vascular resistance and improves cardiac efficiency. The capillary gate component (see above) provides a more efficient and effective explanation of hemodynamic physiology, because capillary surface area is vastly greater than that of all other vessels combined; capillary pressure, turbulence, and flow are minimal; and blood turbulence explains atherosclerosis, blood pressure, and the palpable pulse.

A more recent impediment to anesthesia theory is the idea that opioids promote cancer. Older studies in both humans and animals have proved that cancer is not contagious. Transplants from cancer victims to healthy individuals neither induce cancer nor reduce life span. Furthermore, there is abundant evidence that analgesia prevents cancer and reduces surgical complications (Mangano *et al.* 1992; Myles *et al.* 2002; Exadaktylos *et al.* 2006). However, recent studies have demonstrated that opioids can temporarily prolong the survival of transplanted malignant tissues (Shavit *et al.* 2004). These studies are seriously flawed, because the animals were prematurely sacrificed. Had the test animals been allowed to live, the cancer transplants would no doubt have been rejected with no effect on the life span of the transplant recipients. The studies thus failed to produce direct evidence that opioids promote cancer, and claims that opioids promote cancer are speculative, unsubstantiated, and unscientific. Nevertheless, the older studies are nowadays ignored, and these recent studies have discouraged opioid research and clinical use at the expense of patient comfort and safety (Mangano *et al.* 1992; Myles *et al.* 2002). This is unfortunate, because the ability of opioid analgesia to reduce cancer and heart disease when added to anesthesia has never been properly evaluated. Perhaps the most subtle and pervasive factor frustrating anesthesia research and theory is carbon dioxide (CO_2) management. To appreciate this, one must understand the history of anesthesia. During the "golden era of ether", anesthesia machines were equipped with "bypass valves" for CO_2 supplementation (Lundy 1925). These valves enabled $FICO_2$ supplementation that stimulated respiratory drive, increased cardiac output, enhanced tissue oxygenation, accelerated ether uptake, and reduced induction times. Unfortunately, these bypass valves enabled hazardous CO_2 elevations that occasionally caused convulsions, cyanosis, and death (Waters 1933). The valves disappeared after the danger was recognized, but anesthesiologists have subsequently regarded CO_2 as a "toxic waste gas" that must be rid from the body. Pre-existing beliefs about CO_2 toxicity have subsequently perturbed anesthesia research. For example, Boniface and Brown mistakenly attributed decreases in cardiac work to CO_2 toxicity even though their own data demonstrated beneficial reductions in blood viscosity that enhanced cardiac efficiency and explained the decreased cardiac work observed when dogs were exposed to elevated CO2 levels (Boniface and Brown 1953). Another example is the study of Eisele and colleagues, where dogs were exposed to elevated $FICO_2$ (Eisele *et al.* 1967). Their studies demonstrated that "CO_2 toxicity" occurs at $FICO_2$ levels only slightly higher than those that induce "CO_2 narcosis" and that both are accompanied by sharp decreases in pH in both blood and cerebrospinal fluid. This study inexplicably failed to report associated pO_2 blood levels, even though arterial cannulae were installed in all the dogs to facilitate blood gas sampling. The oversight is unfortunate, because there is no evidence that CO_2 reacts chemically with any substances in the living vertebrate body, and hypoxemia potentially explains all manifestations of both CO_2 toxicity and CO_2 narcosis. These and other studies are commonly cited to justify iatrogenic hypocarbia via mechanical hyperventilation, which is arguably more dangerous and insidious than hypercarbia (Coleman 2006; Coleman 2010; Coleman 2011). With the introduction of curare, mechanical hyperventilation to prevent CO_2 toxicity became a de facto "standard of practice", so that practitioners and researchers ignore its harmful effects. Hyperventilation persists despite abundant evidence of its hazards as well as the benefits of mild "permissive" hypercapnia, and the universal availability of capnography (Prys-Roberts *et al.* 1967; Salvatore *et al.* 1969; Cartwright *et al.* 1983; Akca 2006). Hyperventilation increases blood viscosity, which reduces cardiac output and decreases tissue and organ perfusion and oxygenation. It damages lung tissues, depletes CO_2 tissue reserves, obtunds respiratory chemoreceptors, and undermines respiratory drive. It necessitates prolonged postoperative ventilator therapy when combined with effective opioid treatment. Hyperventilated patients breathe adequately after anesthesia provided opioids are judiciously minimized, but only because conscious awareness confers a form of respiratory drive that is independent of chemoreceptor function. However, occult chemoreceptor paralysis persists for hours, especially in geriatric patients, and causes unexpected respiratory arrest when patients are treated with seemingly innocuous doses of opioids and sedatives that promote sleep. The problem is known as "opioid hypersensitivity"(Coleman 2006; Coleman 2010; Coleman 2011). These misunderstood problems have perturbed opioid research and clinical utilization at the expense of patient comfort, safety, stress control, and theory development. Meanwhile, critical care specialists re-discovered the clinical benefits of CO_2 more than 30 years ago. They routinely utilize "permissive hypercarbia" outside the operating room to prevent lung damage, reduce blood viscosity, increase cardiac output, improve tissue perfusion, and protect organ function. Mild hypercarbia conserves CO_2 tissue reserves, preserves respiratory chemoreceptor function, enhances respiratory drive, accelerates opioid clearance, and enables effective opioid analgesia without necessitating prolonged respiratory support.

Anesthesia and Stress Theory

Selye's ideas provided the most promising hope for a theory of anesthesia in the recent past. They imply that surgery induces stress mechanism hyperactivity that causes the "surgical stress syndrome." This consists of pathological symptoms that appear distant from the time and location of surgery, including fever, tachycardia, hypertension, mental disorders, myocardial infarction, stroke, malignancy, heart disease, allodynia, inflammation, edema, bowel ileus, and so forth. Selye's theory further implies that the benefits of anesthesia derive from its ability to prevent stress mechanism hyperactivity, and that anesthesia technique can be modified to optimize surgical outcome.

The introduction of halothane and curare synergized with Selye's ideas and produced an era of ferment, change, and stress-related anesthesia research that lasted roughly from 1960 to 1990. This ended the "golden age of ether" and inspired new ideas, equipment, and improvements in anesthetic safety and surgical convenience. Explosive agents were eliminated. Mechanical ventilation, pulse oximetry, capnography, and invasive monitoring were introduced. Fresh evidence corroborated Crile's observation that analgesia added to general anesthesia improves outcome. Opioids and local analgesics were commonly combined with general anesthesia to optimize surgical stress control. However, all these techniques required additional skill and time, or entailed increased difficulties, risks, and inconvenience. For example, hyperventilated patients require prolonged respiratory support after effective opioid dosage. Without a theory that explains the confusing and overlapping effects of anesthesia and analgesia, stress control strategies have been largely abandoned.

Ironically, critical care practitioners re-discovered the benefits of "permissive hypercarbia" only a few years after the end of the era of anesthesia stress research. Capnography was simultaneously implemented as a means to detect lethal esophageal intubation and cardiac arrest, but its ability to safely enable the benefits of mild hypercarbia during anesthesia has yet to be appreciated (Coleman 2011). It is unfortunate that the era of anesthesia stress research occurred at a critical juncture when the benefits of hypercarbia during anesthesia were just forgotten, mechanical hyperventilation had become a de-facto standard of practice, and capnography remained a rare and expensive research tool. Mechanical hyperventilation causes "opioid hypersensitivity" that precludes generous opioid administration without prolonged "weaning" from mechanical ventilation. Entrenched dogma thus precluded the development of a practical and safe opioid-based anesthesia technique that inhibits surgical stress. However, there is growing anesthesia awareness of the dangers of mechanical hyperventilation and the benefits of mild hypercarbia. Perhaps it is only a matter of time before the full potential of capnography is utilized to enhance patient comfort, mitigate morbidity, reduce mortality, encourage stress theory, and revolutionize anesthesia.

The recent discovery of the SRM enables the long-sought theory of anesthesia and analgesia that enables the alteration of anesthesia technique to optimize surgical outcome, and it promises the next significant advance in surgical safety and patient comfort. The SRM explains the surgical stress syndrome. Surgery simultaneously and synergistically activates all three SRM pathways, causing positive feedback in accord with the duration and degree of surgical tissue disruption and surgical nervous stimulation (Warr *et al.* 1990; Weissman 1990; Hampton *et al.* 1991; Samama *et al.* 2001; Adembri *et al.* 2004; Modesti *et al.* 2009). This manifests as symptoms distant from the location and time of surgery (McDaniel *et al.* 1984;

Chernow *et al.* 1987; Kavarana *et al.* 2003; Adembri *et al.* 2004; Inoue *et al.* 2004; Monk *et al.* 2005; Liberzon *et al.* 2006; Garvin *et al.* 2010; Modesti *et al.* 2009). Anesthesia controls the cognitive pathway, and analgesia controls the spinal pathway. Either anesthesia or analgesia can independently reduce positive feedback and surgical stress to the point that most patients survive surgery (Anand *et al.* 1987; Anand *et al.* 1990; Anand and Hickey 1992; Abram and Yaksh 1993, 1994), but outcome is substantially enhanced if synergistic combinations of anesthesia and analgesia are maintained continuously throughout surgery to minimize positive feedback caused by capillary gate component activation (Crile and Lower 1914; Steffey *et al.* 1977; Klassen *et al.* 1980; Dubois *et al.* 1982; Hecker *et al.* 1983; Anand *et al.* 1987; Cousins 1989; Ben-Shlomo *et al.* 1990; Huang *et al.* 1990; Kissin *et al.* 1990; Hickey and Hansen 1991; Mangano *et al.* 1991; Anand and Hickey 1992; Mangano *et al.* 1992; Ben-Shlomo *et al.* 1993; Breslow *et al.* 1993; Brunner *et al.* 1994; Vinik *et al.* 1994; Rakaric-Poznanovic *et al.* 1995; Bromage 1996; Glass *et al.* 1997; Akca *et al.* 1999; Mallinder *et al.* 2000; Negishi *et al.* 2000; Sielenkamper *et al.* 2000; Beattie *et al.* 2001; Schneemilch and Bank 2001; Von Dossow *et al.* 2001; Myles *et al.* 2002; Valverde *et al.* 2004; Pypendop and Ilkiw 2005; Exadaktylos *et al.* 2006; Zhang *et al.* 2007; Zhang *et al.* 2007). Such combinations beneficially minimize positive feedback (Suo *et al.* 2003). They reduce blood viscosity and coagulability, improve tissue perfusion and oxygenation, protect organ function, enhance cardiac efficiency, reduce blood pressure, increase ejection fraction, slow heart rate via the Starling mechanism and minimize fever, tachycardia, hypertension, dysrhythmias, infarction, mental confusion, malignancy, heart disease, and other manifestations of positive feedback in the aftermath of surgery (Raymond S. Sinatra 1972; Haldemann *et al.* 1977; Klassen *et al.* 1980; Kono *et al.* 1981; Murphy and Hug 1982; Moffitt *et al.* 1986; Skarvan and Schwinn 1986; Cahalan *et al.* 1987; Hall *et al.* 1987; Vermeyen *et al.* 1989; Huang *et al.* 1990; McEwan *et al.* 1993; O'Connor and Abram 1994; Stefano *et al.* 1995; Stefano *et al.* 1996; Scott 1998; Kapral *et al.* 1999; Sielenkamper *et al.* 2000; Kehlet and Holte 2001; Schneemilch and Bank 2001; Myles *et al.* 2002; Kabon *et al.* 2003; Lee *et al.* 2003; Lessa *et al.* 2004; Shavit *et al.* 2004; Monk *et al.* 2005; Lessa and Tibirica 2006; Rowlingson 2006; Kang *et al.* 2008).

Many anesthesiologists deliberately employ multiple hypnotic medications based on the belief that anesthesia involves multiple drug receptors, and each hypnotic agent controls a different receptor. The SRM explains why this polypharmacy increases toxicity, undermines predictability, and confers no benefit. Only one anesthetic and one analgesic, continuously maintained during surgery, are necessary to control the capillary gate component and optimize outcome. Their synergistic interaction enables reduced dosages of both, which minimizes toxicity and residual effects, improves predictability, and speeds emergence.

No medication or technique is presently available to control the tissue pathway. Theoretically, continuous control of the spinal and cognitive pathways plus neutralization of tissue factor released into blood during surgery should abolish the surgical stress syndrome altogether (Edde 1981; Taylor *et al.* 1987; Fleck *et al.* 1990; Kuitunen *et al.* 1993; Welty-Wolf *et al.* 2001; Healy 2002).

Blood Pressure and Anesthesia Management

The SRM explains why blood pressure is a confusing, counterintuitive, and counterproductive standard of anesthesia monitoring. Blood pressure does not directly measure the cardiac force that propels blood. Therefore, it is not directly related to cardiac contractility, cardiac output, tissue perfusion, tissue oxygenation, stress, anesthesia, and patient well being as commonly assumed. The heart is often regarded as the "Charles Atlas" of the body, but it more closely resembles a 90 lb weakling. The secret of mammalian is efficiency rather than power and force. Red blood cell morphology minimizes systolic flow resistance and enables the heart to move large quantities of blood with remarkable efficiency (see "Turbulence Mechanism" above). The force that propels blood is very weak, and barely adequate for brain perfusion. This explains why the head of most vertebrates is usually located a short distance above the heart. Exceptions to this rule, such as the giraffe, require a disproportionately large heart to propel blood to the brain. Brain perfusion can be compromised even though blood pressure appears adequate. This explains why the "sitting" or "beach chair" position is deceptively dangerous during surgery (Anesthesia Patient Safety Foundation 2009).

Before the onset of surgical stress, anesthesia induction inhibits the cognitive pathway, and blood viscosity declines. This alters blood turbulence in favor of turbulent mixing effects at the expense of turbulent lateral forces, and blood pressure declines. The subsequent onset of surgical stress activates the spinal pathway and increases blood viscosity and blood pressure despite effective anesthetic inhibition of the cognitive pathway. Based on the mistaken assumption that anesthetic agents possess analgesic properties, anesthesiologists traditionally employ anesthetic "overpressure" to control surgical hypertension. Unfortunately, anesthesia confers no benefit beyond its ability to inhibit the cognitive pathway. Instead, the toxic effects of anesthetic overpressure harmfully reduce cardiac contractility, which reduces diastolic turbulent lateral forces, and blood pressure declines. This creates a hazardous combination of depressed cardiac contractility, increased blood viscosity, and capillary hemostasis (capillary gate closure) that impairs cardiac output and tissue perfusion. Under these circumstances, hypotension is a harbinger of impending disaster.

Occult spinal pathway nociception also causes "wind up" syndrome during surgery that produces problematic muscle tension and unexpected movements. Anesthesia cannot prevent these problems. Muscle relaxants control the symptoms of wind up syndrome, but do not inhibit the cause, and occult spinal pathway nociception continues to release VWF and increase blood viscosity. This spinal pathway activity becomes acutely problematic during anesthetic emergence, when the restoration of conscious awareness causes a sudden increase in capillary gate component activity that increases the risk of infarction (Mangano *et al.* 1991; Mangano *et al.* 1992). Meanwhile, tissue factor is released into systemic circulation by surgery. This activates the tissue repair component, which interacts with the capillary gate component to induce positive feedback that does not reach peak intensity for several hours after surgery (Adembri *et al.* 2004; Modesti *et al.* 2009). Combinations of anesthesia and analgesia that effectively control the capillary gate component can minimize this positive feedback and mitigate the symptoms of the surgical stress syndrome. Unfortunately, there is no presently available means to inhibit the tissue repair component, so surgical stress cannot be completely abolished. However, the SRM potentially indicates that directed pharmaceutical research should be able to develop a safe and effective antidote for tissue factor in blood circulation that would enable the complete elimination of surgical stress.

Anesthesia practitioners often employ fibrinogenic pharmaceuticals to maintain blood pressure at "awake" levels in the misguided belief that this maintains tissue perfusion; instead, these drugs exaggerate blood pressure at the further expense of tissue perfusion and oxygenation. Many practitioners administer crystalloid and colloid solutions to maintain blood pressure and tissue perfusion, but this elevates blood pressure by altering blood turbulence in favor of turbulent lateral forces at the expense of turbulent mixing. This harmful effect soon dissipates when crystalloids and colloids diffuse into extravascular tissues (Ruttmann *et al.* 2007; Chappell *et al.* 2008).

In contrast, the addition of analgesia to anesthesia produces a genuine low stress state comparable to natural sleep that is counterintuitively characterized by mild hypotension and bradycardia. This prevents stress hormone release, reduces sympathetic tone and blood viscosity, promotes cardiac efficiency and tissue perfusion, protects organ function, prevents infarction, discourages infection, inhibits atherosclerosis, and minimizes positive feedback that causes malignancy and heart disease in the distant aftermath of surgery.

Disseminated Intravascular Coagulation (DIC)

The conversion of fibrinogen to soluble and insoluble fibrin is a complex process that involves several enzymes and precursors. DIC illustrates how this process can go awry in several ways. DIC is caused by the abnormal entry of tissue factor into systemic blood circulation due to surgery, trauma, sepsis, and amniotic fluid embolus. This activates factor VII, overwhelms inhibitory mechanisms (protein C, TFPI, and ATIII), and initiates excessive intravascular generation of thrombin, soluble fibrin, and insoluble fibrin. The risk and severity of DIC is exaggerated by sensory stresses that activate factor VIII. Insoluble fibrin reduces blood turbulence below a threshold, whereupon spontaneous systemic coagulation suddenly begins (Warr *et al.* 1990; Wada *et al.* 1996; Toh and Dennis 2003; Wada *et al.* 2003). This rapidly consumes and depletes coagulation enzymes and precursors and distorts the coagulation process. Thrombin converts fibrinogen to soluble fibrin, which depletes fibrinogen (Bowie and Owen 1983; Tran *et al.* 1984). Exaggerated factor VIII activity converts factor X to factor XIII to convert soluble fibrin to insoluble fibrin, but this depletes factor VIII and factor X (Tamaki and Aoki 1981, 1982; Tran *et al.* 1984; Dufner and Marbet 2002). Factor XIII installs "cross-links" of fibronectin and plasminogen to soluble fibrin to generate insoluble fibrin, and this consumes both factor XIII and fibronectin (Wada *et al.* 1996; Wada *et al.* 2003). Shortages of factor XIII and fibronectin cause soluble fibrin to accumulate to excessive blood levels (Wettstein *et al.* 2004). Fibronectin exhaustion also causes factor XIII to produce defective forms of insoluble fibrin with inadequate fibronectin "cross-links"(Schoots *et al.* 2004). These imbalances cause soluble fibrin to form abnormal attachments to the pathological clots to produce "microthrombi". Soluble fibrin also deposits on arterial walls (Hardaway *et al.* 1965; Zerbino and Lukasevich 1982, 1983). The abnormal coagulation activity reduces circulating red cell mass, which exaggerates blood turbulence and further inhibits effective coagulation. These abnormalities characterize DIC (Hardy *et al.*

2004; Hardy *et al.* 2005, 2006). The combined imbalances cause a generalized failure of hemostasis.

DIC most often occurs in patients who undergo extensive surgical intervention in the immediate aftermath of major trauma and massive blood loss (Avikainen 1977; Osterud and Bjorklid 2001; Coleman 2007). Trauma and surgery both release tissue factor into systemic circulation and increase factor VII activity, causing SRM hyperactivity and positive feedback (Tran *et al.* 1984; Cheras *et al.* 1997; Suzuki and Morishita 1998; Khatun *et al.* 1999; Laudes *et al.* 2002; Federici 2003; Singh *et al.* 2003; Hardy *et al.* 2004; Hardy *et al.* 2005; von Kanel *et al.* 2006). In addition, trauma patients are typically subjected to starvation, sepsis, hypothermia, fear, pain, hypoxia, and iatrogenic hyperoxia, and these additional forms of stress exaggerate positive feedback and SRM hyperactivity (Ruttmann *et al.* 2007; Chappell *et al.* 2008).

Misguided treatments can confuse and aggravate DIC. Crystalloids, colloids, and starch solutions alter blood turbulence and dilute coagulation precursors and enzymes (Tous *et al.* 2004). DIC removes red cells from circulation, causing anemia that exaggerates blood turbulence and inhibits coagulation (Dintenfass 1965). Blood transfusion corrects the anemia, reduces blood turbulence, and increases blood coagulability, but excessive transfusion with washed, packed red cells devoid of plasma can reduce blood turbulence below a critical threshold and aggravate the problem. Reduction of body temperature even slightly below normal mammalian body temperatures causes lipoprotein solidification, which increases blood viscosity (Khatun *et al.* 1999). Hypothermia activates the SRM and increases blood levels of insoluble fibrin, which also increases blood viscosity (Hardy *et al.* 2006). Severe hypothermia impairs SRM enzymes, and inhibits hemostasis (Dirkmann *et al.* 2008). Metabolic acidosis and hypothermia synergistically impair hemostasis (Scholtes *et al.* 1983).

Eclampsia and Amniotic Fluid Embolus

Like DIC, ARDS, MOFS and malignancy, eclampsia is a manifestation of SRM hyperactivity caused by combinations of stresses that stimulate the three pathways of SRM activity. Normal pregnancy is a stressful condition characterized by elevated blood levels of factor VIII and insoluble fibrin that increase blood viscosity and coagulability (Thornton and Bonnar 1977; Scholtes *et al.* 1983; Tran *et al.* 1984; Frank and Palomino 1987; Angelov 1989; Roberts *et al.* 1989; Rath *et al.* 2000). This is partially offset by hemodilution that increases blood turbulence. Stressful conditions such as diabetes, obesity, and sepsis (commonly caused by occult urinary tract infections during pregnancy) can increase the risk of eclampsia by elevating SRM hyperactivity above the level of normal pregnancy (Mannucci *et al.* 1971; Angelov 1989, 1989; Warr *et al.* 1990; Lockwood *et al.* 1991; Lau and Chui 1994; Osterud and Bjorklid 2001). Eclampsia increases the risk of DIC, in the presence of amniotic fluid embolus. Amniotic fluid contains large concentrations of tissue factor, so that amniotic fluid embolus causes a sudden increase in factor VII activity (Lockwood *et al.* 1991; Lau and Chui 1994; Osterud and Bjorklid 2001; Toh and Dennis 2003).

When this occurs in the presence of pre-existing factor VIII hyperactivity, it causes blood viscosity and coagulability to suddenly rise above the critical threshold where DIC begins (Lind and Janmey 1984; Janmey *et al.* 1985; Lind *et al.* 1986, 1988; Orbach *et al.* 2007).

Sickle Cell Anemia

Sickle cell anemia is caused by a structural weakness in red blood cells that renders them unable to withstand the physical stresses induced by pulsatile blood turbulence. Biconcave mammalian red blood cells spontaneously form "aggregate patterns" during systolic acceleration that inhibit systolic turbulent flow resistance. This explains how the mammalian heart efficiently accelerates blood from 0 to 125 cm/s and ejects its contents in a tenth of a second. As diastolic deceleration disintegrates aggregate patterns, the kinetic energy of speeding blood converts to a burst of turbulent energy that moves rapidly proximal to distal, halting blood flow as it moves and generating lateral forces that account for blood pressure and the palpable pulse. It simultaneously generates turbulent mixing forces that mobilize particulate deposits from the inner walls of arteries to retard atherosclerosis.

Blood levels of insoluble fibrin fluctuate in accord with stressful stimuli that activate the capillary gate component. Insoluble fibrin binds to red cells and interferes with the formation of aggregate patterns during systole, which increases systolic blood turbulence and subjects the red cells to exaggerated turbulent forces as they are accelerated during systole (Giovanardi *et al.* 1998; Tous *et al.* 2004; Bogar *et al.* 2005; Schilling *et al.* 2006). Insoluble fibrin also alters the balance between turbulent mixing forces and turbulent lateral forces during the burst of turbulence that subsequently occurs during diastole. These turbulent forces do not harm normal red blood cells, but they damage the structurally weak red cells of sickle cell patients. The turbulent forces induced by insoluble fibrin explain how stress causes the sudden "sickling" phenomenon (Devine *et al.* 1986; Famodu 1988; Francis 1989). It likewise explains why sickle cell crises affect blood levels of fibrin split products (Salvaggio *et al.* 1963) and why long-term treatment with anticoagulants reduces the severity and frequency of sickle cell crises (Morgan 2008; Solomon 2008). Opioids mitigate the sickle cell crisis by minimizing capillary gate component activity and reducing blood levels of insoluble fibrin.

Pharmacology and the SRM

In 1965, Holemans reported that all "vasoactive" drugs increase fibrin turnover, and that "vasoconstrictors" cause greater fibrin turnover than "vasodilators" (Holemans 1965). The significance of these observations remained unappreciated in the absence of a logical explanation. The effects of vasoactive drugs are generally attributed to drug-induced vascular smooth muscle contraction and relaxation that regulates vascular flow resistance. However, this explanation has to be revised, because the ability of vascular smooth muscle to sustain contraction is energy-intensive, limited in duration, and soon followed by obligatory relaxation, so that it cannot explain sustained elevations of vascular resistance such as occurs in essential hypertension. The capillary gate component provides an improved explanation of these effects. "Vasoconstrictor" drugs promote fibrinogenesis (insoluble fibrin generation) that elevates blood viscosity, closes the capillary gate, decreases tissue and organ perfusion, and increases diastolic turbulent lateral forces at the expense of turbulent mixing. Fibrinogenic drugs therefore increase systemic vascular resistance and blood pressure, accelerate atherosclerosis, and increase blood coagulability. "Vasodilator" drugs promote fibrinolysis (the disintegration of insoluble fibrin) that opens the capillary gate, reduces blood viscosity, enhances tissue and organ perfusion, and increases turbulent mixing at the expense of turbulent lateral forces. They reduce systemic vascular resistance and blood pressure, inhibit atherosclerosis, and decrease blood coagulability. The terms "vasoconstrictor", "vasodilator", and "vasoactive" are therefore misnomers, for they suggest an explanation that is at odds with known facts. Drugs that affect vascular resistance are better described as "fibrinogenic" and "fibrinolytic."

Ca^{2+} levels affect thrombin activity that is essential for fibrinogenesis (Sakata and Aoki 1980; Zuccala *et al.* 1997; Zuccala *et al.* 2000; James and Roche 2004). Low calcium levels inhibit thrombin activity, and thereby interfere with both the generation and the stabilization of insoluble fibrin, which impairs capillary hemostasis and clot formation, and causes bleeding (James and Roche 2004). Trisodium citrate and ethylenediaminetetraacetic acid (EDTA) bind strongly to calcium and halt fibrinogenesis, and are used for blood preservation. Their effects are reversed by the addition of calcium (Murdoch *et al.* 1994). Calcium chloride and calcium gluconate elevate serum Ca^{2+} levels, increase thrombin activity, promote fibrinogenesis, close the capillary gate, and cause sharp but short-lived increases in systemic vascular resistance that increase blood pressure and reduce cardiac index (Barinov *et al.* 1989; Amano *et al.* 1994). Nitroprusside (NTP) and nitroglycerine exert their fibrinolytic effects by releasing nitric oxide from the vascular endothelium that binds to calcium and reduces thrombin activity (Erodi 1973; Menzel *et al.* 1985; Seelig 1990; Assaley *et al.* 1998).

MgSO4 competitively inhibits calcium and promotes fibrinolysis (Rukshin *et al.* 2002). It prevents stent thrombosis (Wu *et al.* 1998; Gerber *et al.* 2000), reduces mortality after myocardial infarction (Ruttmann *et al.* 2007), offsets the hypercoagulability of blood caused by rapid crystalloid infusion (Fuentes *et al.* 1995), and mitigates the manifestations of eclampsia by inhibiting the generation of soluble fibrin that disrupts organ function (Chohan *et al.* 1977; Weksler *et al.* 1977; Genovese *et al.* 1980; Chiariello *et al.* 1983; Brugger *et al.* 1985; Berglund *et al.* 1988; Weiss 1988; Grant 1990; Coffman 1991; Rich *et al.* 1992; Guo *et al.* 1993; Singh *et al.* 1993; Ito *et al.* 1999; Ciardella 2004).

Beta-blockers, furosemide, and "calcium channel blocker" drugs such as nifedipine and verapamil all have fibrinolytic properties that are best explained by their ability to bind Ca^{2+} (Stoltz *et al.* 1999). Their beneficial effects may best be explained by their ability to reduce both pulmonary and systemic vascular resistance and improve cardiac efficiency and organ perfusion (Cremer *et al.* 1984; Weiss 1988; Rich *et al.* 1992; Zuccala *et al.* 1997; Zuccala *et al.* 2000; Naeije and Vachiery 2001). Calcium channel blocker drugs also inhibit platelet activity, promote bleeding, and improve pulmonary hypertension (especially when combined with "anticoagulant" medications), and these effects can be explained by their ability to inhibit thrombin activity (Hampton *et al.* 1991). Vasopressin promotes beneficial fibrinolysis by activating plasmin (Grant 1990).

Epinephrine releases von Willebrand's factor from the vascular endothelium to induce capillary fibrinogenesis and capillary gate closure, and this explains how it increases systemic vascular resistance and blood pressure (Hudetz 1997; Kim *et al.* 2003). Astrocytes protect brain perfusion from epinephrine effects, which explains why the use of epinephrine during cardiac arrest does not cause brain damage (Undas *et al.* 2001). Salicylates exert their anti-inflammatory and anti-platelet effects by interfering with thrombin generation (Vlahos *et al.* 2003). Glucocorticoids inhibit the cellular effects of thrombin (Hassoun *et al.* 1989; Rich *et al.* 1992; Archer and Rich 2000). Anticoagulant medications have no direct effect on vascular smooth muscle, but they interfere with thrombin production and fibrinogenesis, and this explains how they inhibit atherosclerosis, mitigate hypertension, and prevent sickle cell anemia crisis (Itakura *et al.* 1977; Luostarinen *et al.* 1981).

The effects of local anesthetics are explained by their ability to block the function of exposed sympathetic nerve endings that directly innervate the vascular endothelium in addition to their ability to block nerve conduction (Mannucci *et al.* 1971; Luostarinen *et al.* 1981; Orr *et al.* 1986; Tobias *et al.* 1996; Tobias *et al.* 1999; Sielenkamper *et al.* 2000; Hahnenkamp *et al.* 2002; Federici 2003; Weinberg *et al.* 2004; Kuo *et al.* 2006; Sen *et al.* 2006). They block the sympathetic nerve endings that induce the release of von Willebrand's factor from the vascular endothelium, and inhibit the capillary gate component (Luostarinen *et al.* 1981; Modig *et al.* 1983; Modig *et al.* 1983; Modig 1985; Orr *et al.* 1986; Kennedy and Strom 1990; Liu *et al.* 1995; Moore *et al.* 1995; Tobias *et al.* 1996; Kapral *et al.* 1999; Tobias *et al.* 1999; Sielenkamper *et al.* 2000; Temple and Timms 2001; Hahnenkamp *et al.* 2002; Lee *et al.* 2003; Filimonovic *et al.* 2005). Local anesthetics increase capillary flow and reduce coagulability and surgical stress whether administered via intravenous, tissue infiltration, epidural or spinal routes (Cooke *et al.* 1977; Groeben *et al.* 1996; Groudine *et al.* 1998; Lee *et al.* 1998; Hahnenkamp *et al.* 2002; Weinberg *et al.* 2004). When administered intravenously, they reduce blood coagulability, bronchial hyper-reactivity, and surgical stress (Luostarinen *et al.* 1981; Kennedy and Strom 1990; Temple and Timms 2001). When infiltrated into tissues, they increase capillary flow and inhibit capillary hemostasis (Chohan *et al.* 1974; Epstein *et al.* 1976; Bartsch *et al.* 1989; Friedman *et al.* 1997; Fenton *et al.* 1998; Goldsack *et al.* 1998; Watkins *et al.* 2000; Webb *et al.* 2000; Przyklenk and Kloner 2001; Zhang *et al.* 2001; Archiniegas *et al.* 2004; Das *et al.* 2004; Trachte *et al.* 2005; Caruso *et al.* 2006; Korom *et al.* 2006; Swallow and Anderson 2006; Ali and Rakkah 2007; Ayala *et al.* 2007; Behr-Roussel *et al.* 2007; Fagenholz *et al.* 2007; Lewis *et al.* 2007; Parker *et al.* 2007; Schafer *et al.* 2008).

Sildinafil mimics parasympathetic activity by releasing nitric oxide from the vascular endothelium to promote capillary fibrinolysis and organ and tissue perfusion. This explains why it synergizes the effects of nitroglycerin, enhances organ transplantation, increases peristalsis, and treats high altitude pulmonary edema (HAPE), pulmonary and systemic hypertension, congestive heart failure, diabetes, achalasia as well as erectile dysfunction (Hojo *et al.* 2001). The ability of angiotensin converting enzyme (ACE) inhibitors to control hypertension is attributed to their effects on angiotensin, but is also explained by their reduction of von Willebrand factor levels (Drenth and Nagengast 2000; Fujita *et al.* 2000; Veyradier *et al.* 2001; Warkentin *et al.* 2003; Leibovitz *et al.* 2004). The reduction of von Willebrand factor explains how they increase cardiac output and reduce systemic vascular resistance, why they cause unpredictable tissue edema and swelling that is analogous to angioneurotic edema, and why they are contra-indicated in patients with aortic valve replacements and aortic outflow obstruction (Chesebro *et al.* 1995). The SRM indicates that fibrinolysis and thrombin inhibition should improve outcome in organ transplantation, spinal injuries, burns, ARDS, MSOF, and malignancy.

Infarction

The presently prevailing explanation of infarction is plaque disruption that releases debris, obstructs distal flow, and initiates occlusive thrombus formation (Mangano *et al.* 1991; Mangano *et al.* 1992; Landesberg *et al.* 2001). This hypothesis does not explain myocardial infarction that occurs during anesthetic emergence that does not involve thrombus formation and is prevented by analgesia (Kloner *et al.* 1974; Ito and Iwakura 1998; Morishima *et al.* 2000; Rezkalla and Kloner 2002). It likewise fails to explain the "no-reflow" phenomenon, wherein stent installation restores arterial flow but fails to restore capillary perfusion in infarcted tissues (Kent and Epstein 1976; Klassen *et al.* 1980; Gasser *et al.* 1995; Wu *et al.* 1998; Roe *et al.* 2001; Hellstrom 2002, 2003; Danson and Paterson 2006). It also fails to explain why infarction symptoms, autonomic imbalance, and microvascular flow disturbances appear long before thrombus formation (Nees 1989; Wu *et al.* 1998; Gerber *et al.* 2000; McDonagh and Hokama 2000; Hellstrom 2002, 2003); why anticoagulants must be administered before thrombus formation to prevent myocardial damage; and why opioids, which have no anticoagulant properties, mitigate infarction symptoms and severity (Neuhof *et al.* 1975; Gasser *et al.* 1995; Wu *et al.* 1998; Tatu-Chitoiu *et al.* 2004). The reductions in systemic vascular resistance and blood pressure that accompany successful treatment with anticoagulants such as streptokinase and urokinase remain unexplained, as anticoagulants do not affect muscular vasculature (Wu *et al.* 1998).

The simplest explanation of early stages of myocardial infarction is that capillary gate hyperactivity inhibits tissue perfusion and oxygenation (Kent and Epstein 1976), causing a vicious cycle of angina that elevates SNS activity and aggravates capillary gate closure in the affected tissues (Neuhof *et al.* 1975). The beneficial effects of anticoagulants are best explained by rapid fibrinolysis that opens the capillary gate, restores capillary perfusion to infarcted tissues, and reduces systemic vascular resistance and blood pressure (Kranenburg *et al.* 2002; Tatu-Chitoiu *et al.* 2004). Tissue plasminogen activator (TPA) has largely supplanted urokinase and streptokinase as treatments for acute infarction. It causes less dramatic reductions in systemic vascular resistance and blood pressure, but it is probably less potent as a treatment, because it only indirectly accelerates the disintegration of insoluble fibrin by increasing plasmin activity (Kent and Epstein 1976; Wu *et al.* 1998).

Opioids lack direct effects on either muscular vasculature or coagulation; they mitigate myocardial infarction damage via their ability to control infarction angina, reduce SNS tone and activity, open the capillary gate, and restore perfusion in afflicted tissues (Sotiriou and Cheng 2000; Rim *et al.* 2001; Krysiak *et al.* 2003). The ability of "statin" drugs to prevent myocardial infarction can best be explained by their ability to lower VWF levels, inhibit insoluble fibrin generation, reduce viscosity, retard atherosclerosis and promote capillary perfusion (Genovese *et al.* 1983; Pardo Mindan and Panizo 1993). However, these drugs undermine capillary gate function and can cause lethal angioneurotic edema. Nitroglycerin and nitroprusside prevent angina and infarction by releasing nitric oxide from the vascular endothelium, which opens the capillary gate (see above). The exaggerated vulnerability of geriatric patients to infarction is caused by capillary senescence that compromises tissue and organ perfusion. This is reflected by the presence of capillary bed "filling defects" in healthy geriatric patients (Phillip *et al.* 2003).

Rheumatoid Disease

Rheumatoid disease is usually attributed to "autoimmune" activity, but the cause is unknown. SRM dysfunction that generates amyloid protein explains these diseases. Amyloid deposits are universally present in afflicted organs and tissues in rheumatoid disease (Frank and Palomino 1987; O'Hara *et al.* 2004). Rheumatoid nodules consist of amyloid deposits (Powell *et al.* 2003; EshKalback *et al.* 2004). Amyloid deposits are present in 90% of type II diabetics, and they destroy pancreatic islet cells (Sahoo *et al.* 2003). Lymphomas and diabetes cause amyloid tumor formation (Furie *et al.* 1977; Greipp *et al.* 1981; Gastineau *et al.* 1991; Liebman *et al.* 1992; Marcatti *et al.* 1995; Gamba *et al.* 1999; Gamba *et al.* 2000; Neuhaus *et al.* 2002; Uprichard and Perry 2002; Nilsson 2004; Palmero Marti *et al.* 2004; Smith *et al.* 2004; Takamori *et al.* 2004; Wiland *et al.* 2004). Amyloidosis explains the symptoms and relationships of rheumatoid diseases, diabetes, Parkinson's disease, vitamin D depletion, and infectious "prions" (Schwartz 1975; Jacquot *et al.* 1981; Jabor *et al.* 2006). Surgery and other forms of stress aggravate amyloidosis (Janmey *et al.* 1992; Nilsson 2004). Fibrillar actin protein interacts with insoluble fibrin, and disrupts the tissue repair function of the viscoelastic clot. This causes a "vicious cycle" that consumes and depletes factor X and vitamin D, accelerates atherosclerosis, and generates amyloid protein that forms disruptive deposits in organs and tissues.

Amyloidosis is a disorder of protein conformation caused by "misfolding" in which normally soluble proteins are deposited extracellularly as insoluble fibrils that impair tissue structure and function (San Biagio *et al.* 1999; Hirschfield and Hawkins 2003; Page *et al.* 2004). Over 20 unrelated proteins form amyloid fibrils in vivo, with fibrils sharing a lamellar cross-beta sheet structure composed of non-covalently associated protein or peptide subunit s(Yood *et al.* 1983; Liebman *et al.* 1992; Beardell *et al.* 1997; Mumford *et al.* 2000; Choufani *et al.* 2001; Uprichard and Perry 2002; Buhl *et al.* 2003). Disorders of actin metabolism cause the actin molecule to undergo conformational changes to form amyloid protein (Schwartz 1976; Furie *et al.* 1977; Neuhaus *et al.* 2002; Powell *et al.* 2003; Clark and Nilsson 2004; Hall and Edskes 2004; Ho *et al.* 2004; Palmero Marti *et al.* 2004; Tanaka *et al.* 2004).

Amyloidosis depletes factor X, which disturbs clot permeability and disrupts tissue repair (Smith *et al.* 1993; Smith *et al.* 1996; Sinz *et al.* 2002; Smith *et al.* 2004). Disturbances in clot permeability explain the chronic inflammation, cell proliferation, and increased immune cell activity observed in rheumatoid diseases (Sane *et al.* 1989; Mizutani and Ward 1990; Kaiserling and Krober 1995; Van Nostrand *et al.* 2000). Amyloidosis causes bleeding by damaging blood vessels (Chernow *et al.* 1987; Roher *et al.* 2003; Hall and Edskes 2004; Tian *et al.* 2004; Whitaker *et al.* 2004). Amyloid and/or actin may increase blood viscosity and accelerate atherosclerosis by inhibiting the normal disintegration of insoluble fibrin, and this may explain the strong associations between rheumatoid disease, diabetes, amyloidosis, and atherosclerosis (Kaiserling and Krober 1995; San Biagio *et al.* 1999; Hirschfield and Hawkins 2003; Foguel and Silva 2004).

Like insoluble fibrin, actin is a "fibrillar" molecule that polymerizes into strands (Lind *et al.* 1988; Janmey *et al.* 1992; Erukhimov *et al.* 2000). It is the most abundant protein in the vertebrate body. It is present in all cells, and is released into the blood by cell damage (Janmey *et al.* 1985; Janmey *et al.* 1985; Janmey and Lind 1987; Lind and Smith 1991, 1991; Janmey *et al.* 1992). It becomes entangled with insoluble fibrin in the viscoelastic clot. It binds to the "kringle" portions of the plasmin molecule and inhibits plasmin activity that disintegrates the insoluble fibrin molecule into fibrin split products (Janmey *et al.* 1985; Lind *et al.* 1988; Lind and Smith 1991; Janmey *et al.* 1992). It thus interferes with the normal disintegration of insoluble fibrin by plasmin, which disturbs clot permeability, blood viscosity, and tissue repair (Kaiserling and Krober 1995; Souto *et al.* 1995; Krishnan and Korzenik 2002). Actin triggers a "vicious cycle" that generates amyloid protein, consumes factor X, depletes vitamin D, and accelerates atherosclerosis. This explains the close associations between and among amyloidosis, atherosclerosis, Alzheimer's disease, rheumatoid arthritis, systemic lupus erythematosis, diabetes, Parkinson's disease, infectious "prion" release, inflammatory bowel disease (Schwartz 1976; Chernow *et al.* 1987; Mangano *et al.* 1992; Schwarzinger *et al.* 1992; Inoue *et al.* 2004; Savareux *et al.* 2004; Tian *et al.* 2004; Grant 2006), and other pathologies (Liu and Li 2004). Actin that is released from damaged red blood cells during bypass surgery explains SIRS (systemic inflammatory response syndrome) that is observed in these patients (Kawasaki *et al.* 2004).

Gelsolin and vitamin D neutralize actin and its effects (Lind *et al.* 1986; Janmey and Lind 1987; Erukhimov *et al.* 2000). Actin is metabolized in two stages (Smith *et al.* 1987; Smith *et al.* 1988; Smith *et al.* 1988). In the first stage, the fibrillar actin molecule is rapidly reduced to inert subunits by the blood enzyme gelsolin (Lind and Janmey 1984). Gelsolin binds avidly to fibronectin, so that it becomes concentrated in the viscoelastic clot (Janmey *et al.* 1985; Janmey and Lind 1987; Lind *et al.* 1987). Thrombin energizes gelsolin (Janmey and Lind 1987; Erukhimov *et al.* 2000; Grant 2006; Orbach *et al.* 2007). In the second stage, actin subunits are metabolized in a slower reaction that consumes vitamin D (Lind and Smith 1991; Kranenburg *et al.* 2002; Laudes *et al.* 2002; Hirschfield and Hawkins 2003; Powell *et al.* 2003; Clark and Nilsson 2004; EshKalback *et al.* 2004; Foguel and Silva 2004; Hall and Edskes 2004; Ho *et al.* 2004; Nilsson 2004; Orbach *et al.* 2007). This explains why depletion of gelsolin and Vitamin D aggravates the chronic inflammatory effects and exaggerated immune activity that occur in rheumatoid diseases as well as in the aftermath of cardio-pulmonary bypass (systemic inflammatory response syndrome), major surgery (surgical stress syndrome), severe injury (multi-organ failure syndrome) and sepsis (Frank and Palomino 1987; Grant 2006; Smedby *et al.* 2006; Orbach *et al.* 2007).

Hypertension and Diabetes

Essential hypertension (EH) is elevated blood pressure of unknown cause that increases the risk for cerebral, cardiac, and renal events (Lip *et al.* 1997; Buhl *et al.* 2003). It begins with unexplained proteinuria and insulin resistance, while blood pressure remains deceptively normal at rest, but increases to unexpected levels during exercise and emotion. As the disease progresses, blood pressure eventually remains continuously elevated even at rest, and organ failure ensues. Pre-eclampsia patients exhibit similar progression from occult proteinuria and insulin resistance to overt hypertension (Cousins 1989; Kawut *et al.* 2005).

Essential hypertension is usually attributed to arteriolar "stiffness," reductions in the caliber and number of arterioles, and impaired arterial compliance (Lip *et al.* 1995; Zlokovic 1997; Buhl *et al.* 2003; Messerli *et al.* 2007). This explanation fails to explain glucose intolerance and elevations of VWF, D-dimer (fibrin split products), insoluble fibrin, factor VII and factor VIII activity, increased blood viscosity and coagulability, systemic inflammatory effects, and accelerated atherosclerosis that occurs in both systemic and pulmonary forms of hypertension (Winniford 1990; Kario *et al.* 1996; Friedman *et al.* 1997; Kario *et al.* 1997; Matsuo *et al.* 1997; Kario *et al.* 1998; Matsuo *et al.* 1998; Matsuo *et al.* 1998; Mazzone *et al.* 2001; Bogar 2002; Chang *et al.* 2002; Hlubocka *et al.* 2002; Kario *et al.* 2003; Hao *et al.* 2005; Kato *et al.* 2006; Messerli *et al.* 2007). It also fails to explain how hypertension increases the risk of stroke and myocardial infarction, because these pathologies are paradoxically thrombotic rather than hemorrhagic (Genovese *et al.* 1980; Genovese *et al.* 1982; Genovese *et al.* 1983; Genovese *et al.* 1983). Hypertension can be successfully treated with anticoagulants, and successful treatment is characterized by reductions in VWF levels (Genovese *et al.* 1980; Genovese *et al.* 1982; Genovese *et al.* 1983; Genovese *et al.* 1983). The hypercoagulable state also explains the association between essential hypertension, amyloidosis, and accelerated atherosclerosis, none of which are explained by stiffness, impaired compliance, and reduced arteriole numbers (Phillip *et al.* 2003).

The SRM explains essential hypertension and diabetes and their close relationships. Direct parasympathetic innervation opens the capillary gate in visceral organs by releasing nitric oxide from the vascular endothelium (van Zwieten and Doods 1995; Hudetz 1997; Si and Lee 2002; Hudetz 2003; Wojtarowicz *et al.* 2003; Dijkstra *et al.* 2004; Toda *et al.* 2005; Anderson *et al.* 2006). Parasympathetic stimulation also releases insulin from the pancreas into flowing blood. Insulin releases nitric oxide from capillary walls and opens the capillary gate in peripheral tissues that lack direct parasympathetic innervation (Wamhoff *et al.* 1976; Belcaro *et al.* 1992; Morita-Tsuzuki *et al.* 1993; Watkins *et al.* 2000; Martin *et al.* 2001; Kvist-Reimer *et al.* 2002; Vincent *et al.* 2003; Colantuoni *et al.* 2005; Ahmed 2006; Ali and Rakkah 2007; Ayala *et al.* 2007; Behr-Roussel *et al.* 2007). This explains why insulin prolongs bleeding time, reduces systemic vascular resistance, increases cardiac index, aggravates angina, and counteracts "vasopressor" (fibrinogenic) drugs (Wamhoff *et al.* 1976; Figueras *et al.* 1979; Rich *et al.* 1992; Singh *et al.* 1993; Baron 1994; Lee *et al.* 2000; Carr 2001; Ciardella 2004; Parker *et al.* 2007); why allostatic load inhibits insulin effects (Brandi *et al.* 1990); and why diabetes and hypertension are closely related (Schneider 1949; Hassoun *et al.* 1989; He 1990; Penny *et al.* 1991; Boudier 1999; Cicco *et al.* 1999; Vicaut 1999; Yi *et al.* 1999; Lee *et al.* 2000; McDonagh and Hokama 2000; Veyradier *et al.* 2000; Esler *et al.* 2001; Long *et al.* 2001; Naeije and Vachiery 2001; Bogar 2002; Hlubocka *et al.* 2002; Muller *et al.* 2002; Adamiec *et al.* 2003; Choi 2005; Colantuoni *et al.* 2005; Kawut *et al.* 2005; Kawut *et al.* 2005; Khan *et al.* 2005; Wallis *et al.* 2005; Caruso *et al.* 2006; Caruso *et al.* 2006; Savoia and Schiffrin 2006; Messerli *et al.* 2007; Schafer *et al.* 2008). Nitric oxide is also bactericidal, so that PNS activity inhibits infection as well as enhances tissue perfusion and oxygenation (Saraiva *et al.* 2011).

Capillary beds naturally deteriorate with age, and this increases both vascular resistance and insulin requirements (Genovese *et al.* 1983; Genovese *et al.* 1983; Fan *et al.* 2000; Fornek *et al.* 2007). Both diabetes and hypertension involve accelerated capillary senility that increases vascular resistance and blood viscosity, elevates blood pressure, impairs tissue perfusion and glucose uptake, and increases insulin requirements. Inadequate insulin release causes type I diabetes. Type II diabetes is caused by accelerated capillary senility that impairs glucose uptake in peripheral tissues and increases insulin requirements. This explains why type II diabetes occurs in older persons. Chemical destruction of sympathetic nerve endings in the pancreas has cured type I diabetes in a rat model, which refutes the hypothesis that autoimmune activity causes diabetes (Kvist-Reimer *et al.* 2002).

Environmental and chemical stress accelerates both capillary senility and atherosclerosis, and aggravates both diabetes and hypertension (Genovese *et al.* 1983; Genovese *et al.* 1983; Fan *et al.* 2000; Wilson 2001; Fornek *et al.* 2007). Emotional stress, such as earthquakes and job stress, accelerates both atherosclerosis and capillary senility by increasing SNS activity that elevates blood viscosity (Khomulo *et al.* 1976; Gutstein and Parl 1978; Khomulo *et al.*

1980; Ranjbar *et al.* 2007). For example, Carroll Shelby of car racing fame employed nitroglycerin treatment to sustain his emotionally stressful career, and ultimately underwent heart replacement surgery twice. The baboons used by NASA for rocket sled tests developed hypertension and died prematurely (Wolfe 1979). Uninjured earthquake victims exhibit infarctions, strokes, and elevations of blood pressure, von Willebrand factor, factor VIII, blood viscosity, and blood coagulability that persist for months (Kario and Matsuo 1995; Kario *et al.* 1998; Kario *et al.* 2003). The simplest explanation is that emotional and environmental stress causes occult SRM hyperactivity that generates thrombin, soluble fibrin, and insoluble fibrin.

Thrombin induces inflammatory effects. Soluble fibrin causes proteinuria and insoluble fibrin increases blood viscosity. Their combined effects insidiously undermine organ function, accelerate atherosclerosis and capillary senility, and increase insulin requirements and vascular resistance (Figueras *et al.* 1979; Belcaro *et al.* 1992; Baron 1994; Lee *et al.* 2000; Long *et al.* 2001; Hlubocka *et al.* 2002; Vincent *et al.* 2003; Colantuoni *et al.* 2005; Wallis *et al.* 2005; Ahmed 2006). In the early stages, exercise increases cardiac output and emotional stress exaggerates pre-existing abnormal flow resistance, so that both cause exaggerated elevations of the blood pressure. Blood pressure and insulin resistance gradually increase as the disease progresses. Chronically increased blood viscosity increases cardiac work and deteriorates cardiac performance, and it inexorably induces cardiomyopathy that is characterized by myocyte hypertrophy, extracellular collagen deposition, and increased cardiac wall thickness. Ultimately the heart suddenly "balloons" in size, cardiac walls become thin, and overt congestive heart failure ensues (Belcaro *et al.* 1992; Bredbacka *et al.* 1994; Cicco *et al.* 1999; Akassoglou *et al.* 2000; Lee *et al.* 2000; Akassoglou and Strickland 2002; Akassoglou *et al.* 2002; Vincent *et al.* 2003).

Athletic Conditioning

Exercise conditioning produces several unexplained beneficial effects (Eichner 1983; Schmermund 2004). It ameliorates the pathological effects of chronic hypertension, coronary artery disease, atherosclerosis, and diabetes (Carr 2001; Choi 2005; Zanesco and Antunes 2007). It produces resting bradycardia and reduced blood pressure that is usually attributed to increased vagal tone, but this explanation is weak (Sandercock *et al.* 2005; Zanesco and Antunes 2007). Capillary gate operation offers an improved explanation for exercise conditioning. Exercise increases SRM activity (van den Burg *et al.* 2000). It induces both arteriogenesis (collateral vessel enlargement and recruitment) and angiogenesis (capillary proliferation) in the muscles that are subjected to regular exercise, and this reduces systemic vascular resistance (Wijnen *et al.* 1994; Moser and Patterson 2003; Prior *et al.* 2003; Lloyd *et al.* 2005).

The reduction in systemic vascular resistance lowers blood pressure at rest, when metabolic demands and nervous stimulation of the cardiovascular system are both minimal, and facilitates increased ejection fraction, so that heart rate is reduced in accord with the Frank-Starling principle. The alleviation of hypertension is also explained by the reduction in systemic vascular resistance. The improvement in diabetes is explained by the angiogenesis in skeletal muscle that improves muscle cell exposure to glucose and facilitates glucose uptake (Baron 1994; Yi *et al.* 1999; Lee *et al.* 2000; Long *et al.* 2001).

Organ Function and the Capillary Gate

Autonomic balance governs organ function by controlling organ perfusion. SNS activity "closes" the capillary gate, reduces organ perfusion, and decreases organ function; while PNS activity "opens" the capillary gate, increases organ perfusion, and enhances organ function (Kent and Epstein 1976; Itakura *et al.* 1977). Parasympathetic activity increases capillary flow in the lung (Kondo *et al.* 2004), which can result is capillary engorgement that manifests as "bronchoconstriction". It increases brain blood flow in accord with brain activity (Morita-Tsuzuki *et al.* 1993; Hudetz 1997; Si and Lee 2002). It enhances esophageal peristalsis (Zhang *et al.* 2001), which decreases food transit time (Beyak *et al.* 2000; Zhang *et al.* 2001; Beyak *et al.* 2003) and increases saliva production by enhancing salivary gland perfusion (Anderson *et al.* 2006). It increases penis perfusion to enable erection (Toda *et al.* 2005, 2007), enhances intestinal peristalsis and digestive fluid production (Martin *et al.* 2001; Dijkstra *et al.* 2004), increases the activity of beta cells and the release of insulin from the pancreas. SNS activity opposes all these PNS effects by closing the capillary gate. Severe increases in SNS tone can cause death from myocardial infarction or stroke by disrupting the perfusion of these vital tissues (Kent and Epstein 1976; Wu *et al.* 1998; Lip *et al.* 2002; Kario *et al.* 2003).

Direct SNS innervation is present throughout all body tissues, but direct PNS innervation is limited to internal organs (Itakura *et al.* 1977). Insulin primarily affects those peripheral tissues that are devoid of PNS innervation, such as skeletal muscle (Kvist-Reimer *et al.* 2002). It opens the capillary gate by releasing nitric oxide (McDonagh and Hokama 2000; Vincent *et al.* 2003; Wallis *et al.* 2005), and thereby increases cell exposure to glucose and facilitates glucose uptake (Wamhoff *et al.* 1976; Lee *et al.* 2000). This explains why insulin causes a prolonged bleeding time (Wamhoff *et al.* 1976; Figueras *et al.* 1979), reduces systemic vascular resistance, increases cardiac index and stroke volume about 20 minutes after a meal (Baron 1994), and opposes the effects of "vasopressors"(Itakura *et al.* 1977; Zlokovic *et al.* 1995; Hudetz 1997; Zlokovic 1997; Lee *et al.* 2000; Si and Lee 2002; Kim *et al.* 2003; Wang and Reiser 2003, 2003).

Astrocytes release nitric oxide and thrombomodulin in response to PNS stimulation to protect oxygen-sensitive brain tissue from the harmful effects of capillary hemostasis (Hudetz 1997; Zlokovic 1997). They proliferate in the presence of thrombin elevations (Wang and Reiser 2003, 2003). Their presence explains why brain tissue bleeds readily (Grant 1990; Schwertz *et al.* 2004). It also explains why epinephrine, which releases VWF and increases systemic vascular resistance in accord with SNS activity, does not ordinarily cause brain damage when used in medical emergencies (Fleck *et al.* 1990). Astrocyte activity also explains the abundance of tissue factor in brain tissue that is necessary to supplement capillary hemostasis in brain tissues (Feigl *et al.* 1987). Severe head injuries release tissue factor into systemic circulation, which increases morbidity and mortality (Ungerstedt *et al.* 2003).

Sildenafil is a recently introduced drug that appears to have the unique ability to mimic the effects of the PNS. It releases nitric oxide and promotes organ function in capillary beds in the same manner as parasympathetic stimulation (Przyklenk and Kloner 2001). Penile erection normally occurs because of PNS stimulation that opens the capillary gate in penile tissues (Webb *et al.* 2000). Sildenafil synergizes this effect in the clitoris as well as the penis (Caruso *et al.* 2006), but its useful effects are not limited to this aspect (Friedman *et al.* 1997; Trachte *et al.* 2005; Lewis *et al.* 2007). It has proved to be useful for treating pulmonary edema, pulmonary hypertension, congestive heart failure (Chohan *et al.* 1974; Das *et al.* 2004; Swallow and Anderson 2006; Fagenholz *et al.* 2007), Diabetes (Caruso *et al.* 2006; Ali and Rakkah 2007; Ayala *et al.* 2007; Behr-Roussel *et al.* 2007; Schafer *et al.* 2008), high altitude pulmonary edema (HAPE) (Zhang *et al.* 2001; Swallow and Anderson 2006), achalasia (Zhang *et al.* 2001), peristalsis (Watkins *et al.* 2000; Korom *et al.* 2006), and organ transplants (Korom *et al.* 2006; Parker *et al.* 2007). Sildenafil synergizes the hypotensive effects of nitroglycerine, which is often assumed to be dangerous (Epstein *et al.* 1976), but the risk is probably exaggerated because both drugs exert their effects by opening the capillary gate, improving tissue perfusion, reducing systemic vascular resistance, and improving cardiac efficiency (Przyklenk and Kloner 2001). Their additive effects are thus beneficial despite the fact that they reduce blood pressure (Epstein *et al.* 1976; Fenton *et al.* 1998; Goldsack *et al.* 1998; Archiniegas *et al.* 2004; Parker *et al.* 2007).

Medical Treatments for Stress-related Pathologies

SRM hyperactivity can be lethal, and it is stubbornly resilient because of its redundant, synergistic pathways. For example, the worldwide influenza epidemic of 1918 killed millions of young, healthy victims but paradoxically spared the very young, the very old, and the weak (Taylor *et al.* 1987; Healy 2002; Idell 2002; van der Poll *et al.* 2005; Robriquet *et al.* 2006). Similarly, asthma afflicts young, healthy victims who generate excessive soluble fibrin in airway passages exposed to inhaled antigens (Mattick 2003, 2004). Control of the SRM is expected to improve outcome in these and numerous other conditions, including severe burns, MOFS, ARDS, eclampsia, acute spinal cord injury, acute brain injury, and so forth. Treatments for many forms of SRM activity have long been available, but their effective use is hampered by the lack of effective theory that explains how and why they work, and how they can best be applied.

Heparin and Plavix inhibit factor VIII but do not interfere with the interaction of factors VII and X and tissue factor that is essential for tissue maintenance, tissue repair, and embryological development. They are thus relatively safe for use in pregnant women, surgery patients, and for prolonged treatment to prevent infarction and retard atherosclerosis. In contrast, warfarin interferes with the interaction of factors VII and X and tissue factor, so that it disrupts embryological development, wound healing and tissue maintenance, and is dangerous when used for prolonged treatment. For the same reason, it inhibits malignancy, which involves tissue repair hyperactivity.

Trisodium citrate and MgSO4 inhibit thrombin activation by Ca^{2+}, so that they could be useful in a wide variety of situations where acute reduction in SRM hyperactivity is needed, such as asthma, pneumonia, influenza, eclampsia, mis-matched blood transfusion, acute spinal cord injury, infarction, organ transplants, severe burns, ARDS, MOFS, and malignancy. Sildenafil mimics the effects of PNS activity and promotes organ function in a wide variety of conditions by releasing nitric oxide from the vascular endothelium. It thus provides an effective treatment for HAPE, achalasia, digestive disorders, diabetes, and hypertension as well as sexual dysfunction.

Pharmaceutical research to develop safe treatments that neutralize tissue factor in blood circulation or mimic the effects of stoichiometric antithrombin III, protein C, and tissue factor pathway inhibitor would undoubtedly be useful. The addition of fibrinogen, fibronectin, and vitronectin to intravenous fluids should improve their safety and effectiveness. Non-invasive monitors of blood viscosity would provide a useful means to detect SRM hyperactivity during and after surgery.

Evolution, Embryology and the SRM

Most DNA information derives from prokaryotic (i.e. bacterial) cell research. Prokaryotic cells are easy to study. They employ their outer membrane for respiration, which limits them to single-cell existence, small size, and a few shapes that optimize surface area. They have simple internal structures and only one type of DNA that floats free in the cytoplasm and transmits its genetic information via a straightforward mechanism that employs RNA templates to generate proteins. Multi-cellular animals consist of eukaryotic cells that are vastly more complex than prokaryotic cells. They utilize mitochondria for respiration, which enables them to become much larger, assume diverse shapes, and build complex multicellular life forms. Their internal structure is complex. Their DNA is enclosed within a nucleus in the form of chromosomes that divide when the cell replicates. Their cytoplasm contains structurally distinct "organelles" with specific functions. Many of these organelles have their own DNA that replicates independent of the nuclear DNA. Eukaryotic cells are thus believed to have originated when a "parent" cell somehow engulfed other types of previously free-living single-cell organisms that subsequently became symbiotic organelles. The nuclear membrane of the parent cell isolates its DNA from the cytoplasmic DNA of the organelles.

The nuclear DNA of complex animals transmits its genetic information via mechanisms that are not yet fully understood. It consists of short protein-encoding segments that are interspersed with large sections of "junk" DNA that remains inert in the mature individual. "Junk" DNA was initially assumed to have no function, but recent research reveals that it consists at least in part of "introns" that somehow control stem cell maintenance, cell proliferation, and apoptosis to enable embryological tissue development. However, the introns do not produce proteins. These observations have led the current generation of cell researchers to hypothesize that "junk" DNA transmits its information via an unknown cytoplasmic mechanism to enable embryological development (Mahajan *et al.* 2000; Mattick 2003, 2004, 2004).

The previous generation of stress researchers held a similar viewpoint. They knew that the DNA mechanism does not explain embryological development. They believed that the stress mechanism postulated by Hans Selye acts as a "companion mechanism" that works closely with DNA to convert genetic information into cell proliferation and differentiation to generate embryological structures, and that the stress mechanism remains active throughout life to maintain and repair mature structures, while DNA itself becomes quiescent once embryological development is complete.

Both viewpoints may be correct. Thrombin receptors are present on the outer surface of all animal cells thus far tested, and they determine how cells respond to thrombin (Kirschner and Gerhart 2005; Luo *et al.* 2005; Tantivejkul *et al.* 2005). Mature cells have stable configurations of thrombin receptors that characterize their type, but cells can change their thrombin receptors during tissue repair and malignancy, and thereby alter their responses to thrombin. It is hypothesized that "introns" regulate thrombin receptors at precise time intervals to govern cell proliferation and differentiation during embryological development, and that they release tissue factor to induce thrombin generation by the SRM to energize embryological development. Such a mechanism would explain how "introns" control three-dimensional cell proliferation, differentiation, apoptosis, and other cell activities necessary for structural development. It would explain why "introns" do not produce proteins, and why they remain quiescent once embryological development is complete, while the SRM remains active for the duration of life to maintain and repair mature structures. It would explain why defects in tissue factor and factors VII and X and medications such as Coumadin and thalidomide, which disrupt their function, cause death or disruption during embryological development, while heparin and other anticoagulants that affect only factor VIII do not disturb embryological development, because factor VIII is not essential for embryological development.

The SRM appears to be highly conserved in nature, and it provides insight to the nature of evolution. The sudden appearance of the SRM/introns mechanism explains the "Cambrian Explosion" of complex animal forms some 540 million years ago, because it enables complex animal structures. It explains how DNA preserves genetic information that enables adaptation to environmental changes (Kirschner and Gerhart 2005).

Fresh definitions enabled by the SRM

Definitions of stress-related phenomena remain imprecise because of the inability to explain them. For example, the *International Association for the Study of Pain* defines pain as "an unpleasant sensory or emotional experience associated with actual or potential tissue damage." It defines analgesia as "absence of pain in response to stimulation, which would normally be painful" and it defines nociception as "the neural process of encoding noxious stimuli" (Loeser 1994). The *American Institute of Stress* states "stress is difficult for scientists to define because it is a subjective sensation associated with varied symptoms that differ for each of us" (Rosch *n.d.*). The SRM enables improved definitions as follows:

Stress is any force or stimulus that activates the SRM.

Nociceptors are nervous tissue disruption sensors in the skin and internal organs that activate the SRM in accord with mechanical, chemical, and thermal changes above a set threshold.

Nociception is nociceptor activation that stimulates increased SNS activity via peripheral sensory nerves and spinal cord internuncial neurons that communicate with sympathetic ganglia. Nociception also communicates with the corticofugal structures in the brain that generate conscious awareness. Descending cortical pathways inhibit nociception pathways in the spinal cord. Nociception is effectively controlled by analgesia, but is ineffectively controlled by anesthesia in clinically safe and reasonable doses.

Allostasis is the automatic alteration of autonomic balance and the generation of rage, apprehension, and fear in accord with subconscious memories of prior sensory input. The brain maintains audiovisual, olfactory, emotional, and sensory memories of all waking moments. During sleep the memory recording process halts while the dreaming process compares, contrasts, exaggerates and suppresses existing memories so as to enhance the ability of vertebrates to pre-emptively recognize dangerous circumstances and facilitate "fight or flight".

Pain is the perception of nociception by conscious awareness and/or a subconscious memory of nociception that represents a form of allostasis. The perception of pain can be exaggerated or minimized by emotional mechanisms in accord with subconscious memories of prior experiences as a manifestation of allostasis. Pain activates the SNS via hypothalamic pathways that are independent of spinal cord function, and this grossly exaggerates the SNS activity caused by nociception alone. Pain can be controlled either by analgesics that inhibit nociception or anesthetics that inhibit conscious awareness.

Anesthesia is the reversible inhibition of corticofugal and emotional mechanisms that generate conscious awareness. Anesthetic agents include intravenous drugs such as propofol, alcohol, benzodiazepines, barbiturates, etomidate, droperidol, ketamine, and volatile inhalation agents including halothane, ether, ethrane, chloroform, cyclopropane, isoforane, desflurane, and sevoflurane. All anesthetics are hypnotic agents that exert their benefits by inhibiting conscious awareness, which prevents SNS activation by fear and pain. Small doses of anesthetic agents can eliminate the perception of pain without completely abolishing conscious awareness. Ether readily illustrates this effect, because it has a high blood/gas solubility coefficient and takes effect slowly. During the early onset of ether effects, patients lose the ability to perceive pain even though they continue to speak coherently. Greater doses of ether abolish conscious awareness altogether. Modern inhalation agents such as isoforane have low blood/gas solubility coefficients and take effect so quickly that these nuances cannot be readily observed. However, neither ether nor any other anesthetic agent can inhibit nociception in safe and practical doses. Furthermore, anesthetic agents may indirectly exaggerate nociception by inhibiting descending brain pathways that suppress spinal cord pathways.

Analgesia is the inhibition of nociception. NSAID analgesics inhibit inflammation that activates nociceptors. Lidocaine, bupivacaine, and other "local anesthetics" (which should logically be called "local *analgesics*") interfere with the function of peripheral sensory nerves and/or spinal cord pathways that transmit nociceptor signals to the SNS. Opioid analgesics inhibit nociception pathways in the spinal cord. By inhibiting nociception, analgesia eliminates the ability of conscious awareness to perceive pain, but it does not prevent other forms of sensation that are perceived by conscious awareness, including auditory, tactile, visual and olfactory stimuli that cause conscious awareness to activate the SNS via hypothalamic pathways even in the absence of nociception and pain. For example, a patient undergoing hernia repair under spinal analgesia may be frightened to death in the event that a fire or earthquake occurs during the surgery, because his perception of danger via sight, sound, vibration, and smell activates the SNS.

Conclusion

In his book *"The Structure of Scientific Revolutions"*, Thomas Kuhn describes how scientific progress occurs in a predictable pattern (Kuhn 1996). Prolonged periods of "ordinary science" prevail during the intervals between scientific revolutions. During these quiet intervals, patient research toil produces fresh evidence that is perceived in terms of prevailing theory. As fresh information accumulates, inconsistencies appear that cannot be explained by the prevailing paradigm. Researchers employ strained and speculative rationalizations to explain these inconsistencies in terms of the prevailing paradigm, and new theories appear. Researchers and experts seldom propose revolutionary theories. Instead, amateurs or persons working outside the specialty are the usual source of important new theories. Eventually, there is a "paradigm shift" as large numbers of researchers and experts embrace a new theory that provides a better explanation of available evidence. Nevertheless, many adhere to the old paradigm long after most have embraced the new concept.

DNA history illustrates Kuhn's principles. Before the discovery of DNA, most experts believed that proteins were the medium of genetic inheritance. Vernon Avery provided convincing evidence to the contrary, but prevailing opinion was little affected until Watson and Crick described the testable DNA mechanism. Both Watson and Crick were young amateurs with no research experience or formal training in cell biology. Watson was a graduate student in ornithology, and Crick was a mathematician who had participated in war research. They gleaned information from published reports and from x-ray diffraction photographs surreptitiously smuggled from the laboratory of Rosalind Franklin, a talented researcher. Crick utilized his mathematical expertise to calculate the angles of DNA atoms, and Watson employed this information to construct models of the DNA molecule. Their description of the DNA molecule was revolutionary, because it provided a convincing testable mechanism that explains how the DNA molecule stores and transmits genetic information. Nevertheless, many experts and researchers stubbornly adhered to the old belief that proteins are the medium of genetic inheritance long after the majority had embraced DNA theory.

Scientific history suggests that DNA theory has reached the limit of its utility, and will soon be either replaced or reinvigorated by a new scientific paradigm. DNA has dominated biological science and research for more than 60 years, but it has failed to explain either embryological development or adult biology. There is growing frustration with the lack of theoretical progress in the biological sciences (Gibbs 2003). Attempts to explain incompatible evidence in terms of the prevailing DNA paradigm have become strained, speculative, and complex (Shomron *et al.* 2009). The Genome Project illustrates this failure. It promised dramatic advances in medicine and biology. It cost billions of dollars and produced a complete description of the gene sequences in human and animal DNA as planned, but it failed to inspire even a single medical treatment (Pontin 2010).

Stress theory represents the most obvious successor to the DNA paradigm. The ability to explain disparate phenomena is the hallmark of an effective theory, and stress theory has always offered the simplest (and therefore best) explanation of adult biology. It complements and extends DNA theory. It explains embryological development as well as physiology, pathology, and stress. It enables a Unified Theory of Medicine. It has never been refuted, and it remains as potent as ever. The SRM description remains crude, but it provides the long-sought mechanism needed to enable, test, and confirm stress theory, unleash its enormous promise, and introduce a new era of scientific progress.

Medicine is the most conservative of sciences, and change comes slowly. Nevertheless, it is now poised at the threshold of the most revolutionary advance in its venerable history. Once the SRM has been tested and confirmed, stress theory will transform medicine from an art based on experiment to a genuine science founded on theory. It will provide a universe of opportunities for research, pharmaceutical development, diagnosis, and treatment at least as vast as current practice, and it will introduce a new era of health, longevity, productivity, and freedom from the scourge of disease.

References

Abraham, E. (1991) Physiologic stress and cellular ischemia: relationship to immunosuppression and susceptibility to sepsis. *Critical Care Medicine*, 19, pp. 613-618.

Abram, S.E. and Yaksh, T.L. (1993) Morphine, but not inhalation anesthesia, blocks post-injury facilitation. The role of preemptive suppression of afferent transmission. *Anesthesiology*, 78, pp. 713-721.

Abram, S.E. and YAKSH, T.L. (1994) Systemic lidocaine blocks nerve injury-induced hyperalgesia and nociceptor-driven spinal sensitization in the rat. *Anesthesiology*, 80, pp. 383-391.

Adamiec, R. *et al.* (2003) Contribution of selected factors of inflammatory creative process in the vascular endothelial damage in the diabetes patients [Polish]. *Polskie Archiwum Medycyny Wewnetrznej*, 110, pp. 683-689.

Adembri, C. *et al.* (2004) Pulmonary injury follows systemic inflammatory reaction in infrarenal aortic surgery. *Critical Care Medicine*, 32, pp. 1170-1177.

Ades, P.A. *et al.* (1996) Skeletal muscle and cardiovascular adaptations to exercise conditioning in older coronary patients. *Circulation*, 94, pp. 323-330.

Ahmed, M.H. (2006) Chloroquine-induced nitric oxide improves insulin sensitivity in rheumatoid arthritis. *Medical Hypotheses*, 66, pp. 208-209.

Ahmed, W. *et al.* (2001) Cardiovascular complications of weight reduction diets. *American Journal of the Medical Sciences*, 321, pp. 280-284.

Akassoglou, K. *et al.* (2003) Fibrin is a regulator of Schwann cell migration after sciatic nerve injury in mice. *Neuroscience Letters*, 338, pp. 185-188.

Akassoglou, K. *et al.* (2000) Tissue plasminogen activator-mediated fibrinolysis protects against axonal degeneration and demyelination after sciatic nerve injury. *Journal of Cell Biology*, 149, pp. 1157-1166.

Akassoglou, K. and strickland, S. (2002) Nervous system pathology: the fibrin perspective. *Biological Chemistry*, 383, pp. 37-45.

Akassoglou, K. *et al.* (2002) Fibrin inhibits peripheral nerve remyelination by regulating Schwann cell differentiation. *Neuron*, 33, pp. 861-875.

Akca, O. (2006) Optimizing the intraoperative management of carbon dioxide concentration. *Current Opinion in Anaesthesiology*, 19, pp. 19-25.

Akca, O. *et al.* (1999) Postoperative pain and subcutaneous oxygen tension. *Lancet*, 354, pp. 41-42.

Alexandrov, A.V. *et al.* (2004) Ultrasound-enhanced systemic thrombolysis for acute ischemic stroke. *New England Journal of Medicine*, 351, pp. 2170-2178.

Ali, S.T. and rakkah, N.I. (2007) Neurophysiological role of sildenafil citrate (Viagra) on seminal parameters in diabetic males with and without neuropathy. *Pakistan Journal of Pharmaceutical Sciences*, 20, pp. 36-42.

Aluoch, J.R. (1998) Fibrinolytic activity in adult Kenyan patients with sickle cell disease. *East African Medical Journal*, 75, pp. 351-352.

Amano, M. *et al.* (1994) Differential inhibition of platelet aggregation and calcium mobilization by nitroglycerin and stabilized nitric oxide. *Journal of Cardiovascular Pharmacology*, 24, pp. 860-866.

Anand, K.J. *et al.* (1990) Hormonal-metabolic stress responses in neonates undergoing cardiac surgery. *Anesthesiology*, 73, pp. 661-670.

Anand, K.J. and HICKEY, P.R. (1992) Halothane-morphine compared with high-dose sufentanil for anesthesia and postoperative analgesia in neonatal cardiac surgery. *New England Journal of Medicine*, 326, pp. 1-9.

Anand, K.J. *et al.* (1987) Randomised trial of fentanyl anaesthesia in preterm babies undergoing surgery: effects on the stress response. *Lancet*, 1, pp. 62-66.

Anderson, L.C. *et al.* (2006) The influence of gender on parasympathetic vasodilatation in the submandibular gland of the rat. *Experimental Physiology*, 91, pp. 435-444.

Angelov, A. (1989) Intracranial venous thrombosis in relation to pregnancy and delivery. *Pathology, Research and Practice*, 185, pp. 843-847.

Angelov, A. (1989) Intravascular coagulation in amniotic fluid embolism [Bulgarian]. *Akusherstvo i Ginekologiia*, 28, pp. 24-29.

Angelov, A. (1989) Intravascular coagulation in relation to pregnancy and delivery. *Zentralblatt fur Gynakologie*, 111, pp. 1169-1175.

Anim-NYAME, N. *et al.* (2003) Evidence of impaired microvascular function in pre-eclampsia: a non-invasive study. *Clinical Science (London)*, 104, pp. 405-412.

Antovic, J.P. *et al.* (2002) Overall haemostatic potential can be used for estimation of thrombin-activatable fibrinolysis inhibitor-dependent fibrinolysis in vivo and for possible follow-up of recombinant factor VIIa treatment in patients with inhibitors to factor VIII. *Haemophilia*, 8, pp. 781-786.

Anesthesia Patient Safety Foundation (2009) *Cerebral Perfusion Experts Share Views on Management of Head-Up Cases* [WWW] APSF Newsletter. Available from: www.apsf.org/ newsletters/html/2010/winter/01_workshop.htm [accessed 1/23/12].

Archer, S. and RICH, S. (2000) Primary pulmonary hypertension: a vascular biology and translational research "Work in progress". *Circulation*, 102, pp. 2781-2791.

Archiniegas, E. *et al.* (2004) Thrombin and its protease-activated receptor-1 (PAR1) participate in the endothelial-mesenchymal transdifferentiation process. *DNA and Cell Biology*, 23, pp. 815-825.

Armstrong, M.T. *et al.* (2000) Regulation of proliferation of the fetal myocardium. *Developmental Dynamics*, 219, pp. 226-236.

Asanuma, K. *et al.* (2004) Thrombin inhibitor, argatroban, prevents tumor cell migration and bone metastasis. *Oncology*, 67, pp. 166-173.

Asero, R. *et al.* (2006) Plasma of patients with chronic urticaria shows signs of thrombin generation, and its intradermal injection causes wheal-and-flare reactions much more frequently than autologous serum. *Journal of Allergy and Clinical Immunology*, 117, pp. 1113-1117.

Assaley, J. *et al.* (1998) Effects of magnesium sulfate infusion upon clotting parameters in patients with pre-eclampsia. *Journal of Perinatal Medicine*, 26, pp. 115-119.

Audu, P. *et al.* (2006) The impact of tissue factor pathway inhibitor on coagulation kinetics determined by thrombelastography. *Anesthesia and Analgesia*, 103, pp. 841-845.

Augustin, H.G. *et al.* (1995) Ovarian angiogenesis. Phenotypic characterization of endothelial cells in a physiological model of blood vessel growth and regression. *American Journal of Pathology*, 147, pp. 339-351.

Avikainen, V. (1977) Coagulation disorders in severely and critically injured patients. *Annales Chirurgiae et Gynaecologiae*, 66, pp. 269-277.

Ayala, J.E. *et al.* (2007) Chronic treatment with sildenafil improves energy balance and insulin action in high fat-fed conscious mice. *Diabetes*, 56, pp. 1025-1033.

Bajaj, M.S. *et al.* (2001) Structure and biology of tissue factor pathway inhibitor. *Thrombosis and Haemostasis*, 86, pp. 959-972.

Baker, S.B. and Worthley, L.I. (2002a) The essentials of calcium, magnesium and phosphate metabolism: part I. Physiology. *Critical Care and Resuscitation*, 4, pp. 301-306.

Baker, S.B. and Worthley, L.I. (2002b) The essentials of calcium, magnesium and phosphate metabolism: part II. Disorders. *Critical Care and Resuscitation*, 4, pp. 307-315.

Barbagallo, M. *et al.* (2007) Magnesium metabolism in hypertension and type 2 diabetes mellitus. *American Journal of Therapeutics*, 14, pp. 375-385.

Barinov, V.G. *et al.* (1989) Analysis of whole blood viscosity in patients with acute myocardial infarction using a rotation viscosimeter [Russian]. *Laboratornoe Delo*, pp. 25-27.

Barnhart, M.I. (1978) Platelet responses in health and disease. *Molecular and Cellular Biochemistry*, 22, pp. 113-137.

Baron, A.D. (1994) Hemodynamic actions of insulin. *American Journal of Physiology*, 267, pp. E187-202.

Bartsch, P. *et al.* (1989) Coagulation and fibrinolysis in acute mountain sickness and beginning pulmonary edema. *Journal of Applied Physiology*, 66, pp. 2136-2144.

Bartsch, P. *et al.* (1987) Enhanced fibrin formation in high-altitude pulmonary edema. *Journal of Applied Physiology*, 63, pp. 752-757.

Baskurt, O.K. and Meiselman, H.J. (2003) Blood rheology and hemodynamics. *Seminars in Thrombosis and Hemostasis*, 29, pp. 435-450.

Baskurt, O.K. and Meiselman, H.J. (2007) Hemodynamic effects of red blood cell aggregation. *Indian Journal of Experimental Biology*, 45, pp. 25-31.

Baskurt, O.K. and Meiselman, H.J. (2008) RBC aggregation: more important than RBC adhesion to endothelial cells as a determinant of in vivo blood flow in health and disease. *Microcirculation*, 15, pp. 585-590.

Baskurt, O.K. *et al.* (2004) Modulation of endothelial nitric oxide synthase expression by red blood cell aggregation. *American Journal of Physiology - Heart and Circulatory Physiology*, 286, pp. H222-229.

Bassiouny, H.S. *et al.* (1994) Hemodynamic stress and experimental aortoiliac atherosclerosis. *Journal of Vascular Surgery*, 19, pp. 426-434.

Basso, I.N. and Keeling, D. (2004) Myocardial infarction following recombinant activated factor VII in a patient with type 2A von Willebrand disease. *Blood Coagulation and Fibrinolysis*, 15, pp. 503-504.

Baum, M. *et al.* (2005) Does surgery unfavourably perturb the "natural history" of early breast cancer by accelerating the appearance of distant metastases? *European Journal of Cancer*, 41, pp. 508-515.

Beardell, F.V. *et al.* (1997) Normalization of plasma factor X levels in amyloidosis after plasma exchange. *American Journal of Hematology*, 54, pp. 68-71.

Beattie, W.S. *et al.* (2001) Epidural analgesia reduces postoperative myocardial infarction: a meta-analysis. *Anesthesia and Analgesia*, 93, pp. 853-858.

Behar, M. (2007) *Can Fear Be Forgotten* [WWW] Popular Science. Available from: http://www.popsci.com/scitech/article/2007-12/can-fear-be-forgotten [accessed on 4/16/10].

Behr-ROUSSEL, D. *et al.* (2007) Daily Treatment with Sildenafil Reverses Endothelial Dysfunction and Oxidative Stress in an Animal Model of Insulin Resistance. *European Urology*, 53, pp. 1272-1280.

Belcaro, G. *et al.* (1992) Fibrinolytic enhancement in diabetic microangiopathy with defibrotide. *Angiology*, 43, pp. 793-800.

Ben-Shlomo, I. *et al.* (1990) Midazolam acts synergistically with fentanyl for induction of anaesthesia. *British Journal of Anaesthesia*, 64, pp. 45-47.

Ben-Shlomo, I. *et al.* (1993) Propofol and fentanyl act additively for induction of anaesthesia. *Anaesthesia*, 48, pp. 111-113.

Ben Amor, N. *et al.* (2005) Caspases 3 and 9 are translocated to the cytoskeleton and activated by thrombin in human platelets. Evidence for the involvement of PKC and the actin filament polymerization. *Cellular Signalling*, 18, pp. 1252-1261.

Bergamaschini, L. *et al.* (1995) Posttransfusion anaphylactic reactions in a patient with severe von Willebrand disease: role of complement and alloantibodies to von Willebrand factor. *Journal of Laboratory and Clinical Medicine*, 125, pp. 348-355.

Bergamaschini, L. *et al.* (1996) Study of complement-mediated anaphylaxis in humans. The role of IgG subclasses (IgG1 and/or IgG4) in the complement-activating capacity of immune complexes. *Journal of Immunology*, 156, pp. 1256-1261.

Berglund, U. *et al.* (1988) Platelet function and plasma fibrinogen and their relations to gender, smoking habits, obesity and beta-blocker treatment in young survivors of myocardial infarction. *Thrombosis and Haemostasis*, 60, pp. 21-24.

Beyak, M.J. *et al.* (2003) Release of nitric oxide in the central nervous system mediates tonic and phasic contraction of the cat lower oesophageal sphincter. *Neurogastroenterology and Motility*, 15, pp. 401-407.

Beyak, M.J. *et al.* (2000) Central nervous system nitric oxide induces oropharyngeal swallowing and esophageal peristalsis in the cat. *Gastroenterology*, 119, pp. 377-385.

Bhatia, S. *et al.* (1996) Breast cancer and other second neoplasms after childhood Hodgkin's disease. *New England Journal of Medicine*, 334, pp. 745-751.

Biais, M. *et al.* (2008) Cardiac output measurement in patients undergoing liver transplantation: pulmonary artery catheter versus uncalibrated arterial pressure waveform analysis. *Anesthesia and Analgesia*, 106, pp. 1480-1486.

Biondi, B. and Klein, I. (2004) Hypothyroidism as a risk factor for cardiovascular disease. *Endocrine*, 24, pp. 1-13.

Biondi, B. *et al.* (2002) Effects of subclinical thyroid dysfunction on the heart. *Annals of Internal Medicine*, 137, pp. 904-914.

Birkenbach, M. *et al.* (1993) Epstein-Barr virus-induced genes: first lymphocyte-specific G protein-coupled peptide receptors. *Journal of Virology*, 67, pp. 2209-2220.

Bobe, R. *et al.* (2003) Evidence for ERK1/2 activation by thrombin that is independent of EGFR transactivation. *American Journal of Physiology - Heart and Circulatory Physiology*, 285, pp. H745-754.

Bobek, V. and Kovarik, J. (2004) Antitumor and antimetastatic effect of warfarin and heparins. *Biomedicine and Pharmacotherapy*, 58, pp. 213-219.

Bogar, L. (2002) Hemorheology and hypertension: not "chicken or egg" but two chickens from similar eggs. *Clinical Hemorheology and Microcirculation*, 26, pp. 81-83.

Bogar, L. *et al.* (2005) Erythrocyte transport efficacy of human blood: a rheological point of view. *European Journal of Clinical Investigation*, 35, pp. 687-690.

Bonacci, J.V. *et al.* (2003) Collagen-induced resistance to glucocorticoid anti-mitogenic actions: a potential explanation of smooth muscle hyperplasia in the asthmatic remodelled airway. *British Journal of Pharmacology*, 138, pp. 1203-1206.

Boniface, K.J. and Brown, J.M. (1953) Effect of carbon dioxide excess on contractile force of heart, in situ. *American Journal of Physiology*, 172, pp. 752-756.

Boudier, H.A. (1999) Arteriolar and capillary remodelling in hypertension. *Drugs*, 58, pp. 37-40.

Bouma, B.N. and Mosnier, L.O. (2006) Thrombin activatable fibrinolysis inhibitor (TAFI)-how does thrombin regulate fibrinolysis? *Annals of Medicine*, 38, pp. 378-388.

Bovill, J.G. *et al.* (1983) The influence of sufentanil on endocrine and metabolic responses to cardiac surgery. *Anesthesia and Analgesia*, 62, pp. 391-397.

Bovill, J.G. *et al.* (1984) Opioid analgesics in anesthesia: with special reference to their use in cardiovascular anesthesia. *Anesthesiology*, 61, pp. 731-755.

Bowie, E.J. and OWEN, C.A. (1983) The clinical pathology of intravascular coagulation. *Bibliotheca Haematologica*, pp. 217-224.

Bradlow, H.L. et al. (1997) Preface. Annals of the New York Academy of Sciences, 833, p. ix.

Brandi, L.S. *et al.* (1990) Insulin resistance after surgery: normalization by insulin treatment. *Clinical Science (London)*, 79, pp. 443-450.

Brass, E.P. *et al.* (1976) Fibrin formation: the role of the fibrinogen-fibrin monomer complex. *Thrombosis and Haemostasis*, 36, pp. 37-48.

Brass, E.P. *et al.* (1978) Fibrin formation: effect of calcium ions. *Blood*, 52, pp. 654-658.

Brass, L.F. and Molino, M. (1997) Protease-activated G protein-coupled receptors on human platelets and endothelial cells. *Thrombosis and Haemostasis*, 78, pp. 234-241.

Bredbacka, S. *et al.* (1986) Per- and postoperative changes in coagulation and fibrinolytic variables during abdominal hysterectomy under epidural or general anaesthesia. *Acta Anaesthesiologica Scandinavica*, 30, pp. 204-210.

Bredbacka, S. *et al.* (1994) Soluble fibrin: a predictor for the development and outcome of multiple organ failure. *American Journal of Hematology*, 46, pp. 289-294.

Bredbacka, S. and Edner, G. (1994) Soluble fibrin and D-dimer as detectors of hypercoagulability in patients with isolated brain trauma. *Journal of Neurosurgical Anesthesiology*, 6, pp. 75-82.

Breslow, M.J. *et al.* (1993) Determinants of catecholamine and cortisol responses to lower extremity revascularization. The PIRAT Study Group. *Anesthesiology*, 79, pp. 1202-1209.

Bretschneider, E. *et al.* (1999) Evidence for proteinase-activated receptor-2 (PAR-2)-mediated mitogenesis in coronary artery smooth muscle cells. *British Journal of Pharmacology*, 126, pp. 1735-1740.

Britton, B.J. *et al.* (1974) Stress-a significant factor in venous thrombosis? *British Journal of Surgery*, 61, pp. 814-820.

Bromage, P.R. (1996) 50 Years on the wrong side of the reflex arc. *Regional Anesthesia*, 21, pp. 1-4.

Brostrom, M.A. *et al.* (2003) Ca^{2+} dynamics of thrombin-stimulated rat heart-derived embryonic myocytes: relationship to protein synthesis and cell growth. *International Journal of Biochemistry and Cell Biology*, 35, pp. 1573-1587.

Brugger, W. *et al.* (1985) Effect of nitroglycerin on blood rheology in healthy subjects. *European Journal of Clinical Pharmacology*, 29, pp. 331-336.

Bruhn, H.D. *et al.* (1983) Influences of thrombin, factor XIII and fibronectin on the growth of tumor cells and leukemic cells in vitro. *Klinische Wochenschrift*, 61, pp. 209-211.

Brummel, K.E. *et al.* (1999) An integrated study of fibrinogen during blood coagulation. *Journal of Biological Chemistry*, 274, pp. 22862-22870.

Brummel, K.E. *et al.* (2002) Thrombin functions during tissue factor-induced blood coagulation. *Blood*, 100, pp. 148-152.

Brunner, M.D. *et al.* (1994) MAC reduction of isoflurane by sufentanil. *British Journal of Anaesthesia*, 72, pp. 42-46.

Bryson, C.L. *et al.* (2003) Association between gestational diabetes and pregnancy-induced hypertension. *American Journal of Epidemiology*, 158, pp. 1148-1153.

Buhl, R. *et al.* (2003) Risk of recurrent intracerebral hemorrhages. *Neurological Research*, 25, pp. 853-856.

Burnstock, G. and Ralevic, V. (1994) New insights into the local regulation of blood flow by perivascular nerves and endothelium. *British Journal of Plastic Surgery*, 47, pp. 527-543.

Butenas, S. *et al.* (2003) How factor VIIa works in hemophilia. *Journal of Thrombosis and Haemostasis*, 1, pp. 1158-1160.

Butenas, S. *et al.* (2002) Mechanism of factor VIIa-dependent coagulation in hemophilia blood. *Blood*, 99, pp. 923-930.

Butenas, S. *et al.* (2003) Influence of factor VIIa and phospholipids on coagulation in "acquired" hemophilia. *Arteriosclerosis, Thrombosis, and Vascular Biology*, 23, pp. 123-129.

Butenas, S. and MANN, K.G. (2002) Blood coagulation. *Biochemistry*, 67, pp. 3-12.

Butenas, S. *et al.* (2000) Models of blood coagulation. *Blood Coagulation and Fibrinolysis*, 11[Suppl 1], pp. 9-13.

Cahalan, M.K. *et al.* (1987) Narcotics decrease heart rate during inhalational anesthesia. *Anesthesia and Analgesia*, 66, pp. 166-170.

Campagna, J.A. *et al.* (2003) Mechanisms of actions of inhaled anesthetics. *New England Journal of Medicine*, 348, pp. 2110-2124.

Cao, Q.Z. *et al.* (2005) In vitro growth inhibition of human colonic tumor cells by Verapamil. *World Journal of Gastroenterology*, 11, pp. 2255-2259.

Carr, M.E. (2001) Diabetes mellitus: a hypercoagulable state. *Journal of Diabetes and Its Complications*, 15, pp. 44-54.

Cartwright, P. *et al.* (1983) Ventilatory depression related to plasma fentanyl concentrations during and after anesthesia in humans. *Anesthesia and Analgesia*, 62, pp. 966-974.

Caruso, S. *et al.* (2006) Sildenafil improves sexual functioning in premenopausal women with type 1 diabetes who are affected by sexual arousal disorder: a double-blind, crossover, placebo-controlled pilot study. *Fertility and Sterility*, 85, pp. 1496-1501.

Caruso, S. *et al.* (2006) Changes in clitoral blood flow in premenopausal women affected by type 1 diabetes after single 100-mg administration of sildenafil. *Urology*, 68, pp. 161-165.

Casonato, A. *et al.* (2003) Fainting induces an acute increase in the concentration of plasma factor VIII and von Willebrand factor. *Haematologica*, 88, pp. 688-693.

Casonato, A. *et al.* (2001) Plasma and platelet von Willebrand factor abnormalities in patients with uremia: lack of correlation with uremic bleeding. *Clinical and Applied Thrombosis/Hemostasis*, 7, pp. 81-86.

Castellino, F.J. (1981) Recent Advances in the Chemistry of Fibrinolytic system. *Chemical Reviews*, 81, pp. 431-446.

Castoldi, E. and ROSING, J. (2004) Factor V Leiden: a disorder of factor V anticoagulant function. *Current Opinion in Hematology*, 11, pp. 176-181.

Chalmers, C.J. *et al.* (2003) Thrombin inhibits Bim (Bcl-2-interacting mediator of cell death) expression and prevents serum-withdrawal-induced apoptosis via protease-activated receptor 1. *Biochemical Journal*, 375, pp. 99-109.

Chambless, L.E. *et al.* (2003) Coronary heart disease risk prediction in the Atherosclerosis Risk in Communities (ARIC) study. *Journal of Clinical Epidemiology*, 56, pp. 880-890.

Chang, S.J. *et al.* (2002) Job characteristics and blood coagulation factors in Korean male workers. *Journal of Occupational and Environmental Medicine*, 44, pp. 997-1002.

Chanson, M. *et al.* (2005) Gap junctional communication in tissue inflammation and repair. *Biochimica et Biophysica Acta*, 1711, pp. 197-207.

CHAPMAN, C.R. *et al.* (2008) Pain and stress in a systems perspective: reciprocal neural, endocrine, and immune interactions. *Journal of Pain*, 9, pp. 122-145.

Chappell, D. *et al.* (2008) A rational approach to perioperative fluid management. *Anesthesiology*, 109, pp. 723-740.

Chen, J. and Goligorsky, M.S. (2006) Premature senescence of endothelial cells: Methusaleh's dilemma. *American Journal of Physiology - Heart and Circulatory Physiology*, 290, pp. H1729-1739.

Cheras, P.A. *et al.* (1997) Hypercoagulability and hypofibrinolysis in primary osteoarthritis. *Clinical Orthopaedics and Related Research*, 334, pp. 57-67.

Chernow, B. *et al.* (1987) Hormonal responses to graded surgical stress. *Archives of Internal Medicine*, 147, pp. 1273-1278.

Chesebro, J.H. *et al.* (1995) Acute Myocardial Infarction and the Role of Aspirin, Heparin, and Warfarin. *Journal of Thrombosis and Thrombolysis*, 1, pp. 231-235.

Chiariello, M. *et al.* (1983) Dilazep-induced reduction of ischemic necrosis in rats with coronary artery occlusion. *International Journal of Cardiology*, 2, pp. 339-348.

Chinni, C. *et al.* (1999) Thrombin, a survival factor for cultured myoblasts. *Journal of Biological Chemistry*, 274, pp. 9169-9174.

Chohan, I.S. *et al.* (1974) Fibrinolytic activity at high altitude and sodium acetate buffer. *Thrombosis et Diathesis Haemorrhagica*, 32, pp. 65-70.

Chohan, I.S. *et al.* (1984) Influence of noise on blood coagulation. *Thrombosis and Haemostasis*, 51, pp. 22-23.

Chohan, I.S. *et al.* (1977) Effect of furosemide on plasma fibrinolytic activity and urokinase excretion. *Experimental Hematology*, 5, pp. 153-157.

Choi, C.Q. (2005) Pressure Sensitive. *Scientific American*, 293, pp. 98.

Choi, S.H. *et al.* (2003) Thrombin induces nigral dopaminergic neurodegeneration in vivo by altering expression of death-related proteins. *Neurobiology of Disease*, 14, pp. 181-193.

Choufani, E.B. *et al.* (2001) Acquired factor X deficiency in patients with amyloid light-chain amyloidosis: incidence, bleeding manifestations, and response to high-dose chemotherapy. *Blood*, 97, pp. 1885-1887.

Woodyard, C. *et al.* (2006) *BP Spill Highlights Aging Oil Field's Increasing Problems* [WWW] *USA Today*. Available from: http://www.usatoday.com/money/industries/energy/2006-08-14-bp-cover-usat_x.htm?POE=click-refer [accessed 3/9/10].

Christopherson, R. *et al.* (1993) Perioperative morbidity in patients randomized to epidural or general anesthesia for lower extremity vascular surgery. Perioperative Ischemia Randomized Anesthesia Trial Study Group. *Anesthesiology*, 79, pp. 422-434.

Christopherson, R. *et al.* (1996) Control of blood pressure and heart rate in patients randomized to epidural or general anesthesia for lower extremity vascular surgery. Perioperative Ischemia Randomized Anesthesia Trial (PIRAT) Study Group. *Journal of Clinical Anesthesia*, 8, pp. 578-584.

Ciardella, A.P. (2004) Partial resolution of diabetic macular oedema after systemic treatment with furosemide. *British Journal of Ophthalmology*, 88, pp. 1224-1225.

Ciavarella, D. *et al.* (1987) Clotting factor levels and the risk of diffuse microvascular bleeding in the massively transfused patient. *British Journal of Haematology*, 67, pp. 365-368.

Cicco, G. *et al.* (1999) Hemorheology in complicated hypertension. *Clinical Hemorheology and Microcirculation*, 21, pp. 315-319.

Cinar, Y. *et al.* (1999) Effect of hematocrit on blood pressure via hyperviscosity. *American Journal of Hypertension*, 12, pp. 739-743.

Cirillo, P. *et al.* (2004) Tissue factor binding of activated factor VII triggers smooth muscle cell proliferation via extracellular signal-regulated kinase activation. *Circulation*, 109, pp. 2911-2916.

Clark, A. and NILSSON, M.R. (2004) Islet amyloid: a complication of islet dysfunction or an aetiological factor in Type 2 diabetes? *Diabetologia*, 47, pp. 157-169.

Coderre, T.J. and Melzack, R. (1987) Cutaneous hyperalgesia: contributions of the peripheral and central nervous systems to the increase in pain sensitivity after injury. *Brain Research*, 404, pp. 95-106.

Coffman, J.D. (1991) Raynaud's phenomenon: An update. *Hypertension*, 17, pp. 593-602.

Colantuoni, A. *et al.* (2005) Protective effects of insulin during ischemia-reperfusion injury in hamster cheek pouch microcirculation. *Journal of Vascular Research*, 42, pp. 55-66.

Coleman, L. (2007) A Testable Stress Mechanism Explains Both Unified Stress Theory and Capillary Gate Theory. *FDA Anesthesia and Life Support Drugs Advisory Committee pp239-243 3/29/07.*

Coleman, L.S. (2005) A capillary hemostasis mechanism regulated by sympathetic tone and activity via factor VIII or von Willebrand's factor may function as a "capillary gate" and may explain angiodysplasia, angioneurotic edema, and variations in systemic vascular resistance. *Medical Hypotheses*, 66, pp. 773-775.

Coleman, L.S. (2005) An improved explanation of atherosclerosis. *PLoS Medicine*, 2, e98.

Coleman, L.S. (2005) Insoluble fibrin may reduce turbulence and bind blood components into clots. *Medical Hypotheses*, 65, pp. 820-821.

Coleman, L.S. (2006) Atherosclerosis may be caused by inadequate levels of turbulence and mixing. *World Journal of Surgery*, 30, pp. 638-639.

Coleman, L.S. (2006) Should soda lime be abolished? *Anesthesia and Analgesia*, 102, pp. 1290-1291.

Coleman, L.S. (2006) A testable hypothesis that may explain the morbidity and mortality caused by surgical stress. *Anesthesia and Analgesia*, 103, pp. 1589.

Coleman, L.S. (2007) A hypothesis: Factor VII governs clot formation, tissue repair and apoptosis. *Medical Hypotheses*, 69, pp. 903-907.

Coleman, L.S. (2010) *Intraoperative Hyperventilation May Contribute to Postop Opioid Hypersensitivity* [WWW] Anesthesia Patient Safety Foundation Newsletter. Available from: http://www.apsf.org/newsletters/ html/2010/winter/12_hypervent.htm [accessed 2/5/2012].

Coleman, L.S. (2010) A stress repair mechanism that maintains vertebrate structure during stress. *Cardiovascular and Hematological Disorders Drug Targets*, 10, pp. 111-137.

Coleman, L.S. (2011) A call for standards on perioperative CO(2) regulation. *Canadian Journal of Anaesthesia*, 58, pp. 473-474.

Cooke, E.D. *et al.* (1977) Intravenous lignocaine in prevention of deep venous thrombosis after elective hip surgery. *Lancet*, 2, pp. 797-799.

Couch, P. and STUMPF, J.L. (1990) Management of uremic bleeding. *Clinical Pharmacy*, 9, pp. 673-681.

Cousins, M.J. (1989) John J. Bonica distinguished lecture: Acute pain and the injury response: immediate and prolonged effects. *Regional Anesthesia*, 14, pp. 162-179.

Coussens, L.M. and Werb, Z. (2002) Inflammation and cancer. *Nature*, 420, pp. 860-867.

Cremer, K.F. *et al.* (1984) Effects of diltiazem, dipyridamole, and their combination on hemostasis. *Clinical Pharmacology and Therapeutics*, 36, pp. 641-644.

Crile, G.W. and Lower, L.W. (1914) *Anoci-association*. Philadelphia: Saunders.

Dalen, P. *et al.* (1999) Warfarin can have a negative effect on bone formation [Swedish]. *Lakartidningen*, 96, pp. 3074.

Danson, E.J. and Paterson, D.J. (2006) Reactive oxygen species and autonomic regulation of cardiac excitability. *Journal of Cardiovascular Electrophysiology*, 17[Suppl 1], pp. 104-112.

Dargaud, Y. *et al.* (2005) Evaluation of thrombin generating capacity in plasma from patients with haemophilia A and B. *Thrombosis and Haemostasis*, 93, pp. 475-480.

Darmoul, D. *et al.* (2003) Aberrant expression and activation of the thrombin receptor protease-activated receptor-1 induces cell proliferation and motility in human colon cancer cells. *American Journal of Pathology*, 162, pp. 1503-1513.

Das, B.B. *et al.* (2004) High-altitude pulmonary edema in children with underlying cardiopulmonary disorders and pulmonary hypertension living at altitude. *Archives of Pediatrics and Adolescent Medicine*, 158, pp. 1170-1176.

Davies, M.S. *et al.* (1997) Calcium alginate as haemostatic swabs in hip fracture surgery. *Journal of the Royal College of Surgeons of Edinburgh*, 42, pp. 31-32.

Davies, P.F. (1995) Flow-mediated endothelial mechanotransduction. *Physiological Reviews*, 75, pp. 519-560.

Davis, D. (2007) *The Secret History of the War on Cancer*. New York: Perseus Books Group.

Davis, R.F. *et al.* (1986) Thoracic epidural anesthesia reduces myocardial infarct size after coronary artery occlusion in dogs. *Anesthesia and Analgesia*, 65, pp. 711-717.

Day, J.R. *et al.* (2006) Aprotinin inhibits proinflammatory activation of endothelial cells by thrombin through the protease-activated receptor 1. *Journal of Thoracic and Cardiovascular Surgery*, 131, pp. 21-27.

De Vos, J. *et al.* (2001) Identifying intercellular signaling genes expressed in malignant plasma cells by using complementary DNA arrays. *Blood*, 98, pp. 771-780.

Dedhia, H.V. and BANKS, D.E. (1994) Pulmonary response to hyperoxia: effects of magnesium. *Environmental Health Perspectives*, 102[Suppl 10], pp. 101-105.

Devine, D.V. *et al.* (1986) Fragment D-dimer levels: an objective marker of vaso-occlusive crisis and other complications of sickle cell disease. *Blood*, 68, pp. 317-319.

Dijkstra, G. *et al.* (2004) Targeting nitric oxide in the gastrointestinal tract. *Current Opinion in Investigational Drugs*, 5, pp. 529-536.

Dintenfass, L. (1965) Some Observations on the Viscosity of Pathological Human Blood Plasma. *Thrombosis et Diathesis Haemorrhagica*, 13, pp. 492-499.

Dirkmann, D. *et al.* (2008) Hypothermia and acidosis synergistically impair coagulation in human whole blood. *Anesthesia and Analgesia*, 106, pp. 1627-1632.

Donders, S.H. *et al.* (1993) Coagulation factors and lipid composition of the blood in treated and untreated hypertensive patients. *Scandinavian Journal of Clinical and Laboratory Investigation*, 53, pp. 179-186.

Dorges, V. *et al.* (2002) The effect of midazolam on stress levels during simulated emergency medical service transport: a placebo-controlled, dose-response study. *Anesthesia and Analgesia*, 95, pp. 417-422.

Drenth, J.P. and Nagengast, F.M. (2000) Aortic stenosis and intestinal blood loss from angiodysplasia: valve replacement is a therapeutic option [Dutch]. *Nederlands Tijdschrift Voor Geneeskunde*, 144, pp. 2237-2240.

Dubois, M. *et al.* (1982) Effects of fentanyl on the response of plasma beta-endorphin immunoreactivity to surgery. *Anesthesiology*, 57, pp. 468-472.

Dufner, G.S. and MARBET, G.A. (2002) Factor XIII in man: a review [German]. *Hamostaseologie*, 22, pp. 11-19.

Dvorak, H.F. (1986) Tumors: wounds that do not heal. Similarities between tumor stroma generation and wound healing. *New England Journal of Medicine*, 315, pp. 1650-1659.

Edde, R.R. (1981) Hemodynamic changes prior to and after sternotomy in patients anesthetized with high-dose fentanyl. *Anesthesiology*, 55, pp. 444-446.

Eichner, E.R. (1983) Exercise and heart disease. Epidemiology of the "exercise hypothesis". *American Journal of Medicine*, 75, pp. 1008-1023.

Eisele, J.H. *et al.* (1967) Narcotic properties of carbon dioxide in the dog. *Anesthesiology*, 28, pp. 856-865.

Elikowski, W. *et al.* (2006) Multifocal ischaemic stroke and myocardial infarction in a woman with occult lung cancer complicated with chronic DIC and thrombotic endocarditis [Polish]. *Neurologia i Neurochirurgia Polska*, 40, pp. 530-535.

Elin, R.J. (1988) Magnesium metabolism in health and disease. *Disease-a-Month*, 34, pp. 161-218.

Elsharnouby, N.M. and Elsharnouby, M.M. (2006) Magnesium sulphate as a technique of hypotensive anaesthesia. *British Journal of Anaesthesia*, 96, pp. 727-731.

Epstein, S.E. *et al.* (1976) Protection of ischemic myocardium by nitroglycerin: experimental and clinical results. *Circulation*, 53, pp. I191-198.

Erodi, A. (1973) Magnesium-an anticoagulant physiological electrolyte [German]. *Medizinische Klinik*, 68, pp. 216-219.

Erukhimov, J.A. *et al.* (2000) Actin-containing sera from patients with adult respiratory distress syndrome are toxic to sheep pulmonary endothelial cells. *American Journal of Respiratory and Critical Care Medicine*, 162, pp. 288-294.

Eshkalback, W. *et al.* (2004) Atherosclerosis, vascular amyloidosis and brain hypoperfusion in the pathogenesis of sporadic Alzheimer's disease. *Neurological Research*, 26, pp. 525-539.

Esler, M. *et al.* (2001) Sympathetic nerve biology in essential hypertension. *Clinical and Experimental Pharmacology and Physiology*, 28, pp. 986-989.

Esmon, C.T. (2004) Crosstalk between inflammation and thrombosis. *Maturitas*, 47, pp. 305-314.

Exadaktylos, A.K. *et al.* (2006) Can anesthetic technique for primary breast cancer surgery affect recurrence or metastasis? *Anesthesiology*, 105, pp. 660-664.

Fagenholz, P.J. *et al.* (2007) Treatment of high altitude pulmonary edema at 4240 m in Nepal. *High Altitude Medicine and Biology*, 8, pp. 139-146.

Fairley, J.K. *et al.* (1983) Protein composition of urinary casts from healthy subjects and patients with glomerulonephritis. *British Medical Journal (Clinical Research Edition)*, 287, pp. 1838-1840.

Famodu, A.A. (1988) Plasma fibrinolytic activity in sickle cell disease. *Tropical and Geographical Medicine*, 40, pp. 331-333.

Fan, J. *et al.* (2000) Priming for enhanced alveolar fibrin deposition after hemorrhagic shock: role of tumor necrosis factor. *American Journal of Respiratory Cell and Molecular Biology*, 22, pp. 412-421.

Farber, E. (1995) Cell proliferation as a major risk factor for cancer: a concept of doubtful validity. *Cancer Research*, 55, pp. 3759-3762.

Farkas, K. *et al.* (2005) Impairment of skin microvascular reactivity in hypertension and uraemia. *Nephrology, Dialysis, Transplantation*, 20, pp. 1821-1827.

Fazio, S. *et al.* (2004) Effects of thyroid hormone on the cardiovascular system. *Recent Progress in Hormone Research*, 59, pp. 31-50.

Federici, A.B. (2003) The factor VIII/von Willebrand factor complex: basic and clinical issues. *Haematologica*, 88, EREP02.

Fehlinger, R. *et al.* (1986) Rheographic indications for reduced cerebral vasoconstriction after oral magnesium medication in tetanic patients, a double-blind, placebo-controlled trial. *Magnesium*, 5, pp. 60-65.

Feigl, E.O. *et al.* (1987) Adrenergic coronary vasoconstriction during myocardial underperfusion. *Circulation*, 75, pp. I1-5.

Fenton, J.W., 2ND *et al.* (1998) Thrombin and antithrombotics. *Seminars in Thrombosis and Hemostasis*, 24, pp. 87-91.

Fernandez, F. *et al.* (1985) Low haematocrit and prolonged bleeding time in uraemic patients: effect of red cell transfusions. *British Journal of Haematology*, 59, pp. 139-148.

Ferrell, W.J. *et al.* (1983) Comparative study of blood clotting factors in anaphylactic and primary and secondary endotoxin shock. *Annals of Clinical Laboratory Science*, 13, pp. 291-298.

Fidler, I.J. and Kripke, M.L. (1977) Metastasis results from preexisting variant cells within a malignant tumor. *Science*, 197, pp. 893-895.

Figueras, J. *et al.* (1979) Haemodynamic and electrocardiographic accompaniments of resting postprandial angina. *British Heart Journal*, 42, pp. 402-409.

Filimonovic, J. *et al.* (2005) Anesthesia for radical prostatectomy. *Acta Chirurgica Iugoslavica*, 52, pp. 113-117.

Fink, S. (2005) Beyond bad: new ways of considering the stress response. *New York Academy of Sciences Magazine,* 205, p. 2.

Fiorucci, S. *et al.* (2004) PAR1 antagonism protects against experimental liver fibrosis. Role of proteinase receptors in stellate cell activation. *Hepatology*, 39, pp. 365-375.

Fisk, N.M. *et al.* (2001) Effect of direct fetal opioid analgesia on fetal hormonal and hemodynamic stress response to intrauterine needling. *Anesthesiology*, 95, pp. 828-835.

Fitzgerald, R.H., JR. (1979) Laboratory diagnosis of postoperative sepsis of the musculoskeletal system. *Orthopedic Clinics of North America*, 10, pp. 361-374.

Fleck, R.A. *et al.* (1990) Localization of human tissue factor antigen by immunostaining with monospecific, polyclonal anti-human tissue factor antibody. *Thrombosis Research*, 59, pp. 421-437.

Foguel, D. and SILVA, J.L. (2004) New insights into the mechanisms of protein misfolding and aggregation in amyloidogenic diseases derived from pressure studies. *Biochemistry*, 43, pp. 11361-11370.

Fornek, J.L. *et al.* (2007) Use of functional genomics to understand influenza-host interactions. *Advances in Virus Research*, 70, pp. 81-100.

Francis, R.B., JR. (1989) Elevated fibrin D-dimer fragment in sickle cell anemia: evidence for activation of coagulation during the steady state as well as in painful crisis. *Haemostasis*, 19, pp. 105-111.

Frank, J.M. and Palomino, N.J. (1987) Primary amyloidosis with diffuse splenic infiltration presenting as fulminant pneumococcal sepsis. *American Journal of Clinical Pathology*, 87, pp. 405-407.

Franzoni, F. *et al.* (2004) Plasma antioxidant activity and cutaneous microvascular endothelial function in athletes and sedentary controls. *Biomedicine and Pharmacotherapy*, 58, pp. 432-436.

Freeman, L.J. *et al.* (1987) Psychological stress and silent myocardial ischemia. *American Heart Journal*, 114, pp. 477-482.

Fricchione, G.L. *et al.* (1996) Neuroimmunologic implications in coronary artery disease. *Advances in Neuroimmunology*, 6, pp. 131-142.

Friedman, R. *et al.* (1997) Continuous infusion of prostacyclin normalizes plasma markers of endothelial cell injury and platelet aggregation in primary pulmonary hypertension. *Circulation*, 96, pp. 2782-2784.

Fuentes, A. *et al.* (1995) The effect of magnesium sulfate on bleeding time in pregnancy. *American Journal of Obstetrics and Gynecology*, 173, pp. 1246-1249.

Fujita, H. *et al.* (2000) Diffuse angiodysplasia of the upper gastrointestinal tract in a patient with hypertrophic obstructive cardiomyopathy. *Internal Medicine*, 39, pp. 385-388.

Furie, B. *et al.* (1977) Syndrome of acquired factor X deficiency and systemic amyloidosis in vivo studies of the metabolic fate of factor X. *New England Journal of Medicine*, 297, pp. 81-85.

Galland, L. (1991) Magnesium, stress and neuropsychiatric disorders. *Magnesium and Trace Elements*, 10, pp. 287-301.

Gamba, G. *et al.* (2000) Clotting alterations in primary systemic amyloidosis. *Haematologica*, 85, pp. 289-292.

Gamba, G. *et al.* (1999) Abnormalities in thrombin-antithrombin pathway in AL amyloidosis. *Amyloid*, 6, pp. 273-277.

Ganzel, B.L. *et al.* (2010) Allostasis and the human brain: Integrating models of stress from the social and life sciences. *Psychological Review*, 117, pp. 134-174.

Garcia, J.G. *et al.* (1995) Vascular endothelial cell activation and permeability responses to thrombin. *Blood Coagulation and Fibrinolysis*, 6, pp. 609-626.

Garrison, R.N. *et al.* (1998) Microvascular changes explain the "two-hit" theory of multiple organ failure. *Annals of Surgery*, 227, pp. 851-860.

Gartner, H.V. (1994) Nephropathy in pregnancy-an endothelial lesion? [German]. *Zentralblatt fur Gynakologie*, 116, pp. 123-137.

Garvin, S. *et al.* (2010) Postoperative activity, but not preoperative activity, of antithrombin is associated with major adverse cardiac events after coronary artery bypass graft surgery. *Anesthesia and Analgesia*, 111, pp. 862-869.

Gasser, R. *et al.* (1995) Cyclic phenomena in early myocardial infarction. *Acta Medica Austriaca*, 22, pp. 69-72.

Gastineau, D.A. *et al.* (1991) Inhibitor of the thrombin time in systemic amyloidosis: a common coagulation abnormality. *Blood*, 77, pp. 2637-2640.

Genovese, A. *et al.* (1980) Inhibition of hypoxia-induced cardiac hypertrophy by verapamil in rats. *Basic Research in Cardiology*, 75, pp. 757-763.

Genovese, A. *et al.* (1980) Effects of antiplatelet and calcium antagonist drugs on infarct size in rats. *Acta Cardiologica*, 35, pp. 419-427.

Genovese, A. *et al.* (1983) Bilateral ventricular hypertrophy in rats exposed to acute or chronic hypobaric hypoxia. *Respiration*, 44, pp. 289-293.

Genovese, A. *et al.* (1982) Regression of myocardial hypertrophy in the rat following removal of acute or chronic hypobaric hypoxia. *European Heart Journal*, 3[Suppl A], pp. 161-164.

Genovese, A. *et al.* (1983) Response of the left ventricular connective tissue to hypoxia. *Research in Experimental Medicine*, 183, pp. 111-115.

Gerber, B.L. *et al.* (2000) Microvascular obstruction and left ventricular remodeling early after acute myocardial infarction. *Circulation*, 101, pp. 2734-2741.

Gibbs, W.W. (2003) Untangling the roots of cancer. *Scientific American*, 289, pp. 56-65.

Gibson, C.M. *et al.* (1999) Relationship between TIMI frame count and clinical outcomes after thrombolytic administration. Thrombolysis In Myocardial Infarction (TIMI) Study Group. *Circulation*, 99, pp. 1945-1950.

Giddens, D.P. *et al.* (1993) The role of fluid mechanics in the localization and detection of atherosclerosis. *Journal of Biomechanical Engineering*, 115, pp. 588-594.

Giesecke, K. *et al.* (1988) High- and low-dose fentanyl anaesthesia: hormonal and metabolic responses during cholecystectomy. *British Journal of Anaesthesia*, 61, pp. 575-582.

Giovanardi, P. *et al.* (1998) Erythrocytosis in patients with hepatocarcinoma in alcoholic cirrhosis: ectopic production of erythropoietin? [Italian]. *Recenti Progressi in Medicina*, 89, pp. 250-252.

Glagov, S. *et al.* (1995) Pathobiology of plaque modeling and complication. *Surgical Clinics of North America*, 75, pp. 545-556.

Glagov, S. *et al.* (1988) Hemodynamics and atherosclerosis. Insights and perspectives gained from studies of human arteries. *Archives of Pathology and Laboratory Medicine*, 112, pp. 1018-1031.

Glass, P.S. *et al.* (1997) Drug interactions: volatile anesthetics and opioids. *Journal of Clinical Anesthesia*, 9[Suppl 6], pp. 18-22.

Gleick, J. (1988) *Chaos: Making a New Science*. London: Penguin.

Glembotski, C.C. *et al.* (1993) Myocardial alpha-thrombin receptor activation induces hypertrophy and increases atrial natriuretic factor gene expression. *Journal of Biological Chemistry*, 268, pp. 20646-20652.

Goldsack, N.R. *et al.* (1998) Thrombin. *International Journal of Biochemistry and Cell Biology*, 30, pp. 641-646.

Gong, Y. *et al.* (2005) Complement inhibition attenuates brain edema and neurological deficits induced by thrombin. *Acta Neurochir Suppl*, 95, pp. 389-392.

Gorbacheva, L.R. *et al.* (2005) Proteinase-activated type 1 receptors are involved in the mechanism of protection of rat hippocampal neurons from glutamate toxicity. *Bulletin of Experimental Biology and Medicine*, 140, pp. 285-288.

Gordon, J.B. *et al.* (1989) Atherosclerosis influences the vasomotor response of epicardial coronary arteries to exercise. *Journal of Clinical Investigation*, 83, pp. 1946-1952.

Goudemand, M. (1983) Plasma fibronectin [French]. *Revue Francaise de Transfusion et Immuno-Hematologie*, 26, pp. 279-298.

Grant, P.J. (1990) Hormonal regulation of the acute haemostatic response to stress. *Blood Coagulation and Fibrinolysis*, 1, pp. 299-306.

Grant, W.B. (2006) Epidemiology of disease risks in relation to vitamin D insufficiency. *Progress in Biophysics and Molecular Biology*, 92, pp. 65-79.

Greipp, P.R. *et al.* (1981) Factor-X deficiency in amyloidosis: a critical review. *American Journal of Hematology*, 11, pp. 443-450.

Griffin, J.H. *et al.* (2007) Activated protein C. *Journal of Thrombosis and Haemostasis*, 5[Suppl 1], pp. 73-80.

Groban, L. *et al.* (2004) Intrathecal morphine reduces infarct size in a rat model of ischemia-reperfusion injury. *Anesthesia and Analgesia*, 98, pp. 903-909.

Groebe, K. (1996) Precapillary servo control of blood pressure and postcapillary adjustment of flow to tissue metabolic status. A new paradigm for local perfusion regulation. *Circulation*, 94, pp. 1876-1885.

Groeben, H. *et al.* (1996) Intravenous lidocaine and bupivacaine dose-dependently attenuate bronchial hyperreactivity in awake volunteers. *Anesthesiology*, 84, pp. 533-539.

Groeben, H. *et al.* (1994) High thoracic epidural anesthesia does not alter airway resistance and attenuates the response to an inhalational provocation test in patients with bronchial hyperreactivity. *Anesthesiology*, 81, pp. 868-874.

Groudine, S.B. *et al.* (1998) Intravenous lidocaine speeds the return of bowel function, decreases postoperative pain, and shortens hospital stay in patients undergoing radical retropubic prostatectomy. *Anesthesia and Analgesia*, 86, pp. 235-239.

Grunewald, M. *et al.* (2002) Paradoxical hyperfibrinolysis is associated with a more intensely haemorrhagic phenotype in severe congenital haemophilia. *Haemophilia*, 8, pp. 768-775.

Grunewald, M. *et al.* (2002) Absence of compensatory platelet activation in patients with severe haemophilia, but evidence for a platelet collagen-activation defect. *Platelets*, 13, pp. 451-458.

Guo, X.Q. *et al.* (1993) Inhibitory effect of intraventricular administration of morphine on the hyperviscosity and elevation of blood pressure induced by stress in the rat [Chinese]. *Sheng Li Xue Bao*, 45, pp. 270-278.

Gurrieri, M.A. (1990) Thrombin-fibrinogen interaction: release of fibrinopeptides and the effects of ATP [Italian]. *Medicina (Firenze)*, 10, pp. 51-52.

Gutstein, W.H. (1988) The central nervous system and atherogenesis: endothelial injury. *Atherosclerosis*, 70, pp. 145-154.

Gutstein, W.H. *et al.* (1978) Neural factors contribute to atherogenesis. *Science*, 199, pp. 449-451.

Gutstein, W.H. and PARL, F. (1978) Neural factors in experimental degenerative arteriopathy. *Lipids*, 13, pp. 380-382.

Haas, S. (2002) Future potential indications for an oral thrombin inhibitor [German]. *Hamostaseologie*, 22, pp. 36-43.

Hahnenkamp, K. *et al.* (2002) The effects of local anesthetics on perioperative coagulation, inflammation, and microcirculation. *Anesthesia and Analgesia*, 94, pp. 1441-1447.

Haldemann, G. *et al.* (1977) Anaesthesia with flunitrazepam (rohypnol) and fentanyl for geriatric patients [German]. *Anaesthesist*, 26, pp. 168-171.

Hall, D. and EDSKES, H. (2004) Silent prions lying in wait: a two-hit model of prion/amyloid formation and infection. *Journal of Molecular Biology*, 336, pp. 775-786.

Hall, R.I. *et al.* (1987) The enflurane-sparing effect of alfentanil in dogs. *Anesthesia and Analgesia*, 66, pp. 1287-1291.

Hampton, K.K. *et al.* (1991) Haemostatic responses and vasopressin release during colonoscopy in man. *Clinical Science (London)*, 81, pp. 257-260.

Hao, Z. *et al.* (2005) Stimulated release of tissue plasminogen activator from artery wall sympathetic nerves: implications for stress-associated wall damage. *Stress*, 8, pp. 141-149.

Hardaway, R.M. *et al.* (1965) Histologic evidence of disseminated intravascular coagulation in clinical shock. *Vascular Diseases*, 2, pp. 254-265.

Hardy, J.F. *et al.* (2005) The coagulopathy of massive transfusion. *Vox Sanguinis*, 89, pp. 123-127.

Hardy, J.F. *et al.* (2006) Massive transfusion and coagulopathy: pathophysiology and implications for clinical management. *Canadian Journal of Anaesthesia*, 53, pp. S40-58.

Hardy, J.F. *et al.* (2004) Massive transfusion and coagulopathy: pathophysiology and implications for clinical management. *Canadian Journal of Anaesthesia*, 51, pp. 293-310.

Harskamp, R.E. and Zeeman, G.G. (2007) Preeclampsia: at risk for remote cardiovascular disease. *American Journal of the Medical Sciences*, 334, pp. 291-295.

Hassoun, P.M. *et al.* (1989) Effect of heparin and warfarin on chronic hypoxic pulmonary hypertension and vascular remodeling in the guinea pig. *American Review of Respiratory Disease*, 139, pp. 763-768.

He, G.Z. (1990) Study on the fibrin fibrinogen degradation products levels and it's significance in the phlegm of the patients with chronic cor pulmonale through monoclonal antibodies [Chinese]. *Zhonghua Jie He He Hu Xi Za Zhi*, 13, pp. 154-156, 191.

He, S. *et al.* (2003) The role of recombinant factor VIIa (FVIIa) in fibrin structure in the absence of FVIII/FIX. *Journal of Thrombosis and Haemostasis*, 1, pp. 1215-1219.

Healy, D.P. (2002) New and emerging therapies for sepsis. *Annals of Pharmacotherapy*, 36, pp. 648-654.

Hecker, B.R. *et al.* (1983) The decrease of the minimum alveolar anesthetic concentration produced by sufentanil in rats. *Anesthesia and Analgesia*, 62, pp. 987-990.

Hedner, U. (2002) General haemostatic agents-fact or fiction? *Pathophysiol Haemost Thromb*, 32[Suppl 1], pp. 33-36.

Hellstrom, H.R. (2002) Coronary microvascular spasm in patients with vasospastic angina. *Journal of the American College of Cardiology*, 40, pp. 573-574.

Hellstrom, H.R. (2003) Can the premises of the spasm of resistance vessel concept permit improvement in the treatment and prevention of ischemic heart disease? *Medical Hypotheses*, 60, pp. 36-51.

Henriksen, R.A. *et al.* (1997) Thrombin-induced thromboxane synthesis by human platelets. Properties of anion binding exosite I-independent receptor. *Arteriosclerosis, Thrombosis, and Vascular Biology*, 17, pp. 3519-3526.

Henson, J.H. *et al.* (2002) Wound closure in the lamellipodia of single cells: mediation by actin polymerization in the absence of an actomyosin purse string. *Molecular Biology of the Cell*, 13, pp. 1001-1014.

Herrero, J.F. *et al.* (2000) Wind-up of spinal cord neurones and pain sensation: much ado about something? *Progress in Neurobiology*, 61, pp. 169-203.

Hesselvik, J.F. *et al.* (1989) Coagulation, fibrinolysis, and kallikrein systems in sepsis: relation to outcome. *Critical Care Medicine*, 17, pp. 724-733.

Hickey, P.R. and Hansen, D.D. (1991) High-dose fentanyl reduces intraoperative ventricular fibrillation in neonates with hypoplastic left heart syndrome. *Journal of Clinical Anesthesia*, 3, pp. 295-300.

Himber, J. *et al.* (2003) Inhibition of tissue factor limits the growth of venous thrombus in the rabbit. *Journal of Thrombosis and Haemostasis*, 1, pp. 889-895.

Hirschfield, G.M. and Hawkins, P.N. (2003) Amyloidosis: new strategies for treatment. *International Journal of Biochemistry and Cell Biology*, 35, pp. 1608-1613.

Hjortoe, G.M. *et al.* (2004) Tissue factor-factor VIIa-specific up-regulation of IL-8 expression in MDA-MB-231 cells is mediated by PAR-2 and results in increased cell migration. *Blood*, 103, pp. 3029-3037.

Hlubocka, Z. *et al.* (2002) Is mild essential hypertension without obvious organ complications and risk factors associated with increased levels of circulating markers of endothelial dysfunction? Effect of ACE inhibitor therapy [Czech]. *Vnitrni Lekarstvi*, 48, pp. 718-723.

Ho, L. *et al.* (2004) Diet-induced insulin resistance promotes amyloidosis in a transgenic mouse model of Alzheimer's disease. *FASEB Journal*, 18, pp. 902-904.

Hobson, J.A. (1997) Dreaming as delirium: a mental status analysis of our nightly madness. *Seminars in Neurology*, 17, pp. 121-128.

Hof, B. *et al.* (2004) Experimental observation of nonlinear traveling waves in turbulent pipe flow. *Science*, 305, pp. 1594-1598.

Hoffmeister, A. *et al.* (2003) Moderate alcohol consumption and plasma concentration of sensitive markers of inflammation. Comment on an atheroprotective relationship [German]. *Deutsche Medizinische Wochenschrift*, 128, pp. 2237-2241.

Hojo, Y. *et al.* (2001) Effect of angiotensin converting enzyme inhibitor on plasma von Willebrand factor level in patients with coronary artery disease. *Cardiovascular Drugs and Therapy*, 15, pp. 91-92.

Holemans, R. (1965) Enhancement of fibrinolysis in the dog by injection of vasoactive drugs. *American Journal of Physiology*, 208, pp. 511-520.

Holm, B. *et al.* (1985) Purification and characterization of 3 fibrinogens with different molecular weights obtained from normal human plasma. *Thrombosis Research*, 37, pp. 165-176.

Holt, J.P. *et al.* (1968) Ventricular volumes and body weight in mammals. *American Journal of Physiology*, 215, pp. 704-715.

Holzheimer, R.G. (2004) Low-molecular-weight heparin (LMWH) in the treatment of thrombosis. *European Journal of Medical Research*, 9, pp. 225-239.

Hong, S.L. and Levine, L. (1976) Stimulation of prostaglandin synthesis by bradykinin and thrombin and their mechanisms of action on MC5-5 fibroblasts. *Journal of Biological Chemistry*, 251, pp. 5814-5816.

Hoppensteadt, D.A. *et al.* (2001) Endogenous release of tissue factor pathway inhibitor by topical application of an ointment containing mucopolysaccharide polysulfate to nonhuman primates. *Thrombosis Research*, 103, pp. 157-163.

Hornstra, G. (1981) Platelet - vessel wall interaction: role of blood clotting. *Philosophical Transactions of the Royal Society of London. Series B: Biological Sciences*, 294, pp. 355-371.

Hornstra, G. and Hemker, H.C. (1979) Clot-promoting effect of platelet-vessel wall interaction: influence of dietary fats and relation to arterial thrombus formation in rats. *Haemostasis*, 8, pp. 211-226.

Hovinga, J.A. *et al.* (2007) Adamts-13, von Willebrand factor and related parameters in severe sepsis and septic shock. *Journal of Thrombosis and Haemostasis*, 5, pp. 2284-2290.

Howell, D.C. *et al.* (2001) Direct thrombin inhibition reduces lung collagen, accumulation, and connective tissue growth factor mRNA levels in bleomycin-induced pulmonary fibrosis. *American Journal of Pathology*, 159, pp. 1383-1395.

Howells, G.L. *et al.* (1993) Peripheral blood lymphocytes express the platelet-type thrombin receptor. *British Journal of Haematology*, 84, pp. 156-160.

Hu, V.W. and Xie, H.Q. (1994) Interleukin-1 alpha suppresses gap junction-mediated intercellular communication in human endothelial cells. *Experimental Cell Research*, 213, pp. 218-223.

Hua, Y. *et al.* (2003) A thrombin inhibitor reduces brain edema, glioma mass and neurological deficits in a rat glioma model. *Acta Neurochirurgica Supplementum*, 86, pp. 503-506.

Huang, F.Y. *et al.* (1990) Microvascular perfusion and resistance in extracorporeal cardiopulmonary bypass under hypothermia with high-dose narcotic anesthesia-animal model. *Ma Zui Xue Za Zhi*, 28, pp. 1-8.

Huang, Y.Q. *et al.* (2000) Thrombin inhibits tumor cell growth in association with up-regulation of p21(waf/cip1) and caspases via a p53-independent, STAT-1-dependent pathway. *Journal of Biological Chemistry*, 275, pp. 6462-6468.

Hudetz, A.G. (1997) Regulation of oxygen supply in the cerebral circulation. *Advances in Experimental Medicine and Biology*, 428, pp. 513-520.

Hudetz, A.G. (2003) The cerebral microcirculation in ischemia and hypoxemia. The Arisztid G. B. Kovach Memorial Lecture. *Advances in Experimental Medicine and Biology*, 530, pp. 347-357.

Idell, S. (2002) Adult respiratory distress syndrome: do selective anticoagulants help? *Am J Respir Med*, 1, pp. 383-391.

Idell, S. (2002) Endothelium and disordered fibrin turnover in the injured lung: newly recognized pathways. *Critical Care Medicine*, 30, pp. S274-280.

Imamura, T. (2004) Tissue factor expression at the site of inflammation: a cross-talk between inflammation and the blood coagulation system [Japanese]. *Rinsho Byori (Japanese Journal of Clinical Pathology)*, 52, pp. 342-349.

Inglis, T.C. *et al.* (1982) Haemostatic and rheological changes in normal pregnancy and pre-eclampsia. *British Journal of Haematology*, 50, pp. 461-465.

Inoue, K. *et al.* (2004) Surgical stress in ARDS open-lung biopsy. *Chest*, 126, pp. 1383-1384.

Itakura, T. *et al.* (1977) Central dual innervation of arterioles and capillaries in the brain. *Stroke*, 8, pp. 360-365.

Ito, H. and Iwakura, K. (1998) Assessing the relation between coronary reflow and myocardial reflow. *American Journal of Cardiology*, 81, pp. 8G-12G.

Ito, H. *et al.* (1996) Myocardial perfusion patterns related to thrombolysis in myocardial infarction perfusion grades after coronary angioplasty in patients with acute anterior wall myocardial infarction. *Circulation*, 93, pp. 1993-1999.

Ito, H. *et al.* (1999) Intravenous nicorandil can preserve microvascular integrity and myocardial viability in patients with reperfused anterior wall myocardial infarction. *Journal of the American College of Cardiology*, 33, pp. 654-660.

Jabor, A. *et al.* (2006) Serum amyloid A as an effective marker for the assessment of surgical trauma and risk of post-operative complications [Czech]. *Ceska Gynekologie*, 71, pp. 131-136.

Jacquot, C. *et al.* (1981) Dramatic aggravation of renal amyloidosis after surgery. Three cases [French]. *Nouvelle Presse Medicale*, 10, pp. 3389-3390, 3395.

Jadhav, M. and Warrier, I. (2000) Anaphylaxis in patients with hemophilia. *Seminars in Thrombosis and Hemostasis*, 26, pp. 205-208.

Jaeger, B.R. and Labarrere, C.A. (2003) Fibrinogen and atherothrombosis: vulnerable plaque or vulnerable patient? [German]. *Herz*, 28, pp. 530-538.

James, M.F. and Cronje, L. (2004) Pheochromocytoma crisis: the use of magnesium sulfate. *Anesthesia and Analgesia*, 99, pp. 680-686.

James, M.F. and Roche, A.M. (2004) Dose-response relationship between plasma ionized calcium concentration and thrombelastography. *Journal of Cardiothoracic and Vascular Anesthesia*, 18, pp. 581-586.

Janmey, P.A. *et al.* (1985) Interactions of gelsolin and gelsolin-actin complexes with actin. Effects of calcium on actin nucleation, filament severing, and end blocking. *Biochemistry*, 24, pp. 3714-3723.

Janmey, P.A. *et al.* (1992) Effects of actin filaments on fibrin clot structure and lysis. *Blood*, 80, pp. 928-936.

Janmey, P.A. and LIND, S.E. (1987) Capacity of human serum to depolymerize actin filaments. *Blood*, 70, pp. 524-530.

Janmey, P.A. *et al.* (1985) Effects of semi-dilute actin solutions on the mobility of fibrin protofibrils during clot formation. *Biochimica et Biophysica Acta*, 841, pp. 151-158.

Jee, S.H. *et al.* (2005) Fasting serum glucose level and cancer risk in Korean men and women. *JAMA*, 293, pp. 194-202.

Jeng, J.H. *et al.* (2004) Protease-activated receptor-1-induced calcium signaling in gingival fibroblasts is mediated by sarcoplasmic reticulum calcium release and extracellular calcium influx. *Cellular Signalling*, 16, pp. 731-740.

Jern, C. *et al.* (1989) Changes of plasma coagulation and fibrinolysis in response to mental stress. *Thrombosis and Haemostasis*, 62, pp. 767-771.

JIN, E. *et al.* (2003) Protease-activated receptor (PAR)-1 and PAR-2 participate in the cell growth of alveolar capillary endothelium in primary lung adenocarcinomas. *Cancer*, 97, pp. 703-713.

John, E.R. and Prichep, L.S. (2005) The anesthetic cascade: a theory of how anesthesia suppresses consciousness. *Anesthesiology*, 102, pp. 447-471.

Juhan-Vague, I. and Hans, M. (2003) From fibrinogen to fibrin and its dissolution [French]. *Bulletin de l Academie Nationale de Medecine*, 187, pp. 69-82.

Juster, R.P. *et al.* (2010) Allostatic load biomarkers of chronic stress and impact on health and cognition. *Neuroscience and Biobehavioral Reviews*, 35, pp. 2-16.

Kabon, B. *et al.* (2003) Thoracic epidural anesthesia increases tissue oxygenation during major abdominal surgery. *Anesthesia and Analgesia*, 97, pp. 1812-1817.

Kabon, B. *et al.* (2004) Obesity decreases perioperative tissue oxygenation. *Anesthesiology*, 100, pp. 274-280.

Kadar, J.G. *et al.* (2007) IgE-mediated anaphylactic reaction to purified and recombinant factor VIII in a patient with severe haemophilia A. *Haemophilia*, 13, pp. 104-105.

Kaiserling, E. and Krober, S. (1995) Massive intestinal hemorrhage associated with intestinal amyloidosis. An investigation of underlying pathologic processes. *General and Diagnostic Pathology*, 141, pp. 147-154.

Kang, J.G. *et al.* (2008) A prospective, randomized comparison of the effects of inhaled sevoflurane anesthesia and propofol/remifentanil intravenous anesthesia on salivary excretion during laryngeal microsurgery. *Anesthesia and Analgesia*, 106, pp. 1723-1727.

Kapral, S. *et al.* (1999) The effects of thoracic epidural anesthesia on intraoperative visceral perfusion and metabolism. *Anesthesia and Analgesia*, 88, pp. 402-406.

Kario, K. and MATSUO, T. (1995) Increased incidence of cardiovascular attacks in the epicenter just after the Hanshin-Awaji earthquake. *Thrombosis and Haemostasis*, 74, p. 1207.

Kario, K. *et al.* (1998) Earthquake-induced cardiovascular disease and related risk factors in focusing on the Great Hanshin-Awaji Earthquake. *Journal of Epidemiology*, 8, pp. 131-139.

Kario, K. *et al.* (1996) Factor VII hyperactivity and endothelial cell damage are found in elderly hypertensives only when concomitant with microalbuminuria. *Arteriosclerosis, Thrombosis, and Vascular Biology*, 16, pp. 455-461.

Kario, K. *et al.* (1997) Earthquake-induced potentiation of acute risk factors in hypertensive elderly patients: possible triggering of cardiovascular events after a major earthquake. *Journal of the American College of Cardiology*, 29, pp. 926-933.

Kario, K. *et al.* (2003) Disasters and the heart: a review of the effects of earthquake-induced stress on cardiovascular disease. *Hypertension Research*, 26, pp. 355-367.

Karp, J.M. *et al.* (2005) Thrombin mediated migration of osteogenic cells. *Bone*, 37, pp. 337-348.

Kato, T. *et al.* (2006) Short-term passive smoking causes endothelial dysfunction via oxidative stress in nonsmokers. *Canadian Journal of Physiology and Pharmacology*, 84, pp. 523-529.

Katritsis, D. *et al.* (2007) Wall shear stress: theoretical considerations and methods of measurement. *Progress in Cardiovascular Diseases*, 49, pp. 307-329.

Kaunitz, H. (1977) The significance of dietary fat in arteriosclerosis. An outmoded theory? [German]. *MMW. Munchener Medizinische Wochenschrift*, 119, pp. 539-542.

Kaushal, V. *et al.* (2004) Thalidomide protects endothelial cells from doxorubicin-induced apoptosis but alters cell morphology. *Journal of Thrombosis and Haemostasis*, 2, pp. 327-334.

Kavarana, M.N. *et al.* (2003) Gastric hypercarbia and adverse outcome after cardiac surgery. *Intensive Care Medicine*, 29, pp. 742-748.

Kawada, H. *et al.* (2003) Coagulation activity in the airways of asthmatic patients [Japanese]. *Nihon Kokyuki Gakkai Zasshi*, 41, pp. 620-625.

Kawasaki, J. *et al.* (2004) Electron microscopic evaluations of clot morphology during thrombelastography. *Anesthesia and Analgesia*, 99, pp. 1440-1444.

Kawut, S.M. *et al.* (2005) New predictors of outcome in idiopathic pulmonary arterial hypertension. *American Journal of Cardiology*, 95, pp. 199-203.

Kawut, S.M. *et al.* (2005) von Willebrand factor independently predicts long-term survival in patients with pulmonary arterial hypertension. *Chest*, 128, pp. 2355-2362.

Kehlet, H. and Holte, K. (2001) Effect of postoperative analgesia on surgical outcome. *British Journal of Anaesthesia*, 87, pp. 62-72.

Kennedy, K.S. and Strom, C.G. (1990) A comparison of postoperative bleeding incidence between general and local anesthesia tonsillectomies. *Otolaryngology - Head and Neck Surgery*, 102, pp. 654-657.

Kenny, L.C. *et al.* (2002) The role of gap junctions in mediating endothelium-dependent responses to bradykinin in myometrial small arteries isolated from pregnant women. *British Journal of Pharmacology*, 136, pp. 1085-1088.

Kensey, K.R. (2003) The mechanistic relationships between hemorheological characteristics and cardiovascular disease. *Current Medical Research and Opinion*, 19, pp. 587-596.

Kent, K.M. and Epstein, S.E. (1976) Neural basis for the genesis and control of arrhythmias associated with myocardial infarction. *Cardiology*, 61, pp. 61-74.

Khan, T.M. *et al.* (2005) Comparison of plasma viscosity and fibrinogen concentration in hypertensive and normotensive diabetics. *Journal of Ayub Medical College Abbottabad*, 17, pp. 45-47.

Khatun, S. *et al.* (1999) Induction of hypercoagulability condition by chronic localized cold stress in rabbits. *Thrombosis and Haemostasis*, 81, pp. 449-455.

Khomulo, P.S. *et al.* (1980) Development of atherosclerosis in alternating prolonged electrostimulation of the negative and positive hypothalamic emotiogenic zones [Russian]. *Kardiologiia*, 20, pp. 104-108.

Khomulo, P.S. *et al.* (1976) Atherosclerosis in rabbits induced by prolonged electrical stimulation of the hypothalamus [Russian]. *Biulleten Eksperimentalnoi Biologii i Meditsiny*, 82, pp. 1294-1296.

Kim, K.J. *et al.* (1997) Fibrinogen and fibrinolytic activity in CAPD patients with atherosclerosis and its correlation with serum albumin. *Peritoneal Dialysis International*, 17, pp. 157-161.

Kim, J.A. et al. (2003) Astrocyte regulation of human brain capillary endothelial fibrinolysis. Thrombosis Research, 112, pp. 159-165.

Kipnis, E. *et al.* (2004) Massive alveolar thrombin activation in Pseudomonas aeruginosa-induced acute lung injury. *Shock*, 21, pp. 444-451.

Kirschner, M.W. and Gerhart, J.C. (2005) *The Plausibility of Life: Resolving Darwin's Dilemma*. Binghamton: Vail-Ballou Press.

Kissin, I. *et al.* (1990) Alfentanil potentiates midazolam-induced unconsciousness in subanalgesic doses. *Anesthesia and Analgesia*, 71, pp. 65-69.

Klassen, G.A. *et al.* (1980) Effect of acute sympathectomy by epidural anesthesia on the canine coronary circulation. *Anesthesiology*, 52, pp. 8-15.

Klementsen, B. and Jorgensen, L. (1997) Mechanisms involved in the early interaction between HeLa cells, platelets and endothelial cells in vitro under the influence of thrombin. Effects of acetylsalicylic acid and Na-salicylate. *APMIS*, 105, pp. 391-401.

Klingel, R. *et al.* (2002) Rheopheresis for age-related macular degeneration: a novel indication for therapeutic apheresis in ophthalmology. *Therapeutic Apheresis*, 6, pp. 271-281.

Kloner, R.A. *et al.* (1974) The "no-reflow" phenomenon after temporary coronary occlusion in the dog. *Journal of Clinical Investigation*, 54, pp. 1496-1508.

Koch, B. *et al.* (1984) Physical fitness in children with hemophilia. *Archives of Physical Medicine and Rehabilitation*, 65, pp. 324-326.

Kocsis, E. *et al.* (2000) Hyperglycaemia alters the endothelium-dependent relaxation of canine coronary arteries. *Acta Physiologica Scandinavica*, 169, pp. 183-187.

Koenig, W. (2003) Fibrin(ogen) in cardiovascular disease: an update. *Thrombosis and Haemostasis*, 89, pp. 601-609.

Koenig, W. *et al.* (2001) Plasma fibrin D-dimer levels and risk of stable coronary artery disease: results of a large case-control study. *Arteriosclerosis, Thrombosis, and Vascular Biology*, 21, pp. 1701-1705.

Kondo, H. *et al.* (2004) A role for L-glutamate ionotropic receptors in the development of rat neurogenic pulmonary edema. *European Journal of Pharmacology*, 499, pp. 257-263.

Kondo, H. *et al.* (2002) Hematology tests of blood anticoagulated with magnesium sulphate. *Southeast Asian Journal of Tropical Medicine and Public Health*, 33 Suppl 2, pp. 6-9.

Kono, K. *et al.* (1981) Renal function and stress response during halothane or fentanyl anesthesia. *Anesthesia and Analgesia*, 60, pp. 552-556.

Korom, S. *et al.* (2006) Sildenafil extends survival and graft function in a large animal lung transplantation model. *European Journal of Cardio-Thoracic Surgery*, 29, pp. 288-293.

Korte, S.M. *et al.* (2005) The Darwinian concept of stress: benefits of allostasis and costs of allostatic load and the trade-offs in health and disease. *Neuroscience and Biobehavioral Reviews*, 29, pp. 3-38.

Koscielny, J.K. *et al.* (2000) Capillary microscopic and rheological dimensions for the diagnosis of von Willebrand disease in comparison to other haemorrhagic diatheses. *Thrombosis and Haemostasis*, 84, pp. 981-988.

Koumbarelis, E. *et al.* (1994) Epidemiology of haemophilia in Greece: an overview. *Thrombosis and Haemostasis*, 72, pp. 808-813.

Kranenburg, O. *et al.* (2002) Tissue-type plasminogen activator is a multiligand cross-beta structure receptor. *Current Biology*, 12, pp. 1833-1839.

Krishnan, A. and KORZENIK, J.R. (2002) Inflammatory bowel disease and environmental influences. *Gastroenterology Clinics of North America*, 31, pp. 21-39.

Krysiak, R. *et al.* (2003) Effects of HMG-CoA reductase inhibitors on coagulation and fibrinolysis processes. *Drugs*, 63, pp. 1821-1854.

Ku, D.N. *et al.* (1985) Pulsatile flow and atherosclerosis in the human carotid bifurcation. Positive correlation between plaque location and low oscillating shear stress. *Arteriosclerosis*, 5, pp. 293-302.

Kuhn, T.S. (1996) *The Structure of Scientific Revolutions*. Chicago: University of Chicago Press.

Kuitunen, A. *et al.* (1993) Anaesthesia affects plasma concentrations of vasopressin, von Willebrand factor and coagulation factor VIII in cardiac surgical patients. *British Journal of Anaesthesia*, 70, pp. 173-180.

Kullo, I.J. *et al.* (2000) Novel risk factors for atherosclerosis. *Mayo Clinic Proceedings*, 75, pp. 369-380.

Kuo, C.P. *et al.* (2006) Comparison of the effects of thoracic epidural analgesia and i.v. infusion with lidocaine on cytokine response, postoperative pain and bowel function in patients undergoing colonic surgery. *British Journal of Anaesthesia*, 97, pp. 640-646.

Kurth, A.A. *et al.* (1999) Prevalence, pathophysiology, diagnosis and treatment of von Willebrand syndrome in orthopedic trauma patients [German]. *Orthopade*, 28, pp. 366-374.

Kuznik, B.I. *et al.* (1985) Effect of thrombin on macrophage and lymphocyte functional activity [Russian]. *Biulleten Eksperimentalnoi Biologii i Meditsiny*, 99, pp. 597-598.

Kvasnicka, T. (2003) NO (nitric oxide) and its significance in regulation of vascular homeostasis [Czech]. *Vnitrni Lekarstvi*, 49, pp. 291-296.

Kvist-REIMER, M. *et al.* (2002) Effects of chemical sympathectomy by means of 6-hydroxydopamine on insulin secretion and islet morphology in alloxan-diabetic mice. *Cell and Tissue Research*, 307, pp. 203-209.

Kwaan, H.C. and WANG, J. (2003) Hyperviscosity in polycythemia vera and other red cell abnormalities. *Seminars in Thrombosis and Hemostasis*, 29, pp. 451-458.

Landesberg, G. *et al.* (2001) Myocardial infarction after vascular surgery: the role of prolonged stress-induced, ST depression-type ischemia. *Journal of the American College of Cardiology*, 37, pp. 1839-1845.

Lau, C.S. *et al.* (1991) Factor VIII von Willebrand factor antigen levels correlate with symptom severity in patients with Raynaud's phenomenon. *British Journal of Rheumatology*, 30, pp. 433-436.

Lau, G. and CHUI, P.P. (1994) Amniotic fluid embolism: a review of 10 fatal cases. *Singapore Medical Journal*, 35, pp. 180-183.

Laudes, I.J. *et al.* (2002) Anti-c5a ameliorates coagulation/fibrinolytic protein changes in a rat model of sepsis. *American Journal of Pathology*, 160, pp. 1867-1875.

Laurent, P. *et al.* (2003) Heart rate and pulse pressure amplification in hypertensive subjects. *American Journal of Hypertension*, 16, pp. 363-370.

Lee, R. *et al.* (1998) Retrograde infusion of lidocaine or L-arginine before reperfusion reduces myocardial infarct size. *Annals of Thoracic Surgery*, 65, pp. 1353-1359.

Lee, T.W. *et al.* (2003) High spinal anesthesia for cardiac surgery: effects on beta-adrenergic receptor function, stress response, and hemodynamics. *Anesthesiology*, 98, pp. 499-510.

LEE, Y.H. *et al.* (2000) Microcirculatory changes following reperfusion insult in diabetic rat skeletal muscles. *Microsurgery*, 20, pp. 77-84.

LEIBOVITZ, E. *et al.* (2004) Persistent anemia in otherwise asymptomatic severe aortic stenosis: a possible indication for valve replacement? *Israel Medical Association Journal*, 6, pp. 400-402.

LESSA, M.A. *et al.* (2004) Cardioprotective action of fentanyl in a model of central sympathetic overactivity in rabbits: antiarrhythmic and anti-ischemic effects. *Acta Anaesthesiologica Scandinavica*, 48, pp. 1115-1122.

Lessa, M.A. and Tibirica, E. (2006) Pharmacologic evidence for the involvement of central and peripheral opioid receptors in the cardioprotective effects of fentanyl. *Anesthesia and Analgesia*, 103, pp. 815-821.

Levi, M. *et al.* (2006) Tissue factor in infection and severe inflammation. *Seminars in Thrombosis and Hemostasis*, 32, pp. 33-39.

Lewis, G.D. *et al.* (2007) Sildenafil improves exercise capacity and quality of life in patients with systolic heart failure and secondary pulmonary hypertension. *Circulation*, 116, pp. 1555-1562.

Liberzon, I. *et al.* (2006) Increased psychiatric morbidity after abdominal aortic surgery: risk factors for stress-related disorders. *Journal of Vascular Surgery*, 43, pp. 929-934.

Liebman, H.A. *et al.* (1992) Excessive fibrinolysis in amyloidosis associated with elevated plasma single-chain urokinase. *American Journal of Clinical Pathology*, 98, pp. 534-541.

Lind, S.E. and Janmey, P.A. (1984) Human plasma gelsolin binds to fibronectin. *Journal of Biological Chemistry*, 259, pp. 13262-13266.

Lind, S.E. *et al.* (1987) Reversible binding of actin to gelsolin and profilin in human platelet extracts. *Journal of Cell Biology*, 105, pp. 833-842.

Lind, S.E. and Smith, C.J. (1991) Actin accelerates plasmin generation by tissue plasminogen activator. *Journal of Biological Chemistry*, 266, pp. 17673-17678.

Lind, S.E. and Smith, C.J. (1991) Actin is a noncompetitive plasmin inhibitor. *Journal of Biological Chemistry*, 266, pp. 5273-5278.

Lind, S.E. *et al.* (1986) Role of plasma gelsolin and the vitamin D-binding protein in clearing actin from the circulation. *Journal of Clinical Investigation*, 78, pp. 736-742.

Lind, S.E. *et al.* (1988) Depression of gelsolin levels and detection of gelsolin-actin complexes in plasma of patients with acute lung injury. *American Review of Respiratory Disease*, 138, pp. 429-434.

Lindenfeld, J. *et al.* (1985) Hemodynamic response to normovolemic polycythemia at rest and during exercise in dogs. *Circulation Research*, 56, pp. 793-800.

Lindenfeld, J. *et al.* (2005) Regulation of oxygen delivery during induced polycythemia in exercising dogs. *American Journal of Physiology - Heart and Circulatory Physiology*, 289, pp. H1821-1825.

Lip, G.Y. *et al.* (2002) Baseline abnormalities of endothelial function and thrombogenesis in relation to prognosis in essential hypertension. *Blood Coagulation and Fibrinolysis*, 13, pp. 35-41.

Lip, G.Y. *et al.* (2002) Sequential alterations in haemorheology, endothelial dysfunction, platelet activation and thrombogenesis in relation to prognosis following acute stroke: The West Birmingham Stroke Project. *Blood Coagulation and Fibrinolysis*, 13, pp. 339-347.

Lip, G.Y. *et al.* (1997) Relation of endothelium, thrombogenesis, and hemorheology in systemic hypertension to ethnicity and left ventricular hypertrophy. *American Journal of Cardiology*, 80, pp. 1566-1571.

Lip, G.Y. *et al.* (1995) Soluble adhesion molecule P-selectin and endothelial dysfunction in essential hypertension: implications for atherogenesis? A preliminary report. *Journal of Hypertension*, 13, pp. 1674-1678.

Lip, G.Y. *et al.* (2001) A cross-sectional, diurnal, and follow-up study of platelet activation and endothelial dysfunction in malignant phase hypertension. *American Journal of Hypertension*, 14, pp. 823-828.

Lip, G.Y. *et al.* (2002) Oxidative stress in malignant and non-malignant phase hypertension. *Journal of Human Hypertension*, 16, pp. 333-336.

Lisman, T. *et al.* (2003) Recombinant factor VIIa reverses the in vitro and ex vivo anticoagulant and profibrinolytic effects of fondaparinux. *Journal of Thrombosis and Haemostasis*, 1, pp. 2368-2373.

Liu, S. *et al.* (1995) Epidural anesthesia and analgesia. Their role in postoperative outcome. *Anesthesiology*, 82, pp. 1474-1506.

LIU, Y.G. and LI, C.S. (2004) Coagulation dysfunctions in patients with systemic inflammatory response syndrome [Chinese]. *Zhonghua Nei Ke Za Zhi*, 43, pp. 94-97.

Lloyd, P.G. *et al.* (2005) VEGF receptor antagonism blocks arteriogenesis, but only partially inhibits angiogenesis, in skeletal muscle of exercise-trained rats. *American Journal of Physiology - Heart and Circulatory Physiology*, 288, pp. H759-768.

Lockwood, C.J. *et al.* (1991) Amniotic fluid contains tissue factor, a potent initiator of coagulation. *American Journal of Obstetrics and Gynecology*, 165, pp. 1335-1341.

Loeser, J.D.M. (1994) IASP Taxonomy. In: LOESER, J.D. (ed) *Pain*. Seattle: International Association for the Study of Pain.

London, G.M. *et al.* (2004) Arterial stiffness: pathophysiology and clinical impact. *Clinical and Experimental Hypertension*, 26, pp. 689-699.

Long, Z.F. *et al.* (2001) Relationship between the level of plasma D-dimer and diabetic microangiopathy [Chinese]. *Hunan Yi Ke Da Xue Xue Bao*, 26, pp. 434-436.

Lundy, J.S. (1925) Carbon Dioxide as an Aid In Anesthesia. *JAMA*, 85, p. 1953.

Luo, W. *et al.* (2005) Two types of protease-activated receptors (PAR-1 and PAR-2) mediate calcium signaling in rat retinal ganglion cells RGC-5. *Brain Research*, 1047, pp. 159-167.

Luostarinen, V. *et al.* (1981) Antithrombotic effects of lidocaine and related compounds on laser-induced microvascular injury. *Acta Anaesthesiologica Scandinavica*, 25, pp. 9-11.

Mahajan, V.B. *et al.* (2000) Creatine kinase, an ATP-generating enzyme, is required for thrombin receptor signaling to the cytoskeleton. *Proceedings of the National Academy of Sciences of the United States of America*, 97, pp. 12062-12067.

Malek, A.M. *et al.* (1999) Hemodynamic shear stress and its role in atherosclerosis. *JAMA*, 282, pp. 2035-2042.

Malik, A.B. (1987) Role of fibrin-neutrophil interactions in lung vascular injury. *Progress in Clinical and Biological Research*, 236A, pp. 33-42.

Mallinder, P.A. *et al.* (2000) A comparison of opiate- and epidural-induced alterations in splanchnic blood flow using intra-operative gastric tonometry. *Anaesthesia*, 55, pp. 659-665.

Malyszko, J. *et al.* (2006) Thrombin activatable fibrinolysis inhibitor in hypertensive kidney transplant recipients. *Transplantation Proceedings*, 38, pp. 105-107.

Malyszko, J. *et al.* (2002) A comprehensive study on hemostasis in CAPD patients treated with erythropoietin. *Peritoneal Dialysis International*, 22, pp. 582-592.

Mangano, D.T. *et al.* (1991) Perioperative myocardial ischemia in patients undergoing noncardiac surgery-I: Incidence and severity during the 4 day perioperative period. The Study of Perioperative Ischemia (SPI) Research Group. *Journal of the American College of Cardiology*, 17, pp. 843-850.

Mangano, D.T. *et al.* (1992) Postoperative myocardial ischemia. Therapeutic trials using intensive analgesia following surgery. The Study of Perioperative Ischemia (SPI) Research Group. *Anesthesiology*, 76, pp. 342-353.

Mann, K.G. *et al.* (2003a) The dynamics of thrombin formation. *Arteriosclerosis, Thrombosis, and Vascular Biology*, 23, pp. 17-25.

Mann, K.G. *et al.* (2003b) What is all that thrombin for? *Journal of Thrombosis and Haemostasis*, 1, pp. 1504-1514.

Mannucci, P.M. *et al.* (1971) Nervous regulation of factor-VIII levels in man. *British Journal of Haematology*, 20, pp. 195-207.

Marcatti, M. *et al.* (1995) Unusual bleeding manifestations in a case of primary amyloidosis with factor X deficiency but elevations of in vivo markers of thrombin formation and activity. *Thrombosis Research*, 80, pp. 333-337.

Markakis, P. *et al.* (1984) Fractures in hemophilia patients [German]. *Unfallchirurgie*, 10, pp. 173-176.

Martin, M.J. *et al.* (2001) New issues about nitric oxide and its effects on the gastrointestinal tract. *Current Pharmaceutical Design*, 7, pp. 881-908.

Matsuo, T. *et al.* (1997) Acute myocardial infarction in the 1995 Hanshin-Awaji Earthquake [Japanese]. *Rinsho Byori. Japanese Journal of Clinical Pathology*, Suppl 104, pp. 133-141.

Matsuo, T. *et al.* (1998) Role of biochemical and fibrinolytic parameters on cardiac events associated with Hanshin-Awaji earthquake-induced stress [Japanese]. *Rinsho Byori. Japanese Journal of Clinical Pathology*, 46, pp. 593-598.

Matsuo, T. *et al.* (1998) Hemostatic activation and cardiac events after the 1995 Hanshin-Awaji earthquake. *International Journal of Hematology*, 67, pp. 123-129.

Mattick, J.S. (2003) Challenging the dogma: the hidden layer of non-protein-coding RNAs in complex organisms. *Bioessays*, 25, pp. 930-939.

Mattick, J.S. (2004) The hidden genetic program of complex organisms. *Scientific American*, 291, pp. 60-67.

Mattick, J.S. (2004) The regulatory architecture of the human genome. *Asia Pacific Journal of Clinical Nutrition*, 13, p. S14.

Mazzone, A. *et al.* (2001) Cigarette smoking and hypertension influence nitric oxide release and plasma levels of adhesion molecules. *Clinical Chemistry and Laboratory Medicine*, 39, pp. 822-826.

McCoy, G.D. and Wynder, E.L. (1979) Etiological and preventive implications in alcohol carcinogenesis. *Cancer Research*, 39, pp. 2844-2850.

McDaniel, M.D. *et al.* (1984) Sequential changes in coagulation and platelet function following femorotibial bypass. *Journal of Vascular Surgery*, 1, pp. 261-268.

McDonagh, P.F. and Hokama, J.Y. (2000) Microvascular perfusion and transport in the diabetic heart. *Microcirculation*, 7, pp. 163-181.

McEwan, A.I. *et al.* (1993) Isoflurane minimum alveolar concentration reduction by fentanyl. *Anesthesiology*, 78, pp. 864-869.

McIntosh, J.H. *et al.* (2003) A modified thrombin generation test for the measurement of factor VIII concentrates. *Journal of Thrombosis and Haemostasis*, 1, pp. 1005-1011.

McVey, J.H. (1999) Tissue factor pathway. *Baillieres Best Pract Res Clin Haematol*, 12, pp. 361-372.

Mehta, J. and SINGHAL, S. (2003) Hyperviscosity syndrome in plasma cell dyscrasias. *Seminars in Thrombosis and Hemostasis*, 29, pp. 467-471.

Meiselman, H.J. (1999) Hemorheologic alterations in hypertension: chicken or egg? *Clinical Hemorheology and Microcirculation*, 21, pp. 195-200.

Meiselman, H.J. *et al.* (2007) RBC aggregation: laboratory data and models. *Indian Journal of Experimental Biology*, 45, pp. 9-17.

Melzack, R. and WALL, P.D. (1965) Pain mechanisms: a new theory. *Science*, 150, pp. 971-979.

Menzel, R. *et al.* (1985) Serum magnesium in insulin-dependent diabetics and healthy subjects in relation to insulin secretion and glycemia during glucose-glucagon test. *Experimental and Clinical Endocrinology*, 85, pp. 81-88.

Messerli, F.H. *et al.* (2007) Essential hypertension. *Lancet*, 370, pp. 591-603.

Mizutani, A.R. and Ward, C.F. (1990) Amyloidosis associated bleeding diatheses in the surgical patient. *Canadian Journal of Anaesthesia*, 37, pp. 910-912.

Moalli, R. *et al.* (1989) Fibrinolysis in critically ill patients. *American Review of Respiratory Disease*, 140, pp. 287-293.

Modesti, P.A. *et al.* (2009) Response of serum proteome in patients undergoing infrarenal aortic aneurysm repair. *Anesthesiology*, 111, pp. 844-854.

Modig, J. (1985) The role of lumbar epidural anaesthesia as antithrombotic prophylaxis in total hip replacement. *Acta Chirurgica Scandinavica*, 151, pp. 589-594.

Modig, J. *et al.* (1983) Role of extradural and of general anaesthesia in fibrinolysis and coagulation after total hip replacement. *British Journal of Anaesthesia*, 55, pp. 625-629.

Modig, J. *et al.* (1983) Thromboembolism after total hip replacement: role of epidural and general anesthesia. *Anesthesia and Analgesia*, 62, pp. 174-180.

Modig, J. *et al.* (1983) The value of variables of disseminated intravascular coagulation in the diagnosis of adult respiratory distress syndrome. *Acta Anaesthesiologica Scandinavica*, 27, pp. 369-375.

Moffitt, E.A. *et al.* (1986) Myocardial metabolism and hemodynamic responses with fentanyl-enflurane anesthesia for coronary arterial surgery. *Anesthesia and Analgesia*, 65, pp. 46-52.

Monk, T.G. *et al.* (2005) Anesthetic management and one-year mortality after noncardiac surgery. *Anesthesia and Analgesia*, 100, pp. 4-10.

Moore, C.M. *et al.* (1995) Hormonal effects of thoracic extradural analgesia for cardiac surgery. *British Journal of Anaesthesia*, 75, pp. 387-393.

Morgan, M.T. (2008) Use of meperidine as the analgesic of choice in treating pain from acute painful sickle cell crisis. *Annals of Emergency Medicine*, 51, pp. 202-203.

Mori, Y. *et al.* (1989) Hypercoagulable state in the Watanabe heritable hyperlipidemic rabbit, an animal model for the progression of atherosclerosis. Effect of probucol on coagulation. *Thrombosis and Haemostasis*, 61, pp. 140-143.

Morishima, I. *et al.* (2000) Angiographic no-reflow phenomenon as a predictor of adverse long-term outcome in patients treated with percutaneous transluminal coronary angioplasty for first acute myocardial infarction. *Journal of the American College of Cardiology*, 36, pp. 1202-1209.

Morita-Tsuzuki, Y. *et al.* (1993) Inhibition of nitric oxide synthase attenuates the cerebral blood flow response to stimulation of postganglionic parasympathetic nerves in the rat. *Journal of Cerebral Blood Flow and Metabolism*, 13, pp. 993-997.

Moser, M. and Patterson, C. (2003) Thrombin and vascular development: a sticky subject. *Arteriosclerosis, Thrombosis, and Vascular Biology*, 23, pp. 922-930.

Mosesson, M.W. (2005) Fibrinogen and fibrin structure and functions. *Journal of Thrombosis and Haemostasis*, 3, pp. 1894-1904.

Mosnier, L.O. *et al.* (2007) Activated protein C mutant with minimal anticoagulant activity, normal cytoprotective activity, and preservation of thrombin activable fibrinolysis inhibitor-dependent cytoprotective functions. *Journal of Biological Chemistry*, 282, pp. 33022-33033.

Mukamal, K.J. *et al.* (2004) Alcohol consumption and inflammatory markers in older adults: the Cardiovascular Health Study. *Atherosclerosis*, 173, pp. 79-87.

Muller, A.M. *et al.* (2002) Expression of von Willebrand factor by human pulmonary endothelial cells in vivo. *Respiration*, 69, pp. 526-533.

Mullins, E.S. *et al.* (2009) Genetic elimination of prothrombin in adult mice is not compatible with survival and results in spontaneous hemorrhagic events in both heart and brain. *Blood*, 113, pp. 696-704.

Mumford, A.D. *et al.* (2000) Bleeding symptoms and coagulation abnormalities in 337 patients with AL-amyloidosis. *British Journal of Haematology*, 110, pp. 454-460.

Murakami, K. *et al.* (1995) Thrombin induces GRO alpha/MGSA production in human umbilical vein endothelial cells. *Thrombosis Research*, 79, pp. 387-394.

Murdoch, I.A. *et al.* (1994) Perioperative haemodynamic effects of an intravenous infusion of calcium chloride in children following cardiac surgery. *Acta Paediatrica*, 83, pp. 658-661.

Murphy, M.R. and Hug, C.C., JR. (1982) The anesthetic potency of fentanyl in terms of its reduction of enflurane MAC. *Anesthesiology*, 57, pp. 485-488.

Mussoni, L. *et al.* (2001) Magnesium inhibits arterial thrombi after vascular injury in rat: in vivo impairment of coagulation. *Thrombosis and Haemostasis*, 86, pp. 1292-1295.

Myles, P.S. *et al.* (2002) Remifentanil, fentanyl, and cardiac surgery: a double-blinded, randomized, controlled trial of costs and outcomes. *Anesthesia and Analgesia*, 95, pp. 805-812.

Naeije, R. and Vachiery, J.L. (2001) Medical therapy of pulmonary hypertension. Conventional therapies. *Clinics in Chest Medicine*, 22, pp. 517-527.

Nakase, T. *et al.* (2003) Astrocytic gap junctions composed of connexin 43 reduce apoptotic neuronal damage in cerebral ischemia. *Stroke*, 34, pp. 1987-1993.

Naldini, A. *et al.* (2003) Inhibition of interleukin-12 expression by alpha-thrombin in human peripheral blood mononuclear cells: a potential mechanism for modulating Th1/Th2 responses. *British Journal of Pharmacology*, 140, pp. 980-986.

Naldini, A. *et al.* (2005) Thrombin-mediated IL-10 up-regulation involves protease-activated receptor (PAR)-1 expression in human mononuclear leukocytes. *Journal of Leukocyte Biology*, 78, pp. 736-744.

Naldini, A. and CARNEY, D.H. (1996) Thrombin modulation of natural killer activity in human peripheral lymphocytes. *Cellular Immunology*, 172, pp. 35-42.

Naldini, A. *et al.* (1993) Thrombin enhances T cell proliferative responses and cytokine production. *Cellular Immunology*, 147, pp. 367-377.

Naldini, A. *et al.* (2002) Human alpha-thrombin stimulates proliferation of interferon-gamma differentiated, growth-arrested U937 cells, overcoming differentiation-related changes in expression of p21CIP1/WAF1 and cyclin D1. *Journal of Cellular Physiology*, 191, pp. 290-297.

Naldini, A. *et al.* (2000) Thrombin regulates the expression of proangiogenic cytokines via proteolytic activation of protease-activated receptor-1. *General Pharmacology*, 35, pp. 255-259.

Naldini, A. *et al.* (2004) The thrombin peptide, TP508, enhances cytokine release and activates signaling events. *Peptides*, 25, pp. 1917-1926.

Naldini, A. *et al.* (2006) Thrombin inhibits IFN-gamma production in human peripheral blood mononuclear cells by promoting a Th2 profile. *Journal of Interferon and Cytokine Research*, 26, pp. 793-799.

Naldini, A. *et al.* (2002) Thrombin enhancement of interleukin-1 expression in mononuclear cells: involvement of proteinase-activated receptor-1. *Cytokine*, 20, pp. 191-199.

Naldini, A. *et al.* (1998) Thrombin receptor expression and responsiveness of human monocytic cells to thrombin is linked to interferon-induced cellular differentiation. *Journal of Cellular Physiology*, 177, pp. 76-84.

Nees, S. (1989) The adenosine hypothesis of metabolic regulation of coronary flow in the light of newly recognized properties of the coronary endothelium. *Zeitschrift fur Kardiologie*, 78[Suppl 6], pp. 42-49.

Nees, S. (1989) Coronary flow increases induced by adenosine and adenine nucleotides are mediated by the coronary endothelium: a new principle of the regulation of coronary flow. *European Heart Journal*, 10[Suppl F], pp. 28-35.

Negishi, C. *et al.* (2000) Alfentanil reduces the febrile response to interleukin-2 in humans. *Critical Care Medicine*, 28, pp. 1295-1300.

Nerem, R.M. and Seed, W.A. (1972) An in vivo study of aortic flow disturbances. *Cardiovascular Research*, 6, pp. 1-14.

Neuhaus, T. *et al.* (2002) Recurrent spontaneous hemorrhage in a patient with light chain immunocytoma [German]. *Schweizerische Rundschau fur Medizin Praxis*, 91, pp. 112-118.

Neuhof, H. *et al.* (1975) Streptokinase therapy in patients with acute myocardial infarction. *Intensive Care Medicine*, 1, pp. 27-30.

Newman, M.G. *et al.* (2001) Cigarette smoking and pre-eclampsia: their association and effects on clinical outcomes. *Journal of Maternal-Fetal Medicine*, 10, pp. 166-170.

Nielsen, V.G. *et al.* (2004) The impact of factor XIII on coagulation kinetics and clot strength determined by thrombelastography. *Anesthesia and Analgesia*, 99, pp. 120-123.

Nilsson, M.R. (2004) Techniques to study amyloid fibril formation in vitro. *Methods*, 34, pp. 151-160.

O'Brien, J.R. (1996) Angiodysplasia, haemostasis and capillaries. A hypothesis. *Thrombosis Research*, 84, pp. 385-387.

O'Brodovich, H.M. *et al.* (1984) Hypoxia alters blood coagulation during acute decompression in humans. *Journal of Applied Physiology*, 56, pp. 666-670.

O'Connor, T.C. and ABRAM, S.E. (1994) Halothane enhances suppression of spinal sensitization by intrathecal morphine in the rat formalin test. *Anesthesiology*, 81, pp. 1277-1283.

O'Donnell, J. *et al.* (2000) Elevation of FVIII: C in venous thromboembolism is persistent and independent of the acute phase response. *Thrombosis and Haemostasis*, 83, pp. 10-13.

O'Donnell, J. *et al.* (2001) Marked elevation of thrombin generation in patients with elevated FVIII:C and venous thromboembolism. *British Journal of Haematology*, 115, pp. 687-691.

O'Hara, R. *et al.* (2004) Local expression of the serum amyloid A and formyl peptide receptor-like 1 genes in synovial tissue is associated with matrix metalloproteinase production in patients with inflammatory arthritis. *Arthritis and Rheumatism*, 50, pp. 1788-1799.

Ofek, H. and Defrin, R. (2007) The characteristics of chronic central pain after traumatic brain injury. *Pain*, 131, pp. 330-340.

Ogawa, T. *et al.* (1983) Possible relationship between the ratio of Factor VIII complex and placental insufficiency in preeclampsia. *Biological Research in Pregnancy and Perinatology*, 4, pp. 155-157.

Okada, M. *et al.* (2006) Detection of up-regulated genes in thrombin-stimulated human umbilical vein endothelial cells. *Thrombosis Research*, 118, pp. 715-721.

Orbach, H. *et al.* (2007) Novel biomarkers in autoimmune diseases: prolactin, ferritin, vitamin D, and TPA levels in autoimmune diseases. *Annals of the New York Academy of Sciences*, 1109, pp. 385-400.

Orr, J.E. *et al.* (1986) A haemorheological study of lignocaine. *British Journal of Anaesthesia*, 58, pp. 306-309.

Orser, B.A. *et al.* (2002) Mechanisms of general anesthesia. *Current Opinion in Anaesthesiology*, 15, pp. 427-433.

Osterud, B. and Bjorklid, E. (2001) The tissue factor pathway in disseminated intravascular coagulation. *Seminars in Thrombosis and Hemostasis*, 27, pp. 605-617.

Page, L.J. *et al.* (2004) Ca^{2+} binding protects against gelsolin amyloidosis. *Biochemical and Biophysical Research Communications*, 322, pp. 1105-1110.

Pagel, C.N. *et al.* (2003) Inhibition of osteoblast apoptosis by thrombin. *Bone*, 33, pp. 733-743.

Palmero Marti, J.L. *et al.* (2004) Secondary vesical amyloidosis [Spanish]. *Actas Urologicas Espanolas*, 28, pp. 238-242.

Pankhurst, T. *et al.* (2004) Malignancy is increased in ANCA-associated vasculitis. *Rheumatology*, 43, pp. 1532-1535.

Pardo Mindan, F.J. and PANIZO, A. (1993) Alterations in the extracellular matrix of the myocardium in essential hypertension. *European Heart Journal*, 14[Suppl J], pp. 12-14.

Park, G. (2002) Rescue is stressful. *Anesthesia and Analgesia*, 95, pp. 263-265.

Parker, E.S. *et al.* (2006) A case of unusual autobiographical remembering. *Neurocase*, 12, pp. 35-49.

Parker, J.D. *et al.* (2007) Safety of intravenous nitroglycerin after administration of sildenafil citrate to men with coronary artery disease: A double-blind, placebo-controlled, randomized, crossover trial. *Critical Care Medicine*, 35, pp. 1863-1868.

PARKER, K.H. (1977) *Instability in Arterial Blood Flow*. Baltimore, Md: University Park Press.

PENNY, W.F. *et al.* (1991) Correlation of circulating von Willebrand factor levels with cardiovascular hemodynamics. *Circulation*, 83, pp. 1630-1636.

Petrovitch, C.T. (2003) An approach to the patient who may have a bleeding disorder. In: *American Society of Anesthesiologists Annual Meeting*. San Francisco: American Society of Anesthesiologists, p. 186.

Pflug, A.E. and Halter, J.B. (1981) Effect of spinal anesthesia on adrenergic tone and the neuroendocrine responses to surgical stress in humans. *Anesthesiology*, 55, pp. 120-126.

Phillip, B. *et al.* (2003) The prevalence of preoperative diastolic filling abnormalities in geriatric surgical patients. *Anesthesia and Analgesia*, 97, pp. 1214-1221.

Pignalberi, C. *et al.* (2002) Psychological stress and sudden death [Italian]. *Italian Heart Journal*, 3, pp. 1011-1021.

Plendl, H. *et al.* (2002) Molecular variants of fibrinogen [German]. *Hamostaseologie*, 22, pp. 36-41.

Pohl, J. *et al.* (1979) Thrombin and fibrin-induced growth of fibroblasts: role in wound repair and thrombus organization. *Klinische Wochenschrift*, 57, pp. 273-277.

Pontin, J. (2010) A Decade of Genomics. In: Pontin J. (ed) *Technology Review*. MIT: MIT, pp. 1.

Poste, G. and GREIG, R. (1982) On the genesis and regulation of cellular heterogeneity in malignant tumors. *Invasion and Metastasis*, 2, pp. 137-176.

Powell, D.S. *et al.* (2003) Apolipoprotein E genotype, islet amyloid deposition and severity of Type 2 diabetes. *Diabetes Research and Clinical Practice*, 60, pp. 105-110.

Powell, J. *et al.* (1987) Raised serum thyrotrophin in women with peripheral arterial disease. *British Journal of Surgery*, 74, pp. 1139-1141.

Prandoni, P. *et al.* (2003) An association between atherosclerosis and venous thrombosis. *New England Journal of Medicine*, 348, pp. 1435-1441.

Price, J. (2008) *The Woman Who Can't Forget: The Extraordinary Story of Living with the Most Remarkable Memory Known to Science-A Memoir*. New York: Free Press - a division of Simon and schuster.

PrioR, B.M. *et al.* (2003) Exercise-induced vascular remodeling. *Exercise and Sport Sciences Reviews*, 31, pp. 26-33.

Prys-Roberts, C. *et al.* (1967) Accidental severe hypercapnia during anaesthesia. A case report and review of some physiological effects. *British Journal of Anaesthesia*, 39, pp. 257-267.

Przyklenk, K. and KLONER, R.A. (2001) Sildenafil citrate (Viagra) does not exacerbate myocardial ischemia in canine models of coronary artery stenosis. *Journal of the American College of Cardiology*, 37, pp. 286-292.

Puckett, L.G. *et al.* (2003) Monitoring blood coagulation with magnetoelastic sensors. *Biosensors and Bioelectronics*, 18, pp. 675-681.

Pypendop, B.H. and Ilkiw, J.E. (2005) The effects of intravenous lidocaine administration on the minimum alveolar concentration of isoflurane in cats. *Anesthesia and Analgesia*, 100, pp. 97-101.

Quaknine-Orlando, B. *et al.* (1999) Role of the hematocrit in a rabbit model of arterial thrombosis and bleeding. *Anesthesiology*, 90, pp. 1454-1461.

Rakaric-Poznanovic, M. *et al.* (1995) Multiorgan dysfunction syndrome (MODS) caused by long bone fractures in young persons [Croatian]. *Lijecnicki Vjesnik*, 117 Suppl 2, pp. 85-87.

Rakusan, K. and Nagai, J. (1994) Morphometry of arterioles and capillaries in hearts of senescent mice. *Cardiovascular Research*, 28, pp. 969-972.

Rampling, M.W. *et al.* (2004) Influence of cell-specific factors on red blood cell aggregation. *Biorheology*, 41, pp. 91-112.

Ranjbar, F. *et al.* (2007) Relaxation therapy in the background of standard antihypertensive drug treatment is effective in management of moderate to severe essential hypertension. *Saudi Med J*, 28, pp. 1353-1356.

RAO, K. *et al.* (2007) Effect of chronic changes in heart rate on congestive heart failure. *Journal of Cardiac Failure*, 13, pp. 269-274.

Rath, W. *et al.* (2000) HELLP syndrome. *Journal of Perinatal Medicine*, 28, pp. 249-260.

Sinatra, R.S. *et al.* (1972) *Acute Pain Mechanisms and Management*. St. Louis, Missouri: Mosby Year-Book, Inc.

Reich, D.L. *et al.* (2002) Intraoperative tachycardia and hypertension are independently associated with adverse outcome in noncardiac surgery of long duration. *Anesthesia and Analgesia*, 95, pp. 273-277.

Rezkalla, S.H. and Kloner, R.A. (2002) No-reflow phenomenon. *Circulation*, 105, pp. 656-662.

Rich, S. *et al.* (1992) The effect of high doses of calcium-channel blockers on survival in primary pulmonary hypertension. *New England Journal of Medicine*, 327, pp. 76-81.

Rim, S.J. *et al.* (2001) Decrease in coronary blood flow reserve during hyperlipidemia is secondary to an increase in blood viscosity. *Circulation*, 104, pp. 2704-2709.

Roberts, J.M. *et al.* (1989) Preeclampsia: an endothelial cell disorder. *American Journal of Obstetrics and Gynecology*, 161, pp. 1200-1204.

Robriquet, L. *et al.* (2006) Intravenous administration of activated protein C in Pseudomonas-induced lung injury: impact on lung fluid balance and the inflammatory response. *Respiratory Research*, 7, pp. 41.

Rodeghiero, F. (2002) von Willebrand disease: still an intriguing disorder in the era of molecular medicine. *Haemophilia*, 8, pp. 292-300.

Rodgers, A. *et al.* (2000) Reduction of postoperative mortality and morbidity with epidural or spinal anaesthesia: results from overview of randomised trials. *British Medical Journal*, 321, pp. 1493.

Rodriguez-Inigo, E. *et al.* (2001) Expression of factor VII in the liver of patients with liver disease: correlations with the disease severity and impairment in the hemostasis. *Blood Coagulation and Fibrinolysis*, 12, pp. 193-199.

Roe, M.T. *et al.* (2001) Shifting the open-artery hypothesis downstream: the quest for optimal reperfusion. *Journal of the American College of Cardiology*, 37, pp. 9-18.

Roguski, J. *et al.* (1964) Incidence of clinical criteria of atherosclerosis in hypo- and hyperthyroidism, polycythaemia vera and chronic cor pulmonale (para- and antiatherosclerotic syndromes). *Cor et Vasa*, 103, pp. 219-230.

Roher, A.E. *et al.* (2003) Circle of willis atherosclerosis is a risk factor for sporadic Alzheimer's disease. *Arteriosclerosis, Thrombosis, and Vascular Biology*, 23, pp. 2055-2062.

Roizen, M.F. (1988) Should we all have a sympathectomy at birth? Or at least preoperatively? *Anesthesiology*, 68, pp. 482-484.

Rosborough, T.K. and Swaim, W.R. (1978) Acquired von Willebrand's disease, platelet-release defect and angiodysplasia. *American Journal of Medicine*, 65, pp. 96-100.

Rosch, P.J. (n.d.) *Stress, definition of stress, stressor, what is stress?, eustress?* [WWW] The American Institute of Stress. Available from: http://www.stress.org/topic-definition-stress.htm [accessed 2/3/2012].

Rosendaal, F.R. *et al.* (1990) Haemophilia protects against ischaemic heart disease: a study of risk factors. *British Journal of Haematology*, 75, pp. 525-530.

Rosenfeld, B.A. *et al.* (1993) The effects of different anesthetic regimens on fibrinolysis and the development of postoperative arterial thrombosis. Perioperative Ischemia Randomized Anesthesia Trial Study Group. *Anesthesiology*, 79, pp. 435-443.

Rosenson, R.S. *et al.* (2001) Elevated blood viscosity in systemic lupus erythematosus. *Seminars in Arthritis and Rheumatism*, 31, pp. 52-57.

Ross, R. (1999) Atherosclerosis-an inflammatory disease. *New England Journal of Medicine*, 340, pp. 115-126.

Rothman, A. *et al.* (1994) Immediate-early gene expression in response to hypertrophic and proliferative stimuli in pulmonary arterial smooth muscle cells. *Journal of Biological Chemistry*, 269, pp. 6399-6404.

Rowlingson, J.C. (2006) Update on Acute Pain Management. In: *80th Clinical and Scientific Congress of the International Anesthesia Research Society*. San Francisco: International Anesthesia Research Society, p. 137.

Roy, K.K. *et al.* (2001) Recurrent eclampsia in a woman with chronic pyelonephritis. *European Journal of Obstetrics, Gynecology, and Reproductive Biology*, 94, pp. 307-308.

Rubin, D.B. *et al.* (1990) Elevated von Willebrand factor antigen is an early plasma predictor of acute lung injury in nonpulmonary sepsis syndrome. *Journal of Clinical Investigation*, 86, pp. 474-480.

Rudnicka, A.R. *et al.* (2006) Associations of plasma fibrinogen and factor VII clotting activity with coronary heart disease and stroke: prospective cohort study from the screening phase of the Thrombosis Prevention Trial. *Journal of Thrombosis and Haemostasis*, 4, pp. 2405-2410.

Rukshin, V. *et al.* (2002) Comparative antithrombotic effects of magnesium sulfate and the platelet glycoprotein IIb/IIIa inhibitors tirofiban and eptifibatide in a canine model of stent thrombosis. *Circulation*, 105, pp. 1970-1975.

Ruttmann, T.G. *et al.* (2007) The coagulation changes induced by rapid in vivo crystalloid infusion are attenuated when magnesium is kept at the upper limit of normal. *Anesthesia and Analgesia*, 104, pp. 1475-1480.

Sabri, A. *et al.* (2000) Signaling properties and functions of two distinct cardiomyocyte protease-activated receptors. *Circulation Research*, 86, pp. 1054-1061.

Sadler, J.E. (1991) von Willebrand factor. *Journal of Biological Chemistry*, 266, pp. 22777-22780.

Sadler, J.E. *et al.* (2006) Update on the pathophysiology and classification of von Willebrand disease: a report of the Subcommittee on von Willebrand Factor. *Journal of Thrombosis and Haemostasis*.

Sahoo, S. *et al.* (2003) Amyloid tumor: a clinical and cytomorphologic study. *Diagnostic Cytopathology*, 28, pp. 325-328.

Sajadi, S. *et al.* (2003) Tissue factor pathway inhibitors as a novel approach to antithrombotic therapy. *Drug News Perspect*, 16, pp. 363-369.

Sakariassen, K.S. *et al.* (1984) Factor VIII-von Willebrand factor requires calcium for facilitation of platelet adherence. *Blood*, 63, pp. 996-103.

Sakata, Y. and AOKI, N. (1980) Cross-linking of alpha 2-plasmin inhibitor to fibrin by fibrin-stabilizing factor. *Journal of Clinical Investigation*, 65, pp. 290-297.

Sala-Serra, M. *et al.* (1996) Cohort study on cancer mortality among workers in the pulp and paper industry in Catalonia, Spain. *American Journal of Industrial Medicine*, 30, pp. 87-92.

Salvaggio, J.E. *et al.* (1963) Long-term anti-coagulation in sickle-cell disease. A clinical study. *New England Journal of Medicine*, 269, pp. 182-186.

Salvatore, A.J. *et al.* (1969) Postoperative hypoventilation and hypoxemia in man after hyperventilation. *New England Journal of Medicine*, 280, pp. 467-470.

Samama, C.M. *et al.* (2001) Perioperative activation of hemostasis in vascular surgery patients. *Anesthesiology*, 94, pp. 74-78.

Sambrano, G.R. *et al.* (2001) Role of thrombin signalling in platelets in haemostasis and thrombosis. *Nature*, 413, pp. 74-78.

San Biagio, P.L. *et al.* (1999) Interacting processes in protein coagulation. *Proteins*, 37, pp. 116-120.

Sandercock, G.R. *et al.* (2005) Effects of exercise on heart rate variability: inferences from meta-analysis. *Medicine and Science in Sports and Exercise*, 37, pp. 433-439.

Sane, D.C. *et al.* (1989) Elevated urokinase-type plasminogen activator level and bleeding in amyloidosis: case report and literature review. *American Journal of Hematology*, 31, pp. 53-57.

Sano, H. and ITOH, H. (1998) Idiopathic insomnia [Japanese]. *Nippon Rinsho (Japanese Journal of Clinical Medicine)*, 56, pp. 361-364.

Saraiva, J. *et al.* (2011) Nanocarriers for nitric oxide delivery. *Journal of Drug Delivery*, 2011, pp. 936438.

Savareux, L. *et al.* (2004) Pyelo-ureteric amyloidosis [French]. *Progres En Urologie*, 14, pp. 406-410.

Savoia, C. and Schiffrin, E.L. (2006) Inflammation in hypertension. *Current Opinion in Nephrology and Hypertension*, 15, pp. 152-158.

Schafer, A. *et al.* (2008) Improvement of vascular function by acute and chronic treatment with the PDE-5 inhibitor sildenafil in experimental diabetes mellitus. *British Journal of Pharmacology*, 153, pp. 886-893.

Scheibe, F. *et al.* (2000) Preventive magnesium supplement reduces ischemia-induced hearing loss and blood viscosity in the guinea pig. *European Archives of Oto-Rhino-Laryngology*, 257, pp. 355-361.

Schiller, H. *et al.* (2002) Thrombin as a survival factor for cancer cells: thrombin activation in malignant effusions in vivo and inhibition of idarubicin-induced cell death in vitro. *International Journal of Clinical Pharmacology and Therapeutics*, 40, pp. 329-335.

Schilling, R.F. *et al.* (2006) Arteriosclerotic events are less frequent in persons with chronic anemia: evidence from families with hereditary spherocytosis. *American Journal of Hematology*, 81, pp. 315-317.

Schmermund, A. (2004) Cardiorespiratory fitness. Importance of exercise for healthiness [German]. *Herz*, 29, pp. 365-372.

Schneemilch, C.E. and BANK, U. (2001) Release of pro- and anti-inflammatory cytokines during different anesthesia procedures [German]. *Anaesthesiologie und Reanimation*, 26, pp. 4-10.

Schneider, R.A. (1949) The relation of stress to clotting time, relative viscosity and certain other biophysical alterations of the blood in the normotensive and hypertensive subject. *Research Publications - Association for Research in Nervous and Mental Disease*, 29, pp. 818-831.

Scholtes, M.C. *et al.* (1983) The factor VIII ratio in normal and pathological pregnancies. *European Journal of Obstetrics, Gynecology, and Reproductive Biology*, 16, pp. 89-95.

Schoots, I.G. *et al.* (2004) Enhancement of endogenous fibrinolysis does not reduce local fibrin deposition, but modulates inflammation upon intestinal ischemia and reperfusion. *Thrombosis and Haemostasis*, 91, pp. 497-505.

Schramm, W. *et al.* (1977) The pathogenesis of postoperative abdominal wound dehiscence. Part II: Hemostasiological checks during the course in selected patient groups [German]. *Munchener Medizinische Wochenschrift*, 119, pp. 690-694.

Schwartz, P. (1975) Amyloidosis, expression and cause of presenile and senile mental and physical regression. A revision of the amyloid problem [German]. *Zentralblatt fur Allgemeine Pathologie und Pathologische Anatomie*, 119, pp. 533-548.

Schwartz, P. (1976) Amyloidosis as a manifestation and origin of presenile and senile degeneration [German]. *Fortschritte der Medizin*, 94, pp. 890-896.

Schwarzinger, I. *et al.* (1992) Recurrent, isolated factor X deficiency in myeloma: repeated normalization of factor X levels after cytostatic chemotherapy followed by late treatment failure associated with the development of systemic amyloidosis. *Thrombosis and Haemostasis*, 68, pp. 648-651.

Schwertz, H. *et al.* (2004) Catecholamine therapy in cardiogenic shock: helpful, useless or dangerous? [German]. *Deutsche Medizinische Wochenschrift*, 129, pp. 1925-1930.

Scott, B.H. (1998) Opioids in cardiac surgery: cardiopulmonary bypass and inflammatory response. *International Journal of Cardiology*, 64[Suppl 1], pp. S35-41.

Sebel, P.S. and BOVIL, J.G. (1982) Cardiovascular effects of sufentanil anesthesia. *Anesthesia and Analgesia*, 61, pp. 115-119.

Seelig, M.S. (1990) Increased need for magnesium with the use of combined oestrogen and calcium for osteoporosis treatment. *Magnesium Research*, 3, pp. 197-215.

Segler, C.P. (2001) Prophylaxis of climbers for prevention of embolic accidents. *Medical Hypotheses*, 57, pp. 472-475.

Selye, H. (1954) Sketch for a unified theory of medicine. *International Record of Medicine and General Practice Clinics*, 167, pp. 181-203.

Selye, H. (1976) *The Stress of Life*. New York: McGraw-Hill.

Sen, S. *et al.* (2006) The analgesic effect of nitroglycerin added to lidocaine on intravenous regional anesthesia. *Anesthesia and Analgesia*, 102, pp. 916-920.

Seo, T. *et al.* (1991) A case of multiple myeloma with heart failure improved remarkably by chemotherapy alone [Japanese]. *Kokyu to Junkan (Respiration and Circulation)*, 39, pp. 601-605.

Sersa, I. *et al.* (2007) A mathematical model for the dissolution of non-occlusive blood clots in fast tangential blood flow. *Biorheology*, 44, pp. 1-16.

Setian, N. *et al.* (2002) Hypopituitarism, deficiency of factors V and VIII and von Willebrand factor: an uncommon association. *Journal of Pediatric Endocrinology and Metabolism*, 15, pp. 331-333.

Shapiro, M.J. and MISTRY, B. (1996) Calcium regulation and nonprotective properties of calcium in surgical ischemia. *New Horizons*, 4, pp. 134-138.

Shavit, Y. *et al.* (2004) Effects of fentanyl on natural killer cell activity and on resistance to tumor metastasis in rats. Dose and timing study. *Neuroimmunomodulation*, 11, pp. 255-260.

Shomron, N. *et al.* (2009) An evolutionary perspective of animal microRNAs and their targets. *Journal of Biomedicine and Biotechnology*, 2009, pp. 594738.

Si, M.L. and Lee, T.J. (2002) Alpha7-nicotinic acetylcholine receptors on cerebral perivascular sympathetic nerves mediate choline-induced nitrergic neurogenic vasodilation. *Circulation Research*, 91, pp. 62-69.

Siegbahn, A. (2000) Cellular consequences upon factor VIIa binding to tissue factor. *Haemostasis*, 30[Suppl 2], pp. 41-47.

Siegbahn, A. *et al.* (2000) Binding of factor VIIa to tissue factor on human fibroblasts leads to activation of phospholipase C and enhanced PDGF-BB-stimulated chemotaxis. *Blood*, 96, pp. 3452-3458.

Sielenkamper, A.W. *et al.* (2000) Thoracic epidural anesthesia increases mucosal perfusion in ileum of rats. *Anesthesiology*, 93, pp. 844-851.

Sielenkamper, A.W. *et al.* (2001) The effects of sepsis on gut mucosal blood flow in rats. *European Journal of Anaesthesiology*, 18, pp. 673-678.

Silber, H.A. *et al.* (2001) The relationship between vascular wall shear stress and flow-mediated dilation: endothelial function assessed by phase-contrast magnetic resonance angiography. *Journal of the American College of Cardiology*, 38, pp. 1859-1865.

Singh, G. *et al.* (1993) Diltiazem reduces whole blood viscosity following trauma-hemorrhagic shock and resuscitation. *Circulatory Shock*, 39, pp. 231-236.

Singh, M.V. *et al.* (2003) Blood gases, hematology, and renal blood flow during prolonged mountain sojourns at 3500 and 5800 m. *Aviation Space and Environmental Medicine*, 74, pp. 533-536.

Sinz, A. *et al.* (2002) Mass spectrometric proteome analyses of synovial fluids and plasmas from patients suffering from rheumatoid arthritis and comparison to reactive arthritis or osteoarthritis. *Electrophoresis*, 23, pp. 3445-3456.

Skarvan, K. and Schwinn, W. (1986) Hemodynamic interaction between midazolam and alfentanil in coronary patients [German]. *Anaesthesist*, 35, pp. 17-23.

Smedby, K.E. *et al.* (2006) Malignant lymphomas in autoimmunity and inflammation: a review of risks, risk factors, and lymphoma characteristics. *Cancer Epidemiology, Biomarkers and Prevention*, 15, pp. 2069-2077.

Smith, D.B. *et al.* (1987) Quantitative measurement of plasma gelsolin and its incorporation into fibrin clots. *Journal of Laboratory and Clinical Medicine*, 110, pp. 189-195.

Smith, D.B. *et al.* (1988) Circulating actin-gelsolin complexes following oleic acid-induced lung injury. *American Journal of Pathology*, 130, pp. 261-267.

Smith, D.B. *et al.* (1988) Decreased plasma gelsolin levels in patients with Plasmodium falciparum malaria: a consequence of hemolysis? *Blood*, 72, pp. 214-218.

Smith, F.B. *et al.* (1993) Localized pleural microdeposition of type A amyloid in a patient with rheumatoid pleuritis. Histologic distinction from pleural involvement in systemic amyloidosis. *American Journal of Clinical Pathology*, 99, pp. 261-264.

Smith, G.R. *et al.* (2004) Etanercept treatment of renal amyloidosis complicating rheumatoid arthritis. *Internal Medicine Journal*, 34, pp. 570-572.

Smith, M.A. *et al.* (1996) The secondary leukemias: challenges and research directions. *Journal of the National Cancer Institute*, 88, pp. 407-418.

Solomon, L.R. (2008) Treatment and prevention of pain due to vaso-occlusive crises in adults with sickle cell disease: an educational void. *Blood*, 111, pp. 997-1003.

Song, S.J. *et al.* (2005) The role of protease-activated receptor-1 in bone healing. *American Journal of Pathology*, 166, pp. 857-868.

Sotiriou, C.G. and Cheng, J.W. (2000) Beneficial effects of statins in coronary artery disease-beyond lowering cholesterol. *Annals of Pharmacotherapy*, 34, pp. 1432-1439.

Souto, J.C. *et al.* (1995) Prothrombotic state and signs of endothelial lesion in plasma of patients with inflammatory bowel disease. *Digestive Diseases and Sciences*, 40, pp. 1883-1889.

Sporn, M.B. (1991) Carcinogenesis and cancer: different perspectives on the same disease. *Cancer Research*, 51, pp. 6215-6218.

Stasko, J. *et al.* (2004) Thrombin activatable fibrinolysis inhibitor (TAFI) and its importance in the regulation of fibrinolysis [Slovak]. *Vnitrni Lekarstvi*, 50, pp. 36-44.

Stefano, G.B. *et al.* (1995) Hyperstimulation of leukocytes by plasma from cardiopulmonary by-pass patients is diminished by morphine and IL-10 pretreatment. *Journal of Cardiovascular Surgery*, 36, pp. 25-30.

Stefano, G.B. *et al.* (1996) Opioid and opiate immunoregulatory processes. *Critical Reviews in Immunology*, 16, pp. 109-144.

Steffey, E.P. *et al.* (1977) Meperidine-halothane interaction in dogs. *Canadian Anaesthetists Society Journal*, 24, pp. 459-467.

Stevens, L.E. *et al.* (1986) Fibronectin in severe sepsis. *Surgery, Gynecology and Obstetrics*, 162, pp. 222-228.

Stewart, A.J. *et al.* (1999) Warfarin-induced skin necrosis. *Postgraduate Medical Journal*, 75, pp. 233-235.

Stoltz, J.F. *et al.* (1999) Influence of a calcium antagonist on blood rheology and arterial compliance in hypertension: comparison with a thiazide diuretic. *Clinical Hemorheology and Microcirculation*, 21, pp. 201-208.

Stuart, J. *et al.* (1981) Haematological stress syndrome in atherosclerosis. *Journal of Clinical Pathology*, 34, pp. 464-467.

Stvrtinova, V. *et al.* (1998) Vascular endothelium as a factor in information transfer between the cardiovascular and immune systems [Slovak]. *Bratislavske Lekarske Listy*, 99, pp. 5-19.

Suo, Z. *et al.* (2003) Persistent protease-activated receptor 4 signaling mediates thrombin-induced microglial activation. *Journal of Biological Chemistry*, 278, pp. 31177-31183.

Sutherland, C.J. and Schurman, J.R. (1987) Complications associated with warfarin prophylaxis in total knee arthroplasty. *Clinical Orthopaedics and Related Research*, pp. 158-162.

Suttner, S. *et al.* (2004) The influence of allogeneic red blood cell transfusion compared with 100% oxygen ventilation on systemic oxygen transport and skeletal muscle oxygen tension after cardiac surgery. *Anesthesia and Analgesia*, 99, pp. 2-11.

Suzuki, S. and Morishita, S. (1998) Hypercoagulability and DIC in high-risk infants. *Seminars in Thrombosis and Hemostasis*, 24, pp. 463-466.

Swallow, T. and Anderson, C. (2006) Phosphodiesterase-5 inhibitors help climbers to achieve new heights. *BJU International*, 97, pp. 672-673.

Takamori, S. *et al.* (2004) Amyloid tumor in the anterior mediastinum: report of a case. *Surgery Today*, 34, pp. 518-520.

Tamaki, T. and Aoki, N. (1981) Cross-linking of alpha 2-plasmin inhibitor and fibronectin to fibrin by fibrin-stabilizing factor. *Biochimica et Biophysica Acta*, 661, pp. 280-286.

Tamaki, T. and AOKI, N. (1982) Cross-linking of alpha 2-plasmin inhibitor to fibrin catalyzed by activated fibrin-stabilizing factor. *Journal of Biological Chemistry*, 257, pp. 14767-14772.

Tanaka, F. *et al.* (2004) Interleukin-18 induces serum amyloid A (SAA) protein production from rheumatoid synovial fibroblasts. *Life Sciences*, 74, pp. 1671-1679.

Tangelder, G.J. *et al.* (1985) Distribution of blood platelets flowing in arterioles. *American Journal of Physiology*, 248, pp. H318-323.

Tantivejkul, K. *et al.* (2005) PAR1-mediated NFkappaB activation promotes survival of prostate cancer cells through a Bcl-xL-dependent mechanism. *Journal of Cellular Biochemistry*, 96, pp. 641-652.

TATE, B.F. and Rittenhouse, S.E. (1993) Thrombin activation of human platelets causes tyrosine phosphorylation of PLC-gamma 2. *Biochimica et Biophysica Acta*, 1178, pp. 281-285.

Tatu-Chitoiu, G. *et al.* (2004) Streptokinase-induced hypotension has no detrimental effect on patients with thrombolytic treatment for acute myocardial infarction. A substudy of the Romanian Study for Accelerated Streptokinase in Acute Myocardial Infarction (ASK-ROMANIA). *Romanian Journal of Internal Medicine*, 42, pp. 557-573.

Tavel, M.E. *et al.* (1969) Korotkoff sounds. Observations on pressure-pulse changes underlying their formation. *Circulation*, 39, pp. 465-474.

Taylor, F.B., JR. *et al.* (1987) Protein C prevents the coagulopathic and lethal effects of Escherichia coli infusion in the baboon. *Journal of Clinical Investigation*, 79, pp. 918-925.

Temple, R.H. and Timms, M.S. (2001) Blood loss reduction during laser turbinectomy. *Rhinology*, 39, pp. 230-232.

Thornton, C.A. and Bonnar, J. (1977) Factor VIII-related antigen and factor VIII coagulant activity in normal and pre-eclamptic pregnancy. *British Journal of Obstetrics and Gynaecology*, 84, pp. 919-923.

Tian, J. *et al.* (2004) Relationships between arteriosclerosis, cerebral amyloid angiopathy and myelin loss from cerebral cortical white matter in Alzheimer's disease. *Neuropathology and Applied Neurobiology*, 30, pp. 46-56.

Tighe, D. *et al.* (1989) Multi-organ damage resulting from experimental faecal peritonitis. *Clinical Science (London)*, 76, pp. 269-276.

Tobias, M.D. *et al.* (1999) Lidocaine and bupivacaine exert differential effects on whole blood coagulation. *Journal of Clinical Anesthesia*, 11, pp. 52-55.

Tobias, M.D. *et al.* (1996) Lidocaine inhibits blood coagulation: implications for epidural blood patch. *Anesthesia and Analgesia*, 82, pp. 766-769.

Toda, N. *et al.* (2005) Nitric oxide and penile erectile function. *Pharmacology and Therapeutics*, 106, pp. 233-266.

Toda, N. *et al.* (2007) Interaction of endothelial nitric oxide and angiotensin in the circulation. *Pharmacological Reviews*, 59, pp. 54-87.

Toh, C.H. and Dennis, M. (2003) Current clinical practice. DIC 2002: a review of disseminated intravascular coagulation. *Hematology*, 8, pp. 65-71.

Tordai, A. *et al.* (1993) Functional thrombin receptors on human T lymphoblastoid cells. *Journal of Immunology*, 150, pp. 4876-4886.

Tous, M. *et al.* (2004) Circulating blood cells modulate the atherosclerotic process in apolipoprotein E-deficient mice. *Metabolism: Clinical and Experimental*, 53, pp. 95-100.

Trachte, A.L. *et al.* (2005) Oral sildenafil reduces pulmonary hypertension after cardiac surgery. *Annals of Thoracic Surgery*, 79, pp. 194-197; discussion 194-197.

Tran, T. and Stewart, A.G. (2003) Protease-activated receptor (PAR)-independent growth and pro-inflammatory actions of thrombin on human cultured airway smooth muscle. *British Journal of Pharmacology*, 138, pp. 865-875.

Tran, T.H. *et al.* (1984) Factor VIII (procoagulant activity VIII:C, and antigen VIII:CAg, related antigen VIIIR:Ag and ristocetin cofactor VIIIR:Cof) in intensive care patients with clinically suspected disseminated intravascular coagulation (DIC). *American Journal of Clinical Pathology*, 82, pp. 565-572.

Treschan, T.A. *et al.* (2003) The effects of epidural and general anesthesia on tissue oxygenation. *Anesthesia and Analgesia*, 96, pp. 1553-1557.

Tsopanoglou, N.E. and Maragoudakis, M.E. (1998) On the mechanism of thrombin-induced angiogenesis: inhibition of attachment of endothelial cells on basement membrane components. *Angiogenesis*, 1, pp. 192-200.

Tsopanoglou, N.E. and Maragoudakis, M.E. (2004) Role of thrombin in angiogenesis and tumor progression. *Seminars in Thrombosis and Hemostasis*, 30, pp. 63-69.

Turgeon, V.L. *et al.* (1998) Thrombin perturbs neurite outgrowth and induces apoptotic cell death in enriched chick spinal motoneuron cultures through caspase activation. *Journal of Neuroscience*, 18, pp. 6882-6891.

Tverskoy, M. *et al.* (1990) Postoperative pain after inguinal herniorrhaphy with different types of anesthesia. *Anesthesia and Analgesia*, 70, pp. 29-35.

Tverskoy, M. *et al.* (1985) Influence of fentanyl and morphine on intestinal circulation. *Anesthesia and Analgesia*, 64, pp. 577-584.

Ueno, A. *et al.* (1996) Thrombin stimulates production of interleukin-8 in human umbilical vein endothelial cells. *Immunology*, 88, pp. 76-81.

Undas, A. *et al.* (2001) Blood coagulation at the site of microvascular injury: effects of low-dose aspirin. *Blood*, 98, pp. 2423-2431.

Ungerstedt, J.S. *et al.* (2003) Clotting onset time may be a predictor of outcome in human brain injury: a pilot study. *Journal of Neurosurgical Anesthesiology*, 15, pp. 13-18.

Uprichard, J. and Perry, D.J. (2002) Factor X deficiency. *Blood Reviews*, 16, pp. 97-110.

Valverde, A. *et al.* (2004) Effect of lidocaine on the minimum alveolar concentration of isoflurane in dogs. *Veterinary Anaesthesia and Analgesia*, 31, pp. 264-271.

Van Den Burg, P.J. *et al.* (2000) Aging, physical conditioning, and exercise-induced changes in hemostatic factors and reaction products. *Journal of Applied Physiology*, 88, pp. 1558-1564.

Van Der Poll, T. *et al.* (2005) Activated protein C inhibits local coagulation after intrapulmonary delivery of endotoxin in humans. *American Journal of Respiratory and Critical Care Medicine*, 171, pp. 1125-1128.

Van Gelder, J.M. *et al.* (1994) The significance of red cell surface area to the permeability of fibrin network. *Biorheology*, 31, pp. 259-275.

Van Mourik, J.A. *et al.* (1999) von Willebrand factor propeptide in vascular disorders: A tool to distinguish between acute and chronic endothelial cell perturbation. *Blood*, 94, pp. 179-185.

Van Nostrand, W.E. *et al.* (2000) Cerebrovascular smooth muscle cell surface fibrillar A beta. Alteration of the proteolytic environment in the cerebral vessel wall. *Annals of the New York Academy of Sciences*, 903, pp. 89-96.

Van Zwieten, P.A. and Doods, H.N. (1995) Muscarinic receptors and drugs in cardiovascular medicine. *Cardiovascular Drugs and Therapy*, 9, pp. 159-167.

Vehar, G.A. and Davie, E.W. (1977) Formation of a serine enzyme in the presence of bovine factor VIII (antihemophilic factor) and thrombin. *Science*, 197, pp. 374-376.

Ventura, H. *et al.* (1984) Impaired systemic arterial compliance in borderline hypertension. *American Heart Journal*, 108, pp. 132-136.

Ventura, J.E. *et al.* (1997) Acute renal failure in pregnancy. *Renal Failure*, 19, pp. 217-220.

Vermeyen, K.M. *et al.* (1989) Low-dose sufentanil-isoflurane anaesthesia for coronary artery surgery. *British Journal of Anaesthesia*, 63, pp. 44-50.

Versteeg, H.H. *et al.* (2004) Coagulation factors VIIa and Xa inhibit apoptosis and anoikis. *Oncogene*, 23, pp. 410-417.

Veyradier, A. *et al.* (2001) Abnormal von Willebrand factor in bleeding angiodysplasias of the digestive tract. *Gastroenterology*, 120, pp. 346-353.

Veyradier, A. *et al.* (2000) Improvement of von Willebrand factor proteolysis after prostacyclin infusion in severe pulmonary arterial hypertension. *Circulation*, 102, pp. 2460-2462.

Vicaut, E. (1999) Microcirculation and arterial hypertension. *Drugs*, 59 Spec No, pp. 1-10.

Vincent, M.A. *et al.* (2003) Molecular and physiologic actions of insulin related to production of nitric oxide in vascular endothelium. *Curr Diab Rep*, 3, pp. 279-288.

Vinckier, F. and Vermylen, J. (1984) Wound healing following dental extractions in rabbits: effects of tranexamic acid, warfarin anti-coagulation, and socket packing. *Journal of Dental Research*, 63, pp. 646-649.

Vinik, H.R. *et al.* (1994) Triple anesthetic combination: propofol-midazolam-alfentanil. *Anesthesia and Analgesia*, 78, pp. 354-358.

Vlahos, R. *et al.* (2003) Differential inhibition of thrombin- and EGF-stimulated human cultured airway smooth muscle proliferation by glucocorticoids. *Pulmonary Pharmacology and Therapeutics*, 16, pp. 171-180.

Von Brecht, J.H. *et al.* (1986) Regional anticoagulation: hemodialysis with hypertonic trisodium citrate. *American Journal of Kidney Diseases*, 8, pp. 196-201.

Von Dossow, V. *et al.* (2001) Thoracic epidural anesthesia combined with general anesthesia: the preferred anesthetic technique for thoracic surgery. *Anesthesia and Analgesia*, 92, pp. 848-854.

Von Kanel, R. *et al.* (2003) Acute procoagulant stress response as a dynamic measure of allostatic load in Alzheimer caregivers. *Annals of Behavioral Medicine*, 26, pp. 42-48.

Von Kanel, R. *et al.* (2006) Altered blood coagulation in patients with posttraumatic stress disorder. *Psychosomatic Medicine*, 68, pp. 598-604.

Von Kries, R. *et al.* (1981) The clinical relevance of factor VIII: C and factor VII R: Ag determination in newborns. *European Journal of Pediatrics*, 137, pp. 189-194.

Von Tempelhoff, G.F. *et al.* (2000) Association between blood rheology, thrombosis and cancer survival in patients with gynecologic malignancy. *Clinical Hemorheology and Microcirculation*, 22, pp. 107-130.

Von Tempelhoff, G.F. *et al.* (2002) Thrombosis-a clue of poor prognosis in primary non-metastatic breast cancer? *Breast Cancer Research and Treatment*, 73, pp. 275-277.

Wada, H. *et al.* (2003) Increased soluble fibrin in plasma of patients with disseminated intravascular coagulation. *Clinical and Applied Thrombosis/Hemostasis* 9, pp. 233-240.

Wada, H. *et al.* (1996) Increased plasma-soluble fibrin monomer levels in patients with disseminated intravascular coagulation. *American Journal of Hematology*, 51, pp. 255-260.

Wall, P.D. and WOOLF, C.J. (1986) The brief and the prolonged facilitatory effects of unmyelinated afferent input on the rat spinal cord are independently influenced by peripheral nerve section. *Neuroscience*, 17, pp. 1199-1205.

Wallis, M.G. *et al.* (2005) Acute glucosamine-induced insulin resistance in muscle in vivo is associated with impaired capillary recruitment. *Diabetologia*, 48, pp. 2131-2139.

Walsh, P.N. and Ahmad, S.S. (2002) Proteases in blood clotting. *Essays in Biochemistry*, 38, pp. 95-111.

Wamhoff, D. *et al.* (1976) Studies on the influence of glucose infusion on parameters of hemostasis [German]. *Zeitschrift fur Die Gesamte Innere Medizin und Ihre Grenzgebiete*, 31, pp. 711-715.

Wang, H. and Reiser, G. (2003) The role of the Ca2+-sensitive tyrosine kinase Pyk2 and Src in thrombin signalling in rat astrocytes. *Journal of Neurochemistry*, 84, pp. 1349-1357.

Wang, H. and Reiser, G. (2003) Thrombin signaling in the brain: the role of protease-activated receptors. *Biological Chemistry*, 384, pp. 193-202.

Wang, K.Y. *et al.* (2000) Expression of functional type 1 protease-activated thrombin receptors by mouse primary palatal mesenchymal cells in vitro. *Archives of Oral Biology*, 45, pp. 819-825.

Wang, X. *et al.* (2005) Ovarian cancer, the coagulation pathway, and inflammation. *Journal of Translational Medicine*, 3, pp. 25.

Wannamethee, S.G. *et al.* (2003) The effects of different alcoholic drinks on lipids, insulin and haemostatic and inflammatory markers in older men. *Thrombosis and Haemostasis*, 90, pp. 1080-1087.

Warkentin, T.E. *et al.* (2003) Gastrointestinal bleeding, angiodysplasia, cardiovascular disease, and acquired von Willebrand syndrome. *Transfusion Medicine Reviews*, 17, pp. 272-286.

Warkentin, T.E. *et al.* (1999) Multicentric warfarin-induced skin necrosis complicating heparin-induced thrombocytopenia. *American Journal of Hematology*, 62, pp. 44-48.

Warr, T.A. *et al.* (1990) Disseminated intravascular coagulation in rabbits induced by administration of endotoxin or tissue factor: effect of anti-tissue factor antibodies and measurement of plasma extrinsic pathway inhibitor activity. *Blood*, 75, pp. 1481-1489.

Waters, R.M. (1933) Toxic effects of carbon dioxide. *JAMA*, 100, p. 519.

Watkins, C.C. *et al.* (2000) Insulin restores neuronal nitric oxide synthase expression and function that is lost in diabetic gastropathy. *Journal of Clinical Investigation*, 106, p. 803.

Webb, D.J. *et al.* (2000) Sildenafil citrate potentiates the hypotensive effects of nitric oxide donor drugs in male patients with stable angina. *Journal of the American College of Cardiology*, 36, pp. 25-31.

Wei, S.J. (1990) The assessment of factor VIII-related antigen in endothelial cells of pulmonary blood vessels in multiple organ failure [Chinese]. *Zhonghua Jie He He Hu Xi Za Zhi*, 13, pp. 346-348, 380.

Weijer, S. *et al.* (2004) Inhibition of the tissue factor/factor VIIa pathway does not influence the inflammatory or antibacterial response to abdominal sepsis induced by Escherichia coli in mice. *Journal of Infectious Diseases*, 189, pp. 2308-2317.

Weinberg, G. *et al.* (2004) The effect of bupivacaine on myocardial tissue hypoxia and acidosis during ventricular fibrillation. *Anesthesia and Analgesia*, 98, pp. 790-795.

Weiner, C.P. and Brandt, J. (1982) Plasma antithrombin III activity: an aid in the diagnosis of preeclampsia-eclampsia. *American Journal of Obstetrics and Gynecology*, 142, pp. 275-281.

Weisel, J.W. (2005) Fibrinogen and fibrin. *Advances in Protein Chemistry*, 70, pp. 247-299.

Weiss, H.J. *et al.* (1989) Evidence for the presence of tissue factor activity on subendothelium. *Blood*, 73, pp. 968-975.

Weiss, K. (1988) Calcium antagonists: anti-atherosclerotic effect by modification of the prostaglandin system [German]. *Wiener Klinische Wochenschrift*, 100, pp. 718-720.

Weissman, C. (1990) The metabolic response to stress: an overview and update. *Anesthesiology*, 73, pp. 308-327.

Weksler, B.B. *et al.* (1977) Effect of propranolol on platelet function. *Blood*, 49, pp. 185-196.

Welty-Wolf, K.E. *et al.* (2001) Coagulation blockade prevents sepsis-induced respiratory and renal failure in baboons. *American Journal of Respiratory and Critical Care Medicine*, 164, pp. 1988-1996.

Wettstein, P. *et al.* (2004) Decreased factor XIII availability for thrombin and early loss of clot firmness in patients with unexplained intraoperative bleeding. *Anesthesia and Analgesia*, 99, pp. 1564-1569.

Whitaker, D.C. *et al.* (2004) Angina with a normal coronary angiogram caused by amyloidosis. *Heart*, 90, pp. e54.

Widdicombe, J.G. (1992) Asthma. Tracheobronchial vasculature. *British Medical Bulletin*, 48, pp. 108-119.

Wijnen, J.A. *et al.* (1994) Effect of exercise training on ambulatory blood pressure. *International Journal of Sports Medicine*, 15, pp. 10-15.

Wiland, P. *et al.* (2004) The prevalence of subclinical amyloidosis in Polish patients with rheumatoid arthritis. *Clinical Rheumatology*, 23, pp. 193-198.

Willert, H.G. *et al.* (1983) Orthopaedic surgery in hemophilic patients. *Archives of Orthopaedic and Trauma Surgery*, 101, pp. 121-132.

Wilmer, M. *et al.* (2002) Methods for the determination of factor XIII/XIIIa [German]. *Hamostaseologie*, 22, pp. 32-42.

Wilson, J. (2001) Chlorine quandry. *Popular Mechanics Magazine,* 178, p. 54.

Winniford, M.D. (1990) Smoking and cardiovascular function. *Journal of Hypertension - Supplement*, 8, pp. S17-23.

Witte, S. (1984) The role of blood coagulation in capillary permeability Vitalmicroscopic contributions. *Biorheology*, 21, pp. 121-133.

Wittstein, I.S. *et al.* (2005) Neurohumoral features of myocardial stunning due to sudden emotional stress. *New England Journal of Medicine*, 352, pp. 539-548.

Wojtarowicz, A. *et al.* (2003) Adrenergic and cholinergic innervation of pulmonary tissue in the pig. *Folia Morphologiica*, 62, pp. 215-218.

Wolak, T. *et al.* (2004) Duplex study of the carotid and femoral arteries of patients with systemic lupus erythematosus: a controlled study. *Journal of Rheumatology*, 31, pp. 909-914.

Wolfe, T. (1979) *The Right Stuff*. New York: Bantam Books.

Wong, K.C. (1983) Narcotics are not expected to produce unconsciousness and amnesia. *Anesthesia and Analgesia*, 62, pp. 625-626.

Woolf, C.J. (1983) Evidence for a central component of post-injury pain hypersensitivity. *Nature*, 306, pp. 686-688.

Woolf, C.J. and Chong, M.S. (1993) Preemptive analgesia-treating postoperative pain by preventing the establishment of central sensitization. *Anesthesia and Analgesia*, 77, pp. 362-379.

Woolf, C.J. and Wall, P.D. (1986) Morphine-sensitive and morphine-insensitive actions of C-fibre input on the rat spinal cord. *Neuroscience Letters*, 64, pp. 221-225.

Wu, K.C. *et al.* (1998) Prognostic significance of microvascular obstruction by magnetic resonance imaging in patients with acute myocardial infarction. *Circulation*, 97, pp. 765-772.

Xia, X. *et al.* (2010) Prostaglandin promotion of osteocyte gap junction function through transcriptional regulation of connexin 43 by glycogen synthase kinase 3/beta-catenin signaling. *Molecular and Cellular Biology*, 30, pp. 206-219.

Yalcin, O. *et al.* (2004) Graded alterations of RBC aggregation influence in vivo blood flow resistance. *American Journal of Physiology - Heart and Circulatory Physiology*, 287, pp. H2644-2650.

Yeager, M.P. *et al.* (1987) Epidural anesthesia and analgesia in high-risk surgical patients by preventing nociception that activates the capillary gate component via the spinal pathway. *Anesthesiology*, 66, pp. 729-736.

Yehuda, R.M. and MCEWEN, B. (eds.) (2005) *Behavioral Stress Response: Protective and Damaging Effects*. New York: New York Academy of Science.

Yi, Y. *et al.* (1999) Changes of nailfold microcirculation in patients of type II diabetes mellitus with diabetic retinopathy. *Chinese Medical Sciences Journal*, 14, pp. 233-236.

Yoo, K. *et al.* (2006) Anesthetic requirements and stress hormone responses in spinal cord-injured patients undergoing surgery below the level of injury. *Anesthesia and Analgesia*, 102, pp. 1223-1228.

Yood, R.A. *et al.* (1983) Bleeding manifestations in 100 patients with amyloidosis. *JAMA*, 249, pp. 1322-1324.

Zain, J. *et al.* (2000) Concentration-dependent dual effect of thrombin on impaired growth/apoptosis or mitogenesis in tumor cells. *Blood*, 95, pp. 3133-3138.

Zanesco, A. and Antunes, E. (2007) Effects of exercise training on the cardiovascular system: Pharmacological approaches. *Pharmacology and Therapeutics*, 114, pp. 307-317.

Zania, P. *et al.* (2006) Blockade of angiogenesis by small molecule antagonists to protease-activated receptor-1 (PAR-1): Association with endothelial cell growth suppression and induction of apoptosis. *Journal of Pharmacology and Experimental Therapeutics*, 318, pp. 246-254.

Zerbino, D.D. and Lukasevich, L.L. (1982) Disseminated intravascular coagulation syndrome: morphological criteria [Russian]. *Arkhiv Patologii*, 44, pp. 29-35.

Zerbino, D.D. and Lukasevich, L.L. (1983) Syndrome of disseminated intravascular coagulation as the principal morphologic manifestation of shock [Russian]. *Arkhiv Patologii*, 45, pp. 13-20.

Zhang, J. *et al.* (2007) The effect of epidural anesthesia with different concentrations of ropivacaine on sevoflurane requirements. *Anesthesia and Analgesia*, 104, pp. 984-986.

Zhang, X. *et al.* (2001) Effect of sildenafil, a phosphodiesterase-5 inhibitor, on oesophageal peristalsis and lower oesophageal sphincter function in cats. *Neurogastroenterology and Motility*, 13, pp. 325-331.

Zhang, Y. *et al.* (2007) Lidocaine, MK-801, and MAC. *Anesthesia and Analgesia*, 104, pp. 1098-1102.

Zhang, Z.G. *et al.* (1999) Cerebral microvascular obstruction by fibrin is associated with upregulation of PAI-1 acutely after onset of focal embolic ischemia in rats. *Journal of Neuroscience*, 19, pp. 10898-10907.

Zhao, S.Z. *et al.* (2002) Inter-individual variations in wall shear stress and mechanical stress distributions at the carotid artery bifurcation of healthy humans. *Journal of Biomechanics*, 35, pp. 1367-1377.

Zhao, S.Z. *et al.* (2000) Blood flow and vessel mechanics in a physiologically realistic model of a human carotid arterial bifurcation. *Journal of Biomechanics*, 33, pp. 975-984.

Zlokovic, B.V. (1997) Antithrombotic, procoagulant, and fibrinolytic mechanisms in cerebral circulation: implications for brain injury and protection. *Neurosurg Focus*, 2, pp. e5.

Zlokovic, B.V. *et al.* (1995) Expression of tissue plasminogen activator in cerebral capillaries: possible fibrinolytic function of the blood-brain barrier. *Neurosurgery*, 37, pp. 955-961.

Zuccala, G. *et al.* (1997) Use of calcium antagonists and need for perioperative transfusion in older patients with hip fracture: observational study. *British Medical Journal*, 314, pp. 643-644.

Zuccala, G. *et al.* (2000) Use of calcium antagonists and hemoglobin loss in hospitalized elderly patients: a cohort study. Gruppo Italiano di Farmacoepidemiologia nell'Anziano (GIFA) investigators. *Clinical Pharmacology and Therapeutics*, 67, pp. 314-322.

Index

A

B

C

D

F

G

H

I

J

K

L

M

N

O

P

Q

R

S

T